THE
33 DOCTORS
OF THE
CHURCH

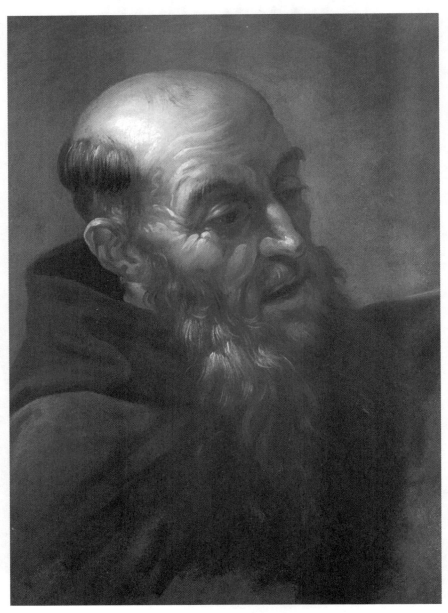

Saint Lawrence of Brindisi
"The Apostolic Doctor"
1559–1619

THE
33 DOCTORS
OF THE
CHURCH

Fr. Christopher Rengers, O.F.M. Cap.

*"But they that are learned shall shine
as the brightness of the firmament: and
they that instruct many to justice, as stars
for all eternity."*
—Daniel 12:3

TAN BOOKS AND PUBLISHERS, INC.
Rockford, Illinois 61105

NIHIL OBSTAT:
Rev. Joseph Mindling, O.F.M. Cap.
Censor Deputatus

IMPRIMI POTEST:
Very Rev. William Wiethorn,
O.F.M. Cap.
Provincial
September 1, 1993

IMPRIMI POTEST:
Very Rev. Paul Kuppe,
O.F.M. Cap.
Provincial
September 25, 2000

NIHIL OBSTAT:
Reverend Isidore Dixon
Censor Deputatus

IMPRIMATUR:
✛ Most Reverend William E. Lori
Vicar General for the Archdiocese of Washington
Washington, D.C.
November 30, 2000

The Nihil Obstat and Imprimatur are official declarations that a book or pamphlet is free of doctrinal or moral error. No implication is contained therein that those who have granted the *Nihil Obstat* and the *Imprimatur* agree with the content, opinions or statements expressed.

ISBN 0-89555-440-2

Library of Congress Control No.: 91-65353

Cover Illustrations: St. John of the Cross—anonymous 17th-c. portrait, Carmel of Valladolid; St. Therese of Lisieux—portrait by her sister Celine, courtesy of Society of the Little Flower, Darien, IL; St. Peter Canisius—portrait by Xavier Dietrich, courtesy of Canisius College, Buffalo, NY. For credits on other cover illustrations, see below or see the credit line on the illustration in the respective chapter.

The following icons have been reproduced in and/or on the cover of this book courtesy of Monastery Icons, Borrego Springs, California (800-729-4952): St. Athanasius (cover and inside) © 1989 by Monastery Icons; St. Ephrem (inside) © 1982 by Monastery Icons; St. Cyril of Jerusalem (inside) © 1994 by Monastery Icons; St. Ambrose (inside) © 1991 by Monastery Icons; St. Jerome (cover and inside) © 1997 by Monastery Icons; St. Augustine (cover) © 1993 by Monastery Icons; St. Cyril of Alexandria (inside) © 1989 by Monastery Icons; St. Leo the Great (inside) © 1994 by Monastery Icons; St. John of Damascus (inside) © 1991 by Monastery Icons.

Printed and bound in the United States of America.

TAN BOOKS AND PUBLISHERS, INC.
P.O. Box 424
Rockford, Illinois 61105
MM

To All My Teachers . . .

Beginning with parents and grandparents, aunts, uncles, cousins, friends;

On to teachers in kindergarten and in wood-working at public schools in Pittsburgh, PA;

To nuns at grade schools in the Pittsburgh Diocese: St. Joseph's, Bloomfield; St. Mary's, 46th St.; St. Mary of the Mount; St. Wendelin's, Carrick;

To Capuchin Friars at Herman, PA; Victoria, Kansas; Washington, D.C.; and in the novitiate at Cumberland, MD;

To Jesuits and lay teachers at St. Louis University; lay and clergy teachers in Adult Ed at Catholic University;

To teachers for special courses at Hays State, KS and Bowling Green State at Bowling Green, OH; and to the chaplains at the V.A. Hospital, Washington, D.C.;

And all along, to bishops, priests and deacons proclaiming and explaining the Gospel and exhorting us to use the Sacraments and lead a good life;

And to the silent teachers speaking in measured voices from many good books—a long and varied list deserving gratitude for being shapers of mind and heart.

May they rest in peace or continue in life
until we all meet happily in Heaven
with the Doctors of the Church,
those most eminent shapers of minds and hearts in
the Church founded by Jesus Christ.

CONTENTS

PREFACE

"O blessed doctor, light of holy Church and lover of God's law, pray to the Son of God for us."

This antiphon—to be recited or sung at the beginning and end of Our Lady's hymn, *The Magnificat*, during vespers for the feast of a Doctor of the Church—was one of the distinguishing marks of the common prayers of the Divine Office for such feasts which were introduced into the liturgy by Pope Boniface VIII (1294-1303) in 1298. The antiphon underscores the connection of a Doctor of the Church with light and love, with God's law, with the Church and with the Son of God.

Today, the word "doctor" would probably conjure up in most people's minds the image of one who is a specialist in caring for physical or mental health. But that was not its original meaning. For one thing, medical practice was not always associated with the term "doctor." In the early days of surgery, for example, one went to the barber, the only person in town who had the kinds of instruments needed for those primitive operations. The red and white poles which hang outside barber shops are hold-overs from that earlier time, their "medical" origins, now mostly forgotten.

The term "doctor" originally derived from the Latin word *docere*, "to teach." It designated anyone whose knowledge qualified him to teach, and therefore not necessarily one who would be skilled in caring for human health. But, as such, "doctors" were experts in promoting a certain kind of health—you might even say the most important kind: that health of soul and spirit which comes from knowing the truth.

"And you shall know the truth, and the truth shall make you free." (*John* 8:32). A human being cannot be free and therefore cannot be wholly human—cannot be personally and spiritually healthy—unless he or she knows the truth. Pontius Pilate asked Jesus: "What is truth?" (*John*. 18:38). If his question was not just one of those cruel taunts which were tossed at Jesus, the silent Lamb, during His Passion, then it shows that Pilate was at least wise enough to know that he did not yet know the truth and that he wanted to find it. Had he been able really to see Jesus for who He is, he would have found the answer to his question. "I am the way, and the truth, and the life." (*John* 14:6). "And the Word was made flesh, and dwelt among us, and we saw his glory, the glory as of the only-begotten of the Father, full of grace and truth." (*John* 1:14).

"Doctors of the Church" are people who have seen the glory of Jesus Christ, full of grace and truth. In addition, by cooperating with God's special graces and by employing as well as possible their unique intellectual and pedagogical gifts, they are persons who have succeeded in an outstanding way in communicating the truth they have contemplated in Jesus. As such they are eminent as *teachers*, which, as we have seen, corresponds precisely to the original meaning of the word "doctor." Moreover, their teaching brings health to the human heart and soul. St. Augustine, one of the first and greatest to be recognized as a Doctor of the Church, recalling the period in his own life when he was becoming disillusioned with the emptiness of the teachings of the professedly Christian group called the Manichaeans, and yet hesitant to accept the teachings of the Catholic Church, wrote:

> By believing I might have been cured, so that the sight of my mind would be clearer and might be somehow or other directed toward Your truth, which is the same forever and in no point fails. But it was the same with me as with a man who, having once had a bad doctor, is afraid to trust himself even to a good one. So it was with the health of my soul; it could not possibly be cured except by believing, but refused to be cured for fear of believing something falser. (*The Confessions of St. Augustine*, Book VI, chapter 4; translated by Rex Warner, New York: Mentor-Omega, 1963, page 117).

For decades now, some of the most popular books published in the United States, and perhaps in other countries as well, have been the so-called "self-help" books. They promise their readers a fuller life by cooking up home remedies for the soul. I have a hunch that the present book by Fr. Christopher could be more effective than all of them together. It is not that his survey presents itself as one more title among the already long list of "self-help" books. In fact, one of the first things upon which the Doctors of the Church would insist is that human beings should not expect to find happiness by "helping themselves." Rather, they must depend on the One whom the book of Wisdom calls the "Lord, who lovest souls." (*Wis.* 11:27). But if the present book succeeds in helping people to come to know some of Christianity's greatest teachers, and even stimulates them to read more about one or another of them and to taste some of their original works, then it will undoubtedly have a truly healing effect upon its readers. I suspect that it will do just that, especially because of the vivid and interesting way in which it presents each of these thirty-three marvelous individuals.

Fr. Christopher has the gift of making these characters come alive. He has uncovered very human anecdotes about them with which any of us can resonate, thus giving a feel for what kind of person each of these "doctors" actually was, even though they are separated from us by a considerable length of time, often by many centuries.

Who could not be struck by the triumphant return from exile of "the empire's most wanted criminal," St. Athanasius, to his diocese of Alexandria, when the whole city turned out to welcome him home, creating such a celebration that for years afterward any particularly grand feast was said to be "like the return of Athanasius"? What refinement and goodness is displayed by St. Francis de Sales who, when pressed by the King of France to accept a diocese in better condition than his own of Geneva—where he could not even live because the Reformation headed by John Calvin had come to dominate that city so completely—replied: "Sire, I have married a poor wife and cannot desert her for a richer."

One will find here some unforgettable deathbed scenes, like that of the ancient scholar Bede the Venerable, who was helped by the young man who had just finished taking his last dictation to sit on the floor of his cell to pray and who died pronouncing the words "Glory be to the Father, and to the Son and to the Holy Ghost." Another such scene, this one especially revelatory of the person involved, is that described in the touching account of the final illness of St. Therese of Lisieux. She had been stroking a picture of one of her favorite saints, St. Theophane Venard, and when asked why, replied: "Because I can't reach him to kiss him." And how can one not receive a lasting impression upon reading that St. Lawrence of Brindisi knelt down in prayer as he wrote out his sermons and undertook long journeys on foot from one European capital to another, all the while singing hymns to the Blessed Mother?

To these wonderful narrative details, sprinkled generously throughout the book, is added in each chapter something of the central doctrinal message of each saint. Thus, life and teaching form a whole, just as should be the case when the topic to be considered is not an abstract doctrine, but that truth which is wisdom. For wisdom is truth put into practice. It is not simply knowing the truth, but living it. Solomon's beautiful prayer for the gift of wisdom (Chapters 8-9 of the book of *Wisdom*) was re-echoed in a most unexpected way by Jesus in the Garden of Gethsemane: "Not my will, but thine be done." (*Luke* 22:42). He lived this wisdom in the paschal mystery of His death and res-urrection, about which St. Paul writes: "We preach Christ cru-cified, unto the Jews indeed a stumbling block, and unto the Gentiles foolishness: but unto them that are called, both Jews and Greeks, Christ the power of God, and the wisdom of God." (*1 Cor.* 1:23-24). St. Paul goes on to add:

> But we speak the wisdom of God in a mystery, a wisdom which is hidden, which God ordained before the world, unto our glory: which none of the princes of this world knew; for if they had known it, they would never have crucified the Lord of glory. But, as it is written: "That eye hath not seen, nor ear heard, neither hath it entered into the heart of man, what things God hath prepared for them that love him." But to us God hath revealed them by his Spirit. (*1 Cor.* 2:7-10).

Pope John Paul II, now at the dawn of a new millennium, has called upon all who live in the countries of North, Central and South America to meet Jesus Christ once again. By encounter-ing the living Jesus Christ, it is possible to be *converted*, to establish and grow in *communion* with the Holy Trinity by grace and with all those who form the Church, and to reach out in *solidarity* toward those who suffer from injustice, poverty and any kind of disadvantage. People from the Americas can dis-cover great examples of conversion, communion and solidarity in the Saints who have grown and lived in their lands over the past centuries—Pope John Paul lists some thirty-five American Saints and Blesseds in paragraph 15 of his apostolic exhorta-tion *Ecclesia in America*. Adding to these American Saints, Fr. Christopher in the present book draws our attention to another thirty-three who belong to the whole Church, on every conti-nent, because they were so outstanding for their healthful teach-ing. He compares them to the star of Bethlehem, for the life and teaching of each of the Saints here presented simply points once again to Jesus. This image reflects very well another antiphon

from the Divine Office for the feast day of a Doctor of the Church—
that assigned to the morning Gospel canticle, the *Benedictus*:

> But they that are learned shall shine as the brightness of
> the firmament: and they that instruct many to justice, as stars
> for all eternity. (*Dan*. 12:3).

Thanks are due to the author of the pages which follow, for
there is much light in this book. May it guide those who today,
like the Magi of old, still seek wisdom by following a star to
meet Jesus Christ, the Light of the Nations, who brings truth,
health and peace to the human heart.

—Fr. William Henn, O.F.M. Cap.
Professor of Theology
Gregorian University, Rome
April 26, 2000

ACKNOWLEDGMENTS

Gratitude is owed to my Capuchin Superiors for encouragement and for arranging a Franciscan and Gospel way of life for me that allowed time for doing a little writing. Thanks are due to my Capuchin confreres who have helped in finding, checking out and returning books, or who have perhaps listened to a noisy old typewriter after dream time. Thanks also to many helpful and patient librarians at St. Louis University, St. Louis Public Library, St. Anthony Friary Library in St. Louis and the Library of Congress—in particular, to Catherine Weidle and her father Ben Weidle, who often brought books from St. Louis University along with their prayerbooks to old St. Charles Borromeo's; to Fr. Raymond Vandergriff, O.P. at Dominican Library in Washington, D.C.; to Fr. Michael Griffin, O.C.D., Carmelite Library, Washington, D.C. and to Sister Mary Virginia Brennan, Visitation Convent, Georgetown, Washington, D.C. Thanks for other help go to Paul Brown, Michael Carrigan, Gloria Villacis, John McElroy, David Georgii, Fr. Walter Burgholdt, S.J.; to Latinist Tom Lawler; confreres Manuel Mendez and Eric Gauchet; Mrs. Brian Norwood (Lorice), librarian at Capuchin College, Washington, D.C.; to Emilio Biosca, O.F.M. Cap., who did the chart on the Office of Readings for this book; and to Fr. Joseph Mindling, O.F.M. Cap., the Censor Deputatus. Thanks also to our former Provincial, Fr. William Wiethorn, O.F.M. Cap. and Msgr. William J. Kane, former Vicar General, Washington, D.C., who gave the manuscript approval before St. Therese was made a Doctor.

Thanks go also to my brother Gerard Rengers and his wife Helen and their family for refraining from going on a clean-up spree, thereby preserving carbon copies of these chapters and saving the day after five of the originals in my possession had strayed away and found happy repose in some chosen nook of a forgetful borrower.

Finally, thanks go to Thomas Nelson, publisher, and associates Carol Wilcox and Mary Frances Lester. One hand can do the script, but it takes many to do the book. May Mary and Joseph and the prayers of the 33 Doctors help all of the helpers.

BIBLIOGRAPHICAL NOTE

In 1959 Pope John XXIII named the Capuchin St. Lawrence of Brindisi to the list of Doctors of the Church. This signalled for me a new challenge: It stirred the ambition to write on all the Doctors. This task has been a grace—long, interesting and arduous. My chapters on the Doctors were substantially finished about 1967; then two more were written in 1971 after Pope Paul VI added St. Teresa of Avila and St. Catherine of Siena, and the 33rd was written after St. Therese of Lisieux became a Doctor of the Church in 1997.

Capuchin friary libraries and the libraries of St. Louis University had ample research materials, except in a few cases. St. Anthony of Padua's *Sermons* were in the friary library of St. Anthony's Parish in St. Louis. Washington University in St. Louis had some of the just-published volumes of St. Lawrence of Brindisi, and the Library of Congress supplied a needed book on St. Ephrem. Patrologies of Quasten, Althaner and Tixeront were good guides for fundamentals on the early Doctors. All (magazine) articles on individual Doctors were checked in English-language magazines such as the *American Ecclesiastical Review, Irish Ecclesiastical Review, Irish Ecclesiastical Record, The Tablet* (London), *Homiletic and Pastoral Review, The Priest, Thought, Catholic World, Liguorian, Messenger of the Sacred Heart, Clergy Review, Catholic Mind, Catholic Digest, Review for Religious, Catholic Historical Review,* and *The Pope Speaks.* In Latin, the *Acta Sanctae Sedis* and the *Acta Apostolicae Sedis* had all the pertinent documents for anniversary encyclicals, Doctor declarations and other noteworthy Papal statements on the Doctors. Jacques Paul Migne's Latin volumes on Latin and Greek authors and Ludwig von Pastor's *History of the Popes* provided samples of writing and historical background. Anniversary or other special issues of periodicals on Doctors who were members of religious orders were very helpful. For example, the Discalced Carmelites in Washington sent a copy of the special issue of their magazine when St. Teresa was made a Doctor. The Redemptorists in Rome sent a rare copy of the hymns of St. Alphonsus.

In short, research was careful, but certainly not exhaustive. The research was done in Latin and English sources. Several friends were very helpful:

At St. Louis University Library, Catherine Weidle, in charge of rare books, provided frequent assistance, often bringing books from the general shelves to our sacristy in the early morning. Her father, Ben Weidle, served daily Mass into his eighties at old St. Charles Borromeo Church. Monsignor Martin Hellriegel answered many questions on Church music and liturgy. Dr. Ed Weltin, author on early Christianity and at the time Chairman of Washington University History Department, helped much in supplying a good "feel" for the first centuries, its Councils and problems. Dr. Thomas P. Neill, my own major history professor at St. Louis University, with his sweeping view of western intellectual history, had helped in providing the essential background framework. (He was also a speaker at the Doctoral Declaration Symposium for St. Lawrence of Brindisi held at Catholic University of America.)

One to three months' time was spent in the research and writing on each individual Doctor. A few of the men and the three women Doctors took longer—from six months to a year. The guiding method was to give biographical facts that seemed to be of general interest, plus anecdotes illustrating the Doctor's personality, character and devotional bent. A sprinkling of quotes to set forth the Doctor's place in history, literature, theology and papal documents was also part of the plan. Definite attention was given to the major writings of the Doctors and to what called them forth to meet the crises of their own age, to the import they have had over the centuries, and to what application they may have for our times.

Good St. Joseph and the individual Doctors were great as back-up resources to invoke when the Scriptural advice, "Go to the ant, thou sluggard," was apropos. *Our Sunday Visitor,* which published about 20 of these chapters in a condensed form, also provided incentive. The longer versions of the chapters, published here for the first time, took on a "natural" length. No exact size was aimed for.

Much of what the Doctors wrote is available chiefly or only in Greek and Latin. A good bit of work could be done to put into English more of their writings in a selective, condensed way. Needed too are full-length biographies in English of individual Doctors, especially some of the earlier Doctors.

Two valuable series of writings, not confined to the Doctors, continue to be edited and published: the *Ancient Christian Writers* and *The Fathers of the Church*. The first is published by Newman-Paulist Press, the other by the Catholic University of America Press.

Fr. Walter Burghardt, S.J., Dr. John Dillon and Thomas Comerford Lawler are co-editors of *Ancient Christian Writers*. This series began in 1961 and has no definite "end-zone." Volume 55 of the series came out in 1992; it was the first of five volumes of the *Against the Heresies* of St. Irenaeus of Lyons. Fr. Dominic Unger, O.F.M. Cap., the Capuchins' Scripture professor in the 1940's, did the English translation. The 1700-page typescript is being edited by Dr. John Dillon.

The *Fathers of the Church* series, begun in 1953, aimed originally at a 100-volume set, but this number may be expanded, according to David McGonagle, Director of the Catholic University of America Press. In 1989 a Medieval continuation of the series, not included in the original 100-volume plan, began with a volume of 30 letters of St. Peter Damian. Fr. Thomas P. Halton is the present editorial director.

Writings of Doctors of the Church from these two series, together with biographical facts and explanatory material, provide a ready, convenient source of reference in English. Moreover, entries in the *Catholic Encyclopedia* (1907) and in the *New Catholic Encyclopedia* (1967) and in Butler's *Lives of the Saints* provide easy, ready sources for English readers. (Harper and Row published a concise edition of *Butler's Lives* in 1985, with a soft-cover edition in 1991.) Other easily overlooked sources of information and hints on additional materials are religious communities who have Doctors among their saints. Librarians of such communities are friendly and competent helpers.

A variety of books of short biographies of Saints' lives include some of the Doctors. Bishop Donald Wuerl's *Fathers of the Church* (1982) has Sts. Augustine, Athanasius, Basil, Gregory Nazianzen, Hilary, Ambrose, Leo the Great and Gregory the Great. The most complete book in English about the Doctors used to be *The Fathers and Doctors of the Church* by a New Zealand priest, Fr. Ernest Simmons (Bruce, 1959, 188 pp.). It includes 30 Doctors—all but the three women Doctors. In 1999, there appeared a book by Bernard McGinn entitled *The Doctors of the Church—Thirty-Three Men and Women Who Shaped Christianity* (Crossroad, NY), and in 2000 Alba House published a two-volume work by John F. Fink entitled *The Doctors of the Church.*

At this beginning of the third millennium, there are 17 Doctors from the first millennium and 16 from the second. It is interesting to note that the current number of these chosen men and women who in life and written works portray so well the life and teachings of Jesus Christ equals the traditional number of His 33 years of earthly life. The coincidence also provides a handy way to remember that in the Church's first two millennia there have been declared exactly 33 Doctors of the Church.

—Fr. Christopher Rengers, O.F.M. Cap.
August 2, 2000
Feast of Our Lady of the Angels
of the Portiuncula

INTRODUCTION

If it ever happened that Creator and creature, God and man, were united in one person, all human history would have to center on that person. A God-man necessarily would enter into the warp and woof of human existence. All that is human would have to pivot on him. He would have to have a primacy in every part of human endeavor and achievement. There could be no boundaries separating him from any part of what men do, say or think.

It did happen. Creator and creature, God and man united in one Person. A messenger hurried from Heaven, and soon the only Virgin-Mother in human history hastened to her cousin Elizabeth and proclaimed: "My soul magnifies the Lord, and my spirit rejoices in God my Saviour; because He has regarded the humility of His handmaid; for behold, from henceforth all generations shall call me blessed, because He who is mighty has done great things for me; and holy is His name." (*Luke* 1:46-49).

The Son of Mary soon to be born in Bethlehem would have to be forever the center of the human race. B.C. and A.D. do not simply mark a convenient central spot in the passage of time. They represent a far deeper truth, that Jesus Christ is the essential center of all that is human in time and eternity.

All are called to walk in His path, to follow His way, to listen to His teaching. All are called first to know, then to believe what He said, then to do what He commanded. Mary's response to the Angel: "Behold the handmaid of the Lord; be it done to me according to thy word" (*Luke* 1:38), must find an echo in every human being; each one must respond: "Behold the servant of the Lord."

All are called to love Jesus Christ, for He is more worthy of love than any other. All love for other human beings must bear a certain order, a right relationship to Him, to what He taught and commanded. All other people must be loved in Him.

Because He enters so intimately into all that is human, there has been, there is and there will be an ongoing need, as the horizons of history and human achievement expand, to explain this one supreme Human Being and how His teaching and His life fit into the changing scene. He Himself provided for this need. He left a living teaching authority to speak in His stead.

Twelve Apostles, Teachers with Authority

The Gospel of St. Matthew ends with the four great *Alls*: *all* power, *all* nations, *all* I have commanded, *all* days. Jesus told His Apostles: "All power is given to me in heaven and in earth. Going therefore, teach ye all nations; baptizing them in the name of the Father, and of the Son, and of the Holy Ghost. Teaching them to observe all things whatsoever I have commanded you: and behold I am with you all days, even to the consummation of the world." (*Matt.* 28:18-20).

Jesus, the God-man, chose twelve men to carry His message to the world. He chose one of them in particular to strengthen the faith of and lead the others. The twelve men were Apostles, which means men sent forth. As Jesus had commanded, eleven of them—plus others, about 120 in all—gathered to await strength and enlightenment from the Holy Spirit, whom Jesus had promised would come. "All these were persevering with one mind in prayer with the women, and Mary the Mother of Jesus, and with His brethren." (*Acts* 1:14).

Jesus knew there would be problems and questions. So He left a teaching authority to speak for Him. He built His Church on the Apostles. He promised to send the Holy Spirit to guide His followers to the End of Time. In His always gentle, though sometimes fiery way, the Holy Spirit gives His gifts to people. The fullness of the gifts of guidance and authority He reserves for the successors of the Apostles, and in a particular way for the successor of Peter, the Pope. (*Matthew* 16 and *John* 21).

The *Acts of the Apostles* and the epistles of the New Testament show over and over again that there were problems to be solved and questions to answer in the early Church. In the first millennium, some venerable teachers, towering in wisdom, who explained Jesus Christ and His message, have merited to be called *Fathers of the Church*. A few of this group have been singled out with the special title of *Doctor of the Church*. The title simply grew up as a popular epithet. Later, the Church officially recognized more Doctors. The first women Doctors were St. Teresa of Avila and St. Catherine of Siena. Pope Paul VI proclaimed them Doctors on his own initiative in 1970.

The Doctors Help the Teaching Authority

There are three requisites for this highly distinguished title: holiness of life, importance and orthodoxy of writings, and official recognition by the Church.

The learning of the Doctors enlightens our minds. Their hearts speak to our hearts. They help us to answer the questions about Jesus Christ: who He is, what He taught, what He wants us to do, how to be more like Him. The Doctors were followers of Christ who entered deeply into the questions and problems of their time concerning Him.

The early centuries of the Christian era faced fundamental questions about the nature and person of Jesus Himself. The *Acts of the Apostles* and the New Testament epistles give a conspectus of what to expect. From the beginning there were teachers who distorted the words and acts of Jesus. Warning after warning against aberrations in doctrine comes through the epistles of St. Paul, St. Peter and St. James.

Through the centuries, sparks of controversy have served to light flames in the hearts of champions for the truth. Great teachers and writers have helped to make clear what was being questioned. By preaching, teaching and writing, they took part in the ongoing quest for a deeper understanding of the truth about Jesus Christ. The scope of the questions widened, like a circle of waters rippling away from the center. But the focus was always on Jesus and His message.

The Doctors Are Safe Guides

The Doctors of the Church speak with a clear voice. They tend to cluster around the great Councils. They are champions of orthodox teaching, sounding a clear note in a babble of confusion, paving the way in a time of crisis, pointing out a sure path in times of doubt. Because they have clear vision, they are safe guides. Because they are saints, they are fully human. Often they show this in strong love and affection for family and friends. They give generously to all people, especially to the suffering, the sick and poor and to the poorest of all, sinners rushing on toward spiritual ruin and loss of Heaven.

Often the pages of the Doctors glisten with tears shed over the person they were writing to, or because of their depth of feeling over someone's resistance to truth, seeing how this hindered the cause of Christ and frustrated the cause of His Church. Their writings have a fully human approach, embedded in the history and culture of their time and place. Most often they wrote to answer an immediate need of a person, of the Church, or of civil society. Their writing is thus not abstract or merely intellectual. Especially in earlier times, they were not writing for publication. Their writing has punch and it names names. The Doctors used their pen as a weapon for embattled truth, and the truth involved Jesus Christ and those He suffered and died for.

The individual personalities of the Doctors run the gamut. Some were very tough, some very sensitive. John Chrysostom walked the last weary miles of exile in forgiving silence. Cyril of Alexandria, defender of Our Lady as the Theotokos—the God-bearer—died with a prayer to Mary on his lips. His enemies, against whom he had shown himself very tough, suggested that a very heavy stone be put on his grave so that he would not show himself again. Sensitive Gregory of Nazianzen struggled through many years to forgive another Doctor and his closest friend, Basil the Great. He forgave, but hurt feelings lingered. We also find other memorable relationships among the Doctors: Ambrose who converted Augustine, Albert who taught Thomas Aquinas. The Doctors include choleric St. Jerome and gentle St. Francis de Sales.

The Doctors spoke and wrote with unadorned directness. They were not image-conscious, not camera-conscious, posing for history. They drove hard for the immediate objectives of their writing and preaching.

The Doctors have helped to shape the decrees of the twenty-one General Councils of the Church. Their writings have inspired and shaped the hearts and minds of uncounted millions who follow the God-man. The Doctors bring us an important part of our Christian heritage. In some ways, through the varied channels of world communications, their writings have entered into the proverbs of the people and the literature of the masters of prose and poetry.

The eminence of these thirty-three as Doctors of the Universal Church shines forth as evidence of God's special Providence. Their writings tell us of the ongoing guidance of the Holy Spirit in the Church.

The Questions about Jesus Go On

The early questions about Jesus Christ—who He is, what He did and said, what He wants us to do—have never stopped. The succeeding centuries reveal the old questions hiding under new names. It has to be that way. There was once a Man in the Mediterranean area, visible like all of us. Others could see Him, hear Him, talk to Him, embrace Him or strike Him with a whip; yet He could also say with full truth: I am God.

In one Person He united the eternal Son of God and the human nature received from a human mother. He grew in the dark security of her womb for nine months. He was born and lived for 33 years. He died and rose again. He ascended into Heaven and promised to return one day to judge all humanity.

Even as man He has the full right to do so, for He is King of Creation. He is "the image of the invisible God, the firstborn of every creature. . . . all things were created by Him and in Him. He is before all, and by Him all things consist." (*Col.* 1:15-17). He can claim every throne, every presidency, every position of leadership anywhere. Nothing human in this world lies beyond His control or His possession. It is impossible that questions about Him should not continue to challenge the greatest of minds— or that He should not continue to comfort the weak and confound the proud. As old Simeon said in the Temple at Jerusalem, He is a sign that shall be contradicted. He is set for the fall and for the resurrection of many in Israel. (*Luke* 2:34).

Mary asked the first question about Jesus. The angel Gabriel answered it: "The Holy Ghost shall come upon thee, and the power of the most High shall overshadow thee. And therefore also the Holy One which shall be born of thee shall be called the Son of God." (*Luke* 1:35). Joseph struggled silently with the first question about Mary. He came to the wrong decision and was corrected by an angel in a dream. Elizabeth asked at Ain-Karim in sheer amazement: "And whence is this to me, that the mother of my Lord should come to me?" (*Luke* 1:43).

The questions of Joseph and Elizabeth about Mary were ultimately questions about Jesus. The same is true today in questions about the Blessed Virgin's spiritual maternity of the Church as spouse of the Holy Spirit. Like Joseph's, today's questions may be perplexing and painful. Like Elizabeth's, they may be exclamatory and joyful. It is thus with all the questions that come up regarding the ramifications of Christian doctrine and practice: about Saints and Sacraments, Heaven, Hell, Purgatory, authority, liberty; all are ultimately questions about what Jesus Christ did and said, questions about what He wants, about what He has said is unchangeable and what may be changed.

In the Temple at the age of twelve, Jesus answered the questions of the learned doctors. His mother asked him a direct and pained question: "Son, why hast Thou done so to us? Behold in sorrow Thy father and I have been seeking Thee." He answered by putting to her two more questions: "How is it that you sought Me? Did you not know that I must be about My Father's business?" (*Luke* 2:49).

Mary and Joseph took Jesus home to Nazareth. By silent prayer, by much reflection, by the events and conversation of daily living, they little by little learned more about the Son under their roof—the Son so close to their hearts, so close to them in affection and obedience, yet so elusive to them in His pursuit of the Father's plan in His life.

Jesus on the New Horizons of Today

The explosive expansion of human achievement in the past century—in communications, in travel, in exploration of the universe, in piercing some of the secrets locked in the tiniest pieces of matter—will raise inevitable new questions about Jesus Christ and all that pertains to Him.

Our present era has exciting questions about the consciousness of Jesus, the formative influence on Him by Mary and Joseph, and the relation of His teaching to modern medicine, science, space exploration and to the proper distribution of the territories and goods abundantly supplied by the Creator.

But this is still Christ's universe—even as man. The mystery of Him will become clearer and more intimate, but as in the case of Mary and Joseph, He will remain elusive, for the expansion of horizons will reveal questions about Him on more distant horizons. These will serve to help us understand that in eternity the finite creature will pursue the infinite Creator endlessly—always knowing more, loving more, yet always swept along to more distant vistas. The Day of Eternity is an endless dawn.

A review of the 33 Doctors of the Church will help show us where we have been for 20 centuries and 21 General Councils. The light cast by the Doctors is a beam onto the present and into the future.

A look at the Doctors helps bring understanding of the place of Jesus in the life of our times and, more importantly, in our own lives. The Doctors are specialists among specialists. Collectively their hand is on the pulse of all that is Christian.

They help us understand the need for an immense patience in learning about Jesus. They give us a valuable clue about the ongoing work of the Holy Spirit.

None of the Holy Spirit's work is to be snubbed. It comes through Scripture and Tradition, through the liturgy, through the strong central current of the Faith as it exists in the followers of Jesus, through special gifts given to some persons, and through private revelations, especially those meant for the Church and the world. It comes through the careful sifting of scholars. The mosaic of the Holy Spirit's work continues to be put into place, bit by bit, according to the plans of the Father. But all must be tested, and the final decision is made by those who speak for Jesus Christ in today's world: the Holy Father, successor of Peter, and the bishops collectively as successors of the Apostles.

The Next Doctor?

As time goes on, there can be more Doctors chosen by the Church. We need new champions who guide minds and hearts by the clarity of their teachings.

Who will be the next Doctor of the Church? This is difficult to say. St. Therese of Lisieux's proclamation as a Doctor of the Church came as a surprise to many, if not most Catholics.

One name that has been suggested is that of St. Louis De Montfort (1673-1716), so influential by his writings in promoting the Rosary and total consecration to Our Lady. Most of his writings are now available in a volume entitled *God Alone,* while his Marian writings have become famous: *The Secret of the Rosary, True Devotion to Mary* and *The Secret of Mary.*

Franciscans have long cherished a hope that Duns Scotus (c. 1266-1308) would be canonized and honored by the title of Doctor of the Church. He is honored by Franciscans as a Blessed, and his Cause for Canonization is current.

Another saint whose name has been suggested by speculators is St. John Bosco (1815-1888), the 19th-century wonder-worker known for his prophetic dreams, miracles, deep understanding of Christian education and also for his writings.

Without even knowing it, we may assist at the Mass of a future Doctor of the Church. His hand may have touched us in blessing. A saintly woman writer of today may be a Doctor of the Church tomorrow. But one thing is sure. The 33 Doctors of

the Church have already touched us by helping the Church to
have a deeper understanding of the doctrine we cherish and the
piety we practice. They are all stars of Bethlehem, and each in
some way has pointed out where Jesus is and has invited us to
come and adore Him.

                            —Fr. Christopher Rengers, O.F.M. Cap.

THE
33 DOCTORS
OF THE
CHURCH

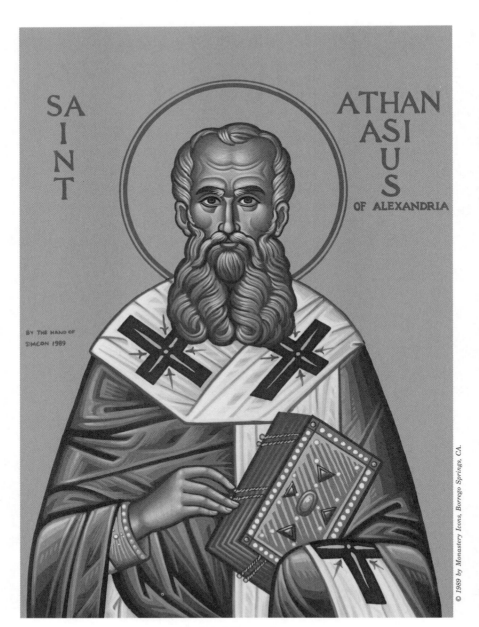

Saint Athanasius

SAINT ATHANASIUS
The Father of Orthodoxy
c. 297-373

A GREAT controversy that involved emperors, popes and bishops, that stirred up intrigue and bloodshed, that shook Christianity to its depths, centered on one simple, sure answer in the Catechism. The answer goes very simply: "The chief teaching of the Catholic Church about Jesus Christ is that He is God made man."

In the providence of God, one man more than any other made the right answer prevail. Because of his championship of this fundamental truth he is called "The Father of Orthodoxy"— "orthodoxy" meaning "right teaching." Cardinal Newman compares him to St. Paul as a defender of Christ's divine Sonship. He calls him "Royal-hearted Athanase, with Paul's own mantle blest."

Counting from the date of his birth, St. Athanasius, defender of Christ's divine Sonship, is the earliest Doctor of the Church. It is fitting that the first man to merit this rare title of honor should have earned it by devotion to a truth of such primary importance. St. Athanasius defended the divine Sonship at the cost of immense personal discomfort, suffering and danger. His whole life was shaped around his defense of the divinity of Christ at a time when powerful imperial forces, and perhaps even the majority of churchmen, had fallen into the Arian Heresy. This situation is summed up in the famous saying: *Athanasius contra mundum*—"Athanasius against the world." At a famous meeting at Milan between the Emperor Constantius and Pope Liberius, the Emperor had challenged the Pope: "Who are you to stand up for Athanasius against the world?" St. Athanasius' life was a life of high adventure that developed precisely from his firm adherence to and clear exposition of the doctrine that Christ is the true Son of God.

From the Emperor Julian's description of St. Athanasius as a "manikin," we gather that he was not very tall. In earlier years his hair was auburn, later turning white. He was energetic in manner, bright and pleasing of countenance, with vivacious eyes; he was engaging and pleasing in conversation. St. Gregory Nazianzen said that St. Athanasius was

> hospitable to strangers, kindly to suppliants, accessible to all, slow to anger, pleasant in conversation, still more pleasant in temper, effective alike in discourse and in action, assiduous in devotions, helpful to Christians of every class and age . . . a theologian with the speculative, a comfort to the afflicted, a staff to the aged, a guide of the young, a physician to the sick . . . a prelate as St. Paul described by anticipation, when in writing to Timothy he showed what a bishop ought to be.

"The Father of Orthodoxy"

St. Athanasius first attracted considerable attention at the First Council of Nicaea, in 325 A.D., where he had accompanied Alexander, then Patriarch of Alexandria. Here the term *homoousios*, "of one substance," was formally introduced to describe the consubstantiality of God the Son with God the Father. The term *homo-ousios*, or "consubstantial," was to become the watchword and standard of orthodoxy. Here the creed known as the Nicene Creed was essentially formulated, though not yet completely. St. Athanasius championed the doctrine of the divinity of Christ, explaining with clarity and force why the Son was equal to and consubstantial with the Father. The First Council of Nicaea anathematized the teaching of Arius, but the Arian struggle was to continue for 50 years.

Five months after the Council of Nicaea, Alexander, Patriarch of Alexandria, died. The bishops of Egypt, spurred on in part by the enthusiastic cries of the people: "Give us Athanasius! He will be a bishop indeed," elected the youthful Athanasius to be the Bishop of Alexandria. He was then just about 30 years old. The exact date of his birth is not known. He was born about 297 A.D. and died on May 2, 373. Nothing is known of his family. From the thoroughness of his education, it is presumed that he came from well-to-do parents who could afford a good education. But he could have received much of this through the influence of Alexander, who very likely took early notice of him and brought him into the episcopal household.

The Empire's Most-Wanted "Criminal"

When one thinks of a bishop, one pictures him as residing in his diocese, directing its affairs. If he is banished or martyred, that is the dramatic end of the story. St. Athanasius was the Bishop of Alexandria, Egypt for almost 47 years. During that time he was driven into exile not once, but five times, and by four different Roman emperors: Constantine, Constantius, Julian and Valens.

His banishment by Julian lasted as he had predicted, just a short time. The first exile—that under Constantine—was from February 5, 336 until November 23, 337. The time spent away from his see under Constantius and Valens covered at least 10 actual years. The gathering storms that led to his flights or banishments covered many of the other years of his life. In between, he did have some periods of relative calm in which to administer his patriarchate.

But the bitter enemies that sought to destroy him were always at work plotting, at times trying to have him discredited and condemned by Church councils, at times whispering lies against him into the ears of the Emperor, trying—and at times succeeding—in having him removed from his bishopric. For some time he was officially condemned to death. He was often in danger of being killed by fierce personal enemies. The roughness of the times is shown by the fact that two usurpers to his see of Alexandria, Gregory and George, both met violent ends. The latter was kicked to death by the pagans of the city, who disliked him so much that his body was then burned and his ashes flung into the sea.

Both these usurping bishops were Arians. They followed Arius, the tall, pale heresiarch who denied that Christ is really God. Arius was a priest of Alexandria. The most active persecutor of St. Athanasius, however, was the Arian bishop, Eusebius of Nicomedia. This powerful, scheming diplomat never gave up. He invented one false charge after another against Athanasius; he won over the Emperor Constantius II to the Arian viewpoint and made him the "scourge and torment" of Athanasius. Constantius said that he would prize a victory over Athanasius more than over Silvanus or Magnentius, his political enemies.

Constantius II eventually stood alone as undisputed ruler of the empire. He had overcome all opposition. Even Hosius of Cordova, who had been the presiding bishop at Nicaea, when beyond the age of 100 was browbeaten and literally beaten into signing an Arian creed (357 A.D.).

Appeals to Rome

When St. Athanasius, who was Patriarch of an important Eastern diocese, was deposed by Eastern Arian bishops, he appealed to Rome. Writing to the Emperor, he said: "When I left Alexandria, I did not go to your brother's headquarters or to any other persons, but only to Rome; and having laid my case before the Church (for this was my only concern), I spent my time in the public worship." (Quoted in *Upon This Rock*, Stephen Ray, ed., Ignatius Press, 1999, p. 201).

In his correspondence, St. Athanasius has also preserved for posterity the celebrated letter of Pope St. Julius I, which defended Athanasius and restored the bishopric from which he had been wrongfully deposed. The letter of Julius called the action of the Arian bishops a *novel* action, indicating that earlier practice had been to refer such cases to Rome. Instead, the bishops had deposed Athanasius and then sent legates to ask approval for their action. Pope St. Julius writes:

> Why was nothing said to us [Pope Julius and the Roman Church] concerning the Church of the Alexandrians in particular? Are you ignorant that the custom has been for word to be written first to us, and then for a just decision to be passed from this place? If then any such suspicion rested upon the Bishop there, notice thereof ought to have been sent to the Church of this place [Rome]; whereas, after neglecting to inform us, and proceeding on their own authority as they pleased, now they desire to obtain our concurrence in their decisions, though we never condemned him. Not so have the constitutions of Paul, not so have the traditions of the Fathers directed; this is another form of procedure, a novel practice. I beseech you, readily bear with me; what I write is for the common good. For what we have received from the blessed Apostle Peter, that I signify to you; and I should not have written this, as deeming that these things were manifest unto all men, had not these proceedings so disturbed us. (Quoted in *Upon This Rock*, pp. 199-200).

On a less happy note, we have the equally famous (though disputed) signature of Pope Liberius on a weak Christological statement, known in history as "the fall of Liberius." Though historians are not unanimous, it is widely agreed that, under duress, Pope Liberius signed an Arian or semi-Arian formula—which he later retracted—and that at one point he signed a condemnation or excommunication of St. Athanasius. This temporary lapse on the part of Pope Liberius is referred to by St. Jerome, by St. Athanasius himself, St. Hilary and by the famous 5th-century historian Sozomen. Cardinal Newman treats of the fall of Liberius in his *The Arians of the Fourth Century*. Rev. Alban Butler in his classic *Lives of the Saints* wrote that Pope Liberius "yielded to the snare laid for him, to the great scandal of the Church. He subscribed the condemnation of St. Athanasius and a confession or creed which had been framed by the Arians at Sirmium. . . ."

The document which Pope Liberius signed while in exile was likely that of the first formula of Sirmium. The formula was not heretical, but it was defective and weak because it omitted the term *homo-ousios*. The case of Pope Liberius passed scrutiny at Vatican Council I (1869-1870), which defined papal infallibility. Liberius, strong defender of Athanasius and of the doctrine of the Council of Nicaea, but weakened by the rigors of exile and apparently hoping to return to Rome, had signed a defective formula. Athanasius mentions the fact in his history of the Arians (*Apologia contra Arianos*). Pope Liberius' weakness was both preceded and followed by firmness in upholding the true Catholic teaching. The fall of Liberius was a temporary lapse, of which he soon repented, and Liberius is now *Saint* Liberius.

In these times St. Jerome could express his feelings with the sad exaggeration: "The whole world groaned and was amazed to find itself Arian." But the symbol of opposition to Arianism, its powerful antagonist, could not be subdued. When Constantius wanted to end the story by killing him, St. Athanasius escaped into the desert.

The importance of St. Athanasius to the Catholic cause can be judged by the universal opposition of those who wanted to make the world Arian, or at least semi-Arian. It can be judged from the political importance of those who sought to destroy him. When the new Emperor, Julian the Apostate, wanted to restore paganism, his advisers told him that the worship of the gods could not be re-established with the Archbishop of Alexandria on the scene. It was then that Julian contemptuously called St. Athanasius "this manikin" and threatened him with worse than banishment.

The Adventures of Athanasius

St. Athanasius fled Alexandria and was pursued up the Nile. When the imperial officers were gaining on him, he ordered his boat turned around. At the time it was still hidden from the pursuers by a bend in the river. When the two boats crossed paths, the Roman officers, not personally knowing Athanasius, shouted out, asking if anyone had seen Athanasius. St. Athanasius himself answered them: "He is not very far off." The other boat hastily continued up the river.

Had he wanted to, St. Athanasius could have written a very interesting account of his hairbreadth escapes. He was a fugitive for many years. He is said to have returned at times in disguise to Alexandria. Even if this is not true, the fact that he was the most wanted "criminal" in the Roman Empire for such a long time would have meant a constant dependence upon places of hiding and shelter; it would have meant a great deal of quick thinking to escape arrest.

At one time St. Athanasius was accused of practicing magic. This was a charge not easy to refute, as it immediately stirred up fear. His accusers showed a wooden box holding the blackened, withered hand of a dead man. This, they said, was the hand of Arsenius, the bishop of Hypsele. They claimed he had been poisoned by Athanasius, who had allegedly also cut off his hand and used it in the practice of magic. Even after St. Athanasius had refuted all the other charges levied against him at this particular time, the suspicion of practicing magic lingered. Then, in the presence of a council of bishops at Tyre in 335, St. Athanasius dramatically introduced Arsenius, who was supposed to be dead. Arsenius was clothed in a long-sleeved robe. Athanasius asked him to put forth slowly first one hand, and then the other. "You see," he told the council, "he has two hands. Where is the third, which I cut off? God has created men with two hands only."

It was at this same council that a woman, bribed to accuse St. Athanasius of immorality, was brought forward. On this occasion a priest named Timothy did some quick thinking and stood up to confront the woman: "Do you really accuse me of this crime?" he asked. She replied, "Certainly," thus showing the whole group that she did not even know St. Athanasius by sight.

His Writings

A convenient sample of St. Athanasius' many writings is provided by the eleven Readings used in the *Liturgy of the Hours* as published in 1971. The earliest of the Doctors of the Church greets us on the first day of each year, now observed as the Solemnity of Mary, the Mother of God. The selected Reading II for the day shows his "clarity, precision and simplicity," qualities by which the great patrologist, Johannes Quasten, characterizes the style of St. Athanasius. In this passage St. Athanasius declares:

> Gabriel used careful and prudent language when he announced His [Christ's] birth. He did not speak of "what will be born in you," in order to avoid the impression that a body would be introduced into her womb from outside; he spoke of "what will be born *from* you," so that we might know by faith that her child originated within her and from her . . . What was born of Mary was therefore human by nature, in accordance with the inspired Scriptures, and the body of the Lord was a true body: It was a true body because it was the same as ours. Mary, you see, is our sister, for we are all born from Adam . . . Even when the Word takes a body from Mary, the Trinity remains a Trinity, with neither increase nor decrease. It is forever perfect. In the Trinity we acknowledge one Godhead; and thus one God, the Father of the Word, is proclaimed in the Church. (*Letter to Epictetus*).

St. Athanasius' Letter to Epictetus was written in answer to questions put by Epictetus, Bishop of Corinth. The questions concerned the relationship of the historical Christ to the Eternal Son. The *Letter* gained much respect and would be used by the Council of Chalcedon in 451 A.D. as the expression of its own conclusions. The opening lines of the *Letter* illustrate St. Athanasius' direct attack in fighting for the precious truths called into question.

> What lower region has vomited forth the statement that the body born of Mary is co-essential with the Godhead of the Word? . . . Whoever heard in the Church, or even from Christians, that the Lord wore a body putatively, not in nature?

Reading II for the Solemnity of the Most Holy Trinity is also taken from St. Athanasius. It is addressed to St. Serapion of

Thmuis, who was himself a bishop and an influential writer. The *Four Letters* of St. Athanasius to him are in effect the first formal treatise on the Holy Spirit. The Reading for Trinity Sunday is from the *First Letter to Serapion:*

> It will not be out of place to consider the ancient tradition, teaching and faith of the Catholic Church, which was revealed by the Lord, proclaimed by the Apostles and guarded by the Fathers. For upon this faith the Church is built, and if anyone were to lapse from it, he would no longer be a Christian, either in fact or in name . . . We acknowledge the Trinity, holy and perfect, to consist of the Father, the Son and the Holy Spirit. In this Trinity there is no intrusion of any alien element or of anything from outside, nor is the Trinity a blend of creative and created being. It is a wholly creative and energizing reality, self-consistent and undivided in its active power, for the Father makes all things through the Word and in the Holy Spirit, and in this way the unity of the Holy Trinity is preserved . . .

Strange to say, a long interval of time separates the writing of St. Athanasius' most notable books. *Against the Pagans* was written in 318, and *On the Incarnation of the Word of God* in 323 (both when St. Athanasius was only in his twenties), but his three *Discourses against the Arians* were not written until 368. Among his *Festal Letters*, sent yearly to suffragan bishops to announce Lenten practice and the Easter date, the one for 367 A.D. has special importance. It lists, for the first time we have a record of them, the 27 canonical books of the New Testament. The Old Testament list of St. Athanasius, however, does not include the deutero-canonical books of the Old Testament. Among his other letters, the *Letter Concerning the Decrees of the Nicene Council* defends the non-scriptural expressions in the Nicene Creed.

Some today think that the familiar *Athanasian Creed*, known also as the *Quicumque*, is actually not the work of St. Athanasius, though our tradition has long attributed it to him, and its tone is typical of his strong defense of the Faith and his entire cast of mind. Before the 1971 changes in the Liturgy, the *Athanasian Creed*, consisting of 40 rhythmic statements, had been used in the Sunday Office for over a thousand years. It closes with the words: "This is the Catholic Faith, which, except a man believe faithfully and firmly, he cannot be saved." That the name of St. Athanasius should have been attached to it attests to his renown as a teacher of orthodoxy, that is, of a fully correct belief in what Jesus Christ teaches, as given to us in Scripture, Tradition and liturgical practice.

Evidence of Early Devotion to Mary

Because of his great defense of Christ as true God and true man, St. Athanasius was also a strong defender of Mary, His Mother. One cannot define Jesus and His place in God's plan without defining Mary and her place in God's plan.

But St. Athanasius also had a warm, devotional attitude to Mary. A remarkable passage from one of his homilies makes this clear. And since a homily also reflects the heart and mind of the people, the passage also points to early popular devotion to our Blessed Mother.

> O noble Virgin, truly you are greater than any other greatness. For who is your equal in greatness, O dwelling place of God the Word? To whom among all creatures shall I compare you, O Virgin? You are greater than them all. O [Ark of the New] Covenant, clothed with purity instead of gold! You are the Ark in which is found the golden vessel containing the true manna, that is, the flesh in which divinity resides. Should I compare you to the fertile earth and its fruits? You surpass them, for it is written: "The earth is my footstool." (*Is.* 66:1). But you carry within you the feet, the head, and the entire body of the perfect God.
>
> If I say that heaven is exalted, yet it does not equal you, for it is written: "Heaven is my throne" (*Is.* 66:1), while you are God's place of repose. If I say that the angels and archangels are great—but you are greater than them all, for the angels and archangels serve with trembling the One who dwells in your womb, and they dare not speak in His presence, while you speak to Him freely.
>
> If we say that the cherubim are great, you are greater than they, for the cherubim carry the throne of God (cf. *Ps.* 80:1; 99:1), while you hold God in your hands. If we say that the seraphim are great, you are greater than them all, for the seraphim cover their faces with their wings (cf. *Is.* 6:2), unable to look upon the perfect glory, while you not only gaze upon His face but caress it and offer your breasts to His holy mouth. . . .
>
> As for Eve, she is the mother of the dead, "for as in Adam all die, even so in Christ shall all be made alive." (*1 Cor.* 15:22). Eve took [fruit] from the tree and made her husband eat of it

along with her. And so they ate of that tree of which God had told them: "The day you eat of it, you shall die." (*Gen.* 2:17). Eve took [fruit] from it, ate some of it, and gave some to her husband [that he might eat] with her. He ate of it, and he died.

In you, instead, O wise Virgin, dwells the Son of God: He, that is, who is the tree of life. Truly He has given us His body, and we have eaten of it. That is how life came to all, and all have come to life by the mercy of God, your beloved Son. That is why your spirit is full of joy in God your Savior! (Quoted in Luigi Gambero, S.M., *Mary and the Fathers of the Church*, Ignatius Press, 1999, pp. 106-107).

His Place in People's Hearts and in History

If St. Athanasius had bitter enemies, he also had loyal, devoted friends. The affection of the Alexandrians for their bishop never lessened during his many vicissitudes. His returns from exile were unmitigated triumphs. Hundreds of thousands of people streamed out of the city to meet him on his second return, in 346. Carpets and tapestries were spread out. Palms were waved. Shouting and clapping rolled out in a continuous wave of sound. The event became proverbial to describe a festive occasion. If there was a really extraordinary celebration, it was "like the return of Athanasius." Moreover, the Patriarch's return did not wear itself out in one big demonstration. Such was his influence that the vigorous pursuit of prayer and holiness continued on in homes and churches.

Besides his many writings setting forth the doctrine of the Incarnation and giving the history of the Arians and refuting them, St. Athanasius wrote the famous *Life of St. Antony* (of the Desert). His authorship of this book, once attacked, is now considered certain. *The Life of St. Antony* had much importance in making known the early history of monasticism and in helping to develop it. St. Augustine in his *Confessions* speaks of the *Life of St. Antony* as a deciding influence in his own conversion. One of the strange twists of history is that St. Antony has stirred the imagination of many artists, who have represented him in sculpture and paintings; whereas, St. Athanasius himself, who made St. Antony known and who had a more influential and interesting career, is unknown to art.

St. Athanasius was a careful user of words. His comment about his own works on the divinity of Christ is a good example: "That which I wrote was unequal to the imperfect shadow of the truth which existed in my conceptions." Erasmus compared St. Athanasius to other early Church writers and considered him free from their various faults. He said that St. Athanasius was "clear, acute, reasonable, appropriate; in short, fitted in all ways for teaching." Cardinal Newman says: . . . "In my own judgment, no one comes near him but Chrysostom and Jerome."

Such praise from two classicists of the stature of Erasmus and Cardinal Newman is high indeed. It is, however, only fitting that the defender of the most important teaching about Christ in the Catechism should be a writer of the highest skill.

A number of Fathers of the Church have pointed out that there is a kind of divine judgment in the names of heretical factions. In their very names they show their origins. St. Jerome says, for instance, "If you ever hear those who are called Christians named, not from the Lord Jesus Christ, but from someone else, say, Marcionites, Valentinians, Montanists, Campestrians, know that it is not Christ's Church, but the synagogue of Anti-Christ."

Pacian pointed out that the word "Catholic" is not borrowed from man. He wrote, "Christian is my name, Catholic my surname." The Arians tried to pin a name on Catholics, calling them "Athanasians." The name did not stick; it was used only by Arians. But the attempt to use it is an unintentional tribute to St. Athanasius.

Today, unfortunately, there is not much general knowledge about St. Athanasius. He is not what we call a popular saint. It would be well if he *were* a popular saint, for we need his spirit and his arguments once again in the Church. For the divinity of Christ is again under attack today, as are many other dogmas. When our present-day champions of the Faith speak out, they indeed stand on the shoulders and in the tradition of St. Athanasius. He is, as Cardinal Newman says, "a principal instrument, after the Apostles, by which the sacred truths of Christianity have been conveyed and secured to the world." His feast day occurs on May 2.

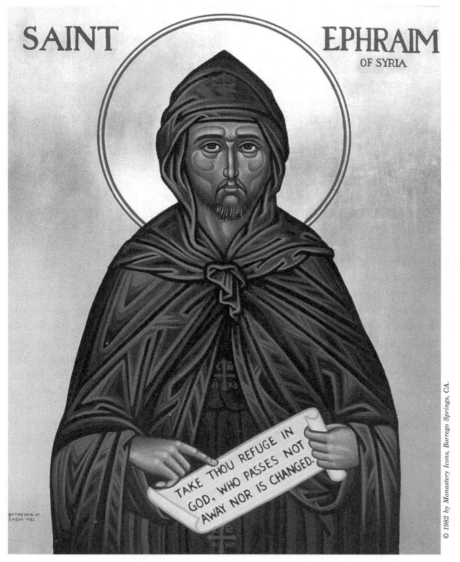

SAINT EPHRAIM OF SYRIA

TAKE THOU REFUGE IN GOD, WHO PASSES NOT AWAY NOR IS CHANGED.

Saint Ephrem

2

SAINT EPHREM

Harp of the Holy Ghost
Mary's Own Singer
Father of Hymnody
c. 306-c. 373

There lie those who improved their complexions,
And artfully disguised their faces;
There lie those who painted their eyelids,
And the worm corrodes their eyes . . .
There lie those who were enemies,
And their bones are mingled together.

THE writer of the above is not a modern poet meditating on death in a cemetery. He is a fourth-century Doctor of the Universal Church, who seems strikingly modern in much of what he says. His fellow countrymen have given him many titles. He is variously called "The Pillar of the Church," "The Doctor of the World," "The Eloquent Mouth," "The Poet of God," "The Prophet of the Syrians," "Mary's Own Singer" and the "Harp of the Holy Ghost."

It is inevitable that St. Ephrem (his name is also spelled Ephraem and Ephraim), the greatest poet of Syria and the one who inspired such titles, would also inspire a large overlay of legend regarding the facts of his life. Thus, there are many stories and details that are hard to prove in the ancient lives of this Saint. Yet, from what we do know and from the evidence of the large remnant of his writings still extant, we could easily employ any of the above titles as a heading in relating his life. St. Ephrem was an extraordinary person, one who is too little known.

From distant and dim fourth-century Syria, his words about the Holy Eucharist, Penance, the primacy of Peter, about the Blessed Virgin and the sufferings of Christ come down to us like bright rays of light. They strike the present and fit in perfectly with our way of thinking and our bent of devotion, which has gradually developed through many centuries. His outlook on the Passion of Christ, for instance, giving attention to the details of Our Lord's suffering, is very much like that of St. Francis of Assisi in the thirteenth century. It is St. Francis who is chiefly credited with shaping our modern outlook on these sufferings.

St. Ephrem wrote of the Scourging at the Pillar:

> A man whom He had formed wielded the scourge. He who sustained all creatures with His might submitted His back to their stripes. He who is the Father's Right Arm yielded His own arms to be extended . . . Savage dogs did bark at the Lord who with His thunder shakes the mountains; they sharpened their teeth against the Son of Glory.

Regarding the Sacrament of Penance, St. Ephrem wrote: "Consider that without the most venerable priesthood, remission of sins is not granted to mortals."

A 20th-century poet would have a hard time summarizing with more clarity and feeling or more concisely and tenderly the Mass and the priest's role in it than does St. Ephrem when he says:

> Blessed is the priest who in the sanctuary
> Offers to the Father the Son of the Father,
> The Fruit that is plucked from our tree,
> Though it be wholly of the Divine Majesty!
> Blessed the hands that are hallowed and offer Him!
> And the lips that are spent in kissing Him.

"The Deacon of Edessa"

St. Ephrem is known to history as "The Deacon of Edessa." There is little doubt that he remained only a deacon, and if so, he is the only male Doctor of the Church who did not become a priest or bishop. Most likely he did not receive even the diaconate until he was past 60. He had gone eagerly to see and to hear St. Basil the Great in Caesarea of Cappadocia (on the south shore of the Black Sea in what is now northern Turkey). According to this view, St. Basil ordained him a deacon at that time but Ephrem refused the higher dignity of the priesthood. The Church historian, Sozomen, says that St. Basil later sent messengers to summon St. Ephrem to consecration as a bishop.

But St. Ephrem feigned madness, putting on such a good show that the shocked messengers went back to report to St. Basil that the man he had chosen was out of his mind. But St. Basil exclaimed: "O hidden pearl of price whom the world knows not! Ye are the madmen and he the sane!"

St. Ephrem's name is associated with Edessa in Syria (Urfa today), where he spent the last ten years of his life and did most of his writing. He actually lived outside of the city as a hermit on Mount Edessa. It is here in the Armenian monastery of St. Sergius that his tomb is still shown today.

St. Ephrem was born at Nisibis in Mesopotamia, about 306 A.D., the date of the beginning of the reign of Constantine. Most of his long life was spent in and around this city. He indicates a Christian parentage when he writes: "I was born in the way of truth: though my boyhood understood not the greatness of the benefit, I knew it when trial came." Ephrem may have accompanied St. James, Bishop of Nisibis, to the Council of Nicaea in 325, and after the return home may have become the headmaster of the episcopal school at Nisibis.

Dissolved in Tears

The life of St. Ephrem was touched by military adventure, since he lived at Nisibis during the three sieges of that city by Sapor, King of Persia, in 338, 346 and 350. Ephrem's account in his Nisibean hymns of how Sapor flooded the land around Nisibis corresponds in detail with the account given by Julian the Apostate. In 363, when the Emperor Jovian surrendered the city to the Persians, St. Ephrem joined most of the Christians in leaving the territory. He came south to Edessa, and except for the trip to see St. Basil and perhaps a journey to Egypt, he lived there until his death about the year 373.

At Edessa, too, there was an invasion. The Huns came to murder and pillage. St. Ephrem is said to have written the history of this attack, but the writing has been lost. In the final year of his life, he came from his retreat outside the city to direct the distribution of grain during a severe famine and to attend to the care of the sick and the burial of the dead. Worn out by these unusual exertions, he died a month after returning to his hermit's cell. "God gave him this occasion that therein he might win the crown in the close of his life."

St. Ephrem led a very austere life, eating little, but praying and working much. He is described as being bald, beardless and of short stature. Gregory of Nyssa tells us that St. Ephrem wept constantly.

As one samples St. Ephrem's writings and thinks over the facts of his life, the impression emerges of an intensely pure, mystical soul. If he wept often or constantly, it was not because he was simply sad. It was, rather, the body's reaction to an over-whelmingly active mind that swept constantly back and forth, viewing the depths of man's misery and God's goodness, that exulted in the simple joys of this life and trembled before the justice of God. St. Ephrem's tears must have been more than tears of repentance. Quite often they must have been tears of joy at recognizing the glory of God and His handiwork. He was simply a soul dissolved in tears.

A Most Prolific Writer

Whenever comment is made by biographers about St. Ephrem's writings, they always use such terms as "most copious," "innumerable," "endless abundance." St. Ephrem wrote commentaries on almost all of Sacred Scripture, besides many homilies and hymns. A great many of his writings are not preserved or at least not known to be still extant, yet a large selection still remains to us. Two Popes, Gregory XIII and Benedict XIV, took pains to have his works collected. The scholars engaged in this work were Vossius (1603) and Assemanus (1732-46). Further manuscripts were discovered in the 19th century. The revised (1971) Liturgy of the Hours takes four Readings from the pen of St. Ephrem. One is the Reading for his own feast day, June 9. (In the earlier breviary, the homily for St. Ephrem's feast day, June 18, was taken from his "Sermon on Monastic Life and Practice.")

Most people who write—including some of the best authors—have to chew on a pencil or gaze for some time at a half-filled page, waiting for a new idea. On the contrary, the great Syrian Doctor had to pray that the flow of his ideas would be slowed down. St. Gregory of Nyssa tells us this in his *Encomium on Ephrem*: "It may be a good idea to call on Ephrem when lost for an idea and ask him to send one he has prayed away."

The unbounded fertility of St. Ephrem's mind and its full, overflowing companion, emotion, drive his busy pen across page after page. His sentences march with clipped, epigrammatic briskness like a vast army in review. Many of them seem almost like soldiers in uniform. They may seem redundant to the Western mind, yet if one reads through any of the Epiphany hymns, for instance, he can see that through the measured sameness there is a constant building up of new ideas and new detail. The hymns give the impression of a great mind that sees some sacred truth or event in all its fullness, and then at once explodes, sending the message in a showering spray, to be gathered gradually into the vessel of the reader's mind.

In some spots it does seem that St. Ephrem is repetitious. But despite this, he packs unusual intensity and beauty into a short space. The clever balancing of phrases and the rhythm of thought and wording is often amazing. It would be a challenge indeed to shorten a passage like the following Christmas message without dropping images or losing meaning.

> To Eve, our mother, a man gave birth, who himself had had no birth. How much more should Eve's daughter [Mary] be believed to have borne a Child without a man! The virgin earth bore that Adam that was head over the earth. The Virgin bore today the Adam that was Head over the heavens. The staff of Aaron budded, and the dry wood yielded fruit.

"Mary's Own Singer"

In the hymns of St. Ephrem on the Nativity and Epiphany one finds the ideas and figures that poets of Mary have used throughout the ages. He keeps coming back to the wonder of her virginity and divine motherhood. In Hymn IV of the Nativity series, Mary speaks: "Who hath given me, the barren, that I should conceive and bring forth this One, that is manifold; a little One, that is great; for that He is wholly with me and wholly everywhere?"

The following excerpt from Hymn XII of the same series has an especially lilting quality:

> The babe that I carry carries me, saith Mary, and He has lowered His wings, and taken and placed me between His pinions, and mounted into the air; and a promise has been given me that height and depth shall be my Son's . . . [O Lord Jesus,] In her virginity Eve put on the leaves of shame: Thy Mother put on in her virginity the Garment of Glory that suffices for all. She gave the little vest of the body to Him that covers all.

Blessed is she in whose heart and mind Thou wast! A King's palace she was by Thee, O Son of the King, and a Holy of Holies by Thee, O High Priest! She had not the trouble nor vexation of a family, or a husband.

In his encyclical proclaiming St. Ephrem a Doctor of the Church (*Principi Apostolorum Petro*, October 5, 1920), Pope Benedict XV asks: "But who can ever explain well enough his filial love for the Virgin Mother of God. Without doubt this 'Harp of the Holy Ghost' never renders sweeter tones than when the composition is the singing of the praises of Mary or the celebrating of her inviolate virginity, her divine maternity or her generous and merciful protection."

As we read St. Ephrem's words about Mary, about her divine maternity, we cannot forget that his words, which strike us as so true and natural, are 16 centuries old. St. Ephrem's Catholic insight and understanding were true, unerring and deep, and that is why he fits in so well with our own forms of expression about the Blessed Virgin Mary.

"The Father of Hymnody"

St. Ephrem was not a poet riding on a cloud, distant from humanity. He wrote for people, the common people, to instruct them and to defend them from error. His anonymous Syrian biographer writes:

And the blessed Ephrem, seeing that all men were led by music, rose up and opposed the profane games and noisy dances of the young people, and established the daughters of the convent and taught them odes and scales and responses . . . He, like a father, stood in the midst of them, a spiritual harper, and arranged for them different kinds of songs . . . until the whole people was gathered to him, and the party of the adversary was put to shame and defeated.

St. Ephrem's poems, as the biographer says, were put to music and were sung. He organized choirs of young women and taught them himself. He soon won over the people from the songs that proclaimed false teachings.

St. Ephrem's immediate incentive for this work came from the disciple of Bardesanes, a Syrian writer of the early third century who had popularized heretical teachings in 150 hymns (recalling the number of Psalms). Harmodius, his son, set these to music. St. Ephrem wrote his own words, setting forth the truth, and borrowed the melodies of Harmodius. The force of truth, superior style and organization combined to make people adopt these hymns and forget those of Bardesanes.

Many of the hymns of St. Ephrem have endured as part of the Syrian liturgy. The rich hymnody of this liturgy has evoked the proper ideas and sentiments in Syrian Christians for 16 centuries. The people hear the appropriate hymn at all the important spiritual events of life, from Baptism to the funeral blessing. As the shaper of this hymnody, St. Ephrem has brought his deep mystical mind and strong, tender feelings to millions of people. He has helped to shape minds and direct emotions in the paths of the Faith.

Following the Syrian model, the churches of eastern Christianity have also developed early a rich hymnody, which lent flavor and instruction to liturgical functions.

The contribution of St. Ephrem to Church music has not received enough attention. It still requires study and defining. Pope Benedict XV asks pointedly: "Does our liturgical music itself, with its chants and ceremonial hymns, which Chrysostom imported to Constantinople and Ambrose to Milan, whence it spread throughout Italy, have any other originator [than St. Ephrem]?" Pope Benedict said further that the Church music which so moved St. Augustine and which Pope St. Gregory the Great refined has its origins in the Syrian antiphonary, or book containing the choral parts of the Divine Office.

It was St. Ephrem who played the leading role in the formation of that antiphonary. With good reason, then, we can call St. Ephrem the Father of Hymnody in the Catholic Church.

The Poet

St. Ephrem was no ethereal mystic, nor was he a recluse with stunted emotions. Henry Burgess, a translator of some of his hymns, comments on this: "In the shorter pieces, especially those on the subject of death, there is a tender spirit displayed which makes us feel that the monastic habits of Ephrem had induced no unnatural sternness nor choked up one fountain of human feeling and kindliness."

His poems about children show his close contact with humanity and his tender heart. On the death of a child he writes:

. . . The sound of thy sweet notes
Once moved me and caught mine ear,
And caused me much to wonder;
Again my memory listens to it,
And is affected by the tones
And harmonies of thy tenderness.

When St. Ephrem dwells on the shortness of life and the mortality of the body, he speaks of the body's corrupting in the grave. That this was not an unbalanced view and that he was not minimizing the body but merely giving expression to one side of a truth, he shows in the following stanza:

O my body, my temporary home,
Remain here in peace;
And in the day of the resurrection
I shall see thee rejoicing.

St. Ephrem, Doctor of Unity

The previously mentioned encyclical of Pope Benedict XV has for its opening phrase: "To Peter, the Prince of the Apostles." This sets the theme and emphasizes the leading idea of the Holy Father. He considered St. Ephrem to have been a strong defender of the primacy of Peter and of the papacy. He hoped that St. Ephrem might be a bond to help re-unite the Eastern churches with Rome. In fact, the Pope did not leave the matter in doubt, but later in the Encyclical made it very specific.

He quoted a hymn of St. Ephrem in which Christ is speaking to His vicar:

Simon, My disciple, I have made you the foundation of the holy Church; I have called you the rock, that you might support the whole building. You are the inspector of those who build the Church for Me on earth. If they wish to build what is reprobate, forbid them. You are the head of the fountain from which My doctrine issues. You are the head of My disciples, and through you I will give drink to all nations.

As he recalled these strong words of St. Ephrem, that great Father of the Syrian Church, the Pope said that he besought God with tears to lead back those Eastern churches separated from the Chair of Peter. St. Ephrem, in fact, offers a special witness to the traditions of the early Church in the East. He lived in Syria, which was to a large extent independent in its development of theology and devotion. Syria was not in the mainstream of Greek and Roman philosophy. Christianity had come to Syria from nearby Palestine, and in many ways this country must represent the most primitive and original traditions.

Stephen L. Ray in his excellent book, *Upon This Rock*, quotes from one of the poems of St. Ephrem. It indicates the authority of St. Peter and his successors in the See of Rome. Ephrem's testimony is especially valuable, for it is early and he is from the East, not likely to be biased in favor of papal claims by a bishop in the West.

> Simon, My follower, I have made you the foundation of the holy Church. I betimes called you Peter [Kefa or *Rock*, in the original text] because you will support all its buildings. You are the inspector of those who will build on earth a Church for Me. If they should wish to build what is false, you, the foundation, will condemn them. You are the head of the fountain from which My teaching flows; you are the chief of My disciples. Through you I will give drink to all peoples. Yours is that life-giving sweetness which I dispense. I have chosen you to be, as it were, the firstborn of My institution, and so that, as the heir, you may be executor of My treasures. I have given you authority over all My treasures. (Quoted in *Upon This Rock*, Stephen K. Ray, ed., Ignatius Press, 1999, pp. 194-195).

St. Ephrem himself was a man of one book, the Bible, and considered it alone worthy of explanation and study. He wrote in Syro-Chaldaic, the language used by Christ, the Blessed Virgin, St. Joseph and the Apostles in everyday life. Using this language, knowing it as his own mother tongue, gave him an insight into their way of thinking, into their finer modes of expression and meaning.

The full force of St. Ephrem's mind and the full power of his poetic and mystical insight were turned to bringing to others the truth drawn from the purest of sources: Scripture and the Apostolic Tradition. To Catholics this helps explain why his voice reaches us today with such clarion distinctness. For Protestants, this must prove a strong attraction, for in St. Ephrem they will find a Gospel simplicity allied to deep sincerity and feeling.

That he could say these things about Catholic doctrines still largely undefined shows that he saw deeply into the essence of Christianity. And the fact that so much of what St. Ephrem says sounds striking and alive also shows that he saw deeply into the human heart.

Perhaps the more we come to know St. Ephrem, the more we will recognize his universal appeal to the Christian heart. The more really Christian we are, the more likely is "The Harp of the Holy Ghost" to strike a responsive chord in our own hearts. The humble deacon of Edessa could possibly become the Doctor of Christian Unity.

St. Ephrem's feast day is celebrated on June 9 (June 18 in the 1962 calendar).

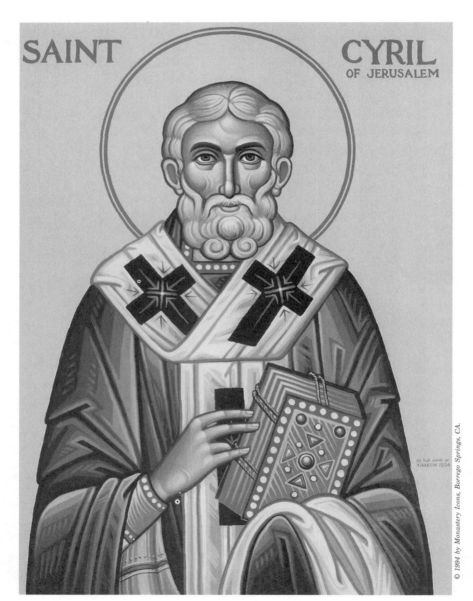

SAINT CYRIL OF JERUSALEM

Saint Cyril of Jerusalem

3

SAINT CYRIL OF JERUSALEM
Doctor of Catechesis
c. 315-386

ALMOST anyone can tell you whose feast is March 17: St. Patrick. Most Catholics will know too that March 19 is the feast of St. Joseph. But how many can name the Saint whom the Church honors on the day in between? Although not too well known in the popular sense, the Saint whose feast day is March 18 belongs to the small and select group honored as Doctors of the Church.

He is the only Doctor who was a bishop in the land of Christ's earthly life. For about 38 years (348-386), he was the Bishop of Jerusalem; for that reason he is known to us as St. Cyril of Jerusalem.

St. Cyril may have actually been born there, in the Holy City, but nobody can say for sure either the place of his birth or the exact year. Some say he was born to the north, in Caesarea. They connect him with this city of northern Palestine because there is some evidence that Cyril was a protege of Eusebius, the Bishop of Caesarea who is called "The Father of Church History." Later, too, Cyril consecrated Gelasius, his sister's son, to be Bishop of Caesarea.

There is more direct evidence, however, that St. Cyril spent his youth in Jerusalem. (He speaks as an eyewitness about the sacred spots of Christ's death and burial as they looked before they were altered in conjunction with the buildings put up by Constantine.) As a keen-eyed, reflective youth, he had very likely watched the workmen prepare the low ridge called Golgotha for the erection of a church. He would have watched this structure-later called "the Martyry" rise from the ground. It covered part of Golgotha, but not the spot later pointed out as the "little mount of the Cross," which was a little to the west, where relics of the True Cross were venerated. The Martyry was dedicated in 335 A.D.

As a boy, he had watched this first church on Calvary rise, tier on tier, built out of cut stone and polished to elegance; later, in 350 A.D., he stood within it as the Bishop of Jerusalem. When he was preparing catechumens for Baptism, delivering his famous *Catechetical Lectures,* he recalled the scene as it had looked in his youth: "For though it has now been most highly adorned with royal gifts, yet formerly, it was a garden, and the signs and the remnants of this remain." (14, 5). He recalled the outer cave that used to be in front of the Holy Sepulchre: "Now it is not to be seen, since the outer cave was cut away at that time for the sake of the present adornment. For before the decoration of the sepulchre by the royal munificence, there was a cave in front of the rock." (14, 9).

St. Cyril was born about 315 A.D., and he died on March 18, 386. Since he never mentions being converted, it is presumed that his parents were Christian. He also speaks with gratitude of parents who place no obstacle to godliness in our way, seeming to include himself among those whose godly parents had taught them to follow Christ.

Three Exiles

St. Cyril's long term as bishop was interrupted by three depositions: He was sent into exile in 358 and again in 360, for a short period each time; the third exile lasted 11 years, from 367-378. Basically, the cause of all these troubles arose from opposition by Arians, especially Acacius, Bishop of Caesarea. The beginning of these troubles for Cyril, however, arose not over doctrine, but over the rights of the Apostolic See of Jerusalem.

As is usual in such cases, even the good a person does is turned against him. Acacius accused St. Cyril of selling a precious robe for profane use. Acacius told the Emperor Constantius that Cyril had sold a sacred garment given by his (Constantius') father, Constantine, which was supposed to be used by the Bishop when baptizing. After a time the robe came into the possession of a dancer at the theater, who fell while dancing in the robe, injured himself and died. The way the story was told made St. Cyril seem guilty of both ingratitude and irreverence. But even if it were true that St. Cyril had sold the garment, this proves only that in a time of need he would not hesitate to sell Church property to help the poor. There had been a famine in Jerusalem a few years before, and at the time, St. Cyril had done all he could to help feed those who were starving.

Two Notable Events

Two events that find mention in most histories of St. Cyril happened at Jerusalem during his time as its bishop. Regarding the first of these events, he wrote a letter to the Emperor Constantius on May 7, 351:

> . . . About the third hour, a gigantic cross made of light appeared in the sky above holy Golgotha, stretching out as far as the holy Mount of Olives. It was not seen by just one or two, but was most clearly displayed before the whole population of the city. Nor did it, as one might have supposed, pass away quickly like something imagined, but was visible to sight above the earth for some hours, while it sparkled with a light above the sun's rays. Of a surety, it would have been overcome and hidden by them had it not exhibited to those who saw it a brilliance more powerful than the sun, so that the whole population of the city made a sudden concerted rush into the martyry, seized by a fear that mingled with joy at the heavenly vision.

The explanation now commonly given for this miraculous shining cross is that it was a "parhelion," a natural phenomenon caused by atmospheric conditions. At the time it was held to be a favorable sign sent by God.

The second event was the attempted restoration of the Temple in 363 A.D. by order of the Emperor, Julian, known in Church history as Julian the Apostate. The Christians in Jerusalem looked upon this as an impious defiance of the prophecy of Christ that the Temple would be destroyed and that Jerusalem would be under the sway of the Gentiles until the End of Time. (*Luke* 21:6, 24).

The work began, but it was soon stopped because of difficulties encountered. A modern Jewish history says that gases trapped in the subterranean passages below the ruins of the old Temple ignited on contact with the air as the site was being cleared, burning the workers. Ancient Christian writers speak of balls of fire coming from the earth, and of earthquakes. Just what St. Cyril had to do with the event is not known, though he has often been credited with prophesying that nothing would come of the attempted re-building.

St. Cyril Thoroughly Catholic

The chief writings of St. Cyril are his *Catechetical Lectures,* which number 24 in all, and his *Collected Letters.* Nineteen of the *Catechetical Lectures* were given during Lent, and the remaining five during the week after Easter. They show St. Cyril as a man strongly upholding the divinity of Christ and zealously defending the Church. He warns against going to the churches of those who teach false doctrines:

> Should you ever be staying in some strange town, do not just ask, "Where is the church?" seeing that all those sects of the ungodly would have their dens called "churches." And do not be content to ask where the church is, but ask where is the Catholic Church. For this is the peculiar name of this Holy Church, the mother of us all, which is the spouse of our Lord Jesus Christ. (18, 26).

St. Cyril also explains why the Church is called "Catholic":

> The Church, then, is called "Catholic" because it is spread through the whole world, from one end of the earth to the other, and because it never stops teaching in all its fullness every doctrine that men ought to be brought to know: and that regarding things visible and invisible, in Heaven and on earth. It is called "Catholic" also because it brings into religious obedience every sort of men, rulers and ruled, learned and simple, and because it is a universal treatment and cure for every kind of sin, whether perpetrated by soul or body, and possesses within itself every form of virtue that is named, whether it expresses itself in deeds or words or in spiritual graces of every description. (18, 23).

St. Cyril was a man of directness and simplicity when teaching divine truths. He did not bother the neophytes he was instructing with problems which theologians were disputing and which even many learned and good men could not quite solve. Therefore, he never used the word—so much in dispute at the time—"consubstantial" (*homo-ousios* in Greek) when speaking of Christ's divinity. The wording of the Creed, as he taught it at Jerusalem, did not include this adjective. Therefore, St. Cyril avoided needless controversy in teaching the rudiments of the Faith by leaving it out of his explanations. Neither did he mention Arius, the infamous heresiarch, or Arianism, his pernicious doctrine.

But St. Cyril so abundantly, clearly and undeniably proves to his prospective converts that Christ is God that it is foolish to try to label him anything but undeniably and completely Catholic. "And as I have said," he told his listeners,

> He [God the Father] did not bring forth the Son from non-existence into being, nor take the non-existent into sonship; but the Father, being Eternal, eternally and ineffably begat one Only Son, who has no brother. Nor are there two first principles; but the Father is the head of the Son; the beginning is One. For the Father begat the Son, very God, called "Emmanuel"; and "Emmanuel," being interpreted, is "God with us." (11, 14).

In explaining the text, "I am in the Father, and the Father in me" (*John* 14:11), St. Cyril says:

> One they are because of the dignity pertaining to the Godhead, since God begat God . . . One because the creative works of Christ are no other than the Father's; for the creation of all things is one, the Father having made them through the Son . . . The Son then is very God, having the Father in Himself, not changed into the Father . . .

Victim of Misunderstanding

In his own lifetime and through many centuries, even to our own day, St. Cyril has been criticized as leaning toward Arianism. One reason is the omission of the word "con-substantial" from his teaching. The other is the harsh view given of him by St. Jerome, who charged him with self-interest and connivance in obtaining the bishopric of Jerusalem. The circumstances of how St. Cyril succeeded St. Maximus as Bishop of Jerusalem are still clouded a bit for lack of historical information, but there is no proof that at any time in his life St. Cyril was a shady character. The Church historian, Theodoret, writing in the following century, says of Cyril's succession simply: "When he [Maximus] was called to enter upon a higher state of existence, his bishopric was conferred upon Cyril, a zealous defender of the apostolic doctrines." (11, 26).

At the First Council of Constantinople in 381, St. Cyril proved the correctness of his faith by officially approving, with the other bishops, the use of the term "con-substantial" (*homo-ousios*) in the Creed. This was not an act of repentance, as some ancient historians suggest, but a reaffirmation of what he had held and taught since the beginning of his long episcopate. At the Synod of Constantinople held the next year, the letter sent by the assembled bishops to Pope Damasus and the bishops assembled in Rome praised St. Cyril: "We must apprise you that the revered and pious Cyril is bishop of the church of Jerusalem, which is the mother of all the churches, that he was ordained according to law by the bishops of the province, and that he has in various places withstood the Arians." (*Theo.*, ch. 9). This is the last particular incident recorded in St. Cyril's life.

St. Jerome's criticism of St. Cyril is a lesson in both the frailty and the fallibility of even holy and learned men. St. Cyril's writings and the definite clearing of his name by the Synod of Constantinople offer strong proof of his correctness in doctrine and holiness of life.

Compared to St. Athanasius

A modern writer says, "The life of St. Cyril of Jerusalem may be described as a kind of abridged edition of that of St. Athanasius." The Church has indicated some resemblance between the two by choosing the same homily for the feast days of both Doctors. It is one written by St. Athanasius.

Athanasius and Cyril were both expelled from their bishoprics—not once but several times. In the case of St. Cyril it was three times, and with St. Athanasius it was five times. Both were expelled because of the machinations of Arian bishops. In the case of Cyril, his arch enemy was Acacius, the Arian Bishop of Caesarea in Palestine. Both St. Athanasius and St. Cyril suffered much for their adherence to the True Faith.

There is a difference, however, in the way they had to endure censure. St. Athanasius has always been historically acknowledged as a champion of the True Faith. His case was clear-cut, and he was persecuted precisely because he stood for the Faith. But St. Cyril, taking a course of moderation and conciliation, was lambasted by both sides. For the Arians, he appeared too inclined toward orthodoxy; and for some of the strictly orthodox, like St. Jerome, he appeared to lean toward heresy.

Cardinal Newman, writing during his Anglican days, sums up very well the essential agreement of the criticized St. Cyril with St. Athanasius, the acknowledged champion of the Faith:

There is something very remarkable, and even startling, to the reader of St. Cyril, to find in a divine of his school such a perfect agreement, for instance, as regards the doctrine of the Trinity, with those Fathers who in his age were more famous as champions of it. Here is a writer, separated by whatsoever cause from what, speaking historically, may be called the Athanasian school, suspicious of its adherents, and suspected by them; yet he, when he comes to explain himself, expresses precisely the same doctrine as that of Athanasius or Gregory, while he merely abstains from the particular theological term in which the latter Fathers, agreeably to the Nicene Council, conveyed it. Can we have a clearer proof that the difference of opinion between them was not one of ecclesiastical and traditionary doctrine, but of practical judgment . . . (Preface to the *Library of the Fathers of the Church*).

Evidence that St. Cyril was a man who could make a practical judgment, approach a question or a subject in a freely chosen definite way and stick to it is provided by his only complete extant sermon. His approach to Scripture in the *Sermon on the Paralytic* is completely different from that displayed in the *Catechetical Lectures*. The *Lectures* use Scripture in a scientific way to prove doctrine. The *Sermon* uses Scripture in a mystical and more subjective way to describe the deeper movements of the soul. A modern scholar says that this sermon may provide a surer clue to St. Cyril's cast of mind and spiritual formation than the more famous *Lectures*. (Stephenson in *Theological Studies*, 1954, pp. 573-93)

Thus, St. Cyril was not the type of man who could approach a subject only in one way, but he had a balance and versatility of mind that allowed him to adapt to different purposes. At such a man, who could be a master of a studied approach, there can be no accusing fingers pointed when he omits a term like "consubstantial" from his *Catechetical Instructions*, which were not intended to be theological treatises.

Attuned to His Listeners

St. Cyril was a man who had contact with his pupils, who was aware of his relationship to them and of their feelings. After speaking for some time, giving his Fourth Lecture, St. Cyril must have detected some motion in the class equivalent to the modern "looking at one's watch." He said:

> Yes, I know that I am giving a long lecture and that it is
> already getting late, but what ought we to think about as much
> as salvation? . . . If your teachers think it no small gain for
> you to learn these things, surely you who are learning them
> ought gladly to welcome a copious instruction!

Having given this teacherly admonition, St. Cyril proceeded
logically to keep his word. The lecture runs on for an additional
time just as long.

He considers the fast learners and explains why they should
be patient and continue to listen:

> And let the more advanced of the present company bear with
> this arrangement ("having their senses more exercised to dis-
> cern both good and evil" and yet), having to listen to instruc-
> tion fitter for children, and to a course of spoon-feeding: just
> so, that at one and the same time, those that have need of the
> instruction will benefit, while those who know it all already
> may have the memory refreshed of things the knowledge of
> which they have gained previously. (4, 3).

We may wonder whether, as he spoke of "those who know it
all already," the saintly Bishop did not give a surreptitious wink
to one of the priests standing by, or perhaps pause for a silent
prayer of forgiveness for exaggerating.

As we read the *Catechetical Lectures* we can picture the scene
of St. Cyril's instruction. The people are gathered in the church
called the Martyry, built just a few years before by Constantine
over the hill of Calvary. Some there are already baptized; most
of these will be sponsors. But the lectures are directed to those
preparing for Baptism at Easter, the *protozomenoi*, or "catechumens." They are seated in a semi-circle, the men on one side,
the women on the other. The energetic young Bishop, zealous
and anxious to pass on the fruits of his own overflowing study
and meditation, earnestly addresses them.

Directness of Speech

The lectures we have are from notes taken by hearers, and
they show that Bishop Cyril spoke with clarity and amazing
directness of speech. There is a constant interweaving of the
speaker's own words with texts from Scripture. His mind ranged
easily over the Scriptures, especially the New Testament, and

he chose now an appropriate phrase, now a sentence, and again a whole passage to illustrate his point.

For directness of speech, how can we improve on this proof of God's power to resurrect the body:

> Tell me, for example, where do you suppose you were a hundred or more years ago? Out of how very small and inconsiderable a primal matter have you grown up to such large stature and such dignity of form? Well then, cannot He that brought a nothing into being raise up what for a while had being and perished again? (4, 30).

Concerning chastity, St. Cyril says:

> . . . Let us not for a short pleasure defile so great, so noble a body: for short and momentary is the sin, but the shame for many years and forever. Angels walking upon earth are they who practice chastity: the virgins have their portion with Mary the Virgin. Let all vain ornament be banished, and every hurtful glance, and all wanton gait, and every flowing robe, and perfume enticing to pleasure. But in all, for perfume let there be the prayer of sweet odor, and the practice of good works and the sanctification of our bodies: that the Virgin-born Lord may say even of us, both men who live in chastity and women who wear the crown, "I will dwell in them and walk in them, and I will be their God, and they shall be My people." (12, 34).

St. Cyril neatly pricks the bubble of self-deception:

> Will any then among those present boast that he entertains friendship unfeigned towards his neighbor? Do not the lips often kiss, and the countenance smile, and the eyes brighten forsooth, while the heart is planning guile, and the man is plotting mischief with words of peace?

Although not having the advantage of coming to us in the original Greek, St. Cyril's words still hit us with much more force and directness than those of many good writers of the present day.

St. Cyril on the Eucharist

The doctrine of the Real Presence is clearly affirmed by St. Cyril: "Since He Himself has declared and said of the bread:

'This is My Body,' who shall dare to doubt any more? And when He asserts and says: 'This is My Blood,' who shall ever hesitate and say it is not His Blood?"

He also writes,

> Do not think it mere bread and wine, for it is the Body and Blood of Christ, according to the Lord's declaration. [Moreover,] Having learned this and being assured of it, that what appears to be bread is not bread, though [so] perceived by the taste, but the Body of Christ, and what appears to be wine is not wine, though the taste says so, but the Blood of Christ . . . strengthen thy heart, partaking of it as spiritual [food], and rejoice the face of thy soul.

There are 12 selections from St. Cyril's writing in the Readings of the revised 1971 Liturgy of the Hours. The Reading for Saturday within the Octave of Easter is on the Eucharist. When reading it a person may wonder whether St. Thomas Aquinas, who wrote the Office and Mass Proper for the Feast of Corpus Christi, did not take his inspiration from St. Cyril. In the *Tantum Ergo*, the most familiar part of St. Thomas' famous hymn, the *Pange Lingua*, we sing of the defect of the senses for which faith must supply. St. Cyril had told the newly baptized, 900 years earlier,

> Consider therefore the Bread and the Wine not as bare elements, for they are, according to the Lord's declaration, the Body and Blood of Christ; for even though sense suggests this to thee, yet let faith establish thee. Judge not the matter from the taste, but from faith be fully assured without misgiving that the Body and Blood of Christ have been vouchsafed to thee. (22, 6).

The Catechetical Lectures

According to the account of Etheria, the noble lady from the West who visited Jerusalem toward the end of the fourth century (*Pilgrimage of Etheria*), the lectures during Lent started at six in the morning and continued for three hours. They were given for forty days. Lent was observed at that time in Jerusalem for eight weeks. Saturday and Sunday were not included, so there were forty days made up by eight weeks of five days each.

After Easter, when the candidates were baptized, the five lectures on the Sacraments were given. These are known as the Mystagogical Lectures, since they concerned the heart of the Mysteries of Christianity. They were given only to those already baptized, initiating them further into the meaning of this Sacrament, Confirmation and the Holy Eucharist, and the manner of receiving Holy Communion.

At the time of Etheria's visit, about 10 years after St. Cyril's death, the Mystagogical Catecheses were given again, this time in the Chapel of the Holy Sepulchre. When St. Cyril first gave them, most likely as a bishop in 350, this little domed chapel, known as the Anastasis (place of the Resurrection), had very likely not yet been built, and the Sepulchre was still uncovered and in the open. The Sepulchre was situated to the west of the place of the Crucifixion.

There is no evidence before the fourth century of an observance of Lent, although there was an observance of a forty hours' fast to commemorate the time Christ was in the tomb. But the practice of the season of Lent developed quickly in the fourth century as the number of applicants for Baptism grew and instructions had to be given less to individuals and more to groups. Lent was the time for such instruction. As the number of faithful grew, there was likewise a need for a period of discipline among those already baptized, to help them maintain the purity of the Faith. The historical beginning of Lent, then, appears to have stemmed primarily from the need for organized instruction or catechising of people in larger groups.

Mary's Place in Catechetics

St. Cyril points an early finger to Mary's place in relation to the Church and basic doctrine. His catechetical instructions have a Mariological value, says noted Marian scholar Luigi Gambero, because "they allow us to see clearly how doctrine about the Virgin Mary fits into the structure of the teaching imparted to fourth-century catechumens as they prepared for baptism." St. Cyril says, for instance: "Believe that this only begotten Son of God came down from heaven to earth for our sins, taking our own same humanity, subject to trials like our own. He was born of the holy Virgin and the Holy Spirit." (Quoted in Luigi Gambero, S.M., *Mary and the Fathers of the Church*, Ignatius Press, 1999, p. 132).

Cyril explains further:

He was made man, not in appearance only or as a phantasm, but in a real way. He did not pass through the Virgin, as if through a channel; rather He truly took flesh from her and by her was truly nursed, really eating and really drinking just as we do. For if the Incarnation were a mere appearance, such would be our redemption as well. In Christ there were two aspects: man, who was visible in Him, and God, who remained invisible . . . (Gambero, p. 133)

The reality of Jesus as man, as fully human, had to be explained to catechumens with precision because the true teaching was questioned in various ways by heretical opinions very prevalent at the time.

St. Cyril makes a unique, indeed a startling statement, about Mary and how she has raised the place of all women. Gambero says the statement could be a starting point for a theology of woman. It deserves study by contemporary theologians. "At first, the feminine sex was obligated to give thanks to men, because Eve, born of Adam but not conceived by a mother, was in a certain sense born of man. Mary, instead, paid off the debt of gratitude: she did not give birth by means of a man, but by herself, virginally, through the working of the Holy Spirit and the power of God." (Gambero, p. 139).

St. Cyril's Importance

St. Cyril's writings are comparatively short. But he is very important for several reasons. He supplies the first complete and simple exposition of the ancient creed as used at Jerusalem. This creed is very similar to the Nicene Creed recited at Mass. All that St. Athanasius and St. Hilary and other great Fathers of the Church said in more detail and in more technically theological language, St. Cyril has given us in summary and limpidly clear form.

Secondly, St. Cyril, particularly in the last five (Mystagogical) *Lectures*, has given us the earliest detailed account of the rites of Baptism, Confirmation and the Holy Eucharist, and has afforded us a clear insight into the Eucharist as a sacrifice.

It is fitting that the *Catechetical Lectures*, containing such a clear summary of the Faith, should have been delivered on the sacred ground of Calvary, where the gift of faith was won for men. It is even more fitting that the strong testimony to the Holy Eucharist and to its nature as a sacrifice should have been given at the spot where Christ's Body was laid after He had completed the Sacrifice of the Cross.

Thirdly, in the twilight years of his life St. Cyril very likely had a strong and guiding influence on the development of our liturgy, especially that of Holy Week.

St. Gregory of Nyssa, visiting Jerusalem in 378, near the end of St. Cyril's long 11-year exile, was extremely discouraged at the strife and immorality there. He wrote, ". . . There is no form of uncleanness that is not perpetrated among them: rascality, adultery, theft, idolatry, poisoning, quarreling, murder are rife."

Thus when St. Cyril returned from his long exile in 379, there was a need for reorganization and direction to remedy the sad situation described by St. Gregory of Nyssa. St. Cyril, beloved by the people of Jerusalem, respected for his long labors for the Faith, and wise from long combat and study, was the man who could restore the Church in the Holy City and bring it to new glory. Within a few short years, there were marvelous changes. When the lady Etheria visited Jerusalem about fifteen years after St. Cyril's return, there was peace and cooperation among the churches of the city. The practice of Holy Week was observed; Good Friday was commemorated as a day of special observance; there were processions to the sacred spots of Christ's suffering and death. In their turn, these changes in Jerusalem had a lasting effect on the Liturgy in the development of a "Proper of the Seasons," and in particular of the observance of Holy Week. Logic points to St. Cyril as the chief agent.

St. Cyril was a man maligned and misunderstood in high places. But he was engaging in manner and beloved by the people. While he was in exile at Tarsus, the people there did not want to allow him to return to Jerusalem—so well did he win their affections in the short time of his stay.

He did not write much; at least, not much has been preserved. But his *Catechetical Lectures* are one of the great treasures of early Christianity. It is very reassuring to read their clear, forthright explanations. Those who teach catechism and who give convert instructions might pray to St. Cyril to help them achieve his fine combination of depth and simplicity in knowledge and explanation of the Faith.

It was because he was a teacher of catechism par excellence that, on July 28, 1882, the Church proclaimed St. Cyril of Jerusalem a Doctor of the Church. His feast day, as stated above, is March 18.

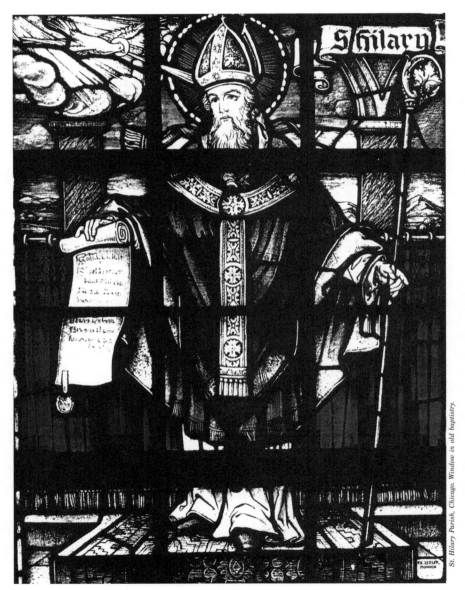

St. Hilary Parish, Chicago. Window in old baptistry.

Saint Hilary of Poitiers

— 4 —
SAINT HILARY OF POITIERS
The Athanasius of the West
c. 315-c. 368

THE youngster in the early grades answers very readily: "Yes, Jesus Christ is true God." The little pupil would hardly know how much the people in the United States—and in all countries whose Catholic inheritance stems from Western Christendom— owe their knowledge of that right answer to a man who lived in the fourth century. We are very much indebted for our belief in the divinity of Christ to the "Athanasius of the West," St. Hilary of Poitiers. Just as St. Athanasius was the champion of Christianity against Arianism in the Eastern Roman Empire, so St. Hilary was its leading defender in the Latin countries.

The Arian heresy wanted to make Christ only a man—the greatest of men, the most renowned of prophets, perhaps similar to God. But this greatest of heresies said that He still was not the true Son of God, equal to and consubstantial with the Father.

The Task Measures the Man

God the Holy Spirit will of course always preserve all divinely revealed truths. So when in the course of history these are challenged or distorted by some men, others meet the challenge by a clear and courageous stating of the truth. The effort to state the truth forcefully and convincingly takes the highest kind of intellect and scholarship. Because passions and conflicting worldly interests are often involved, the champions of truth must be men of courage, willing to endanger life and liberty to tell the truth.

God always raises up such men in times of need. The greatness of St. Hilary can be measured by the magnitude of the challenge of Arianism, which to the people of that time seemed to engulf the whole Church. The fact that God chose this man to defend and explain such a fundamental truth as the divinity of Christ gives us his truest measure. St. Hilary must always stand in the front line, even among the greatest champions of truth.

Arianism was at its height in the decade 350-360 A.D. In 357, at the second Synod of Sirmium, the aged and venerable Hosius, Bishop of Cordova, who had presided at the Council of Nicaea, was forced to sign an Arian creed. The same Synod wrung from Pope Liberius a temporary condemnation of St. Athanasius. In 359, at the Councils of Rimini in the West and Seleucia in the East, the majority of participating bishops succumbed to intrigue and political pressure and agreed to heretical Arian creeds. It was after these twin councils that St. Jerome wrote, "The world groaned in amazement to find itself Arian."

St. Hilary tells us that in 355 he had been a bishop "some little time." This was in the middle of that decade of supreme trial for the Church. The probable date of his election as bishop is 353.

The people of Poitiers, at that time an unimportant diocese in Gaul (France), chose St. Hilary as bishop by popular acclaim. They wanted him to be the bishop just as the people also chose St. Cyprian, St. Ambrose and St. Martin of Tours. The spontaneous testimony of the people among whom he lived tells us much about St. Hilary. It bespeaks a man of reputed holiness, of strong character and the natural virtues of graciousness, kindness and moderation that endear a man to his contemporaries.

Peaceful Years

Before his election as bishop, not much can be said with certainty of St. Hilary. He was born at Poitiers, probably of wealthy, pagan parents. An early biographer, however, Venantius Fortunatus, says that his parents were Christian. The same writer has also said without contradiction that Hilary was married, led a happy domestic life, and was very fond of his daughter, Abra. It is certain that St. Hilary was baptized as an adult, for in the beginning of his greatest work, *On the Trinity*, he describes the process by which he came to believe in Christianity.

He had begun by examining the teachings of pagan philosophers. But their influence worked with an inverse effect, for he rejected most of their teachings. Of these writers he tells us:

> Many of them introduced numerous families of uncertain deities, and imagining that the male and female sex was present in the divine natures, spoke about the birth and the successions of gods from gods. Others proclaimed that there were greater and lesser gods and gods differing in power. . . .

A friend introduced him to the Old Testament, where he found the self-description of God: "I Am Who Am." (*Exodus* 3:14). Later he found the words of St. John, "In the beginning was the Word, and the Word was with God; and the Word was God." (*John* 1:1). St. Hilary's soul, longing for such essence of divine truth and beauty, embraced it with solid certitude and tender feeling.

Meanwhile, the hidden forces of history were already at work that would bring him to the masterful and full expression of this faith which he had found in mature life.

St. Hilary spent the early, peaceful years of his episcopate in composing a commentary on the Gospel of St. Matthew. In a way, this is a pioneer work, since it is the first adequate and continuous commentary on a book of the New Testament by a Latin writer. After his exile he again composed a commentary, this time on the Psalms. His treatment, while inspirational and elevated, favors the allegorical rather than the critical evaluation of meanings.

St. Hilary may also be called the first hymnologist among the Latin Fathers of the Church. He wrote many hymns after returning from exile in the East, in order to introduce into the West the congregational singing he had found there. It is difficult now to say of any one extant hymn that it was composed by St. Hilary, although both the *Gloria in Excelsis* and *Te Deum* have been ascribed to him.

Trying Years

Between two short peaceful periods in his episcopacy, St. Hilary spent eight very active, fruitful and trying years. During most of that time he was absent from his See at Poitiers. Four years were spent in exile (356-360) and a full year in returning; after this, St. Hilary went to Italy to carry on the fight against Auxentius, the Arian bishop of Milan. He left Milan in 364 at the command of the Emperor Valentinian.

St. Hilary's troubles began when he opposed Saturninus, the Metropolitan Bishop of Arles in southern France, a city then styled "the little Rome of Gaul." Saturninus was Metropolitan of all the Gallic bishops, and his position far outranked that of St. Hilary, but unfortunately he was an Arian, and a man of little character and of mediocre intellect. Still, he had position and the confidence of Constantius, the Emperor.

The Emperor had a very simple definition of Church law and government: "A canon is what I wish." After listening to the poisoned whispering of Saturninus, Constantius "wished" for the exile of St. Hilary. This was in the year 356.

Without any trial and, like the poet Ovid, without even being informed of the alleged reason, St. Hilary was ordered into exile. It is impossible to reply to an unknown charge; all St. Hilary could say in self-defense was that not only had he "never done anything unworthy of the sanctity of a bishop, but nothing even unworthy of the uprightness of a layman."

St. Hilary might well serve as a patron of those who are waiting for answers to letters, because he suffered so much in maintaining a one-way correspondence with the Bishops of Gaul. Most of his letters to these bishops were not answered. Many of them failed to reach their destinations, and others were not answered simply because the Gallic bishops did not know where to send a reply. Just as, almost in despair, he was about to stop sending these letters, he heard from the bishops and learned of the great help his letters had afforded them. This was in 358, a full two years after his exile had started.

Fruitful Exile

Comforted at last by an answer to his letters and greatly renewed in courage, St. Hilary carefully gathered information concerning the many Church councils and creeds. The resulting book of 92 chapters, *De Synodis*, helped to dispel much of the error and doubt caused by many conflicting reports concerning Arianism. The book is also of great historical importance for its accurate account of the whole Arian controversy.

One redeeming feature of St. Hilary's exile was the vast extent of the territory to which he was exiled. He was ordered simply to go into "Asia." He made good use of these wide geographical perimeters and managed to travel about, attending the Council at Seleucia and also going to Constantinople.

His contact with the virulent Arianism flourishing in the East provided St. Hilary with all the material and incentive he needed to wage war against its smaller beginnings in the West. His warnings by letter and by more formal writing put the bishops of Gaul on guard and helped save them from Arianism. The personal influence of St. Hilary and that of his writings spread and later helped to save the other lands in the western part of the Roman Empire from much of the baneful influence of Arianism. Thus it often happens that adversity forges the weapons for great victories.

It was in exile that St. Hilary composed his greatest work, now commonly called *De Trinitate*, "On the Trinity." St. Jerome refers to it as the *Twelve Books against the Arians*. It was also known in earlier centuries as the book *On Faith*. In a sense, it is more correctly styled *On Faith*, because while much space is devoted to the divinity of Christ, little is given to the Holy Spirit.

Writing *On the Trinity* was for St. Hilary not a theological exercise, not a display of speculative acumen, but an earnest effort to help men win salvation. For that reason, he devoted all his energies to composing a clear exposition. He also prayed much that he would write well.

St. Hilary's task was formidable because he had to create new words in Latin to express the close and intricate reasoning already well-developed and expressed in the Greek language. St. Hilary's book, *On the Trinity*, is thus a pioneering effort. Its English translator says of it: "This work of St. Hilary is his masterpiece, and upon it rests his fame as a theologian. It is generally regarded as one of the finest writings that the Arian controversy produced. Augustine and Leo the Great are among the early writers who praise it, and St. Thomas Aquinas frequently appeals to it when settling disputes about the Trinity . . . St. Hilary, therefore, is one of the foundation stones upon which later writers would erect a magnificent theological edifice to pay some measure of honor to their triune God."

In a modern magazine article, Fr. L. J. Daly, S.J., summarizes the work with a modern snap: "Hilary was mainly interested in proving beyond the shadow of a doubt that there is a Trinity, and that the Son is God, co-equal and eternal with the Father. He piles proof upon proof until the weary reader says: 'You win.'"

St. Hilary was so successful in opposing Arianism in the East that the Arians asked the Emperor to send him back to Gaul. The Emperor did so, ending the Saint's exile.

Yours Truly, Emperor

Of special interest and value in showing the character of St. Hilary are his three letters to the Emperor Constantius. The first two are conciliatory and kind in expression. This initial approach was the same that St. Hilary used in dealing with the semi-Arians, trying to lead them gently to the truth. But when St. Hilary, the man of patrician reserve and moderation, of kindly disposition, was aroused fully, he could express himself with undeniable vehemence and biting eloquence. His third letter to Constantius is a good example. It begins:

> It is time to speak; the time for holding my peace has passed by. Let Christ be expected, for Anti-Christ has prevailed. Let the shepherds cry, for the hirelings have fled. Thou art fighting against God, thou ragest against the Church; thou persecutest the Saints; thou hatest the preachers of Christ; thou art annulling religion; thou art a tyrant no longer only in the human, but in the divine sphere . . .

These words are those of a man driven to extremes. Had the Emperor seen them, they would have meant death for St. Hilary. But the Emperor was engaged in fighting Julian, and himself died of a fever on November 3, 361. With the death of Constantius, the persecution of Catholics by the Arians came to an end.

Nobody reading the above words would think that controversy rages as to St. Hilary's writing style. But such is the case. Some think his sentences too long, his style too ornate. Even Erasmus shared this opinion. It is no wonder that St. Jerome, who seems to criticize St. Hilary's style in some instances, also calls him "the Rhone of eloquence," "a trumpet of the Latin tongue," "a flood of eloquence and polished discourse." Perhaps much of the criticism can be traced to the difficulties under which St. Hilary worked. For he had to put involved Greek theology into new Latin terms.

Some of the criticism may be due to a misinterpretation of St. Jerome's apparently adverse allusions. For when St. Jerome, in drawing up a list of Hilary's writings, comes to the last work, the letter against Auxentius (*Contra Auxentium*), he calls it "another elegant little book," thereby throwing a compliment back to those previously cited.

The Faith Above All

St. Hilary ends his book on the Trinity with a prayer that summarizes his faith. He traces his belief in God, known first by His heavens, "these starry circles, the yearly revolutions, the seven stars, and the Morning Star . . ." He concludes with a humble petition to God that he will keep the Faith:

> Keep this piety of my faith undefiled, I beseech Thee, and let this be the utterance of my convictions, even to the last breath of my spirit: that I may always hold fast to that which I professed in the creed of my regeneration, when I was baptized in the name of the Father, and of the Son and of the Holy Spirit . . .

St. Hilary died at Poitiers around the year 368, probably on November 1. His feast day is celebrated on January 13 (January 14 in the 1962 calendar) and is the first Saint's feast day after the Christmas-to-Epiphany liturgical cycle. His name catches the eye as we close the Sanctoral cycle in our missals just before Christmas. It is indeed poetically appropriate for St. Hilary thus to cast his shadow before we begin to celebrate the feasts of the Christmas cycle, starting of course with the Nativity of Our Lord, for St. Hilary was one of the supreme champions of His divinity.

In January, 1852, Pope Pius IX recognized this when he conferred on St. Hilary the title, Doctor of the Church.

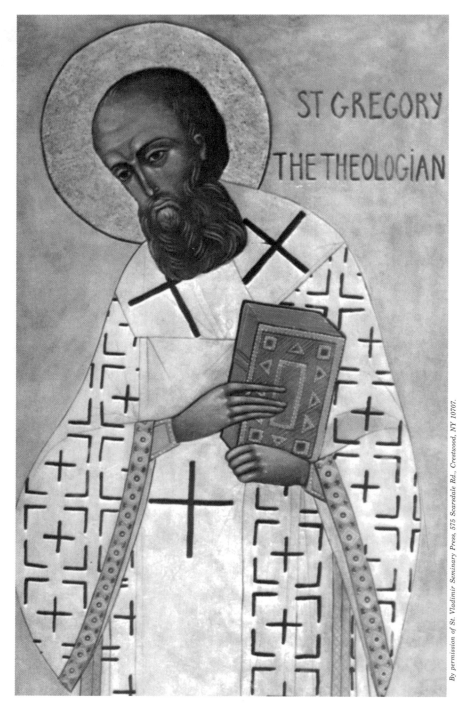

ST GREGORY
THE THEOLOGIAN

By permission of St. Vladimir Seminary Press, 575 Scarsdale Rd., Crestwood, NY 10707.

Saint Gregory Nazianzen

5

SAINT GREGORY NAZIANZEN

The Theologian
The Christian Demosthenes
c. 329-c. 389

PARENTS who name a new son Gregory give the boy a choice of at least 65 Saints and 10 Beati as his patron. Sixteen Popes have borne the name; the thirteenth of them corrected the calendar which hangs on our wall. Even in the small and select circle of the Church Doctors we find two who are called Gregory. One is Pope St. Gregory the Great (540-604) and the other is St. Gregory Nazianzen (Gregory of Nazianzus), called "The Theologian." Indeed the name Gregory is one of the most illustrious in Catholic history.

From a Family of Saints

St. Nonna, the mother of Gregory Nazianzen, is surely one of the great Catholic mothers of Church history. She first converted her husband, also called Gregory, from a strange sect, who then became in time the Bishop of Nazianzus and a saint. Her son St. Caesarius was physician to the Emperor, and he and his sister Gorgonia are also honored as saints.

St. Gregory Nazianzen compares his parents to Abraham and Sara. He tells us that his mother, St. Nonna, did everything with intensity. If she prayed it was as though she never did anything else. When she worked at home, it seemed that she thought only of that. In the funeral oration for his father, St. Gregory says of his mother:

> She increased the resources of her household by her care and practical foresight according to the standards and norms laid down by Solomon for the valiant woman, as though she knew nothing of piety. She devoted herself to God and divine things as though she were completely removed from household cares. In no wise, however, did she neglect one duty in fulfill-

ing the other; rather, she performed both more effectively by making one support the other.

St. Nonna took her firstborn, the future Church Doctor, to the church, and placed his little hands on the altar missal, dedicating him to God's service. Yet despite this early dedication, Gregory was not baptized until young adulthood. During a terrible 20-day storm at sea, Gregory was in agony over the danger to his unbaptized soul. He implored God's mercy, promising to dedicate himself entirely to God if he survived. This he did at his Baptism.

In his youth, St. Gregory had a dream in which Chastity and Temperance bade him follow them, promising to lead him to the light of the Most Holy Trinity. From that time Gregory resolved to practice perpetual continence. He later wrote that to violate a vow of chastity would be death, sacrilege and perfidy.

When St. Gregory compares his parents to Abraham and Sara, what he says of them is at once the highest of tributes to them and also a tribute to his own lifelong filial devotion:

> I believe that, if anyone from the ends of the earth, and from all human stocks, had endeavored to arrange the best possible marriage, a better or more harmonious union than this could not be found. For the best in men and women was so united that their marriage was more a union of virtue than of bodies. Although they surpassed all others, they themselves were so evenly matched in virtue that they could not surpass each other.

Rhetorician and Priest

St. Gregory had been born at Arianzus, the country estate of his well to-do parents, about 329 A.D. The estate was near Nazianzus in Cappadocia, a Roman province of eastern Asia Minor, on the south shore of the Black Sea. Cappadocia and its people had a bad reputation in the ancient world, as exemplified by the epigram, "A viper bit a Cappadocian, and the viper died." It was famous for slavery, avarice and licentiousness. The universality of Gregory's outlook is summed up as he complains of his countrymen, praises their adherence to the True Faith and boasts of the country's fine horses.

St. Gregory was thoroughly educated—first at Caesarea in his native land, then at Caesarea in Palestine, at Alexandria and at Athens. He was in school till the age of 30. He returned to Nazianzus one of the great rhetoricians of his day. Just to please his fellow Nazianzens he gave a few public addresses. As he describes it, he "danced a little, and quitted the stage."

He took his great learning into solitude, joining St. Basil, the great friend of his student days, in the cenobitic (monastic) life. But St. Gregory returned home to help his father, who, untrained in theological terms, had signed the Sirmian Creed promulgated by the Emperor Constantius, who was Semi-Arian.

Respecting his son's great knowledge and knowing his fitness in matters theological, the elder Gregory insisted that his son be ordained a priest, and he performed the ceremony himself on Christmas Day of 361. In an emotional upheaval over what he felt was a kind of tyranny, St. Gregory left on the feast of the Epiphany, 362, to stay with St. Basil in retreat at Pontus. There he came to terms with his priestly vocation and spent time preparing his soul for the heavy responsibilities of the priesthood. He returned to preach his first sermon on Easter.

A second sermon, given soon afterwards, explained the reasons for his leaving the city and laid the foundations for much later writing on the priesthood—including *On the Priesthood* by St. John Chrysostom and *Pastoral Care* by St. Gregory the Great. Such sermons, it may be said, were not of the brevity which the modern congregation is used to, but were long and well-developed treatises.

A Very Painful Episode

When St. Basil, the closest friend of St. Gregory, was having trouble with Anthimus, Bishop of Tyana, St. Gregory offered his assistance. St. Basil, then Metropolitan and Archbishop of Caesarea in Cappadocia, chose St. Gregory as the bishop for what might be described as a "buffer see." This was the dusty, noisy little town of Sasima, located at the meeting place of three roads, and having a transient population. Everything in the highly refined and idealistic Gregory rebelled at the idea of going there, especially since he judged that this bishopric, newly created, was a pawn in an ecclesiastical territorial battle. St. Basil, however, came to Nazianzus and consecrated his reluctant friend in the church built by the elder St. Gregory.

Some of the words of St. Gregory Nazianzen in his letters

about "the illustrious Sasima" are quite strong, indicating the natural reaction of a devoted lover of God who felt himself flung to the ground. In bitterness he wrote to St. Basil that there was one thing he had gained, and that was to trust in God alone.

Cardinal Newman offers, as an explanation of the appointment, that St. Basil considered the post desirable just because it was a place of risk and responsibility and offered the opportunity to manage an important quarrel.

There was little opportunity for using talent or wielding a spiritual influence in the constantly revolving population of Sasima, and St. Gregory left Sasima. The Sasima episode led to a great personal struggle for St. Gregory. After spending some time in solitude, Gregory went back to Nazianzus to act as coadjutor bishop to his father. In 375 he was brought near death by a severe illness; after recovering, he went to spend several years in solitude and a rather penitential convalescence.

His poor health, coupled with the death of his parents, his brother and St. Basil, all within a few years, led him to write to a friend:

> Old age is over my head . . . my friends are faithless; the Church is without pastors. All that is honorable is perishing; evils are naked; our voyage is in the night; there is a beacon nowhere. Christ is sleeping.

St. Gregory's physical appearance about this time, when he was just short of 50 years of age, was not very imposing. He was short, spare and quite pale; his shoulders were stooped. A silvery fringe of thin hair kept him from being completely bald. He was minus his right eye and had a scar on his face.

Constantinople

Yet this man was just about to do the most important and crowning work of his life in Constantinople. He went to this stronghold of Arianism because its few remaining Catholics called for him. He could put his whole congregation in the little chapel which he opened, called Anastasia, the Church of the Resurrection. Cardinal Newman commented that, in his firm and intrepid leadership at Constantinople, St. Gregory—who was by nature gentle and retiring—seems to have received the heroic spirit of St. Basil, who had died a few months previous. And at St. Basil's funeral discourse, St. Gregory was to say: "May we together receive the reward of the warfare which we have waged, which we have endured."

In Constantinople, St. Gregory was the leader of a group that was pitifully small and poor. Moreover, persecution from the Arians was intense, putting Gregory in mortal danger. But his holiness of life, his burning eloquence and brilliant explanation of doctrine, especially regarding the divinity of Christ, gradually won followers and great numbers of converts. St. Jerome, scholarly, eloquent and renowned, came to admire and to listen to him. St. Gregory's clear-cut exposition of truth dealt a crippling blow to Arianism. He was the stylist who could sum up the writings of St. Athanasius, St. Hilary and St. Basil. He was the accomplished orator who could make true doctrine live in the minds of his audience. For this reason he has received the title, "The Christian Demosthenes," after the famous Greek orator.

When the civil power, in the person of the newly baptized Emperor Theodosius, swung to the favor of the Catholic Church, the Arian Bishop of Constantinople, Demophilus, had to leave. Theodosius gave the churches back to the Catholics, forbade the Arians to hold public assemblies and commanded that only those subscribing to the true Faith could call themselves "Catholic."

The First Council of Constantinople chose St. Gregory as Archbishop of the city and president of the Council, much against his will. But after a few months in this office, St. Gregory's great work in Constantinople was done. He had undermined the position of Arianism there and re-established the Catholic Faith, which would flourish strong and hardy in the future. He was not much interested in the organizational work now needed. When opposition to his office arose, he resigned in the interest of peace.

Poet and Friend

St. Gregory Nazianzen was the poet among the great Greek and Latin theologians of the fourth century. As yet, not much of his work has been translated into English or even critically edited in the original Greek. Looking through some of his prose available in English, we notice its fine polish and epigrammatic clarity. The following lines, translated by Cardinal Newman, tell us something about St. Gregory and give us an insight into his quality as a poet, as a man sensitive to words and to deep feeling for another. St. Gregory writes that he and St. Basil

> Had all things in common, and one only
>   soul in lodgement of a double outward frame;
> Our special bond, the thought of God above,
>   And the high longing after holy things.
> And each of us was bold to trust in each
>   Unto the emptying of our deepest hearts.

In his letters, especially to St. Basil, St. Gregory often shows a bantering, playful spirit. At a time when he was living on the family estate in the country and St. Basil was living in the crowded city of Caesarea, St. Gregory replied to a letter of St. Basil which had teased him about living in the mud: "Am I doing wrong because you are pale and breathe with difficulty, and measure your scanty sunlight—while I am fresh with health, and am satisfied and am not circumscribed?" Later, after St. Basil took up residence in the countryside of Pontus, St. Gregory went to share with him his frugal eremitical (hermit) life. Returning to Nazianzus, he wrote about the food that St. Basil had served him: "I have remembrance of the bread and the broth—so they were named—and shall remember them: how my teeth got stuck in your thick lumps, and next lifted and heaved themselves as out of paste." It is rather delightful to find two who would become Doctors of the Universal Church exchanging pleasantries about cooking and about living in the city versus living in the country.

In a letter reflecting on the joys of their days of prayer and work together at Pontus, St. Gregory wrote to St. Basil: "I breathe you more than the air; and I am only alive when I am with you, either in your actual presence or by imagination in your absence."

It was, of course, St. Gregory's very depth of feeling that made the wound of later estrangement so lasting. In his panegyric after St. Basil's death, St. Gregory compares his friend to St. John the Baptist; he says that he imitated the zeal of St. Peter and the energy of St. Paul and the faith of both. Yet in the same speech—21,000 words in length—he still recalls, with an honesty that sounds strange in our day of more form and less honesty, "Basil's extraordinary and unfriendly conduct toward me, of which time has not removed the pain." Gregory refers here to the Sasima episode. "For to this I trace all the irregularity and confusion of my life, and my not being able, or not seeming, to command my feelings." In excuse for Basil, St. Gregory immediately adds that perhaps St. Basil, "knowing how to reverence friendship, then only slighted it when it was a matter of a duty to prefer God and to make more account of the things hoped for than of things perishable."

"The Theologian"

St. Gregory of Nazianzus was not a writer in the sense that he planned and wrote extended commentaries or treatises. He wrote for the immediate occasion: sermons or orations, letters and poems. There are extant 45 orations, about 400 poems and 245 letters. The longest poem, *De Vita Sua*, is autobiographical and is the chief source of information about St. Gregory's life, as well as the classic of this sort of poem in all Greek literature.

Included in the orations are the famous five orations or Theological Discourses delivered at Constantinople in 380 A.D., which earned for him the title of "The Theologian." These are the clear and mature expression of a lifetime of thought about divine truth, and especially the greatest of truths, the Holy Trinity. St. Gregory insisted on the reverence and purity of life which should mark all who deal with these sacred topics. In these Discourses particularly are those words of praise about St. Gregory realized: "In a few pages and a few hours he has summed up and closed the controversy of a whole century." For more than 1,000 years to come, scholars were to write commentaries on the famous five orations.

Due to St. Gregory's intensive thought about the Trinity, we have the proper word to speak of the relation of the Holy Ghost to the Father and the Son. He coined the term in Greek which we translate, "proceed." In his letters to Cledonius, St. Gregory supplied us with clear and correct statements about the human soul of Christ. Theologians studying this subject during the next 100 years found these letters of much value. More than half a century before the final official approval at the Council of Ephesus, St. Gregory strongly defended the term *Theotokos*, "Mother of God."

St. Gregory of Nazianzus was given the title of "The Theologian" or "The Divine" (the theologian) because of his skill and eloquence in upholding the truth of the Divinity of Christ. The title did not have the more exclusive meaning it now has, but it attests to his reputation in the early Church, living as he did as a contemporary of the profound St. Gregory of Nyssa, St. Basil the Great, St. Jerome and others. The title was first mentioned in a sermon ascribed to St. John Chrysostom.

History has given this title only to St. Gregory of Nazianzus and St. John the Evangelist. In the case of St. Gregory, perhaps it is God's way of giving earthly glory to a man who had shunned glory, who hated pomp and display and whose life was marked by recurring flights to the world of solitude, as well as by somewhat pathetic returns to the call of insistent duty.

His Last Years

After resigning from the bishopric of Constantinople, St. Gregory Nazianzen went back to Nazianzus and for a time cared for that diocese, combating heresy. When a worthy successor for his father was found, St. Gregory retired, to spend the last years of his life at Arianzus, the place of his beginning. Here he wrote numerous letters and poems. He was not idle. Though he shunned administrative work, he lived an ascetical, scholarly life, and much of what he wrote was directly aimed at helping others. Many of his poems, for instance, were meant to offset songs like the *Thalia* of Arius, which proclaimed heresy. Others speak of the severe physical and spiritual sufferings which attended the last years of his life.

St. Gregory died at about the end of 389 or the beginning of 390 at Arianzus. Nobody knows the circumstances of his death. He was buried at Nazianzus; later his body was taken to Constantinople, and finally to St. Peter's in Rome.

A Saint Who Struggled

St. Gregory was emotional and sensitive, alive to the details of living and responsive to the actions and opinions of others. It was this sensitiveness which made the exercise of authority and the conduct of business distasteful to him, which drove him at times to solitude and which brought him back to more active life because he wanted to help. His life, in fact, can practically be summed up as a movement back and forth on the checkerboard of life from the "black" of penance, solitude and prayer, to the "white" of active business, oratory and controversy.

He was fundamentally a quiet scholar, a recluse and a poet. But he had intermittent stretches of public activity, especially his three-year stay as bishop at Constantinople, which made him a figure on the world stage. Even though he loved quiet and study, he seemed at times to tire of these and to miss the joys of company. To the end of his days, he felt the burden of temptation and passion. In his late years, he spent an entire Lent in silence, that he might learn better to control a tendency to intemperate speech.

Holiness and Orthodoxy

St. Gregory always emphasized that a good life is necessary in order to understand the truth about God: "Wouldst thou become a theologian? Keep the Commandments. Conduct is the step to contemplation."

He himself is the living example proving this statement. Even his enemies never doubted his holiness. He lived a good life, one devoted to prayer, quiet study and ascetical practices.

St. Gregory Nazianzen saw divine truth so clearly that he became a symbol of orthodoxy. In his own day, it became a byword that if you differed from Gregory, you were in danger of heresy. In the centuries to come, great thinkers would find in his writings a clear guide regarding many difficult questions about religion.

A Doctor of the Church is chosen for holiness of life and eminent learning. St. Gregory Nazianzen held and demonstrated that the one leads to the other. His feast day (May 9 in the 1962 calendar) is now celebrated on January 2, which is also the feast of St. Basil the Great. St. Gregory Nazianzen is one of The Three Cappadocian Fathers, the other two being St. Basil and St. Gregory of Nyssa.

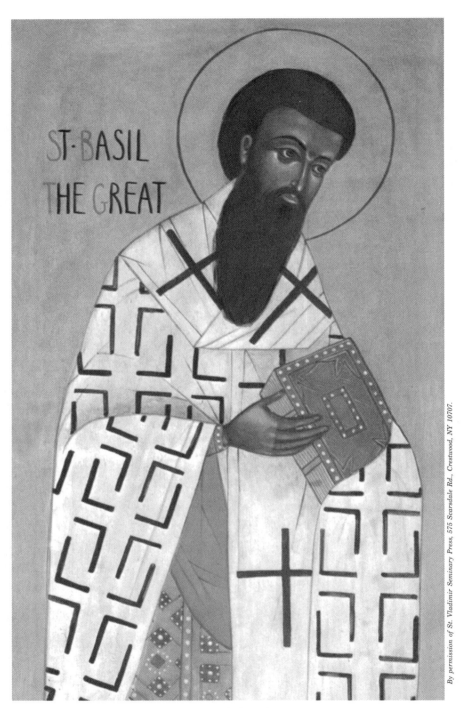

ST·BASIL
THE GREAT

Saint Basil the Great

6

SAINT BASIL THE GREAT

Father of Eastern Monasticism
c. 329-379

THE man in the judge's seat insolently addressed without title the Bishop summoned before him: "What is the meaning of this, you Basil, that you stand out against so great a prince and are self-willed when others yield?" Modestus, the powerful Pretorian Prefect, spoke for the Emperor Valens. The Emperor had sent him to Caesarea in Cappadocia to break down the opposition of St. Basil, its bishop, to the nearly all-pervasive Arian heresy.

St. Basil had refused to communicate with the large group of Arian bishops who accompanied Modestus. Instead, when they assembled in his church, he spoke forthrightly, yet with such moderation that he incurred the wrath of the monks present who wanted to hear a burning condemnation.

Now St. Basil pointed out to Modestus that though he was Prefect, still he was God's creature, and that as such he was the same as any other person in Basil's flock. In anger, Modestus rose from his seat and asked whether Basil did not fear his power. Modestus pointed out that his power could mean for Basil confiscation of his goods, exile, torture and death. To this Basil replied:

> Think of some other threat. These have no influence upon me. He runs no risk of confiscation who has nothing to lose except these mean garments and a few books. Nor does he care about exile who is not circumscribed by place, who makes not a home where he now dwells, but everywhere a home whithersoever he be cast—or rather everywhere God's home, whose pilgrim and wanderer he is. Nor can tortures harm a frame so frail as to break under the first blow. You could but strike once, and death would be gain. It would but send me the sooner to Him for whom I live and labor, nay, am dead rather than live, to whom I have long been journeying.

Modestus objected that nobody had ever yet spoken that way

to the Prefect, St. Basil said: "Perhaps Modestus never yet fell in with a bishop . . ."

Truly a Bishop

There is no doubt that Modestus could hardly meet a bishop more fully deserving the title than the man who was speaking. St. Basil was everything a bishop should be. He was a theologian of depth, an organizer, a good administrator, an eloquent speaker, a stylist in writing. He was an ascetic in personal living and at the same time a keen social thinker and reformer. Many times he reminded the rich: "There would be neither rich nor poor if everyone, after taking from his wealth enough for his personal needs, gave to others what they lacked."

St. Basil emphasized the Scriptures above all, yet he was the first of the Church Fathers to recommend the study of pagan classics. In the midst of the greatest difficulties—raging controversy outside and inside the Church—and personal sickness, he never neglected the details of promoting piety, developing the liturgy, establishing discipline, caring for the spiritual and also the temporal needs of all in his patriarchate.

St. Basil was a bishop for just nine years, from 370 A.D. until his death on January 1, 379. Into that short time he crowded activities that in their variety, scope and lasting value are astounding. When St. Basil was elected bishop, the great St. Athanasius himself wrote to express his pleasure. And well he might, for under St. Basil, the Diocese of Caesarea in Cappadocia (now northern Turkey, along the Black Sea) was to become the solid nucleus of the Catholic Faith in the East.

Defender of the Church against Arianism

After St. Athanasius, St. Basil is recognized as the greatest champion of the Church in the Eastern Roman Empire against Arianism and other fourth-century heresies. He is primarily responsible for the Eastern victory over Arianism, and is rightly known as St. Basil the Great. He laid the broad foundations for the Church's second General Council and its denunciation of Arianism at Constantinople in 381, although he himself did not live to see this victory for the unity of the Catholic Church.

Modestus had failed to shake St. Basil. He reported to Valens: "Emperor, we have been worsted by the bishop of this Church.

He is superior to threats, too firm for arguments, too strong for persuasion. We must try one of the more ignoble. This man will never yield to menaces, or to anything but open force."

The Emperor sent two other emissaries, Count Terentius to try flattery, and Demosthenes the eunuch to threaten with the sword. Finally, the Emperor Valens himself came on Epiphany (January 6) of 372 and entered the church, accompanied by spear-bearers.

The scene is a memorable one. The heretical ruler of state had come to overawe a bishop. His entrance into the church caused no noticeable concern. The people continued to sing the psalms of the liturgy. Behind the altar, facing the people, stood the tall bishop—self-controlled, stern, his beard long, white and flowing, his face lean and pale. He gave no sign at all of seeing the Emperor and his retinue. The fervor of bishop, priests and people, the perfect order and the power of this assembly united in the liturgical sacrifice, had a strong effect on Valens. When he came forward to make his offering, none of the priests made any motion to come to receive it. Waiting to see what St. Basil would do, Valens grew dizzy with emotion and would have fallen had not one of the priests stepped forward to support him. St. Basil took the Emperor's gift and later met with him. When St. Basil spoke, it was as always, with the measured deliberation of one in deep thought, a manner others often tried to imitate. The Emperor left with no concessions from St. Basil; rather, he had signed over the income of his properties in Cappadocia for the poor.

Later, however, Valens, under the influence of his Arian advisors, decided to send St. Basil into exile. Just before the order was to be carried out, the Emperor's only son, Galates, age six, fell suddenly sick. Upon request, St. Basil went to pray for him, and the boy recovered. The promise to have the child baptized as a Catholic was not kept, and he died shortly after baptism by an Arian. Early Church historians tell us that when Valens tried still later to sign decrees banishing St. Basil, the pens split in his hands three times before he could make a mark on the paper.

From a Saintly Family

St. Basil was born about 329 A.D. in Cappadocia, the son of a family thoroughly Christian, refined and wealthy. His father,

St. Basil the Elder, was a renowned teacher of rhetoric in Neo-Caesarea. He held estates in Pontus, Cappadocia and Lesser Armenia. His mother, Emmelia (Emily), was a celebrated beauty who had been much sought after by many suitors. She gave birth to four sons and five daughters. Three of the sons became bishops and saints: St. Basil, St. Gregory of Nyssa, and St. Peter of Sebaste. The eldest daughter, Macrina, founded a convent and is also a Saint. She is known as St. Macrina the Younger, her paternal grandmother being St. Macrina the Elder. Basil's mother is also honored as a Saint. St. Basil, his brother St. Gregory of Nyssa and St. Basil's friend St. Gregory Nazianzen are known as "The three Cappadocian Fathers."

As a young boy, St. Basil was put under the tutelage of his grandmother, Macrina. Later his sister Macrina had a strong influence in directing him to the ascetical life. Few men have had the advantage of having mind and character formed by a grandmother, mother and older sister who would be canonized Saints, and by a father both holy and learned.

Basil studied at Constantinople, and then for nearly five years at Athens, the educational capital of the ancient world. Here his constant companion was St. Gregory Nazianzen. Here, too, he studied and associated with a student named Julian, who was later to become emperor and is now known in Church History as Julian the Apostate. St. Gregory Nazianzen says that when Basil was finished with his studies in Athens, he (Basil) had acquired "all the learning attainable by the nature of man." St. Basil returned to Caesarea to teach rhetoric and plead cases of law. It was about this time that he was shocked by the sudden death of Naucratius, his younger brother. About this time, too, his sister Macrina died. He later journeyed through Egypt, Palestine, Syria and Mesopotamia, learning about the hermits, hermit communities and the nascent monasteries.

On his return, he retired near Annesi, on the banks of the Iris River, to a life of solitude and penance. He gave away his possessions, wore sackcloth by night, a tunic and an outer garment by day, slept on the ground, ate sparingly of bread, vegetables and salt, and drank only water. Others came to join him. St. Basil maintained a similar strict mode of living later on as a priest and bishop. From this time forward, he was an ascetic, and he was to become known for great personal holiness.

Influential Writings

The writings of St. Basil were read by both the Christians and pagans of his own day. They were valued for their style as well as their content. St. Basil's writings flowed directly from the task at hand. He wrote against Arianism and other heresies, composed sermons, made up rules of moral living for ordinary Christians and of ascetical living for monks, and wrote many letters.

St. Basil's doctrinal writings include *On the Holy Spirit, Moralia* and the *Philocalia*, a compilation of Origen's writings which St. Basil and St. Gregory Nazianzen put together. His letters are edited in a series of 365, including some addressed to him by others. Of them it has been said that there is "probably no single source more important for understanding the complex period of Arian controversy than the letters of Basil." (*The Month*, March, 1958).

His Letters Reveal His Personality

It may also be said that these letters provide much insight into the character of St. Basil, complex enough in itself, and yet simple because all the multiple outlets of his efforts and energies came from the single flame of intense and unswerving dedication to God.

The Letters of St. Basil have never rivalled the *Confessions* of St. Augustine in popularity, but they do rival the *Confessions* in uncovering the soul of a man aching over the sins and rebuffs of others and constantly accepting adversities as a punishment for his own sins. They show this man, who was so formidable to his enemies, often groping for strength in his own soul. They have flashes of wit and playfulness. They show that Basil, who could stand alone against all attacks, had such a sensitive spirit that he begged his friends for understanding. The letters indicate that St. Basil, whose ascetical way of living practically ignored the body, was often conscious of the body's ills. He frequently mentions his weakness and sickness. The letters present a picture of one who made all sacrifices in order to put the love of God first, yet who retained deep affections and attachments for others.

A letter written in the summer of 368, two years before he became a bishop, illustrates several of the above points. St. Basil is writing to his friend, Eusebius, Bishop of Samosata:

> . . . I pass over a succession of bodily ills, a tedious winter,
> vexatious affairs of business, all of which are known and have
> previously been explained to Your Excellency. And now, as the
> result of my sins, I have been bereft of the only solace that I
> possessed, my mother. Pray do not deride me for bewailing my
> orphanhood at this time of life, but forgive me for not having
> the patience to endure separation from a soul whose like I do
> not behold among those who are left behind. My ill-health has
> now returned again, and again I lie on my bed, tossing about
> on the anchorage of my little remaining strength and ready at
> almost every hour to accept the inevitable end of life. The
> churches exhibit a condition almost like that of my body: for
> no ground of good hope comes into view, and their affairs are
> constantly drifting toward the worse . . .

Who would expect that the writer of this letter, bewailing the
decline of the Church and sick unto death, would have the spirit,
the energies and the knowledge to be the bulwark of the Catholic
Church in the coming decade? Who would think that a man
approaching 40 and yet calling himself an orphan, would be a
hard driver of men and a leader of the finest courage?

A few years later, St. Basil, so tender-hearted in feeling toward
his family and friends, was to exert the greatest pressure on his
lifelong friend, St. Gregory of Nazianzus. He overrode Gregory's
protests and consecrated him bishop of the wretched town of
Sasima. The word "bishop" may conjure up too exalted a picture. Actually this act was like sending an outstanding orator,
theologian and poet to a rough backwoods parish. St. Gregory
never fully recovered from this blow to their friendship. Even
St. Basil's close friend and admirer, Eusebius, Bishop of Samosata,
was shocked and wrote to St. Basil about it. And St. Basil wrote
in reply that he too "could have wished his brother Gregory [of
Nazianzus] to rule a church adequate to his nature. But this
would have been the whole Church under the sun collected into
one. Since, then, this is impossible, let him be a bishop who
gives dignity to his See, and not one who gains his dignity from
it. For it is the part of a truly great man not only to suffice for
great things but even by his own capacity to make little things
great."

In contrast to these words, hard-polished in literary form and
in sentiment, we may recall St. Basil's playful words to Libanius,

the great rhetorician:

> . . . I have written my letter while covered over with a blanket of snow. When you receive it and touch it with your hands, you will perceive how icy-cold it is in itself and how it characterizes the sender, who is kept inside and is unable to put his head out of the house. (1349).

Pride or Humility?

The strong and complex character of St. Basil is again well indicated by the fact that at one time he fled from a position of influence and a few years later cooperated in winning for himself the bishopric. He left Caesarea when there was a possibility of a schism developing because of his presence. He retired to his solitude and retreat on the Iris. He returned to Caesarea in 365 at the request of his friend, St. Gregory Nazianzen, who had asked him to return because of the new, insistent dangers of Arianism, which old Bishop Eusebius could not cope with. In 370, when Eusebius died, those who loved the cause of the Catholic Church knew that St. Basil was the man to succeed him, to save the Church in that area from the still strongly surging Arianism.

St. Basil had been practically the head of the diocese for the past five years. He was an able theologian, firm in direction, respected for his power, though certainly not loved by all. The wealthy of the city wanted somebody less ascetical, somebody less direct in pointing out their social obligations. Some of the people wanted a bishop who would not always denounce their circus and amphitheater. Some said that Basil's health was too poor. (In reply, the elder St. Gregory Nazianzen asked whether they wanted a bishop or a gladiator.) The suffragan bishops especially disliked St. Basil. Nevertheless, largely through the efforts of the elder Gregory Nazianzen, those who had the power of election were led to choose Basil.

St. Basil was willing to be bishop. Had he not been so and had he not cooperated with those who helped him, the fact could never have been accomplished. Not three bishops could be found among the 50 suffragan bishops (*chor-episcopi*) of Cappadocia to consecrate Basil. The aged Gregory, sick in bed, had himself carried to Caesarea to take part in the consecration.

But St. Basil, often accused of pride by his enemies, and at times even by his friends (St. Jerome being among the accusers), and also of imperiousness, did not want the bishopric for any reason of vanity. He simply knew that he was needed. In this and in other instances of his life, he does not fit the pat picture of humility, i.e., always backing away from influence and honor. Yet perhaps his was the more manly humility of braving charges of pride, and the more complete detachment from self for refusing to hide in the safe compartment of false modesty.

Certainly the bishopric of Caesarea, with its 400,000 inhabitants and its commanding influence over a large part of Asia Minor, was no bed of roses. Not only was there the attack of Arianism from the outside; there was the more heart-rending opposition from within. Of this latter condition St. Basil said in a sermon:

> The bees fly in swarms, and do not begrudge each other the flowers. It is not so with us. We are not at unity. More eager about his own wrath than his own salvation, each aims his sting against his neighbor.

St. Basil was nothing if not plain-spoken.

Even his uncle Gregory, also a Cappadocian bishop, was for a time against him. The disaffected bishops refused to come to Caesarea. But when a false report went out that Basil was dead, they all came into town. He used this occasion to address them, urging peace for the love of the Church.

His Influence on the Liturgy

St. Basil has had a lasting influence on the liturgy. He noticed the weariness of the people at extremely long services and shortened the public prayers. At the same time, he introduced the prayers of Prime and Compline into the monastic office. His providing for eight periods of prayer in his monasteries has helped to determine this number for the hours or periods of prayer of the daily Divine Office, prayed for centuries by priests and many religious. The liturgy of the Orthodox churches even in our time, according to their tradition, is largely that which St. Basil introduced and/or revised at Caesarea. Parts of this liturgy are also in use in present-day Byzantine liturgies.

"Father of Eastern Monasticism"

St. Basil's interest in monasticism was wider than merely a regard for the ascetical life itself. He considered that well-directed monks could be a chief weapon in defending the Church from heresies. The trend of his regulations reflects this general purpose.

St. Basil has had a great and lasting effect in shaping monastic life and spirit. He did not found an order in the strict sense, but he did found many monasteries. For this reason and for his strong formative influence he is rightly called the "Father of Eastern Monasticism." Moreover, since later founders in the West, such as St. Benedict, were able to make use of his writings (in the Latin translation of Rufinus), St. Basil's influence has extended to the whole Church.

The Rules of St. Basil are known as the Long Rules or the Detailed Rules, 55 in number, and the Short Rules, of which there are 313. The Long Rules explain principles and the Short Rules apply them to the daily life of a monk.

Earlier steps in the development of monastic life are represented by St. Antony of the Desert in northern Egypt, who gave direction to other hermits who gathered around him, and by St. Pachomius in southern Egypt, whose monks wore a habit and took vows but were free to arrange much of their daily schedule according to their own wishes. St. Basil introduced the spirit of the common life, in which the day was ordered for all. Thus the element of obedience to a superior became much stronger. Moreover, in Basilian monasteries moderation replaced much of the primitive exaggeration and even rivalry in bodily penance that had sometimes existed. However, St. Basil's standards of moderation still seem very severe compared to our modern practice.

St. Basil also gave a stronger emphasis to work than to bodily penance. In work he saw a discipline for body and will and the means of fulfilling the command of loving one's neighbor. His monks were to help strangers, put up travelers, care for orphans, educate children. They were to learn trades like carpentry and architecture; they were to maintain gardens and farms. St. Basil's fusing of work and prayer gave a direction to monastic practice which to a large extent it has retained. His monks were not to flee from all contact with mankind, but were to raise themselves to spiritual perfection largely by helping others. The exercise of the love of others was to lead to a purer love of God. Yet St. Basil insisted on the primacy of prayer and recollection in order to do this well. He believed, too, in the value of external practices: "For the soul is influenced by outward observances and is shaped and fashioned according to its actions." St. Basil illustrates:

> One regular hour is to be assigned for meals, so that of the twenty-four hours of the day and night, just this one is devoted to the body, the remaining hours to be wholly occupied by the ascetic in the activities of the mind. Sleep should be light and easily broken, a natural consequence of the meagerness of the diet, and it should be deliberately interrupted for meditations on lofty subjects.

The midnight Office may owe something to St. Basil, for he says, "What dawn is to others, this, midnight, is to the men who practice piety."

The Strength of Weakness

It has been said that the later years of St. Basil's life were just one long sickness. Cardinal Newman says of St. Basil that "from his multiplied trials he may be called the Jeremiah or Job of the fourth century . . . He had a very sickly constitution, to which he added the rigor of an ascetic life. He was surrounded by jealousies and dissensions at home; he was accused of heterodoxy in the world; he was insulted and roughly treated by great men; and he labored, apparently without fruit, in the endeavor to restore unity and stability to the Catholic Church." Cardinal Newman does not explicitly say so here, but even Pope St. Damasus suspected St. Basil of heresy. Basil's efforts to have St. Damasus come to the East met with no success, and while Basil's ensuing bitterness indicated his intense dedication to Church unity, it showed too the personal pain of being misunderstood.

St. Basil had been a sickly child to start with, and as mentioned above, much of his later life was spent in illness. He speaks often in his letters of having been laid up for some time. One of his longstanding ailments was liver trouble. Once when St. Basil stood before the tribunal of the sub-prefect of Pontus, the magistrate threatened to tear out his liver. He replied, "Do so, it gives me much trouble where it is." He often mentions that the blows to his spirit from misunderstanding and calumny brought on relapses.

> My heart was constricted, my tongue was unnerved, my hand grew numb, and I experienced the suffering of an ignoble soul . . . I was almost driven to misanthropy. Every line of conduct I considered a matter of suspicion, and I believed that the virtue of charity did not exist in human nature, but that it was a specious word which gave some glory to those using it . . .

But St. Basil did not become embittered by his constant sickness. Instead, he built on the outskirts of Caesarea a large hospital, together with houses for workers, a shelter for travelers, a church and a home for clergy. In one section of the hospital, St. Basil himself received and embraced lepers, just as a decade before he had himself served meals in the soup kitchen which he had organized during a year of famine. Other buildings were situated nearby, so that the area came to be called "The New City." St. Basil also established many other hospitals in his diocese.

St. Basil is truly the bishop par excellence. He devoted himself to everything that pertained to Church life. His supreme interest was the unity of the whole Church, and for this he wrote letters to St. Athanasius, the bishops of the West and to Pope St. Damasus. At the same time, the bodily needs of the poorest man in the city received his energetic attention, and he could take time to write to a tax assessor or a poor widow.

St. Basil's last act before death was to ordain. His last words were, "Into Thy hands I commend my spirit."

At St. Basil's funeral, several people were crushed to death trying to get close to his bier. Today his name clings only to one of the hills of ancient Caesarea (modern Kayseri). The New City is gone. But both the work and the name of St. Basil endure in the Church. He touches our lives at many points. His feast day (June 14 in the 1962 calendar) is now observed in the Roman Rite on January 2, along with that of St. Gregory Nazianzen. The Eastern Rites celebrate St. Basil's feast on January 1, the anniversary of his death. Deservedly has he retained the title first given by his own contemporaries: Basil the Great.

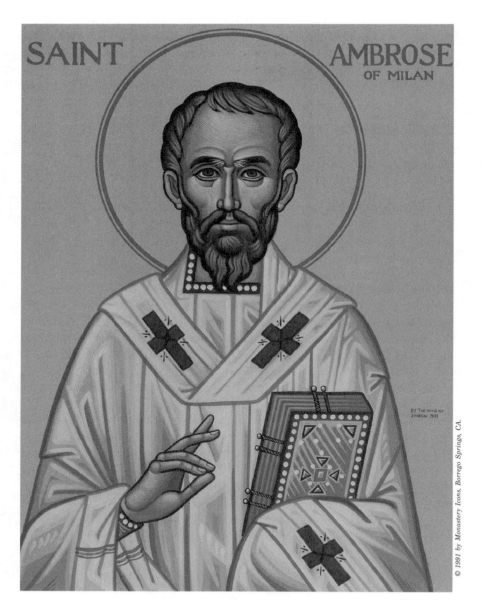

SAINT AMBROSE OF MILAN

© 1991 by Monastery Icons, Borrego Springs, CA.

Saint Ambrose

7

SAINT AMBROSE
Patron of the Veneration of Mary
c. 340-397

THE people of Thessalonica hurried to the circus. There was happy excitement on that day in August of 390 A.D. But those who crowded in to witness the games and races did not know they were walking into a trap. From his country residence the Emperor Theodosius, egged on by vicious counselors, had issued an order for their destruction.

Not long before, a mob in this city had murdered a number of officials including Botheric, its governor, and had dragged his body through the streets. A massacre of the people would be carried out in retribution. Now the Emperor's soldiers were closing in on the circus.

But out in the countryside, his messengers were desperately galloping in toward the city with counter-orders. Theodosius had quickly repented of the rash command. But the news came too late. Seven thousand people were massacred behind the closed gates of the amphitheater.

"A deed has been perpetrated in Thessalonica which has no parallel in history, a deed which I in vain attempted to prevent." From a country retreat, St. Ambrose, Bishop of Milan, wrote to the Emperor Theodosius:

> . . . It grieves me that you, who were an example of singular piety, who exercised consummate clemency, who would not suffer individual offenders to be placed in jeopardy, should not mourn over the destruction of so many innocent persons . . . I dare not offer the Sacrifice if you determine to attend.

If the Bishop could not offer Mass in the presence of the Emperor, that meant Theodosius was excommunicated in the severest way. Yet the Bishop included in his stern letter a note of kindness: "You have my love, my affection, my prayers. If you believe that, follow my instructions . . ."

St. Ambrose wrote in September. After some little delay the Emperor Theodosius did follow his instructions. It is quite likely, however, that even before St. Ambrose wrote, the Emperor had issued an edict on August 18, ruling that all sentences of death must be suspended for a period of 30 days and then re-submitted for final approval. He was repentant as a ruler. But St. Ambrose wanted him as a man to repent of his sin before God. Theodosius was a mighty leader. He was a good man except for sporadic terrible outbursts of temper. He was the last man to unite in his person control of the whole Roman Empire, both East and West. And St. Ambrose demanded that he do public penance.

There is a famous painting by Rubens showing St. Ambrose refusing admittance to Theodosius at the porch of the Basilica. This portrays the story as told by the historian Theodoret but cannot be verified as to detail. The essential story, however, stands. St. Ambrose was stern but very kindly, as his letter shows.

The great Emperor came and took off the imperial purple and all the other signs of imperial power. In the Basilica he confessed the sin of murder and begged the people to pray for him. They wept to see him prostrate and bewailing his sin as any ordinary man before God. At Christmas time he was readmitted to Holy Communion. Theodosius' repentance was not short-lived, but permanent. At his funeral about four years later, St. Ambrose said:

> I loved him because, divesting himself of his regal state, he wept publicly for his sins and asked for pardon with groans and tears. I loved him because, Emperor as he was, he was not ashamed to do the public penance from which many of low degree shrink, and because he deplored his sin every day he lived.

St. Ambrose's bringing of Theodosius to penance is highly significant. For the first time in history, a bishop had claimed and exercised the right of judging, punishing and pardoning a great prince of state. For the first time, an emperor had acknowledged and submitted to a higher power than his own. The penance of Theodosius was a dramatic representation of the principle St. Ambrose had spoken about so clearly a few years before: "The Emperor is within the Church, not over the Church." At that time he had been addressing Valentinian II and his mother, Justina, who were trying to make him give up the Portian Basilica to the Arians.

In bringing Theodosius to penance, in several other dramatic incidents, and in the whole tenor of his relations with the emperors, St. Ambrose set up a pattern of Church-state relationships which would endure for more than a thousand years. His influence on history, therefore, has been deep and important.

Milan, with its 100,000 population, was the capital of the western part of the Roman Empire during most of the fourth century. Before St. Ambrose, however, its bishops had not exerted any great influence. The man who brought Theodosius to penance changed that story.

We might expect to find St. Ambrose powerful in build and robust in health. He was neither. He was short, with a rather long face and high forehead. His hair, probably light brown, was clipped short, and he wore a beard and a drooping moustache. Ordinarily his expression was grave, perhaps verging on melancholic. Considering his ability to play on words, his face must have lit up in conversation when his nimble mind found some happy pun to illustrate a point. St. Ambrose was not handsome, but his manner was courteous and charming.

St. Ambrose came from one of the outstanding families of the Empire, a family which had been Christian for several generations. It is characteristic of his cast of mind that he thought more highly of having a martyr, St. Soteris, in the family history than of its long line of consuls and prefects. At the time of his birth in the Roman city of Trier (Treves) in Germany about 340 A.D., his father, Aurelius Ambrose, was Pretorian Prefect of Gaul. In that capacity he was civil ruler of a territory approximating modern France, Spain, Portugal, Sardinia, Sicily, Corsica and parts of Britain and Germany. The name of St. Ambrose's mother is not known. St. Ambrose was the third child in a family of three. The oldest was his sister, St. Marcellina, and next was his brother, St. Satyrus. His father died when Ambrose was still a child, and the family moved to Rome. Here Marcellina dedicated herself to a life of virginity, living at home, as was the custom in those days before convents. Satyrus and Ambrose received a thorough course in Latin, Greek and rhetoric—which included law.

A Great Orator

Pictures of St. Ambrose sometimes show him with a beehive at his feet. This alludes to the story of his infancy in which his nurse found him asleep, while bees went into and out of his open mouth. She was alarmed and would have tried to chase the bees away, but his father came and told her to wait. Eventually the bees swarmed together and flew high into the sky. The father sighed in relief and said: "If that child lives, he will be something great."

A similar story had also been told of Plato and others. This account is given by Paulinus, St. Ambrose's secretary in the last few years of his life. Paulinus wrote at the request of St. Augustine. The story at least highlights the fact that St. Ambrose became one of the great Christian orators. He spoke with much charm and directness, really using words to convey thought rather than just stringing them together as mere ornaments of speech. While still a pagan, St. Augustine, a great master of words himself, used to listen to St. Ambrose—not because he was interested in Christianity, but because he admired the expressive flow of words and eloquent sincerity of the speaker.

As an example of St. Ambrose's flow of words, we might consider his description of drunkenness—while realizing that a translation does not have the strength and grace of the original:

> From this come also deluding visions, uncertain sight and tottering gait. Often they [the drunken] leap over shadows as if they were pitfalls. The ground sways beneath them; suddenly it seems to be raised and lowered as if it were turning. In terror they fall upon their faces and grasp the ground with their hands; or they imagine that they are being engulfed by mountains rushing upon them. There is rumbling in their ears like the crashing of a tossing sea and shores resounding from the waves. If they see dogs, they think them lions and flee. Some are convulsed with uncouth laughter; others weep with inconsolable grief; others perceive senseless terrors. While awake they sleep, while asleep they quarrel. Life to them is a dream and their sleep is deep.

It was in part St. Ambrose's excellence as a speaker that helped him advance as a young lawyer and quickly rise to the post of Governor of Liguria and Aemilia (northern Italy). His sponsor, Probus, had sent him off with advice meant to encourage mildness, but which would prove prophetic: "Go, act not as a judge, but as a bishop."

So, at the age of 30 or little more, St. Ambrose now sat each morning to listen to the lawyers and to make decisions. He also had powers of administration and the right to the title of "Worshipful." He soon won the respect and confidence of the people.

The People's Choice

In 373 or 374, the Arian Bishop of Milan died. This was the same Auxentius that St. Hilary had tried in vain to oust. There was much discussion about a successor. Arians and Catholics each wanted a bishop after their own manner of thinking. There was in fact danger of a tumult. As governor, Ambrose went to the Basilica to maintain order. He arose and addressed the people. Somewhere in the crowd a voice was heard—according to Paulinus it was the voice of a child: "Ambrose—bishop!" Soon there was a swelling chorus echoing this suggestion.

Both sides respected St. Ambrose and liked him. He was a firm but kind administrator; his personal life was upright and moral.

Nobody in the cathedral was more surprised than Ambrose at the outcry. He had no desire to be a bishop. In fact, he already had an influential position and appeared to be on his way to still higher posts, so he resisted the popular demand. Paulinus supplies details which sound quite dramatic. According to him, during the next few days St. Ambrose tried several ruses aimed at dissuading the popular will. Finally, he went to hide in the country home of a friend named Leontius. However, a letter of approval from the Emperor, Valentinian I, and a threat of punishment for anyone who concealed Ambrose were too much for this friend. Leontius turned over the escaped bishop-elect.

At the time, St. Ambrose was still a catechumen. He had been carefully trained in the Catholic Faith, but the custom in those days was to delay Baptism. This custom seems strange today and indeed was an abuse; still, it gives evidence of the great efforts made by people in the fourth century to keep from mortal sin after Baptism. They considered a lapse after receiving the robe of grace to be a heinous ingratitude. That is also why public penances were so severe.

St. Ambrose was baptized in late November and on successive days received the various minor and major orders of the priesthood. In early December (the first or seventh), he was consecrated a bishop. Even in those days such a rapid advance was against the canons, but the consecrating bishops considered the case very special and deserving of exceptional treatment.

Bishop of Milan

The new Bishop of Milan fully verified the popular judgment. His first act was to dispose of all his properties. He gave his lands to the Church, his silver and gold to the poor, making provision only for his sister, Marcellina. He never had to fear any accusing finger when later he spoke his strong doctrine on social obligation:

> It is not from your own goods that you give largesses to the beggar; it is a portion of his own which you are restoring to him. What was given for all in common, you usurp for your own benefit. The earth belongs to all, not to the rich only. You are consequently paying back a debt; do not go away and think you are making a gift to which you are not bound. (*De Nabuthe* XII, 53).

Balancing this view, we can also mention something St. Ambrose says about beggars:

> Never were there so many beggars as today. We see coming to us strong, hearty fellows, who have no other title but their vagrancy, and who claim the right to despoil the poor of what they earn, and empty their purses. A little does not satisfy them; they must have more. They trick themselves out in a way to render their demands more urgent, and make up false descriptions of their social condition in order to swell the gifts they receive. To give credence too benevolently to their stories means to exhaust in a short time the alms set aside for the subsistence of the poor. There must be, therefore, a limit. Let them not go away empty-handed, but let not him who helps the needy to live become the prey of schemers. Let us not be inhumane, but let us not deprive extreme indigence of all support. (*De Officiis*, II, 16).

Realizing that he was not prepared to teach religion, St. Ambrose began that thorough program of study which was to last through all his 23 years as bishop. He called in the priest

Simplician from Rome to guide him; this was perhaps the tutor of his youth and was to be his successor in the See of Milan. St. Ambrose's knowledge of Greek now helped him to study the Greek Fathers, especially Origen, St. Basil and St. Cyril of Jerusalem. In digesting their works and reworking them into his own orderly presentation of truth, he helped bring the fruits of Eastern theological thought to the West and demonstrated the essential unity of faith in both parts of the Empire.

When St. Ambrose became bishop, his brother St. Satyrus left a promising career in government to take charge of the temporal affairs of the diocese. This assured St. Ambrose the freedom to pursue his studies and to devote himself to the spiritual side of things. There was always a close bond of affection between the two brothers and their sister. When St. Satyrus became seriously ill after being shipwrecked while in pursuit of a defrauder, St. Ambrose also became ill, apparently by way of sympathetic communication. St. Satyrus recovered long enough to return to Italy and see his brother and sister, but he died soon afterwards, in 379. St. Ambrose found the death of his older brother a very heavy blow and preached two beautiful funeral orations in his honor.

The Bishop's Day

St. Ambrose's day began early in the morning with private prayers and Mass. He fasted five days a week, except when entertaining guests. His door was always open. Anybody could come in unannounced and claim his attention. Sometimes people lingered after their business was over to observe him reading. St. Augustine tells us that St. Ambrose immediately began his reading and study when an interview was over. Augustine himself sometimes came and left, not wishing to disturb him. In the evening St. Ambrose did his own writing, practically always in his own hand.

His Writings

Famous among St. Ambrose's many writings are those on virginity (*De Virginibus*). These are chiefly collections and amplifications of sermons on the same subject. In fact, most of his writing is in the same category. Ambrose was primarily one who taught and preached to his own people. To help a wider group, he later wrote out and developed sermons already given.

St. Ambrose played a large part in explicating the high ideals we have in the Church concerning consecrated chastity. He did not do this without criticism in his own day. Many mothers were afraid to allow their daughters to hear him. At that time (as later in history, and even down to our own time), the objection was brought up that the world would be depopulated if all followed his teaching. St. Ambrose asked, with some humor, what young man had ever sought a wife and not found some willing candidate. Moreover, he maintained that the population increases in direct proportion to the esteem in which virginity is held. (*De Virg.*, vii).

In advocating virginity, St. Ambrose often spoke of the peerless Virgin, the Mother of Christ. He often used the Blessed Virgin Mary's life as the pattern in giving people practical direction in habits of virtue. For these reasons St. Ambrose is called the "Patron of the Veneration of Mary."

St. Ambrose is a master of allegory. He wrote extensively about the characters and events of the Old Testament, using them to point out truths in the moral and ascetical order. In all this he shows a mind highly mystical as well as very practical. He is not too much interested in the literal sense of Scripture. Rather, he uses Scripture as a jumping board to set the soul springing in a flight toward God. Then he has the rejuvenated soul drop down with energy to give a new direction to some ordinary affair of life on earth.

St. Ambrose was not a scholar interested in the abstract. He was a bishop interested in stirring his people to piety and a good life. This method, strangely enough, helped the demanding mind of St. Augustine, the great shining light among the converts of St. Ambrose. When he listened to St. Ambrose, the many difficulties of the literal explanations of the Bible vanished for him, and he saw that obscure passages could teach valuable truths. St. Augustine says, "I was pleased to hear Ambrose keep on repeating in his public instructions: 'The letter kills, it is the spirit which gives life.' By removing the veil of mystery enveloping them, he explains in their spiritual meaning those passages which, taken literally, seemed to teach strange errors." St. Augustine would be baptized by St. Ambrose in 387.

There are extant 91 letters of St. Ambrose. In these he offers many explanations of Scriptural passages to those who asked his opinion. His letters give a good picture of the times. It is in one of them that we meet the word "Mass," or "*Missa*," for the first time. In a letter to his sister St. Marcellina, St. Ambrose uses this word to describe the Eucharistic Sacrifice.

The Liturgical Hymn

To St. Ambrose goes most of the credit for bringing the liturgical hymn to the Latin part of the Church. His name became so closely associated with singing that many hymns were called "Ambrosian," even though St. Ambrose did not write them. This would include the well-known *Te Deum*. Four hymns can be surely assigned to his pen. They are: *Aeterne Rerum Conditor; Deus Creator Omnium; Jam Surgit Hora Tertia; Veni, Redemptor Omnium*. The name "Ambrosian" is also given to the ancient liturgy of the church and province of Milan, i.e., "the Ambrosian Rite."

. . . and Its Dramatic Entry

The introduction of hymns into our Church services is connected with an interesting and dramatic episode in the life of St. Ambrose. The Empress Justina, acting for her son, Valentinian II, demanded that St. Ambrose surrender to the Arians the Portian Basilica just outside the walls of Milan. This was the same Justina who some years before had placed Valentinian as a little boy in Ambrose's arms and asked him to act as the boy's ambassador. St. Ambrose had undertaken the mission to Maximus, the usurping Emperor, and saved Italy for Valentinian. With ready forgiveness, Ambrose would go again, at great personal risk, on another mission to Maximus and tell him in favor of Justina and Valentinian, "God bids me defend the widow and the orphan."

But now in the latter part of Lent, 386 A.D., Justina was demanding a church for the Arians. This was a repetition of a similar demand made the year before. This year, however, St. Ambrose was literally besieged in the Basilica. The church and its attached buildings became a kind of fortress. Soldiers stationed outside allowed anybody to enter, but nobody was allowed to leave. So the people just stayed with St. Ambrose over Palm Sunday and on through Holy Week. St. Augustine describes what St. Ambrose did to keep everyone fruitfully occupied:

"The pious people kept watch in the church, ready to die with their bishop. Then it was that the custom arose of singing hymns and psalms, after the use of the Eastern parts, lest the people should wax faint through the tediousness of sorrow; and from that day to this the custom has been retained—many, nay, almost all—of the Christian congregations throughout the rest of the world following herein."

The government relented under popular pressure, but the matter was not settled until June. It was at that time that the people of Milan asked their bishop to obtain the relics of martyrs for a new church, later to be called the Church of St. Ambrose. He directed that excavations be made in the Church of Sts. Felix and Nabor near the tomb of these Saints. After digging for some time in the spot St. Ambrose had pointed out, they found two huge skeletons with the heads severed from the trunks. These were identified as the bones of Sts. Gervase and Protase, who were believed to have suffered under the Emperor Nero.

During the procession bearing the bones to the new church, a blind man of Milan named Severus, formerly a butcher, either touched the pall covering the bier or applied to his eyes a cloth touched to it. He was cured. This, along with the healing of many sick and the delivery of others from evil spirits, caused such a popular wave of approval for St. Ambrose and the Catholic Faith that no more demands were made by the Arians. Cardinal Newman, writing while still an Anglican, dwells on the cure of the blind man as an evident and authentic miracle in an age when the populace and the writers often saw miracles with too much ease.

A Giant in Church and Empire

St. Ambrose was one of the most influential men of the fourth century. He was the friend and confidant of emperors—in fact, the teacher of two of them, the young half-brothers, Gratian and Valentinian II. In 379 he persuaded the Emperor Gratian to outlaw Arianism in the Western Empire. St. Ambrose defeated the last strong effort for the official recognition of paganism when he logically refuted the eloquent plea of Symmachus that the altar of the goddess of victory be placed again in the Senate. Near the end of Ambrose's life, the Emperor Theodosius won an important victory over Arbogastes, thus bringing an end to paganism in the Empire. A few months later, Theodosius died in the arms of Ambrose, and the Saint preached the Emperor's funeral oration. It has well been said of the great St. Ambrose that "more than any other man, he was responsible for the rise of Christianity in the West as the Roman Empire was dying."

Close to God and Man

St. Ambrose combined in himself many divergent qualities. He was a mystic and a man of energetic action; a writer of polished Latin verse as displayed in his hymns, and a person always practical; he was a good administrator, a man of orderly habits, yet anybody could walk into his house for a conference; he was often quite stern and unbending, yet he was extraordinary in his sympathy for the poor and for captives. For these latter he even sold the churchplate and sacred vessels, bringing upon himself the charge of sacrilege.

St. Ambrose was very mortified and austere; he recommended the consecration of human affection to Christ through virginity. Yet at the same time he had an extraordinary love for children, deep friendships, and the warmest of affections for his brother and sister. In his later years he brought up the three grandchildren of a friend, maintaining them in the episcopal residence.

His Holy Death

In February of 397 St. Ambrose became seriously ill. A deputation came to ask him to pray that God would spare his life. Ambrose answered: "I have not so lived among you as to be ashamed to live on; but I am not afraid to die, for Our Lord is good." On Good Friday he lay for some hours with his arms outstretched on the bed in the form of a cross while he prayed silently. He received Holy Viaticum shortly after midnight and died early in the morning of Holy Saturday, April 4.

St. Ambrose was buried near the remains of the two martyrs whose bones he had discovered, Sts. Gervase and Protase. In the ninth century the remains of the three Saints were placed in one sarcophagus. This was opened in 1871. St. Ambrose's bones, together with those of Sts. Gervase and Protase, are now in a silver shrine in the crypt of the Church of St. Ambrose in Milan.

The way St. Ambrose received his vocation is a lesson in the ways of God. We sometimes tend too much to purge out the human elements and to look for some indefinable interior call. God does not always communicate with us openly, as through "the burning bush"; rather, He often speaks through the uncouth and rasping voices of men. Though nominated by men, St. Ambrose was certainly called by God.

Most Saints' feasts are celebrated on the day of their death, their entry into the Kingdom of God. The feast of St. Ambrose, however, is celebrated on the traditional day of his consecration as a bishop, December 7. St. Ambrose is one of the four great Latin Doctors, the others being St. Jerome, St. Augustine and St. Gregory the Great.

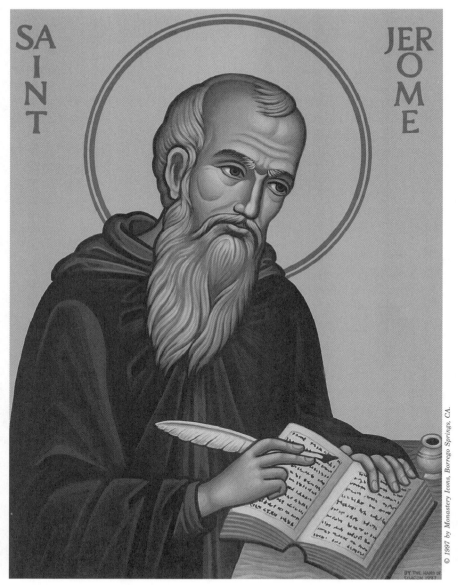

SA INT

JER OME

Saint Jerome

8

SAINT JEROME
Father of Biblical Science
c. 342-c. 420

AS the fourth century turned into the fifth, the ancient world was in turmoil. The Roman Empire was decadent and crumbling. The stir of marching barbaric tribes had begun. A few years later, in 410 A.D., Rome itself would fall to the invading Alaric and his Goths. Deep changes were in progress, whose on-rolling waves would strike the distant shores of a long future. The changes were political and social, cultural and religious. The young adult voice of Christianity spoke out just as the quavering accents of the Old Roman Empire grew faint, although there was not a cause and effect connection between the rise of the one and the fall of the other, as the historian Edward Gibbon has claimed.

It is not surprising, then, that during the fourth and early fifth centuries we witness the appearance of 12 of the Doctors of the Church. They had a large share in the formative influence of the Catholic Church in a period of crisis and change. If asked to choose from among their number the one man who exercised the greatest influence, many scholars would pick St. Jerome. It was just in the years covering the turn of the century (391-406) that he did his most productive and enduring work. During these years, he published his translation into Latin of all the Hebrew books of the Bible.

In his large cave in Bethlehem near the birthplace of Our Lord, St. Jerome, the careful, painstaking scholar, worked on and on for countless hours. He worked day and night, despite trouble with his eyes and not very robust health. A pilgrim wrote: "He is always completely engrossed in his reading and his books. He never rests, day or night. He is reading or writing the whole time." The pilgrim saw a man of pale, ascetic face, with white hair, and a body lean from much fasting and sickness.

The observer might have smiled had he been able to look back half a century and see the learned Jerome as a little boy being pulled from his grandmother's lap to face the hated Orbilius, his first teacher. The pilgrim might have recalled from St. Jerome's own letters the picture of a young man in Rome— eagerly pursuing the classical pagan authors, and between times, almost as eagerly, pursuing the pleasures of the pagans.

For St. Jerome was no ready-made saint, and his early interest as a scholar was in secular fields. He never lost his taste for classical literature. In fact, there is a famous story that St. Jerome had a dream in which an angel asked him to describe himself. Jerome answered that he was a Christian. The Angel denied this and accused St. Jerome of being, rather, a Ciceronian— alluding to the scholar's love for the works of Cicero. The Angel then proceeded to administer a flogging to the Saint. When St. Jerome awoke, the marks of the flogging were still to be seen upon his back. Much chastened, Jerome gave up or at least drastically curtailed his reading of classical pagan authors.

Jerome also never lost his contact with what went on in the world or his deep feelings either for or against other people. To his final years he was vigorously, and often angrily, entering into controversies. He always remained a kind of watchdog for orthodoxy. His warning bark and charging attack scattered and frightened intruders.

The *Vulgate*

St. Jerome was a part of the changing world, but his essential work of translation proceeded. His long training as a classical scholar, his exact knowledge of Hebrew, Greek and Latin, his own passion for exactness fitted him for this supreme task of his life. As the world changed and left behind its ancient molds, St. Jerome was helping to form a new Christian mold that in turn would vastly help to reshape the world.

One of the answers to the question "Why is Latin the language of the Church?" is surely that St. Jerome's mighty translations and revisions of translations of Sacred Scripture helped to establish it as such. He provided a basic, reliable translation of the Bible, a work of appeal and style that could be accepted, referred to and used for meditation as well as for study. This masterpiece is known as the *Latin Vulgate Bible*, or simply as the *Vulgate*, the term deriving from the fact that the work was a translation into the "vulgar" tongue or the common Latin of the people. A Protestant scholar, Dean Millman, says:

> The translation of Jerome created a new language. The inflexible Latin became pliant and expansive, naturalizing Eastern imagery, Eastern modes of expression and thought, and Eastern religious notions most uncongenial to its genius and character, and yet retaining much of its own peculiar strength, solidity and majesty.

St. Jerome's translation from the Hebrew met with much opposition in his own day. Even St. Augustine wrote at first to dissuade him from going directly from the Hebrew. It took about 100 years for St. Jerome's Old Testament translation to find equal favor with other, older versions. Then it gradually grew in favor until, practically speaking, it supplanted all others.

Earlier, St. Jerome had revised the old Latin translation (the old *Itala*) of the Gospels, and perhaps other or all books of the New Testament. Earlier, too, he had twice revised the Psalms. The second of his two previous revisions—known as the Gallican Psalter, from its popularity among the Gauls—found more favor than his later translation directly from the Hebrew. The Gallican Psalter is incorporated into the Vulgate, which is the Latin Bible made up basically of Jerome's translations and revisions of earlier translations. St. Jerome's Gallican Psalter was used until 1945 in reciting the Divine Office. At that time a new Latin text was authorized, though the Gallican Psalter could still be used. Of the Old Testament deuterocanonical books (these seven Old Testament books are not accepted by Protestants), St. Jerome translated only *Judith* and *Tobias*. These were originally written in Chaldaic.

From the Council of Trent (1548-1563) until 1979, the Vulgate was the official Latin Bible of the Catholic Church. (In 1979 Pope John Paul II issued a new Vulgate, the *Nova Vulgata*.) For 800 years before Trent, the Vulgate was the Bible which was most commonly used. In its Fourth Session the Council of Trent decreed:

> Moreover, the same holy council [Trent] . . . ordains and declares that the old Latin Vulgate Edition, which, in use for so many hundred years, has been approved by the Church, be in public lectures, disputations, sermons and expositions held as authentic, and that no one dare or presume under any pretext whatsoever to reject it. (April 8, 1546).

The Vulgate's influence in shaping the thinking of philosophers and theologians was profound. "No other book has so profoundly influenced the literature of the Middle Ages; books of ceremonies, breviaries, medieval plays, books of devotion, and even the great works of philosophy and theology acknowledge their debt to St. Jerome." (F. Moriarty, S. J.).

St. Jerome tells us of two guiding principles which he followed in translating: First, to go back to the original language; secondly, to remember that

> A slavishly literal translation* from one language into another obscures the sense; the exuberance of the language lessens the yield. For while one's diction is enslaved to cases and metaphors, it has to explain by tedious circumlocutions what a few words would otherwise have sufficed to make plain. (*Letter* 57).

The Traveling Scholar

St. Jerome came from a Christian family that was fairly well-to-do. He was named after his father, Eusebius, but he is commonly called Hieronymus in Latin, or Jerome. There was an only sister and a brother, Paulinian, born 20 years after Jerome. In his many writings St. Jerome speaks very little of his family and never mentions the names of his mother or his sister, an omission which contrasts with his devoted and deep friendships with various holy women whose names and deeds he has preserved. The omission may point to an unhappy home situation.

Jerome was born in Stridon, a town of Venetia-Histria or the northern part of Italy between Dalmatia and Pannonia. The exact site of Stridon is not known, nor is the exact date of St. Jerome's birth. The most likely date is 342. Two dates are given for his death, 419 and 420, the latter being more commonly held.

At an early age he was sent to Rome to be educated. Here he developed a great interest in classical authors and led a life somewhat on the wild side. Yet his many visits to the catacombs and his early Christian training soon brought him to request Baptism, which, as was often the case in those days, had been deferred. He was about 20 years old at the time.

St. Jerome had an active, inquiring mind, a lively facility for making friends and enemies, and a roving, restless nature. All these are especially in evidence during the years following his student days at Rome.

---

* St. Jerome may disclaim being "slavishly" literal; however, his translation of the Bible into Latin is *extremely* literal and highly accurate. —*Publisher*, 2000.

He traveled for three years in Gaul and Italy, having a home base at Treves (Trier) in Germany. It was here that he came to admire St. Hilary of Poitiers and copied two of his books for his friend Rufinus. This was a secondhand introduction to the Bible for the future biblical scholar. He lived for three years at Aquileia, then went on a long journey through Asia Minor, ending at the home of Evagrius in Antioch, the great city of Syria. It was while going through Athens that he saw the inscription: "To the gods of Asia, of Europe and of Africa, to the unknown and wandering gods." Concerning this, he said that St. Paul had quoted loosely when basing his Athenian speech on the text: "To the unknown god." (Cf. *Acts* 17:23). St. Jerome then spent five years as a monk in the desert of Calcis. He was about 30 years old at this time.

During this period he learned Hebrew, in part as a penance and an antidote against severe sensual temptations. The most quoted passage of his writings describes these trials. It occurs in a letter, really a treatise, on virginity, addressed to the young virgin, Eustochium. (*Letter* 22). St. Jerome writes with candor and humility:

> How often when I was living in the desert, in the vast solitude which gives to hermits a savage dwelling place, parched by a burning sun, how often did I fancy myself among the pleasures of Rome! I used to sit alone because I was filled with bitterness. Sackcloth disfigured my unshapely limbs; and my skin, from long neglect, had become as black as an Ethiopian's . . . Now, although in my fear of Hell I had consigned myself to this prison, where I had no companions but scorpions and wild beasts, I often found myself amid bevies of girls. My face was pale and my frame chilled with fasting; yet my mind was burning with desire, and the fires of lust kept bubbling up before me when my flesh was as good as dead. Helpless, I cast myself at the feet of Jesus; I watered them with my tears; I wiped them with my hair; and then I subdued my rebellious body with weeks of abstinence . . . I remember how I often cried aloud all night till the break of day, and ceased not beating my breast till tranquility returned at the chiding of the Lord. I used to make my way alone into the desert. Wherever I saw hollow valleys, craggy mountains, steep cliffs, there I made my oratory, there the house of correction for my unhappy flesh . . . When I had shed copious tears and had strained my eyes towards Heaven, I sometimes felt myself amid angelic hosts . . .

There were other disturbances in the desert, since disputes about doctrine engaged the monks. Jerome left there for the same reason he had left Aquileia, because of controversy. He returned to the home of his friend Evagrius at Antioch.

Paulinus, one of the bishops of this See, which was torn by schism, ordained St. Jerome a priest. Jerome, however, always remained a monk and scholar, and did not exercise the priestly office as a pastor of souls. Drawn by the fame of St. Gregory Nazianzen, he went to Constantinople, spent there a happy period of writing and study, and then left for Rome in 382 at the invitation of Pope St. Damasus I.

In Rome St. Jerome acted as secretary and advisor to the Pope; it is for this reason that art sometimes pictures him in cardinal's robes. St. Jerome's renown grew at this time, and he was often mentioned as a possible candidate for the papacy. Yet, it was only during these two years in Rome that his vast scholarship was given direction and purpose. Pope Damasus asked him to revise the existing Latin version of the Gospels, basing the corrections on the original Greek.

At this same time St. Jerome undertook the instruction and spiritual formation of a group of noble women who met at the home of Marcella on the Aventine. Among these were the widow St. Paula and her four daughters, Blesilla, Paulina, St. Eustochium (whose name was actually Eustochium Julia) and Rufina. Among the other holy women were Lea, Asella and Fabiola. Spurred on by these tasks, St. Jerome's interest in the Scriptures and in the ascetical life continued to grow. The questions asked by the Pope and by Jerome's eager and intelligent pupils gave zest to his studies.

But his very work led him into trouble. There was much criticism of his changes in the wording (translation) of the Gospels to which the people had been accustomed. Moreover, St. Jerome's own blunt criticisms of the lives of some of the Roman clergy and of fashionable Christians stirred up a storm against him. He was summoned before a council of clergy to answer charges of misconduct regarding Marcella and Paula. His friend and protector, Pope Damasus, had died. St. Jerome cleared himself of the charges and then left Rome, which he bitterly called Babylon. Nevertheless, he grieved much when the city was later sacked by the Goths.

Bethlehem, the Journey's End

St. Jerome now traveled throughout Palestine, acquainting himself with the geography of this land of the Bible. After this he went for a while to Egypt. On much of this travel he was accompanied by a sizable group of people who had followed him from Rome, including St. Paula and St. Eustochium. Finally, he settled at Bethlehem. He had seen much that would help him in his work on the Bible. As he said, "Whoever has looked with his own eyes on Judea and knows the associations of its ancient towns and their names, old or new, has a clearer grasp of the Scriptures."

St. Jerome himself lived in a cave near the place of Christ's birth. It can be seen today in the northern part of the crypt of the Basilica of the Nativity. Nearby were built monasteries for men and women and a guest house for pilgrims, so that no pilgrim would be left without shelter as the Blessed Virgin Mary and St. Joseph had been. Later, a school for boys and two more convents were built. St. Paula supplied most of the funds for this work, and St. Jerome used the last of his patrimony.

In Bethlehem, which he called "the most august spot in all the world," St. Jerome spent the remaining 34 years of his life. He was a lonely, laboring, prayerful monk who toiled most of the night, and yet at the same time he was an active director of souls, a teacher and an adviser and helper of pilgrims during much of the day.

Enmity with Rufinus

St. Jerome was a very sensitive man. He was naturally responsive to affection and was quickly hurt by criticism. Besides this, he was a careful scholar, paying much attention to the precise use of words. He could not stand the misinterpretations of Scripture of those less careful. Beyond this he was very devoted to the ideal of the monastic life and to the defense of the traditional teachings of the Church. He rose immediately to refute, in unmistakable and strong terms, and with an overwhelming display of knowledge, anyone who wrote against monastic ideals or the orthodox teachings of the Church. His most sensitive spot of all was for himself to be considered in favor of a doubtful or wrong teaching.

It is easy to see that anyone who devotes his whole life to a

cause suffers most when he is accused of working against that
very cause. This is what happened in the case of St. Jerome's
most celebrated encounter with his former cherished friend,
Rufinus. They had been students together in Rome and had a
high regard for each other. But under pressure from St.
Epiphanius, who wanted Origen condemned, St. Jerome gave his
support and Rufinus did not, nor did John, the Bishop of
Jerusalem, who was a close friend of Rufinus. In the furor that
developed, St. Jerome and his monks and St. Paula's religious
were even deprived of Mass and the Sacraments by John. But
after all this, St. Jerome and Rufinus publicly made up, shak-
ing hands after Mass. This was in 397. When Rufinus left for
the West soon afterwards, St. Jerome, in token of friendship,
went part way with him.

But the controversy about Origen broke out again. Some of
the reports that came back to St. Jerome about Rufinus' attacks
on him were exaggerated. It is true, however, that Rufinus did
point a finger of suspicion at St. Jerome for using the works of
Origen, though now condemning him. Rufinus opened a more
personally delicate topic when he criticized St. Jerome for learning Hebrew from a rabbi and for going back on a promise not
to read pagan authors. Perhaps St. Jerome had used up what
he thought was his last ounce of forgiving patience. His reply
to Rufinus shows hurt and anger. He gave vent to personal abuse
and name-calling. Rufinus became the pig, the scorpion, the hun-
dred-headed hydra, the grunter.

St. Augustine summed up the sadness of the Christian world
over this discord when he wrote to St. Jerome: "I feel most
unhappy that such horrible dissension should have occurred
between people who had been so friendly and intimate and who
almost all the Churches knew to have been linked by the closest of bonds."

In the controversy with Rufinus, St. Jerome cannot be excused.
But some of his language even here must be laid to rhetorical
exaggeration. St. Jerome freely admitted that "to teach a disciple is one thing; to vanquish an opponent, another." (*Letter* 50).
He also said that in fighting a foe you use the sword, but you
likewise feint. (*Letter* 47). St. Jerome knew that the public sees
only black and white, and so he sketched in deep black when
he wanted to ruin the damaging effect of heresy or personal
attack. His method had its effect in fighting Pelagius, "the hulk-
ing brute stuffed with his Scots' porridge," and in silencing

Helvidius, Jovinian and Vigilantius. This is not to say that St. Jerome did not use learning and logic. He did pile proof upon proof, appealing especially to Scripture and to traditional teaching. But he also employed ridicule and satire and plain name-calling. His method is not unlike that of a competent modern statesman who knows his subject, but also considers it necessary to employ the exaggerations of political campaigning.

His Aunt Castorina

St. Jerome's caustic pen and his regrettable enmity with Rufinus have been well-publicized. But a letter to his Aunt Castorina, a little masterpiece of forgiving charity, is hardly ever mentioned. Castorina, his mother's sister, had for some unknown reason become estranged from St. Jerome. He wrote, asking for a reconciliation, and received no answer for a year. Then he wrote again:

> How have we been able in our daily prayers to say, "Forgive us our debts as we forgive our debtors," whilst our feelings have been at variance with our words, and our petition inconsistent with our conduct. Therefore, I renew the prayer which I made a year ago in a previous letter that the Lord's legacy of peace may be indeed ours, and that my desires and your feelings may find favor in His sight.

St. Jerome also recalled that one's gift at the altar is not acceptable unless he be first reconciled with his brother. (*Matt.* 5:23-24). St. Jerome knew more than any of us the duty of forgiveness as explained in Scripture. He also feared the Judgment. In the same letter to Castorina he says, "Soon we shall stand before His judgment seat to receive the reward of harmony restored or to pay the penalty for harmony broken." (*Letter* 13).

Although St. Jerome never publicly expressed sorrow for his enmity with Rufinus, he must have forgiven him. One of the many representations of St. Jerome in art portrays him striking his breast with a stone in a gesture of contrition. Pope Sixtus V one day when passing this picture said: "You do well to hold that pebble in your hand, for without it, the Church would never have canonized you." St. Jerome's penitential life and essential humility would atone and would demand his essential forgiveness.

Deep Friendships

We understand St. Jerome's harsh words to opponents better, too, when we contrast them with his unusually strong words of affection for friends. A quarter-century before their quarrel, St. Jerome had written to Rufinus, calling him "dearest Rufinus":

"Believe me, brother, I look forward to seeing you more than the storm-tossed mariner looks for his haven, more than the thirsty fields long for the showers, more than the anxious mother sitting on the curving shore expects her son."

In the same letter, referring to the death of his friend, Innocent, St. Jerome laments: "I lost one of my two eyes; for Innocent, the half of my soul, was taken away from me by a sudden attack of fever." When Hylas, another companion, died soon afterwards, St. Jerome himself, due as much to sorrow as to the hardships of a journey, fell sick and remained so for much of a year. This was about the year 374.

Writing to console St. Paula on the death of her 20-year-old daughter, the widowed Blesilla, St. Jerome says:

> But what is this? I wish to check a mother's weeping, and I groan myself. I make no secret of my feelings; this entire letter is written in tears . . . Dear Paula, my agony is as great as yours . . . I was her father in the spirit, her foster-father in affection . . . No page shall I write in which Blesilla's name shall not occur. Wherever the records of my utterance shall find their way, thither she too will travel with my poor writings . . .

When St. Paula herself died after 20 years in the convent at Bethlehem, St. Jerome was so stricken that he could not control the pen in his hand, but dictated a long letter to her daughter Eustochium. When Eustochium died in 418, St. Jerome, then in his last years, could not find the strength nor the will to compose a funeral oration. He wrote later:

> The sudden falling asleep of the holy and venerable virgin Eustochium has completely crushed us, and it has almost transformed our way of living, for we can no longer carry out our plans in many things, and the fervor of the mind is frustrated by the infirmities of old age.

Earlier, at the end of a long letter giving advice on how to educate the little Paula, granddaughter of St. Paula, St. Jerome had asked to have a share in her education. He advised sending the little girl to her holy grandmother and to her Aunt Eustochium. They would train her in the ways of holiness and virginity. Then he adds:

> If you will only send Paula, I myself promise to be both a tutor and a foster-father to her. Old as I am, I will carry her on my shoulders and train her stammering lips; and my charge will be a far grander one than that of the worldly philosopher . . .

A Prolific Writer

St. Jerome will always be remembered first for his translation of the Bible. Yet his other works are voluminous. He wrote many Scripture commentaries. Those on the major prophets, done in the final years of his life, had a prolonged influence on Church writers. His letters, about 120 in number, give a very valuable picture of fourth-century society and an intimate glimpse into his own personality. His book of short biographies, entitled *De Viris Illustribus (On Illustrious Men)*—and ending with himself—has preserved much information not otherwise known. It is a good, though not always a reliable source book on 135 ancient writers, most of whom were Christian. St. Jerome dismisses St. Ambrose in *De Viris Illustribus:* "Ambrose, Bishop of Milan, is still writing today; as he is living, I shall avoid giving my judgment in order not to expose myself to the contradictory reproach of too much flattery or too much frankness." St. Jerome did give generous notice to St. Gregory Nazianzen. *De Viris Illustribus* is the sole extant source of information on the lives of Tertullian and Cyprian.

St. Jerome was not very speculative in his writings, but he was the greatest stylist among the Latin Fathers. Throughout his writings are many neat twists of rhetoric, many quotable phrases. He is seldom dull and most often interesting, even today. His words of advice are often surprisingly apt, as when he gives his ideas on educating the infant Paula:

> Have letters made for her, of boxwood or ivory, and let them be called by their names. Let her play with them, and *let the play be part of her instruction* . . . She should have companions in her task of learning, whose accomplishments she may envy and whose praises may spur her sense of shame. Do not scold her if she is slow, but arouse her ambition by praise, so

that she may delight at victory and smart at defeat. Above all, do not allow her to hate her studies, lest the bitterness of them, acquired in childhood, last to her maturer years. The very names wherewith she gradually learns to put words together should be purposely chosen—that is, those of the Prophets and the Apostles, and the whole line of patriarchs, from Adam down, and those of Matthew and Luke, so that while she is engaged in something else, she may be laying up a useful store in her memory. (*Letter* 107).

In *Letter* 68 St. Jerome's words are very much to the point in consoling Castrutius, a blind man:

God's hottest anger against sinners is when He shows no anger. "My jealousy will depart from thee and I will be quiet and will be no more angry . . ." (*Ezech.* 16:42). The master does not correct his disciple unless he sees in him signs of promise. When once the doctor gives over caring for the patient, it is a sign that he despairs.

Letters to St. Augustine

The correspondence with St. Augustine, in which nine letters were written, shows St. Jerome with his fiery eloquence at times smoldering but under control. St. Augustine's first two letters to St. Jerome were delayed and were publicly circulated before Jerome saw them. Besides this irritating factor, their suggestions and criticisms came from a younger man, though a bishop, to an older man already an established and renowned scholar. There was some cause for unfavorable reaction on the part of St. Jerome. He kept silent, however, until he received a third letter. Jerome's first extant letter to St. Augustine is polite and reserved but has muffled undertones of displeasure:

Finally, pray esteem one who esteems you; and in the field of Scripture do not you, a youth, challenge me, an old man . . . See how much I esteem you in the fact that I have been unwilling to answer even when challenged, nor will I believe that a document is yours, which in another I should perhaps blame.

In a later letter St. Augustine explained the people's objection to St. Jerome's substituting "ivy" for the familiar "gourd" in the book of *Jonas* (4:6). He added, "Whence even I think that in some things, you may sometimes have been mistaken." Jerome answered this in a way that showed wounded feeling:

> If you wish either to exercise or to display your learning, seek for youths both eloquent and noble who can dare fight with you . . . And pray attend to my request that, whatever you write to me, you would take the trouble to see that it reaches my hands first.

St. Augustine wrote a soothing apology. Later correspondence shows St. Augustine quite careful, if still free in offering suggestions; and St. Jerome measuring his words, though not above injecting some personal feeling.

Virginity and Marriage

By his writings and example St. Jerome gave a great impetus to the practice of asceticism and chastity. He also gave the monastic life a strong direction toward union with a life of study and teaching.

So strong was St. Jerome's defense of the virginal state that he has often been accused of running down marriage. He defends himself from this charge by offering a good example, comparing virginity to gold and marriage to silver. "Gold is more precious than silver, but is silver on that account the less silver?" (*Letter* 48). It is true that St. Jerome does have individual passages that seem to disparage marriage. But whoever reads St. Jerome must keep remembering that he does not wish to weaken his pleadings by quiet qualifications. He writes with the loud emphasis of the orator. Like a cartoonist who makes his characters grotesque but has a solid message, so writes St. Jerome.

In his most famous letter, that to St. Eustochium (*Letter* 22), St. Jerome shows that he fully knew the true value of virginity as a dedication to a higher love:

> How very difficult it is for the human heart not to love something! Of necessity, our minds and wills must be drawn to some kind of affection. Carnal love is overcome by spiritual love. Desire is extinguished by deeper desire. Whatever is taken from carnal love is given to the higher love.

In the life of St. Jerome himself, human affection was by no means extinguished, but rather developed to an unusual degree and purified. He gained such a control over merely sensual attraction that he was able to develop a deep and tender attachment toward various holy women. His love for Sts. Paula and Eustochium, especially, and their regard for him and interest in his work, sustained and spurred him on in his labors.

Defends Our Lady's Perpetual Virginity

In connection with his high view of virginity, St. Jerome wrote a detailed defense of the perpetual virginity of the Blessed Virgin Mary. "I must entreat God the Father to show that the Mother of His Son, who was a mother before she was a bride, continued a virgin after her Son was born." St. Jerome refuted all the objections of Helvidius, among them those based on Scriptural references to Mary's "firstborn son" and "the brothers of the Lord":

> Every only-begotten son is a firstborn son, but not every firstborn is an only-begotten. By firstborn we understand not only one who is succeeded by others, but one who has had no predecessors.

Referring to the Lord's "brothers," St . Jerome says: "In Holy Scripture there are four kinds of brethren—by nature, race, kindred, love." He gives examples of each and shows that in the case of Christ, the brothers are by kindred; they are His cousins and the nephews of the Blessed Virgin Mary. Finally, St. Jerome in his usual blunt way tells Helvidius: "You neglected the whole range of Scripture and employed your madness in outraging the Virgin."

One very interesting sentence of St. Jerome sweeps clean the first three centuries of Christianity from any charges of not believing in Our Lady's perpetual virginity. "Pray, tell me," he asks Helvidius, "who, before you appeared, was acquainted with this blasphemy? Who thought the theory worth two-pence?"

Adherence to Authority

St. Jerome showed many times his reliance on the supreme authority of the Pope and the weight of traditional teaching to provide the guidance needed in matters of doctrine. His definition of heresy, given in his *Commentary on Titus*, implies a firm support of a divinely instituted Teaching Authority. St. Jerome explains that "'Heresy' comes from a Greek word which means 'choice,' because every heretic chooses what seems to him preferable . . ." St. Jerome urged the reading of Holy Scripture:

> I beg of you, my dear brother, to live among these books, to meditate upon them, to know nothing else." (*Letter* 53 to Paulinus, Bishop of Nola). Yet he cautioned that in the Holy Scriptures you can make no progress unless you have a guide to show you the way . . . The art of interpreting the Scriptures is the only one of which all men everywhere claim to be the masters . . . The chatty old woman, the doting old man, and the worldly sophist, one and all, take in hand the Scriptures, rend them in pieces and teach them before they have learned them . . . They do not deign to notice what prophets and apostles have intended, but they adapt conflicting passages to suit their own meaning, as if it were a grand way of teaching—and not rather the faultiest of all—to misrepresent a writer's views and to force the Scriptures reluctantly to do their will . . .

St. Jerome was writing to a bishop. His controversies with bishops and scholars on matters of faith show that he did not consider them—*as individuals*—to be sure guides in faith. Writing to Vigilantius, who had attacked the honoring of relics, prayer for the Saints' intercession and the practice of virginity, St. Jerome laments:

> Shameful to relate, there are bishops who are said to be associated with him in his wickedness—if at least they are to be called bishops—who ordain no deacons but such as have been previously married . . .

St. Jerome's appeal is to the authority of all (or most of) the churches (dioceses) commonly accepting Catholic doctrine. His appeal is also to the See of Rome. Appealing to Pope St. Damasus to decide the disputed bishopric of Antioch, and asking whether one may speak of three *hypostases* (persons) in the Godhead, St. Jerome wrote:

> My words are spoken to the successor of the Fisherman, to the disciple of the Cross. As I follow no leader save Christ, so I communicate with none but Your Blessedness, that is, with the Chair of Peter. For this I know is the rock on which the Church is built. This is the house where alone the Paschal

Lamb can be rightly eaten. This is the Ark of Noah, and he who is not found in it shall perish when the flood prevails.

In a second letter St. Jerome asserts that when he is asked for a decision about the disputed bishopric he always answers: "He who clings to the Chair of Peter is accepted by me." He adds, "Therefore I implore Your Blessedness, by Our Lord's Cross and Passion—those necessary glories of our Faith—as you hold an apostolic office, to give an apostolic decision."

St. Jerome Still Speaks

St. Jerome was close to age 80 when he died around 420 A.D. During life his great subject of meditation had been death and the divine judgment, which no doubt prepared his soul for these realities when they came. The Rev. Alban Butler says that the following saying is ascribed to St. Jerome:

> Whether I eat or drink, or whatever else I do, the dreadful trumpet of the last day seems always sounding in my ears: "Arise, ye dead, and come to judgment!"

It is said that Paula, granddaughter of St. Paula, closed St. Jerome's eyes upon his death. St. Jerome was buried near St. Paula and St. Eustochium. It is thought that eight centuries later his bones were transferred to Rome; in 1747 a casket said to contain them was found there in the crypt of St. Mary Major.

In St. Jerome we have a good proof that saints are not perfect, but are people striving for perfection. St. Jerome experienced temptations against purity even in his later years:

> When I have been angry, or have had evil thoughts in my mind, or some phantom of the night has beguiled me, I do not dare to enter the basilicas of the martyrs; I shudder all over in body and soul.

This was in the year 406. At times, St. Jerome had to drive himself in order to work, despite his eager, inquiring mind. He sometimes misunderstood people, and they misunderstood him; he sometimes quarreled with them, and they answered back. He was one of the great name-callers of all history. But this was largely a tactic, an attempt to discredit his opponents—not only in their ideas (which he saw as harmful to the Faith), but also in their persons, so that neither they nor their ideas would have any credence with anyone. Yet, he feared the judgment of God and recalled that we must forgive if we are to be forgiven. At the same time, he was penitential, full of love for God and man, zealous for souls, devoted to the pursuit of truth, humbly submissive to Church authority.

The traditional trappings of holiness are not essential. Holiness often has to strive not only against the odds without, but also against the odds within, as apparently in St. Jerome the disparate elements of a personality were fused together by his burning zeal for God and the coming of His Kingdom. In some people the fusing often may not be perfect, but in St. Jerome it was, as his sanctity attests.

Nobody will be shocked at St. Jerome's irascibility who compares his own privately spoken words with those that the Saint more candidly wrote for all to see. St. Jerome loved to upset half-baked opinions. No doubt he is quite happy now to be a saint and thereby to have upset the candied opinion that all saints are easy to get along with and that holiness is always equivalent to mildness.

If St. Jerome were living today, he would have a whole new arsenal of facts and principles to work with in the field of Sacred Scripture. It would be very interesting to hear his conclusions. We can be sure that St. Jerome, whom a pagan writer described as "a man signally Catholic and most skilled in Holy Writ," would at once uphold the Catholic Faith and be a monumental influence on all who value the Scriptures. For in him are combined to an unusually high degree an absolute adherence to the authority of Holy Church and an extreme devotion to and knowledge of the Holy Bible.

Writing in the epochal and lengthy encyclical, *Spiritus Paraclitus*, on the occasion of the fifteenth centenary of the death of St. Jerome, Pope Benedict XV said,

> His voice is now still, though at one time the whole Catholic world listened to it when it echoed from the desert; yet Jerome still speaks in his writings, which "shine like lamps throughout the world." Jerome still calls to us.

St. Jerome's feast day is September 30. He is one of the four great Latin Doctors of the Church—along with St. Ambrose, St. Augustine and Pope St. Gregory the Great.

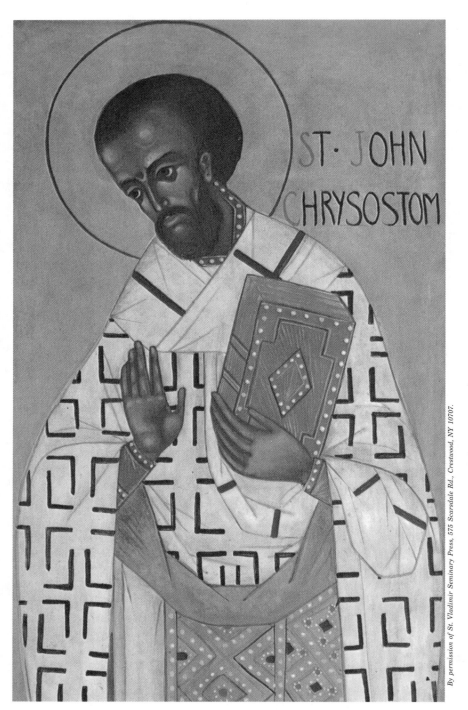

ST· JOHN CHRYSOSTOM

Saint John Chrysostom

By permission of St. Vladimir Seminary Press, 575 Scarsdale Rd., Crestwood, NY 10707.

9

SAINT JOHN CHRYSOSTOM
The Golden-Mouthed
Doctor of the Eucharist
c. 347-407

HE was so good at preaching that pickpockets came to his sermons. While the audience listened intently, they plied their trade with diligence and profit. Two centuries after his death, his reputation had not diminished, but rather had grown. Then the title of *Chrysostom*, or "The Golden-Mouthed" was given him; in succeeding centuries and yet today, men know him by this name more readily than by his baptismal name of John. With as much right as any ecclesiastical orator, St. John Chrysostom can lay claim to the title of the greatest preacher of Christianity.

His appearance did not naturally create the impression of oratorical power, for he was so thin that in his final years he calls himself "spidery." His shortness made it necessary for him to speak from an ambo. A total stranger looking up at the first sound of the not-too-strong voice might have been unimpressed, except for the rather keen look and the high forehead, which men said was like the dome of a church. But as St. John Chrysostom continued and the torrent of balanced phrases poured forth, the stranger, whether highly learned or hardly literate, would find himself lifted above the ordinary. He would be drawn into the flowing, warm stream of thought and emotion of this speaker. In accord with the usage of the day, he might laugh, stamp his feet or cry with the other listeners.

St. John did not fully approve of these customs, and one day he gave the full treatment in reproving the people. He said, moreover, that loud applause gave the sermons too much of a theatrical twist. The people responded by applauding with more enthusiasm than ever.

I avoid as much as possible the treatment of speculative questions. For the people are usually not able to follow these things, and if they are able, still they do not understand them clearly and surely.

St. John stated this principle and lived up to it. He was above all interested in leading men to the fullness of Christian living. He wanted to guide them in a practical way through the problems and difficulties of living in an atmosphere still largely pagan. So he spoke often on moral problems and on the duty of striving for perfection.

Chrysostom was very capable as an exegete, interpreting Scripture in its literal, historical sense. He was also solid in his knowledge of doctrine. But he disliked controversy; he was not like St. Augustine, interested in getting to the bottom of intricate questions of theology; nor like St. Jerome, who was interested in establishing the exact texts of Scripture from a study of many versions. In fact, he knew only one language with any thoroughness, and that was Greek. He accepted the translations of Scripture and the orthodox teachings of theology, and then did his real work in bringing the essential teachings to the people. Especially did he bring the doctrines of Christianity and the events of Scriptural history to bear on the lives of the people, translating them into practical moral and ascetic rules of life.

St. John's contact with his listeners was immediate and complete. It was all of him talking to the all of each one who heard him. "His unrivaled charm," Cardinal Newman says, "as that of every really eloquent man, lies in his singleness of purpose, his fixed grasp of his aim, his noble earnestness." He was a master of the artistry of words and the art of elocution, yet never did he parade these for effect. His whole interest was the moral training and the spiritual uplifting of the people. All was subordinate to this.

And though his thoughts and longings soared to the reaches of Heaven, his feet were always planted on the ground. His sermons are full of references to daily life, to current events, to the weather. He could digress easily, as he did in his fourth homily on *Genesis*, when he chided the congregation for not looking at him but turning to watch the acolyte lighting candles.

Youth in Antioch

St. John Chrysostom was born and spent most of his life in Antioch, the city where the seven Machabees were martyred and where men were first called "Christians." The date was some-time between 344-354 A.D. His father, Secundus, probably of Latin origin, died when St. John was an infant; and his Greek mother, Anthusa, who was left a widow at about the age of 20, devoted herself to her two children, never remarrying. The older child, a daughter, probably died young. John received the best education possible, studying under the great Libanius, rhetorician at Antioch.

In accord with the popular but unsanctioned custom of delaying Baptism, St. John did not receive this Sacrament until he was about 18. Possibly it was conferred by Bishop Meletius of Antioch himself. The same reverential regard for Baptism and the tremendous spiritual change it brought which caused Baptism to be delayed also helped many to persevere in baptismal innocence. The contemporary biography of the Saint, usually attributed to Palladius, says, "After his Baptism, John never cursed or swore or spoke evil of anyone or spoke a lie or wished ill to anyone or tolerated loose talk."

When St. John wished to go with his friend Basilius to live the life of a monk, his mother asked him to stay with her at home and lead an ascetical life there. St. John describes this tender scene in his work, *On the Priesthood*:

> When she perceived that I was meditating this step, she took me into her private chamber, and sitting near me on the bed where she had given birth to me, she shed torrents of tears, to which she added words yet more pitiable than her weeping.

John gave in to his mother's wishes and remained at home. When he did finally leave to lead the monastic life under Diodorus, it is not known whether his mother had died or was still living.

Launched upon His Vocation

For four years St. John lived under Diodorus of Tarsus, and for two years more he lived as a hermit. The location was just outside Antioch. During the last two years, he committed the whole New Testament to memory, an important factor in his ability as a preacher. He also unfortunately undermined his health by too strict a penitential life. Besides his study and his fasts, he never lay down to sleep during those two years, but remained in a sitting position. Prudence measures, but love does not, and it is not always possible to keep the two properly balanced in directing one's life, especially where enthusiasm and single-mindedness are present.

Shortly before Meletius left in 381 to go to the Council of Constantinople, he ordained St. John a deacon. In 386 Flavian, the successor of Meletius as bishop, ordained St. John to the priesthood.

The following year, the city of Antioch trembled for fear of retribution from the Emperor Theodosius after a violent and foolish episode of breaking up imperial statues. This demonstration had been a protest against a new tax. The aged Flavian himself went to beseech the Emperor for clemency. During that Lent of 387 St. John Chrysostom preached to overflowing and fearful congregations. The famous 21 sermons he gave at that time are known as the "Homilies on the Statues."

The 12 years of St. John's priesthood at Antioch were fruitful and happy. He was at the height of his oratorical power and was acclaimed the best speaker in the Empire. Although not immune to praise (and even fearful that he enjoyed it too much), his happiness came from exercising to his fullest ability the office of spiritual director to the people. He enjoyed the love and respect of most of them.

Patriarch of Constantinople

When St. John Chrysostom left Antioch, however, there was no farewell sermon. If there had been, there would have been no farewell, for the people would not have permitted it. He himself left the city thinking he was just going to meet Asterius, the Imperial Governor of Antioch. He accepted a seat in the chariot after meeting Asterius, and while it moved along swiftly, he found out he was not going merely for a short ride, but on to Constantinople, for he had been chosen as its bishop and patriarch. Nectarius, the first Bishop of Constantinople actually to be called Patriarch, had died on September 26, 397.

Strangely, the chief mover in arranging this choice was Eutropius, an unprincipled minister and confidant of the Emperor Arcadius. He had a genuine admiration for Chrysostom and hoped to win him for a friend, as well as make a move popular with the people.

Constantinople was in great turmoil. The ordinary people welcomed St. John Chrysostom as a great and good man. But there was strong opposition to him in circles that were promoting other candidates. Theophilus, Bishop of Alexandria, at first refused to consecrate St. John Chrysostom, but he was forced to do so early in 398 A.D.

The opposition to St. John Chrysostom did not die down, but continued to grow. He was just the opposite of his predecessor, the easy-going Bishop Nectarius. He began to reform immediately and started by "sweeping the stairs from the top down," giving the clergy more work to do, adding nocturnal antiphonal services, denouncing their seeking after wealth, calling them in privately to correct the custom of living with consecrated virgins and other abuses. He required monks to return to their monasteries instead of wandering about, as some of them did. St. John gave no banquets, ate a scanty meal in the evening, dressed poorly, sold the rich furnishings of the bishop's palace and even some of the ornaments of the churches, and gave money and food and clothing to the poor.

There was much murmuring at all this. As he had done at Antioch, St. John continued to preach against the theater and circus and the luxury of the rich in the face of the abject poverty of the lower classes. He made his most influential enemy, however, in the ambitious Empress, Eudoxia. What he said of the vanity and vices of women in general was reported in exaggerated form as though directed against her personally.

Eudoxia had become the chief power in the Eastern Empire, swaying the will of her husband, the Emperor Arcadius. When the imperial minister, Eutropius, who had helped to arrange her marriage in the first place, told her that the hand that had made her could break her, she rushed weeping with two of her babies to the Emperor and secured the deposition of the powerful minister. Having many and powerful enemies, Eutropius ran in fear to the church to cling to the altar for protection. Even there he would not have been safe except that St. John Chrysostom came in just in time to stand between him and the menacing soldiers and mob. "You shall not slay Eutropius unless you first slay me," he declared.

The next day Chrysostom preached what might be called the most dramatic and powerful sermon of his career, and perhaps of all history. When the people assembled, he pulled back a curtain to show the once powerful minister clinging to the altar, telling them, "The altar is more awful than ever, now that it holds the lion chained." At times addressing the wretched Eutropius, at times turning to the congregation, he gave a thrilling exposition of the shortness of earthly glory and the duty of pity and compassion.

Sent into Exile

Intrigue, lies and defamation of character grew until they culminated in the Synod of the Oak, a council of bishops subservient to Bishop Theophilus of Alexandria and inflamed by Bishop Severian, whom St. John had once told to leave Constantinople and return to his own See. The biased synod issued a decree of deposition against St. John Chrysostom and had it ratified by the Emperor.

St. John quietly left the city, but his exile was short, for something happened to make the Empress herself ask for his return. Differing explanations have been given; perhaps it was an earthquake in Constantinople, or perhaps she suffered a miscarriage. In any case, something happened which she took for a Divine judgment. St. John returned like a triumphing hero to the joy and acclaim of a great multitude, who met him carrying candles.

But the fickle heart of the Empress changed, and more constant enemies kept pressing for the Saint's removal. At Easter of 404 there was violence and bloodshed in the cathedral; the 3,000 catechumens St. John was baptizing were driven into the street; the Holy Eucharist was desecrated. In the days that followed, attempts were twice made on St. John's life. On June 20, 404 he left on his second and last exile. On that same day, a fire of mysterious origin burned down the great cathedral and the neighboring Senate House, destroying many priceless works of ancient pagan art. St. John Chrysostom may have seen the flames as he rode away under guard. He did not know what was burning, but soon he knew, as he was made to stand trial for arson.

Those who remained loyal to St. John were known as the Johnites. They were severely persecuted, suffering exile, loss of property, torture, and some even death. On October 6, 404, a few months after St. John had gone into exile, the still young and beautiful Empress Eudoxia died, a fact that has often been seen as a judgment of God.

St. John proceeded to Cucusus in Armenia, his place of exile, which he calls "the most desolate place in the whole world." His sufferings from fever, cold weather and rough treatment are set forth in letters to his friends, addressed to more than a hundred different individuals, 17 being to the deaconess, St. Olympias. Usually he describes these sufferings as past, saying that now everything is going well and nobody should worry.

To Olympias he wrote:

> With a thousand contrivances I could not avoid the mischief which the cold did me; though I had a fire and submitted to the oppressive smoke and imprisoned myself in one room and had coverings without number and never ventured to pass the threshold, nevertheless, I used to suffer in the most grievous way from continual vomitings, headache, disgust at food, and obstinate sleeplessness through the long, interminable nights. But I will not distress you longer with this account of my troubles; I am now rid of them all.

Another letter, after describing similar troubles, concludes by saying: "Do not, then, make yourself anxious about my wintering here, for I feel much easier and better than I did last year."

Death in Exile

After a year at Cucusus, Chrysostom, along with most of the people living there, left the city for fear of the marauding Isaurians. He traveled in the severe cold, fleeing from village to village, and finally came to Arabissus, a fortress. But even from here his enemies drove him, securing a writ of banishment to Pityus, a remote spot on the far coast of the Black Sea. It seems the real object of his further exile was to hasten him mercilessly on his journey and thus secure his death. Already a sick man, he was forced to walk over mountain ranges and under the burning sun without rest.

On the morning of September 14, 407, St. John Chrysostom asked his guards to wait for awhile at the chapel of the martyr Basiliscus, where they had remained overnight. His request was not granted, and he walked on for about three-and-a-half miles. Then, even the guards saw that he could not go on, and they brought him back to the chapel. He received Holy Viaticum from a priest there, and shortly afterwards said what he had so often said in affliction: "Glory be to God for all things. Amen."

So died St. John Chrysostom, the zealous priest and bishop, the magnificent preacher. Far from both those who loved him and those who hated him, his great soul, loving and forgiving, went forth from his exhausted body. In Heaven it must have received a martyr's welcome.

In 438 St. John's hopeful prediction that he would return to Constantinople came sadly true, as his body was transferred there from the chapel of St. Basiliscus at Comana in Cappadocia. Theodosius II and Pulcheria, the children of Arcadius and Eudoxia, begged God's forgiveness for the wrong their parents had done the great Saint. In 1204 his relics were moved to St. Peter's in Rome.

St. John Chrysostom Still Preaches

Some of St. John Chrysostom's sermons were taken down by tachygraphers; many others he wrote out and perhaps never delivered. His health was not very robust, and many times, even in the sunny climate of Antioch, he had to retire to the country for periods of rest. "Preaching makes me healthy. As soon as I open my mouth all tiredness is gone." When St. John Chrysostom said this in a sermon after an earthquake, he gave some indication of his consuming interest in preaching, as well as of his rather poor health. But the brave little man went on preaching and writing until he had left more volumes than any of the other Fathers of the Church. He wrote some treatises, but mostly there are sermons. These are not random sermons, but are largely series of sermons, which in themselves are full-fledged commentaries on many books of Scripture. So today St. John Chrysostom still preaches, and to a wider audience than ever, as translations of his works multiply.

Dr. Paul Harkins of Xavier University, who translated the 88 homilies of St. John Chrysostom on the Gospel of St. John, said that they have a literary, doctrinal and moral value "excelled by few works in the history of the world." An early admirer, St. Isidore of Pelusium, wrote:

> Who would not render thanks to the Providence of God for having lived after him in order to be able to enjoy the divine accents of that lyre by which, even better than Orpheus, he was able to charm not the beasts, but men with savage instincts?

The Rich and the Poor

One of St. John Chrysostom's favorite themes was the duty of taking care of the poor and unfortunate. Time and again he launches into strong criticism of the rich. He points out the gaping differences between those who loll in luxury and those who lack necessities. It was this forthright criticism which made him such strong enemies. A modern seeker after social justice could hardly improve on this appeal of St. John:

> It is foolishness and a public madness to fill the cupboards with clothing, and allow men, who are created in God's image and our likeness, to stand naked and trembling with the cold, so that they can hardly hold themselves upright . . . Indeed, forgive me, but I almost burst from anger. Only see, you who are large and fat, you hold drinking parties until late at night, and sleep in a warm, soft bed. And do you not think of how you must give an account of your misuse of the gifts of God? The wine does not exist in order that we may get drunk; the food is not given us that we may overeat, nor that we may develop a great belly. On the other hand, you question very closely the poor and the miserable, who are scarcely better off in this respect than the dead; and you do not fear the dreadful and terrible judgment seat of Christ. If the beggar lies, he lies from necessity, because your hard-heartedness and merciless inhumanity force him to such cheating. For who would otherwise be so wretched and pitiable that he would needlessly, for the sake of a little bread, so demean himself as to let himself be struck and mishandled. If we would give our alms gladly and willingly, the poor would never have fallen to such depths.
>
> Indeed, for your charioteers in the circus you are ready to sacrifice your own children, and for your actors you would deliver up your own souls; but for the hungering Christ, the smallest piece of money is too large for you to give. And if you sacrifice a penny for once, it is as if you were giving away your whole property. Truly I am ashamed when I see rich people riding about on horses decorated with gold, and with servants clad in gold coming along behind them. They have silver beds and multitudes of other luxuries. But if they have to give something to a poor man, suddenly they themselves are the poorest of the poor.

As for himself, St. John built a great hospital with the money he had saved on household expenses in his first year as bishop.

John Chrysostom enjoyed the wide freedom that a congregation gives to a preacher whom they know really loves the people and whose words proceed from a heart full of love for them. But when ill will or vanity prevent people from recognizing this, then bitter enmities are spawned. St. Chrysostom found his most bitter enemies in the Empress Eudoxia and others among the rich and the influential who considered his stern words as pointing directly at them. None was so severe as he in correcting, but he was also so sympathetic toward sinners that he earned the name "John of Repentance."

Circus and Theater

Chrysostom calls the circus and theater "this universal school of dissoluteness" and "this training ground of unchastity." He was not alone in his denunciation of the abandoned theatricals and spectacles of the late fourth century. The great pagan Libanius in his youth had written a defense of actors, but in his mature years he wrote against them as an open sore in the city of Antioch and accused them of bringing many to corruption. St. John Chrysostom blamed the theater for spoiling the innocent joys of life.

> If but once the flame of impure lust seizes you in the theater and those impure looks bewitch you, then you wrong the pure and respected comrade of your life. You revile her, you do everything possible to reproach her, even though there is no cause for reproach. You shame yourself in knowing your passion, and in showing your wounds, which you have brought home from there. Therefore, you need excuses, and you seek absurd causes for quarreling; you value cheaply everything you have at home, and you demand only vulgar, impure passion after the example of those who have dealt you those wounds. The tone of their voices you have always in your ears, you see always their forms, their glances, their motions, and whatever else such women have shown you of the art of seduction. At home your wife can no longer do anything to please you.

St. John Chrysostom often preached against the theater, but he seemed to effect little with the majority of the people:

> How often have I preached, how often admonished the frivolous and spoken to them, urging them to stay away from the

stage and all the wantonness that results from it. It has not done any good. To this very day they run after a forbidden look at the dancers, place the devil's assembly in preference to the community of God's Church . . .

St. John says that the theater leads to sin and to taking a person from true contact with self and family. The residue of images is toxic. Compared to the excitement of the wrong kind of theater, home and its people can seem dull.

All Called to Be Perfect

"Is it perhaps only monks who are obliged to please God?" Chrysostom asks. He answers, "No, God wishes that all should become holy and that none should neglect the practice of virtue." St. John Chrysostom did not have the idea that perfection belongs only to monks or to priests. He tried constantly to raise the spiritual sights of the laymen of the Church.

> You make a great mistake, if you think that anything different is required from people in the world than from monks. The one difference is this, that the one takes a wife, the other does not. In all other things, the same reckoning will be demanded from each.

In Homily 5 on the *Statues* he quotes St. Paul: "Be you imitators of me, even as I also am of Christ." Then he asks why they who have been educated in piety from the beginning cannot easily imitate someone converted late in life like St. Paul.

In Homily 20 on the *Acts of the Apostles* he urges the people not only to save themselves, but to help save others.

> Nothing can be more chilling than the sight of a Christian who makes no effort to save others. Neither poverty, nor humble station, nor bodily infirmity can exempt men and women from the obligation of this great duty. To hide our light under pretense of weakness is as great an insult to God as if we were to say that He could not make His sun to shine.

Doctor of the Eucharist

St. John Chrysostom has two claims to the title, "Doctor of the Eucharist." He wrote a famous and much-used treatise on the priesthood; it is in fact his best-known work. Plus, he spoke often in the clearest possible terms about the Mass and the Eucharist.

In his treatise *On the Priesthood*, which is in the form of a dialogue between himself and his friend Basilius, he says:

> The greatness and the dignity of the priesthood rise above all that is earthly and human. For the priestly office is indeed discharged on earth, but it ranks amongst heavenly ordinances; and very naturally so, for neither man nor angel, nor archangel, nor any other created power, but the Paraclete Himself, instituted this vocation and persuaded men, while still abiding in the flesh, to represent the ministry of angels. Wherefore, the consecrated priest ought to be as pure as if he were standing in the heavens themselves in the midst of those powers . . . For when thou seest the Lord sacrificed and laid upon the altar, and the priest standing and praying over the Victim, and all the worshippers empurpled with that Precious Blood, canst thou think that thou art still amongst men and standing on the earth. . . . Oh, what a marvel! What love of God to man!

Concerning especially the priest's powers of baptizing and of forgiving sin through the Sacrament of Extreme Unction, St. John Chrysostom says:

> God has bestowed a power on priests greater than that of our natural parents. The two indeed differ as much as the present and the future life. For our natural parents generate us unto this life only, but the others unto that which is to come.

At the end of the second Homily on the *Statues*, St. John Chrysostom makes this comparison:

> Elias left a sheepskin to his disciple, but the Son of God, ascending, left to us His own flesh! . . . Let us not lament, nor fear the difficulties of the times, for He who did not refuse to pour out His Blood for all and has suffered us to partake of His Blood again—what will He refuse to do for our safety?

St. John Chrysostom asks for charity for the leaders of the Church in Homily 21, 7 on *1 Corinthians:*

> Indeed, one can observe that our spiritual leaders do not

experience so much evil censure and calumny from the pagans as they do from the so-called faithful and those who belong to us. And yet there is nothing, absolutely nothing, that can ruin the Church so easily and surely as when no intimate bond exists anymore between the listeners and the teachers, between the children and their spiritual fathers, between chief and subordinate. Of this I warn you, and I pray you weeping: Cease this wicked custom.

Unaffected Simplicity

Cardinal Newman preferred the Saints of the early Church to those who came later because the former revealed their secret heart in their writings. Even their treatises were not so formal that personal feelings and autobiographical details could not be included. The early Saints made it a practice to be themselves—especially St. John Chrysostom, whom Cardinal Newman calls "this many-gifted Saint, this most natural and human of the creations of supernatural grace."

Chrysostom has revealed his secret heart in treatises, sermons and letters. It is a heart that is bent on the supreme goals adhered to with unswerving simplicity: the glory of God and the salvation of souls. At the same time it is responsive to and aware of all the little elements of daily living. "Possessed though he be by the fire of divine charity, he has not lost one fiber, he does not miss one vibration, of the complicated whole of human sentiment and affection; like the miraculous bush in the desert, which for all the flame that wrapt it round, was not thereby consumed." (Newman).

In reading over the sermons of St. John Chrysostom, one might feel sometimes that he was too severe in his words of correction. This may be so, because he was carried along by the heat and fervor of the moment. At least one time he corrected himself for getting too strong in his expression. He had been urging husbands not to get unduly worked up over the foibles of their wives. Then in describing these foibles, he became unduly worked up himself; finally he paused, admitting that he was himself unwittingly demonstrating just what he had preached against.

There was nothing cold and calculated about St. John's choice of words. He felt deeply, and he thought strongly and clearly. He praised and blamed accordingly. He was the loving father speaking to his children. Few really good fathers could have all their words of advice and reproof to their children classified as always sweetly moderate. Strong love and strong feeling must show themselves in strong language.

A Friend to Friends and to Enemies

St. John Chrysostom was of a sunny, sanguine, optimistic disposition. Though he spoke at times of discouragement, he never gave up. He continued to exhort, to praise, to reprove despite the continued relapses of the people. From exile he wrote the treatise, *That None Can Harm the Man Who Does Not Injure Himself.* In his first letter to St. Olympias from exile he said: "Never be cast down then, for one thing alone is fearful, that is, sin."

St. John Chrysostom was not a man who had a wide circle of close friends. On private contact, some few who did not know him well thought him too cold and reserved. But to great numbers, men and women of all ages, he was accepted on affectionate terms. To those who knew him well he was always cheerful and often playful. He lived in his friends; and despite his stern asceticism, he needed them. "It is not a light effort, but it demands an energetic soul and a great mind to bear separation from one whom we love in the charity of Christ," he wrote while in exile. At that sad time, too, he complained pitifully about not receiving letters. "Do not be backward in writing to me from time to time, nay, very frequently."

> I should write more frequently to you, under a feeling that my letters might be of service; but, as it is, many persons have crossed to this place who might have brought me a letter from you, and it has been a great sorrow that I have received nothing.

Cardinal Newman asked himself the question: "Whence is this devotion to St. John Chrysostom, which leads me to dwell upon the thought of him and makes me kindle at his name, when so many other great saints . . . command my veneration, but exert no personal claim on my heart?" He answers it by saying that Chrysostom's charm lies in his intimate sympathy and compassion for the whole world, not only in its strength, but also in its weakness. St. John Chrysostom has an affectionate regard for each person, just because he is that person, different from all others. His affection is not directed to a group, but always to each person. He can be said to have a devotion to the individual.

St. John Chrysostom preached his most enduring sermon when he went quietly into exile. A short while before, he could have sat in judgment on his powerful and scheming foe, Theophilus, Bishop of Alexandria. He was asked to, but refused. At any point in the developing climax of intrigue, he could with his oratory have roused thousands to support him. But he trusted to God's justice to right things in the long run. He wanted no bloodshed. There were no words of bitterness in his letters from exile; rather, hope and forgiveness breathed through them. And even the forgiveness was subdued and in the background. Many words of forgiveness might have shown him to be too interested in his own feelings. He was really more interested in the ultimate good of the Church and in the present circumstances of his friends. He was a man who looked not back, but ahead.

Along with St. Basil, St. Gregory Nazianzen and St. Athanasius, St. John Chrysostom is counted as one of the four great Eastern Doctors of the Church. In 1909 Pope St. Pius X made him the special patron of all those who preach the word of God. St. John Chrysostom would also be an understanding Saint to call on when it is hard to forgive. For he teaches us not to look backward in bitterness, but to keep looking forward with hope. St. John Chrysostom's feast day in the Roman Rite is now celebrated on September 13 (January 27 in the 1962 calendar).

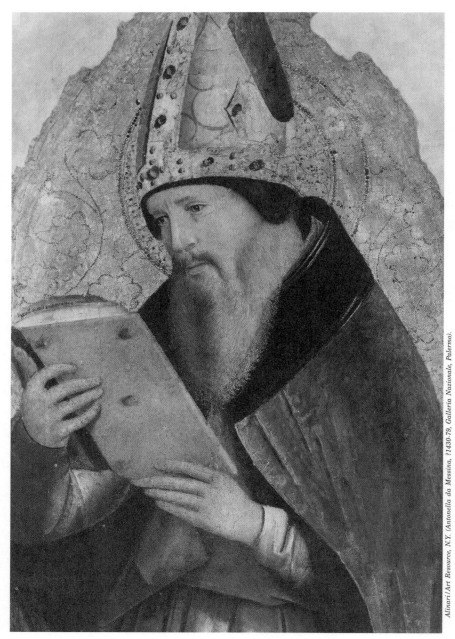

Saint Augustine

— 10 —
SAINT AUGUSTINE
Doctor of Grace
Doctor of Doctors
354-430

THE world's most famous autobiography begins, not by focusing on the writer, but rather on the Divine Author of all things. "Great art Thou, O Lord, and greatly to be praised . . . Thou hast made us for Thyself, O Lord, and our hearts are restless until they rest in Thee."

It was 10 years after his conversion, in about 397 A.D., that St. Augustine wrote his *Confessions*. He was in his early forties and had been a priest for eight years. Just the year before he had succeeded Valerius as Bishop of Hippo, an ancient city on the north coast of Africa, whose ruins now lie about a mile and a quarter southwest of modern Bona in Algeria.

The new bishop of Hippo was gaining renown for learning, for oratorical prowess, and for holiness. He was a man who loved the truth intensely, whose whole life would be spent in seeking out the secrets of nature and of Divine Revelation. He wrote the *Confessions* because he loved the truth; he wanted men to know the kind of man he had been and how much he owed to God's mercy. Later, he said in a letter about his *Confessions*: "See what I was in myself and by myself. I had destroyed myself, but He who made me remade me."

Revelations of personal life are often made to men in order to amuse, interest or shock them. St. Augustine confesses to God. In the very style of his writing, he tells the story to God, and while he relates the facts of the past, he keeps breaking in with the overflowing thanksgivings and petitions of the present.

For a thousand years, or until the publication of the *Imitation of Christ*, St. Augustine's *Confessions* was the most common manual of the spiritual life. In his own lifetime and ever since, his *Confessions* have had more readers than any of his other works. New translations are still appearing in the major languages of the world. New generations of Christians are learning from St. Augustine's own story how to quiet the restless heart of man and bring it closer to God, its real happiness. The long procession of readers still find re-echoing in their wayward hearts St. Augustine's own touching and plaintive words:

> Too late have I loved Thee, O Beauty ever ancient, ever new. Too late have I loved Thee. For behold Thou wert within, and I without, and there did I seek Thee. I, unlovely, rushed heedlessly among the things of beauty which Thou madest. (Bk. 10, 27, 38).

St. Augustine was born at Tagaste, in Northern Africa—now Souk-Ahras, Algeria—50 miles south of Hippo, on November 13, 354. Other children that we know of in the family were a brother, Navigius, and an unnamed sister. She became an abbess of a convent in Hippo. It was shortly after her death that Augustine wrote a letter to her successor, giving advice when questions arose about the government of the convent. This letter is the chief basis of "The Rule of St. Augustine," on account of which St. Augustine ranks as one of the four great founders of religious orders. Augustine's father, Patricius, was a man of quite modest means, ambitious for Augustine's worldly success, but not quite able to pay for a complete education. Patricius was a pagan until shortly before his death.

St. Augustine has painted an enduring picture of his mother, St. Monica, silent under the abuse of a violent-tempered husband, devoted to the service of God and neighbor, never repeating scandals but rather helping to reconcile enemies. St. Augustine's appreciation of this virtue of his mother grew with the years:

> I should have thought this a small virtue if I had not learned by sad experience the endless troubles which, when the horrid pestilence of sins is flowing far and wide, are caused by the repetition of the words of angry enemies and by their exaggeration. It is a man's duty to do his best to alleviate human enmities by kindly speech, not to excite and aggravate them by the repetition of slanders.

St. Augustine's Fall

Because of lack of money, St. Augustine had to leave school during his sixteenth year. Idleness and degenerate companions, plus the strong passions of his youth, combined to lead him into sins of impurity. He resumed school the next year at Carthage, a city of perhaps half a million, which offered fine literary opportunities—but in a degraded moral atmosphere. Augustine continued to frequent the theater, which in those days was grossly immoral and allied to the worship of pagan gods and geared to satisfy human passions. The chief shame he felt was at not joining in with the worst exploits of rowdy gangs. At the age of 17 he entered into a union with a girl with whom he would live for 14 years. Though the union was not a marriage, the parties were faithful to each other, and for Augustine it was a stabilizing influence and most likely a lesser evil than his former practices. One child was born to the couple, the boy Adeodatus ("given by God"), who was extremely bright and highly spiritual, giving high promise until his death in his late teens.

There is something elusively great about this unknown woman who proved an adequate companion to share the richness of Augustine's active and probing mind. There is something poignant about the way she marched off silently at his command, leaving her cherished son and leaving Milan to go back to Africa to spend her final years in chastity until she was laid in an unremembered grave.

> Into the darkness she glides, a silent shame
> And a veiled memory without a name.
> And the world knoweth not what words she prayed,
> With what her wail before the altar wept,
> What tale she told, what penitence she made,
> What measure by her beating heart was kept . . .

Augustine earned his living by teaching. First he taught grammar at his native town of Tagaste, then rhetoric at Carthage, Rome and Milan, spending the longest time, a period of 10 years, at Carthage. He left this city because of the undisciplined conduct of some of the students, especially the accepted practice of bands of outside students coming in and breaking up classes. He left Rome because too many of the students had the unfortunate habit of failing to pay their tuition. Still, he was an esteemed and very successful teacher. At Milan he was beginning to win political favor. He could soon have hoped for some position in the government.

For nine years, from the age of 19 until age 28, Augustine, to the great sorrow of his mother St. Monica, belonged to the sect of the Manicheans. This heretical group, named after the Persian Manes, had a threefold appeal to Augustine. Their teaching of a principle of evil helped to explain to him, and to excuse, his sins. Moreover, they claimed to have scientific explanations unlocking the mysteries of nature. The Manicheans also pleased Augustine's intellectual pride by belittling faith and authority. In substance they argued: "The Church asks you to believe what cannot be supported by reason. We do not force your mind nor threaten you with future punishments. We merely invite you to accept the truths which we first explain." The ever-inquiring mind of Augustine found questions they could not answer, but he was put off with the promise that when he heard their great bishop, Faustus, all would be clear. When Augustine finally heard Faustus, he was charmed by his rhetoric, but very disappointed by his knowledge and logic. Thereafter, he temporarily became a skeptic. These intellectual gropings, along with Augustine's interest for some time in astrology, are very revealing. They show us that even truly great minds require development and, in matters of religion, the guiding hand of active faith.

His Conversion

St. Monica had earlier approached a Catholic bishop, who had himself once been a Manichean, and had asked him to talk to Augustine. He declined, saying it would be of no use. But noting her earnestness and tears he added: "Go and continue to live so; it cannot be that the son of those tears will perish."

The tears and prayers of St. Monica finally did win out. St. Ambrose's sermons, the story of the conversion of Victorinus, a great pagan orator, the reading of St. Paul's epistles, all had a disposing effect on Augustine. But one day a fellow countryman, Pontitian, came to Milan and recounted how some of his associate military officers had vowed a life of chastity after reading St. Athanasius's *Life of St. Antony of the Desert*. St. Augustine was highly affected. Even after sending off his faithful mistress, he had weakly taken another. He had continued his prayer of many years (which was at least an honest one): "Lord, make me pure, but not yet." Now he asked his lifelong friend, Alypius:

"What is this? The unlearned rise and take Heaven by force, and we, with our learning but without heart, see we are rolling ourselves in flesh and blood."

It was then that he rushed out into the garden, flung himself under a fig tree and cried out: "How long, O Lord, how long? Remember not my former sins! Tomorrow and tomorrow—why not now?" About this time, he heard a child's voice sing singing over and over something that sounded like: *Tolle, lege; tolle, lege.* ("Take and read; take and read.") Augustine, remembering how a random opening of the Bible had guided St. Antony, took this for a sign that he should open a book and read the first thing he found. He took up the copy of St. Paul lying by Alypius in the garden and opened it to *Romans* 13:13-14, where he read: ". . . not in rioting and drunkenness, not in chambering and impurities . . . but put ye on the Lord Jesus Christ, and make not provision for the flesh in its concupiscences." This was in the summer of 386. At Easter of 387 he was baptized by St. Ambrose, together with Adeodatus and Alypius.

It seemed that St. Monica's life-work was over; perhaps she had offered her life for the conversion of her son. For she suddenly took sick and died at Ostia, a seaport town a few miles south of Rome. St. Monica was 56, St. Augustine 33. Monica had always wanted to be buried beside her husband in her native Africa. But when her tearful sons asked her, during her last illness, where she wished her last resting place to be, she gave them the following reply, so full of faith in the Mass: "My sons, bury this body where you will; do not trouble yourselves about it. I ask of you only this—remember me whenever you come to the altar of God."

Bishop of Hippo

St. Augustine returned to Africa and lived a quiet, monastic-type life at Tagaste. When he did travel, he purposely avoided towns in which there was a vacant bishopric, fearing to be chosen a bishop, as had Ambrose and many others. He wanted nothing but a monk's life. Then one day he went to Hippo, which had a good, healthy bishop in the person of Valerius. Augustine felt perfectly safe in going into the church and standing with the congregation. But Valerius, a Greek, had been anxious for some time to secure an outstanding priest who could preach in better Latin than himself. With Augustine present, he spoke fervently on the need for a priest to help him. The congregation took up the cue and began to clamor for the ordination of the unsuspecting Augustine. His tears and entreaties could not change their minds; therefore, against his own inclination, but seeing in all this the will of God, he allowed himself to be ordained.

Five years later he was made a bishop, and in the following year, 396, he succeeded Valerius as bishop of Hippo. For 34 years he governed this diocese, giving lavishly of his talent and energy for the spiritual and temporal needs of the people, who were mostly unlearned and simple. At the same time, he wrote constantly to refute the false teachings of the day; he went to the councils of bishops in Africa; and he traveled to neighboring Sees to preach for special occasions. He soon emerged as the leading figure of Christianity in Africa and the most outstanding personality in the whole Church.

In August of 430, St. Augustine took sick. Outside the city walls, the Vandals, under Genseric, were in the third month of a siege. Inside, at Augustine's request, his friends hung on the walls of his room copies of the seven penitential psalms written in large letters. He read them over and over. On August 28, at the age of 76, St. Augustine's soul went forth to rest in God.

His body was buried in Hippo, later moved to Pavia in Italy, and in our present day returned to Bona, in North Africa. After St. Augustine there has been no other bishop of Hippo. The flourishing Church of North Africa which he had spent his life working for and building up was reduced to a mere trace. At St. Augustine's death there were about 500 bishops in the African province. Twenty years later there were less than 20. His immediate work was reduced to ashes, like his body, but his enduring work in the Church, like his immortal soul, has continued through the centuries.

St. Augustine was the greatest contributor of new ideas in the history of the Catholic Church. Excepting St. Paul, he is undoubtedly the Church's greatest convert. In the Latin Rite, only two conversions are observed, that of St. Paul, on January 25, and of St. Augustine, on May 5 (observed in the Augustinian Order).

Defender of Catholic Truth and Unity

St. Augustine's love for truth brought him into contention with the proponents of error. We can divide his long career as priest and bishop, covering about 40 years, into three parts, which correspond to the errors he wrote and spoke against. Counting in round numbers, the first 10 years were employed in fighting against the Manicheans, to which sect he had formerly belonged. The next 10 years were occupied with the Donatist schismatics in Africa. During most of the final two decades of his life, St. Augustine combatted the Pelagians.

The Donatists were very numerous in Africa. They had broken away from the Catholic Church and claimed that they alone were the True Church. In arguing with and writing against them, St. Augustine developed many proofs for the unity, universality and authority of the Catholic Church. He often pointed out to the Donatists that they existed only in Africa, and that all false sects were found chiefly in one geographical location. Therefore, they could not be the true, universal Church. Only one Church was spread about throughout all the nations of the world.

> The Church is spread throughout the whole world: all nations have the Church. Let no one deceive you; it is true, it is the Catholic Church. Christ we have not seen, but we have her; let us believe as regards Him. The Apostles, on the contrary, saw Him, but they believed as regards her. (S. 238).

In another sermon, St. Augustine says: "Indeed, it was precisely in Peter himself that He [the Lord] laid emphasis on unity. There were many disciples, and only to one there is said, 'Feed my sheep . . .'" In a great meeting at Carthage in 412 A.D., with 286 Catholic bishops and 279 Donatist bishops present, St. Augustine played the leading role in refuting the schismatics.

St. Augustine continued to uphold in unmistakable terms the unity of the Church:

> We must hold fast to the Christian religion and to communion with that Church which is Catholic, and is called Catholic, not only by its own members but also by all its enemies. For whether they will or not, even heretics and schismatics, when talking not among themselves but with outsiders, call the Catholic Church nothing else but the Catholic Church. For otherwise they would not be understood unless they distinguished the Church by that name which she bears throughout the whole world. (*Synthesis*, p. 249; from *De vera relig.* 7,12).

St. Augustine sums up very neatly the way in which nuggets of truth are mined from Scripture: "For many things lay hid in the Scriptures, and when the heretics had been cut off, they troubled the Church of God with questions; those things were then opened up which lay hid, and the will of God was understood." (*In Ps.* 54, 22). St. Augustine recognizes this value of controversy, but bewails the loss from the true fold. "Nevertheless, the Catholic mother herself, the Shepherd Himself in her, is everywhere seeking those who are straying and is strengthening the weak, healing the sick, binding up the broken—some from these sects, some from those, which mutually do not know one another."

"Doctor of Grace"

St. Augustine won his title of "Doctor of Grace" especially in combatting the Pelagians. In them he had foes of higher acumen than ever before, and he himself refers to their "great and subtle minds." In explaining Psalm 124, he says: "For you are not to suppose, brethren, that heresies could be produced through any little souls. None save great men have been the authors of heresies."

In God's dealing with men, there is scarcely anything harder to explain than the working together of grace and free will. In fighting the Pelagians, who over-stated the role of free will, St. Augustine made a very strong case for grace and man's complete dependence upon it. In doing this he grappled with problems connected with man's nature—Original Sin, infant Baptism and predestination. He is the great pioneer in this most difficult field, although the common teaching of the Church on grace is more moderate than his system. His severe opinion on the punishment of unbaptized infants, for example, is not generally held. St. Augustine was driven by very powerful foes and perhaps attempted to apply logic beyond its possibilities, as this position was certainly beyond the feelings of his own heart. He has led the Church in most points he held, but the Church has not followed him in every way.

It was in reference to the condemnation of Pelagianism by Pope Zosimus in 418 that the famed expression arose: *Roma locuta est, causa finita est*—("Rome has spoken, the case is closed"). St. Augustine did not say these words in just that way, but he did express the same sense. He said in a sermon (131):

There have already been sent to the Apostolic See two delegations concerning this case, and the answers have come back. The case is finished, and would that the error were also finished.

Interested in Every Person

One of the keys to understanding St. Augustine is to realize his concern for each person. It was his interest in one individual that brought him to Hippo from Tagaste and started the sequence of events that so changed his life, that turned him from the seclusion of penance and study to the active life of priest and bishop. He went to Hippo in response to the request of a man who was considering a life of poverty and renunciation. This man wanted to hear from Augustine's own lips the reasons for doing this. Why should this "agent in God's affairs" not have been expected to go to Augustine? It was certainly the mark of a magnanimous soul, a person interested in each individual, that Augustine left his prayers and studies and traveled 50 miles to help this man.

St. Augustine thought so much of each individual's importance that he said God had some verse or a few verses in Scripture especially for particular people. (*Conf.* 12, 31). The Holy Spirit intended a primary meaning, but He also intended the special and varied aspects of truth that many individuals would see in certain passages. This belief of St. Augustine also gives an insight into his overwhelming sense of Divine Providence.

St. Augustine's books, too, sprang up as answers to the immediate needs of the Church in his time. He was a great speculative philosopher and theologian, but his aims were practical and close at hand. His biographer, Bishop Posidius, when trying to list all of St. Augustine's works, simply classifies them according to the opponents he had encountered. (The *Life* by Posidius in *Early Christian Biographies*, ed. Roy Deferrari, 1952, in the series *Fathers of the Church*).

It was at the request of his friend Marcellinus that St. Augustine started his monumental *City of God*. It began as a fairly simple and short answer to the charge of the pagans that Christianity was responsible for the fall of Rome. St. Augustine continued to write it over the years 413-426 until it ended as a massive theology of history and the best early Christian apologia for the truth of the Catholic Church.

The "City of God" is the Catholic Church. The plans of God will be worked out in history as the organized forces of good in this City gradually overcome the organized forces of the temporal order that war against the will of God.

> So it is that two cities have been made by two loves: the earthly city by love of self to the exclusion of God, the heavenly by love of God to the exclusion of self. The one boasts in itself, the other in the Lord. The one seeks glory from men, the other finds its greatest glory in God's witness to its conscience. The one holds its head high in its own glory, the other calls its God "my glory who raises high my head". . . Thus the one has men wise by human standards, who have made the good things of body, of mind, or of both, their ultimate aim; even those of them who have been able to come to some knowledge of God did not honor Him as God, or give thanks; but they faded away in their own thoughts, and their foolish heart was darkened, calling themselves wise; that is, being eaten with pride and preening themselves on their wisdom, "they became foolish and changed the glory of the incorruptible God into the likeness of the image of corruptible man, and of birds and beasts, and creeping things," in that they either led or followed the populace in the worship of such idols; "and they worshipped and served the creature instead of the Creator," who is blessed forever. (*City of God*, 14, 28).

His Sermons

It has been remarked many times that there is a great difference between St. Augustine's sermons and his more formal written works. The sermons are in a much simpler style, adapted to the congregation at Hippo. He did not try to dazzle, but to instruct and to make himself plain. For this reason his more than 500 extant sermons still have reader appeal today. St. Augustine also showed his awareness of individual needs when he delivered his sermons. He was alive to the reactions of his listeners. He made remarks as he went along, such as, "I see that you do not agree with me." "Perhaps some of you are saying in your hearts, 'Oh, if only he would let us go.'" At other times he said more optimistically, "I see that you approve."

St. Augustine wrote so voluminously that Posidius, after counting up 1,030 of his works, expresses his doubt that any man could ever read all that he wrote. Yet St. Augustine did repeat himself. And he was sensitive to unspoken criticism when he repeated himself.

> Many of you know what I am going to say. But those who do know must put up with the delay; for when two are walking on the road and one goes fast while the other is slower, it is up to the fast walker to secure that they both keep together; for he can wait for the slower man. The person, then, who knows what I am going to say is like the fast walker and must wait for his slower companion.

St. Augustine knew that some of his hearers needed the repetition. Perhaps, too, he at times felt the burden of always coming up with new material. Once he explained: "It should not be necessary for me always to say something new. The real point is that we have to *be* new." In later years he complained that wherever he went, he was always expected to deliver the sermon. After many long years, he would be more content to listen and allow someone else the honor and the burden. In those days, naturally, there were no microphones, and the physical labor involved in making oneself heard was harder than it is today. St. Augustine's basilica in Hippo, when excavated, was found to have been 60 x 129 feet in the central part, with a rounded apse 22 x 25 feet. Therefore, the preacher of sermons in this church would have had to speak quite loudly in order to be heard by all, and such public speaking demands a great deal of energy.

Personal Traits

One incident after another in St. Augustine's life shows him as quite sensitive and alive to his own moods and the moods and opinions of others, as well as to people's physical state. Quite often there is mention of him being in tears. Perhaps social usage today has unnaturally inhibited weeping by men, but St. Augustine and many other men of the fourth and fifth centuries often gave vent to tears. There are not many men of middle age who recall with much emotion the whippings of their childhood, but St. Augustine continued to feel the injustice of beatings from his teachers when he was a boy. After many years, he was also able to recall vividly a severe toothache he had had at Cassiciacum in the early days of his conversion.

It is interesting to note that St. Augustine, who except for

Origen was the most prolific writer among the Church Fathers, disliked the physical labor of using the pen. Also, at an early age he conceived a decided dislike for Greek. Though he later renewed his study of this language, he never acquired a mastery of it.

St. Augustine's health was not robust. He did not make long trips, and after becoming bishop he attended only councils held in Africa. In sermons he at times mentioned that he was tired. Sometimes the sermon would be surprisingly short, although at other times it would be extremely long. Changes in temperature often affected him. "The heat is so great that I cannot say much." More often he was affected by the cold. He found it necessary to wear shoes, though he wanted to do without footgear for love of the poverty and simplicity mentioned in the Gospel.

When St. Augustine was a bishop, his table was very simple. Ordinarily he ate no meat, though he did drink wine. Also, a certain number of cups of wine were allowed to members of his household. Anyone who swore was penalized by losing one cup that day. On the table were inscribed the words: "Whoever likes to chew on the life of one who is absent, let him know that he is not welcome at this table." St. Augustine placed charity above politeness, and one day he pointed out this inscription to a group of offending bishops dining with him.

In trying cases of law, which as a bishop he faithfully did in the mornings, he preferred to pass judgment on strangers rather than on friends. He remembered the saying, "When you judge strangers, you might win one friend, the one who receives the favorable judgment. But when you judge friends, you lose one."

Once St. Augustine had chosen chastity as a way of life, he remained firm. He was also very circumspect about his dealings with women, allowing none in his household, even excluding his own sister and his nieces. He used to say that if they lived within the residence, other women would come to visit and to stay with them.

It seems that St. Augustine enjoyed a bit of praise, and in fact that he felt obliged to combat this inclination. At the same time, his love for truth led him to welcome criticism of his writings. In his final years he carefully went through them and changed and deleted many parts. This evidence of his honesty and love for truth has visible proof in his two volumes summing up the changes, which are called *The Retractations* or *The Retractions*.

A Peerless Spiritual Guide

St. Augustine is a theologian's theologian. His treatises are not for the average reader. Their fruit is better when prepared and selected by experts. But his *Confessions*, sermons and some letters can be used with much profit by all. What he says has great value for spiritual direction. St. Augustine's complete dedication to God and his relentless logic in seeking God everywhere made him reach into the inner fibers of his being to express his thoughts and to lead others on a similar path. Following are a few random cullings:

How can you be proud unless you are empty? For if you were not empty (deflated), you could not be inflated.

Our whole business, therefore, in this life is to restore to health the eye of the heart, whereby God may be seen.

The love of truth requires a holy retiredness, and the necessity of charity a just employment.

Some people, in order to discover God, read books. But here is a great book: the very appearance of created things. Look above you. Look below you. Note it; read it. God, whom you want to discover, never wrote that book with ink; instead, He set before your eyes the things that He had made. Can you ask for a louder voice than that? Why, heaven and earth shout at you: "God made me!"

The whole life of a good Christian is a holy longing. What you long for, as yet you do not see; but longing makes in you the room that shall be filled when that which you are to see shall come. When you would fill a purse, knowing how large a present it is to hold, you stretch wide its cloth or leather: knowing how much you are to put in it, and seeing that the purse is small, you extend it to make more room. So, by withholding the vision, God extends the longing; through longing, He makes the soul extend; by extending it, He makes room in it. So, Brethren, let us long, because we are to be filled.

When men here below throw lively parties to celebrate some occasion, they usually engage a band and have a choir of boys to sing in their houses. And when we hear snatches of it as we pass by, we say, "What's going on here?" And we are told, "They are celebrating; it's a birthday, or a wedding"; some reason to explain the festivities. In the house of God, the festivities go on forever—there are no merely passing occasions for celebrating there. It is an everlasting feast, with choirs of angels to sing at it; with God present in very person, there is joy unflagging, merriment unceasing. And it is from these eternal, everlasting festivities that the ears of our minds catch a something, a sweet melodious echo—but only if the world is not making a din. The man who walks into this tent and turns over in his mind the wonderful things God has done for the redemption of the faithful is struck and bewitched by the sounds of that festival in Heaven, and drawn by them like the stag to the fountain of waters. (*In Ps.* 41).

Sometimes there is a kind of contrariness apparent in the products of hatred and love: hatred may use fair words and love may sound harsh . . . Thus we may see hatred speaking softly and charity prosecuting; but neither soft speeches nor harsh reproofs are what you have to consider. Look for the spring. Search out the root from which they proceed. The fair words of the one are designed for deceiving, the prosecution of the other is aimed at reformation.

A Man of Contrasts

In the life of St. Augustine we have a dramatic summary of the contrasts in human life. We have a picture etched in strong colors of the depths and the heights possible in moral behavior. We realize again that a person can be many-sided, and during one lifetime he can, so to speak, be many persons. There is always an essential unity there, but if the spiritual and intellectual development had been stopped at any of various points along the way, the man would have been quite different.

In reviewing the life of St. Augustine, we gain an insight into the strength and the weakness of even the greatest of minds. Men have often quoted St. Augustine at cross purposes. We gain an insight into the difficulty of understanding any person completely. During his own lifetime and ever since, St. Augustine was and is a man intensely loved and hated. Of course, the same can be said of Christ. And we may wonder if this will not be true of anybody who follows Christ with all his heart. In our day, when we are so conscious of good public relations, we may wonder whether our relations with Christ may not come out second best.

A Giant in the Church

It is the common opinion that St. Augustine was, "with the possible exception of St. Thomas Aquinas, the greatest single intellect the Catholic Church has ever produced." (Delaney, *Dictionary of Saints*). So great was St. Augustine's influence that it dominated the Western world for a thousand years and has put its stamp on Catholic theology to this day.

St. Augustine's theological depth and many-sidedness have at times made him a hero to Protestant as well as to Catholic readers. Even where they disagree with him, they recognize his genius. In the complicated questions of grace and free will, St. Augustine's authority has been claimed, though wrongly, by both Jansenists and Calvinists. This very aspect of his universal appeal springs from his effort to express the complete truth and from the fervor of his profound and complete dedication to God. St. Augustine's greatness of spirit is brought out in the famous saying that has often been attributed to him: *In necessariis unitas, in dubiis libertas, in omnibus caritas*—"In necessary things, unity; in doubtful things, liberty; in all things, charity."

The most common picture of St. Augustine in art does not give a truly correct idea of him. For it shows St. Augustine coming upon a little boy at the seashore who is trying to pour the ocean into a small hole in the sand. Augustine tells the child that this is impossible—and is answered in gentle reproval by the boy, who is really an angel, that it would be easier for him to put the ocean into the little hole than for Augustine to put the mystery of the Blessed Trinity into a small human mind. Versions of this picture have been done by the artists Murillo, Rubens, Van Dyck, Raphael and Dürer. The same legend has been applied to at least three other people besides St. Augustine, although the version featuring St. Augustine is by far the most famous. Though a good story, it is not quite fair to St. Augustine, because he knew full well that many Christian mysteries are incomprehensible. It is this fact which helped to make him a mystic, for he sought illumination from God on these mysteries. He wrote his grand treatise, *On the Trinity*, over a period of 16 years (400-416) and meditated on this mystery daily. But at the same time, while seeking illumination from God and knowing the limits of the mind, he also knew that God had given man reason and that it is to be used to the fullest. He answered one critic who objected to his writings about the Trinity: "Perish the thought that our belief should be such as to prevent us from accepting or looking for reasons! We could not even believe, after all, unless we had reasonable souls." St. Augustine's appreciation of "the great light of reason" made him probably the Church's greatest philosopher and theologian, and he was the forerunner of the Scholastics of the Middle Ages. He is one of the four great Doctors of the Latin Church (the others being St. Ambrose, St. Jerome and St. Gregory the Great).

The truest picture of St. Augustine is that which shows him looking up toward Heaven, a pen in his left hand and a burning heart in his right. For he pursued the knowledge and love of God with mind and heart, with reason and with faith. He pursued truth, moreover, with an intellect guided and protected by the full support of a pure moral life. He speaks to us not only in flowing rhetoric, but heart to heart, as to another human being longing for that "Beauty ever ancient, ever new."

Bossuet calls St. Augustine the "Doctor of Doctors." No higher praise can be spoken for his learning. But when all is said and done, we may wish to accept the judgment of his friend and biographer, Pisidius, who said that we can profit more from a knowledge of St. Augustine's life than from a study of his writings. No higher praise of his holiness can be spoken.

St. Augustine's feast day is August 28.

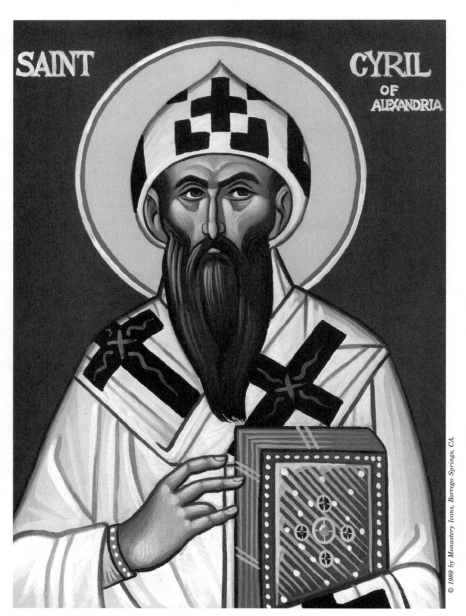

Saint Cyril of Alexandria

11

SAINT CYRIL OF ALEXANDRIA

Doctor of the Incarnation

Seal of the Fathers

c. 376-444

TWO Popes of the twentieth century wrote official letters to the universal Church about St. Cyril of Alexandria and his work. In 1931 Pope Pius XI wrote an encyclical entitled, *The Light of Truth*. It commemorated the Council of Ephesus, 431 A.D., and praised St. Cyril as "that most holy man and champion of Catholic integrity . . . who without question holds the principal place" as the opponent of Nestorianism. In 1944 Pope Pius XII gave us an entire encyclical on St. Cyril. Its opening words, which, as usual, are used as its title, call St. Cyril "the ornament of the Oriental Church." The occasion of this encyclical was the fifteenth centenary of St. Cyril's death.

It is an interesting fact that the encyclical of Pope Pius XI was issued on Christmas Day, and that of Pope Pius XII on Easter. The attention paid to St. Cyril of Alexandria by two twentieth-century popes in official encyclical letters shows not only that he is important, but that he is important in modern times. Both Popes strongly link St. Cyril with their hopes for Christian unity. Pope Pius XII dwells on this quite definitely.

Patron of Unity

Pius XII proposes St. Cyril as a patron of unity among Christians, especially to the Eastern churches which so highly cherish St. Cyril but which are separated from the See of Peter. Pope Pius XII says: "Let this most illustrious Doctor be to them a preceptor and model in the new restoration of unity, with that triple bond which is so strongly recommended as being absolutely necessary, and with which the Divine Founder of the Church wished all His children to be bound together."

Unity will be attained only if these Eastern Christians follow in the footsteps of St. Cyril and sustain the triple and unbreakable bond. The Pope explains what this is:

> There must be union in the one Catholic Faith, in a single love for God and for all men, and finally in a common obedience and submission to the lawful hierarchy constituted by the Divine Redeemer Himself . . . In the task of earnestly pursuing and energetically preserving this genuine unity, we desire that the Patriarch of Alexandria should, at this present time, be to all a master and most illustrious model, even as he was during his own stormy epoch.

In the closing part of the encyclical, Pope Pius XII repeats his hopes for unity under the patronage of St. Cyril:

> It only remains for us, Venerable Brethren, in celebrating this fifteenth centenary of St. Cyril, to implore the benign patronage of this holy Doctor for the whole Church, and especially for those in the East who rejoice in the Christian name, asking above all that in our dissident brethren and sons he may happily accomplish that which he once wrote in the fullness of his joy: "Behold, the lacerated members of the body of the Church have been brought together, and there is no longer any cause of discord which might separate the ministers of the Gospel of Christ."

A Forceful Character

In choosing St. Cyril as a special patron for unity, Pope Pius XII realistically picked a man who basically loved peace, but would put everything on the line to fight for the truth. St. Cyril was a man who came straight to the point whenever the truth of dogma was concerned. He was indeed one who would forthrightly "call a spade a spade."

What could be more curt than St. Cyril's message to the heresiarch Nestorius, telling him that the Council of Ephesus had just deposed him?

> To Nestorius, new Judas. Know that by reason of thine impious preachings and of thy disobedience to the canons, on the 22nd of this month of June [the year 431], in conformity with the rules of the Church, thou hast been deposed by the Holy Synod, and that thou hast now no longer any rank in the Church.

This shows one side of St. Cyril's character and way of thinking. But it does not give the complete picture of the man. One of his early letters in the Nestorian controversy shows that St. Cyril's forcefulness was a logical part of a balance of mind and heart that included true Christian charity.

> I love peace, he wrote; there is nothing that I detest more than quarrels and disputes. I love everybody, and if I could heal one of the brethren by losing all my possessions and my goods, I am willing to do so joyfully because it is concord that I value most . . . But here it is a question of the Faith and of a scandal which concerns all the churches of the Roman Empire. The Sacred Doctrine is entrusted to us . . . How can we remedy these evils? . . .I am ready to endure with tranquillity all blame, all humiliations, all injuries, provided that the Faith is not endangered. I am filled with a love for Nestorius; nobody loves him more than I do . . . If, in accord with Christ's commandment, we must love our very enemies themselves, is it not natural that we should be united in special affection to those who are our friends and brethren in the priesthood? But when the Faith is attacked, we must not hesitate to sacrifice our life itself. . . .

St. Cyril was born about 376 A.D. According to the chronicle of John of Nikiu, his birthplace was a suburb of Alexandria, Egypt—at the time the second largest city in the world. He was a nephew of its archbishop, Theophilus, who is remembered as the learned, powerful and ruthless persecutor of St. John Chrysostom. The first sure date known in Cyril's life is 403 when, as a young priest, he accompanied his uncle to the Synod of the Oaks, which deposed St. John Chrysostom.

Not much can be said of St. Cyril's early years, except that the influence of his uncle was dominant for both good and bad. On the good side, St. Cyril received from his uncle a deep regard for study and a solid foundation in theology. On the other hand, he inherited in particular a bias against St. John Chrysostom, and in general a forcefulness that at times became overbearing—and perhaps a tendency for what may be called holy intrigue in manipulating men and events to secure the good of the Faith.

His enemies called him the "Pharaoh of Egypt." Some historians have not viewed his intrigues as very holy and have attributed personal, selfish reasons to him. A more balanced view is growing that Cyril was always first and foremost for the Faith, though he seems at times to have been too impetuous and hasty. As he grew older, he grew more mellow and prudent.

Before ordination, St. Cyril may have gone to live as a monk for some years in the Nitrian desert. At this time he perhaps came under the direction of St. Isidore of Pelusium. For with the freedom of an old teacher, St. Isidore later wrote to Cyril when he was an archbishop, giving very pointed advice and correction. The ancient *History of the Patriarchs of Alexandria* relates that when St. Cyril came back from the desert he continued to study under Theophilus and that the learned men were astonished at and rejoiced at his beauty of form and sweetness of voice. When the people heard him read, the history continues, they wanted him to continue forever "because he read so sweetly and was so beautiful in countenance."

Later, when St. Cyril was Archbishop of Alexandria, the people enjoyed comparing him to the great St. Athanasius, his predecessor in that See, who had practically carried the Church on his shoulders. Like St. Athanasius, St. Cyril was small and had a modest bearing. His complexion was rose colored; his eyebrows, thick and arched; his hair and beard, turning gray, combined to give him an air of imposing majesty. (*Catholic Mind*, 30, 1-9).

St. Cyril became Archbishop of Alexandria on October 17, 412, just two days after the death of his uncle Theophilus. The forthright Cyril soon closed the churches of the Novations in that city. The Church historian Socrates, tinged by their heresy or at least sympathetic to the Novations, supplies the information. He also tells us that St. Cyril drove all the Jews from Alexandria after they had staged a night of terror in which many Christians were killed. Socrates also relates the murder of the famous pagan woman philosopher, Hypatia, by a group of Christians who thought she was setting the Prefect of Alexandria, Orestes, against St. Cyril. This happened in the fourth year of Cyril's episcopate. St. Cyril himself certainly regretted the murder as much as anyone. But events such as these, the details and implications of which are still not fully understood, tended to besmirch St. Cyril's name during his own lifetime and in succeeding centuries.

The Council of Ephesus

The biggest milestone in the life of St. Cyril came in 431, when he presided at the Council of Ephesus. The bishops of the Empire were summoned by the Emperor, Theodosius II, to gather after Pentecost and settle the troubles stirred up between Alexandria and Constantinople over the term *Theotokos*, "Mother of God." St. Cyril, as patriarch of Alexandria, and Nestorius, as patriarch of Constantinople, had clashed over this term and had already written to Pope Celestine I.

St. Cyril accepted this term as a true description of the Blessed Virgin Mary; Nestorius rejected it. His rejection was based on his view that there were two separate persons in Christ; he held that Mary was mother of the human person but not of the Divine Person. The Catholic teaching, on the contrary, is that while in Christ there are two natures—the Divine and the human—there is in Him only one Person—a Divine Person, the Second Person of the Blessed Trinity. Mary gave birth, according to the flesh, to a Divine Person, therefore she is the Mother of God—though she is not the mother of the Divinity, of God as God.

Nestorius was urged by the Pope, through St. Cyril as his delegate, to recant within 10 days his teaching, which implied that there are two persons in Christ. St. Cyril wrote to Nestorius, telling him this, and adding 12 anathemas for him to subscribe to. With the two most powerful archbishops in the East opposing each other, the Emperor called the Synod. Approved and accepted by the Pope, this "Council of Ephesus" ranks as the Third General Council of the Church.

The bishops gathered in Ephesus, which was the burial place of the Apostle St. John and at that time a flourishing seaport, though now it is an impoverished village. They met in its cathedral, the first in the world to be named St. Mary, after the Blessed Virgin.

It is unfortunate that St. Cyril and Nestorius did not meet each other and talk things over on an informal, friendly basis; it is also unfortunate that the great and respected St. Augustine, summoned to the Council, had just died. Nestorius was garrulous and changeable. Though he spoke openly about never admitting the existence of a "two or three months old God," he also at times said he was willing to accept the term, "Mother of God," though he preferred "Mother of Christ." Interestingly enough, when Nestorius had been called from the monastic life in 428 to be Archbishop of Constantinople, he had said, "I felt that men might more easily launch against me any calumny other than heresy," and he had set himself to vigorous action against all false teachings.

St. Cyril opened the Council before the bishops coming with

John of Antioch had arrived and before the three legates of Pope Celestine I were on hand. Though the time set for opening the Council had already passed, it would have been better for St. Cyril to wait, as urged by many of the bishops. Meeting on June 22, 431, the Council quickly condemned Nestorius and deposed him. The term, *Theotokos,* "Mother of God," was firmly upheld. The people of Ephesus celebrated by a tumultuous torchlight procession, accompanying the bishops from the basilica to the various places where they were residing. To the people it meant a victory for Christ and His Blessed Mother.

When John of Antioch arrived a few days later, he held his own synod, which deposed St. Cyril. When the three papal legates came, they followed instructions and put themselves absolutely under Cyril. In their presence the Council reassembled on July 10 and 11 and confirmed its previous acts.

The Emperor followed the unusual course of accepting the decrees of both synods. He declared both St. Cyril and Nestorius deposed. The aftermath of all this was a temporary schism of the bishops of Antioch and continued hard feelings, which helped to establish Nestorianism. St. Cyril emerged finally as a strong and successful leader, but less impetuous action might have secured a wider victory. Maybe it could have saved Nestorius from heresy and John of Antioch from schism.

Deep-Flowing Spirituality

St. Cyril is called the Doctor of the Incarnation because he fought so hard to establish the truth that Christ is true God and true man and yet only one Person, and because Christ was always the center of his thought. A study of St. Cyril's Old Testament writings says that "it was not in the controversies that he learned of Christ; rather, it was his deep knowledge of the Saviour that drew him into these doctrinal struggles." (Alexander Kerrigan, *St. Cyril of Alexandria: Interpreter of the Old Test.,* Rome: Pontificio Instituto Biblico, 1952).

Another modern scholar (Dominic Unger, O.F.M. Cap., *Franciscan Studies,* 7), in searching the writings of St. Cyril, found that he held the doctrine of the absolute primacy of Christ. This means that from the very beginning, even before the foreseen sin of Adam, God planned Christ as the perfect creature, united to divinity, the "final scope and exemplar and mediator of all creatures." God planned the masterpiece of all Creation, *not after*, but *before* all others. The masterpiece which is Christ is the centerpiece of all God's Creation, the first in the intention or plan of God, divinity substantially united to a creature. This we have in the person of Christ. His humanity is the first step down and the last step up on the beautiful spiral of Creation. It would be the first creature for the eternal God to think about and to want. All others must be related to God and planned by God through this one. It can easily be seen that one who looks at Creation according to this concept has a viewpoint which projects the majesty and goodness of Christ onto everybody and the glow of Him who called Himself "the Light of the World" onto the duller things, making beauty everywhere. Thus the dominant note in the symphony of Creation is a joyful one, and the coming of the Saviour no longer sounds as a minor chord.

St. Cyril was a profound theologian, and at the same time his abstract thought was flavored with the experiences of daily life. He did not compose any devotional work as such, but all his works breathe out the spirit of devotion. Sanctifying grace, the indwelling of the Trinity in the soul, the union of Christ with the soul were his constant preoccupation.

In line with St. Cyril's deep devotion to the mystery of God becoming man is his devotion to the Holy Eucharist. The Roman Breviary, before the 1971 changes, included two of his homilies; one was used on the octave day of Corpus Christi and the other on the Thursday during the octave of the Sacred Heart. In the first of these, St. Cyril sums up in beautiful words our union with Christ in the Eucharist.

> "He that eateth My Flesh and drinketh My Blood abideth in Me and I in him." If into melted wax other wax is poured, the two are certain to get thoroughly mixed, one with the other. In the same way, he who receives the Body and Blood of the Lord is so united with Him that he is in Christ and Christ in him.

In another sermon, St. Cyril's fervor and deep faith are very evident. He expresses his admiration of the Eucharist:

> O tremendous mystery, O ineffable decision of the divine counsel, O humility (*demissionem*) which the mind cannot comprehend! O goodness that cannot be investigated! The Maker offers Himself to the good pleasure of His work. Life Itself gives Itself to mortals to eat and drink. "Come and eat My body," It

exhorts, "and drink the wine which I have mixed for you. I have prepared Myself as food and have set Myself before those who desire." (PG, Vol. 77, p. 1018).

Theotokos

It was St. Cyril's strong emphasis on the place of Christ in the divine plan, his emphasis, too, on the unity of His Person, that made him the champion of the Blessed Virgin Mary. In his second letter to Nestorius, he explained how Mary could be truly called the "Mother of God," which is given in Greek as one word, the famous *Theotokos*.

> He who had an existence before all ages and was born of the Father, is said to have been born according to the flesh of a woman, not as though His divine nature received its beginning of existence in the Holy Virgin, for it needed not any second generation after that of the Father (for it would be absurd and foolish to say that He who existed before all ages, co-eternal with the Father, needed any second beginning of existence), but since for us and for our salvation He personally united to Himself a human body and came forth of a woman, He is in this way said to be born after the flesh; for He was not first born a common man of the Holy Virgin, and then the Word came down and entered into Him, but the union being made in the womb itself, He is said to endure a birth after the flesh, ascribing to Himself the birth of His own flesh.

Nestorius preferred the term "Mother of Christ" and preached against the word *Theotokos*, though it was pointed out to him that he was fighting a windmill, for no sane person would ever imagine that Mary, the creature, was responsible for the birth of the Eternal God in as far as He is God. She simply gave birth to Christ, whose human nature was, already in her womb, substantially united to God. Therefore she is the Mother of God.

St. Cyril pointed out that we speak of the suffering of God, of His death. We may say that God suffered and died for us. Yet we know that this is not to be understood as though God the Word suffered in His divine nature, or that God, the Source of all life, died as God. But it is just because we can say "God suffered and died for us," that our salvation has been won, that infinite honor has been given to God and infinite satisfaction made for sin. If we cannot say that God suffered, meaning the

Second Person of the Trinity substantially united to humanity in Christ, then we cannot say we have been redeemed. Therefore, to deny the title "Mother of God" is to dash to the ground the proper idea of Christ and the concept of how our own salvation was actually won.

St. Cyril concludes his letter to Nestorius, later unanimously adopted by the Council of Ephesus, with an appeal to earlier writers.

> This was the sentiment of the Holy Fathers; therefore, they ventured to call the holy Virgin the "Mother of God," not as if the nature of the Word or divinity had its beginning from the holy Virgin, but because of her was born that holy body with a rational soul, to which the Word being personally united, is said to be born according to the flesh.

St. Cyril did not invent the term *Theotokos*. One of his predecessors, Bishop Alexander of Alexandria, had used it in 320 A.D. in condemning Arianism more than a century before. But the term is forever linked with St. Cyril's name because he championed it. He explained it unmistakably, repeatedly, and at length. In his third letter to Nestorius he says:

> For although visible and a child in swaddling clothes, and even in the bosom of His Virgin Mother, He filled all creation as God and was a fellow-ruler with Him who begat Him, for the Godhead is without quantity and dimension and cannot have limits. We do not divide the God from the man nor separate Him into parts, as though the two natures were mutually united in Him only through a sharing of dignity and authority . . . neither do we give separately to the Word of God the name of Christ and the same name separately to a different one born of a woman, for we know only one Christ, the Word from God the Father with His own flesh.

It is interesting to note that though St. Cyril's theology of Mary was so strong, his somewhat unflattering outlook on the female sex in general weakened his psychology of Mary. "Woman is a twittering, loquacious creature," St. Cyril said, "with a gift for contriving conceit." By inducing man to sin she has become "death's deaconess." St. Cyril's thinking was much influenced by St. Paul (*1 Cor.* 11), who said that "man was not created for woman, but woman for man." The effect of

St. Cyril's general outlook was to cast Mary at the foot of the Cross in a role of weakness and tears. Nevertheless, he gave the most famous Marian sermon of ancient times (at Ephesus in June of 431, during the Council).

Defender of the Papacy

Just as he did not invent the term *Theotokos*, so St. Cyril did not invent the procedure of invoking the Fathers of the Church as proof for doctrine. He did, however, use the method so well and so consistently that he has earned the title, "Seal of the Fathers." To follow the Fathers is to journey along the king's highway, he says; this is the royal way. St. Cyril classifies the teaching of the Fathers (a link with the Apostolic Tradition) along with Scripture as a guide for belief. "We have been taught to hold these things by the holy Apostles and Evangelists, and all the God-inspired Scriptures, and in the true confessions of the blessed Fathers." St Cyril's search for truth in the Fathers has also earned him the title, "Guardian of Accuracy."

His constant appeal to the Fathers makes the writings of St. Cyril a storehouse of information about the teachings of those who preceded him. St. Cyril's reliance on the Fathers of the Church also gives his own teaching greater depth and value as an index of the common, orthodox belief of preceding centuries. This is especially valuable in his position regarding the authority of the Pope. If St. Cyril clearly recognized the position of the Bishop of Rome as visible head of the whole Church, we can be sure that this attitude is a reflection of what he had found in the Fathers of preceding centuries.

Pope Pius XII, in his anniversary encyclical of 1944 about St. Cyril, praises his line of conduct in the Nestorian controversy as upholding the supreme authority of St. Peter and his successors. "Both in defeating the Nestorian heresy and in reaching agreement with the bishops of the province of Antioch, he always acted in the closest possible union with this Apostolic See." Pope Pius XII quotes from St. Cyril's letter to Pope Celestine before the Council of Ephesus: "Since God requires vigilance of us in these matters, and a long established custom of the Churches [i.e., dioceses] directs that questions such as these be communicated to Your Holiness, I write to you, urged thereto by a clear necessity." Later St. Cyril defended his own faith by writing: "Testimony has been borne to the purity of my faith both by the

Roman Church and by the holy synod assembled, I may say, from all the earth which lies under heaven."

Even more convincing proof of St. Cyril's respect for the Apostolic See lies in his accepting the Pope's reversal of his (Cyril's) policy and that of the Council in excommunicating the bishops of the province of Antioch. Pope Celestine I did not approve of this and wrote to St. Cyril, telling him to take steps to bring about peace and concord with these bishops who had sympathized with Nestorius, though not approving his doctrine. St. Cyril immediately made efforts to win back the good will of John of Antioch and his bishops. Peace was established within two years, in 433. At that time, St. Cyril exclaimed in a famous letter: "Let the heavens rejoice and let the earth tremble with gladness! The inner wall of separation has been broken down, the storm which caused such sadness has been stilled, and every occasion of discord has been removed; for Christ, the Saviour of us all, has granted peace to His churches."

At the Council of Ephesus, St. Cyril, along with the other nearly 200 bishops, signed the decrees approving the acts of the Council. Included was a letter read by Philip, a priest who was one of the three papal legates.

> No one doubts, nay, for centuries it has been known that the holy and most blessed Peter, prince and head of the Apostles, pillar of the Faith and foundation of the Catholic Church, received the keys of the kingdom from Our Lord Jesus Christ, the Saviour and Redeemer of the human race, and that to him was given the power of loosing and binding sins: who down even to today, and forever, both lives and judges in his successors. The holy and most blessed Pope Celestine, according to due order, is his successor and holds his place, and us he sent to supply his place in this holy synod, which the most humane and Christian emperors have commanded to assemble, bearing in mind and continually watching over the Catholic Faith.

The dogmatic constitution *Pastor Aeternus* of the first Vatican Council (1870) quotes in part these words of Philip.

Warrior for the Truth

For 32 years St. Cyril was Archbishop of Alexandria, next to Rome the largest diocese in the fifth-century world. After his return from Ephesus, as before, he wrote voluminously. Much of his earlier writing was against Arianism. After the Council of Ephesus, he wrote a great deal against Nestorianism; 20 books were composed to refute the works of the Emperor Julian. Much of his writing has been lost; only about 20 of his sermons survive. Yet, what remains is very considerable and of great value for the history of Christian doctrine.

St. Cyril's style is not attractive; rather, it is too diffuse, but he has a rich, imaginative and speculative mind. He labors to be precise, and his method of giving proofs from the Fathers and from reason makes him, among the Eastern writers, the most eminent forerunner of the Scholastics of the Middle Ages.

St. Cyril died on January 28, 444, with a prayer to the Blessed Virgin Mary on his lips. A bitter letter which circulated in Syria at his death is a reminder of the fierce currents of emotion that swirled about him and of the calibre of some of his enemies:

> Behold, at long last this wicked man is dead . . . His demise brings joy to the living but must terrify the dead; there is danger that they will quickly tire of him and get rid of him. It is imperative to place a very heavy stone on his grave, so that he will not show himself to us again.

From the distance in time and from the current false viewpoint of absolute tolerance for all shades of belief, right or wrong, St. Cyril is hard to understand. But in his day people realized that truth is all-important, that it matters very much—both for the good of the individual and also of organized political society—just what you believe. St. Cyril was a fighter and he fought hard, even considering the tradition of his own time when truth was fought over fiercely, and even considering the accepted social and political approach to religious controversy in his time. He was combatting the forces of a paganism that was outlawed, but on the practical level was still bothersome, insidious in argument and at times positively violent. He knew the upheaval that could be caused by religious teachings at variance with the truth— which he adhered to with all his being—especially when allied with political power. He fought to avoid confusion and division within the Church as well. His very efforts and the force of his action tended to make further division, but after a few years of crisis, peace returned, and for those of good will, it rested on a more secure foundation, thanks in great part to St. Cyril. Yet sadly, soon after his death, his own See fell into the heresy of Monophysitism,* due in part to a misinterpretation of his writings. This sad fact at least bears witness to the reality of the doctrinal dangers that had aroused St. Cyril's fighting spirit. It is also worthy of mention that a "Nestorian Church" still exists today; its members are called "Assyrian Christians."

St. Cyril of Alexandria was a warrior for the truth. He recalled the words of Christ, the Prince of Peace: "Do not think that I came to send peace upon earth: I came not to send peace, but the sword. For I came to set a man at variance against his father, and the daughter against her mother . . ." (*Matt.* 10:34-35). He quoted these words to Nestorius and added,

> For if faith be injured, let there be lost the honor due to parents as stale and tottering, let even the law of tender love toward children and brothers be silenced, let death be better to the pious than living.

St. Cyril knew that the Faith and its truths were all-important. He preferred peace, but he would fight strongly for the truth. At times he seems to have overdone it. But those who would judge St. Cyril should also share his passion for the truth of Christ.

In 1931, Pope Pius XI, on the occasion of the fifteenth centenary of the Council of Ephesus, established a liturgical memorial of this signal event in Church history: He gave to the Universal Church the Feast of the Divine Maternity of Mary, October 11. In 1962 Pope John XXIII chose this feast day as the day on which to open the Second Council of the Vatican, where one of his aims was to promote Christian unity. Therefore, including the great Marian Pope, Pius XII, three popes of the 20th century in succession turned toward the Mother of God in their hopes for unity. Standing in the glow of this new attention to the Divine Maternity of Mary is the embattled and stalwart champion of the *Theotokos*, St. Cyril of Alexandria.

St. Cyril's feast day in the West is June 27 (February 9 in the 1962 calendar).

---

* Monophysitism (or "Monophysism") is the heresy that there is only one nature in Christ, the divine, which opposes the teaching of the Catholic Church that within Christ there are *two* natures, the human *and* the divine. Monophysitism was an extreme reaction against Nestorianism, which had claimed that there are two separate *persons* in Christ.

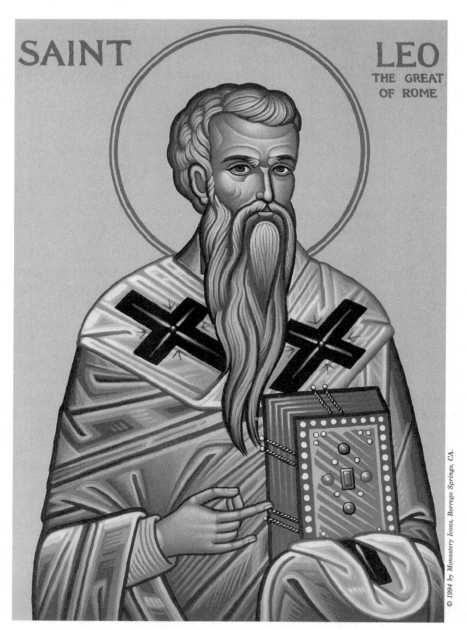

SAINT LEO THE GREAT OF ROME

Pope Saint Leo The Great

12

POPE SAINT LEO THE GREAT
Doctor of the Unity of the Church
c. 400-461

OF all the learned and holy men who have occupied the See of St. Peter, only two have been honored with the title of Doctor. History has chosen the same two for the sobriquet of "Great." They are St. Leo the Great and St. Gregory the Great, in both cases the first among the Supreme Pontiffs to bear those now illustrious names.

In a sermon of October 12, 1952, Pope Pius XII called Pope St. Leo I "the greatest among the great." On November 11, 1961, Pope John XXIII issued an encyclical entitled "The Eternal Wisdom of God" (*Aeterna Dei Sapientia*) commemorating the fifteenth centenary of St. Leo's death. In this encyclical Pius XII stated: "We, called by Divine Providence to occupy the Chair of Peter, which St. Leo the Great made so illustrious with wisdom of government, richness of doctrine, with magnanimity and with his inexhaustible charity, feel it our duty . . . to recall his virtues and immortal merits."

Later in his encyclical letter Pope John recalls St. Leo's strong faith in the Divine origin of the mandate to teach all men and to lead all to salvation. Joining St. Leo, therefore, in his great desire to see all peoples enter on the way of truth, charity and peace, Pope John XXIII says that "it is precisely for the purpose of rendering the Church more capable of accomplishing in our times this great mission that We decided to convene the Second Vatican Ecumenical Council."

"Saviour" of Rome

It has been said that if it were not for the Popes, Rome today would very likely be a mass of ruins like Babylon, Carthage and other ancient cities. Pope Leo the Great is especially remembered for his dramatic part in saving Rome. Twice he went out to meet the leaders of invasions in an effort to turn them back.

The first time was to face the notorious Attila the Hun in 452 A.D., and a few years later, in 455, to face Genseric the Vandal. Although the first meeting, that against Attila, has made a bigger mark in history and art, St. Leo's influence may actually have accomplished more as a result of his meeting with Genseric.

A painting of Raphael shows the encounter with Attila as it has come down to us embellished by legend. The terrible Hun looks above St. Leo and sees Sts. Peter and Paul supporting the Pope's demands. St. Leo had gone out to meet Attila at the request of the Emperor Valentinian and the Roman Senate. He went with two other chosen representatives, the Senators Avienus and Trigetius, to the neighborhood of Mantua. The advancing reinforcements of the Eastern Roman Emperor, Marcian, and Attila's superstitious fear because of the death of Alaric the Goth shortly after sacking Rome, may have helped to back up the courageous words of St. Leo and his companions. In any event, Attila turned back and Rome was spared.

But when Genseric the Vandal came, the Emperor was dead, killed in flight, and no military leader was defending Rome. Only one man could have saved the city at that time, and that was St. Leo the Great. He persuaded Genseric to spare the lives of the people and not to burn the city. The Vandals looted for two weeks, but left the large churches untouched, and did not kill or burn.

This Majestic Man

St. Leo exercised a powerful sway over the minds of his contemporaries. Even before he was Pope, his influence and prestige were widespread. St. Cyril of Alexandria, at the time the leading bishop in the East (431), wrote and explained the bold and unlawful ambitions of Juvenal, Bishop of Jerusalem, to control Palestine, and asked St. Leo to present the matter properly to the Pope. Shortly before this it had been Leo who persuaded St. John Cassian to take up his pen once again—which had been laid aside in favor of a strictly monastic and retired life—and write the treatise, *De Incarnatione* (*Concerning the Incarnation*). Cassian himself acknowledges this: "You, Leo, my honored friend . . . ornament of the Roman Church and of the sacred ministry, have overcome my intention and decision by your praiseworthy zeal and imperious sincerity."

St. Leo was away on a civil mission when he was chosen pope.

He had been sent to bring about peace in France between two of the Roman Empire's military leaders, Aetius and Albinus. It seems that the clergy and people of Rome thought of no other candidate to be their bishop. They sent a delegation to St. Leo, who was then still a deacon and away in France, asking him to return. Forty days after the death of Pope Sixtus III, St. Leo was back in Rome. He was elected Pope unanimously and was consecrated on September 29, 440 A.D., to begin one of the longest pontificates in the ancient Church.

In his Encyclical Pope John XXIII sums up the qualifications and character of St. Leo the Great: "St. Leo shows exceptional gifts as a man of government, that is, an enlightened and supremely practical spirit, a will ready for action, firm in well matured decisions, a heart open to paternal understanding, and full of that charity that St. Paul indicated to all Christians as 'the better way.'"

As one reads the various accounts of St. Leo's life, the word "majestic" keeps cropping up. History, as well as St. Leo's own contemporaries, project an image of him as a strong and principled man whose words of quiet decision must be listened to. During most of the 21 years that St. Leo was Pope, he was the only truly great historical figure in either the Church or the civil order. The great saints and bishops of the East were dead, and the emperors in both East and West were not men of commanding stature. At this time the barbarian nations were pushing in on the frontiers of both the Eastern and Western sections of the Roman Empire. Pope St. Leo the Great was the one man who, by the clarity of his vision of the Church as one and universal and by the force of his own administration, did much to fashion the framework on which European civilization could grow in an essential unity. Because of his pivotal role in history, St. Leo the Great emerges from the pages of time as a truly majestic figure.

The Good Pastor

Yet he was also very much aware of the needs of individual souls. Were we to hear him preach today, his subject matter would sound quite familiar. For he followed the liturgical cycle, and therefore many of his 96 extant sermons deal with Christmas, the Passion, Easter, or Pentecost. In his use of Scripture he differed from most of the early Fathers in not interpreting long

passages or entire books of the Bible. He quoted Scripture liberally, but he used it to explain and inculcate virtues or to exem-
plify a particular divine truth. It is an odd fact that from the
time of St. Peter, the first Pope, to that of St. Leo, the sermons
of the Popes have not been preserved.

Leo's sermons are famous for their clarity of thought and
musical alliteration. Many of the orations used at Mass are
based on them. The way Leo's words reached the common man
may be judged from the way they still reach us today. In Sermon
40, for instance, he says: "For no one's income is small whose
heart is big, and the measure of one's mercy and goodness does
not depend on the size of one's means. The wealth of good will
is never lacking, even in a slender purse."

With directness but with gentleness, he chides his people in
Sermon 84, where he comments on the poor attendance at the
religious observance of the delivery of Rome from the barbarians:

> The fewness of those who were present has of itself shown,
> dearly beloved, that the religious devotion wherewith, in com-
> memoration of the day of our chastisement and release, the
> whole body of the faithful used to flock together in order to
> give God thanks, has on this last occasion been almost entirely
> neglected; and this has caused me much sadness of heart and
> great fear . . . One is ashamed to say it, but one must not keep
> silence: more is spent on demons than upon the Apostles, and
> mad spectacles draw greater crowds than blessed martyrdoms.
> Who was it that restored this city to safety, that rescued it
> from captivity—the games of the circus-goers or the care of the
> Saints?

Jalland, the very capable Protestant biographer of St. Leo the
Great, sums up St. Leo's majestic yet practical nature:

> We are bound to recognize that his words bear the impress
> of a majestic personality, which while supremely conscious of
> the solemn dignity of his office, was bent on working out the
> spiritual and moral salvation of the people committed to his
> charge. It is a personality, the force of which still persists in
> the spirit and outlook of the Roman Church today, and as we
> stand in the pillared nave and aisles of some great basilica,
> we can perhaps still recapture in our imagination the sound
> of the great pope's sonorous voice ringing through its walls.

History's depiction of St. Leo the Great always shows him in some official role. In the first historical information we have of him, he is already a person of some influence in Rome. Possibly he is the Leo mentioned by St. Augustine as a bearer of letters from Pope Zosimus to the bishop of Carthage.

St. Leo was born in Tuscany, in Northern Italy, and his father's name was Quintianus. Very likely the family came to live in Rome while he was young, since he refers to it as his "homeland" (*patria*). The exact date of his birth is not known, but it must have been within a few years of 400 A.D.

Nobody has left an account of his death, which occurred in November of 461, probably on the tenth. He was buried in the entrance passage to the old St. Peter's Basilica. In 688 his remains were removed to a place within the church. When the present St. Peter's Basilica was built, St. Leo's body was placed in its southwest chapel. In 1754 Pope Benedict XIV declared St. Leo the Great a Doctor of the Church. His feast is celebrated on February 18 in the Eastern Churches; in the West his feast (traditionally April 11) is celebrated on November 10.

The Tome

In the stillness of Christmas Eve, as the Church prepares for midnight Mass, she presents to us in the Divine Office the words of St. Leo: "Recognize, O Christian, your dignity, and having been made a partner of the divine nature, do not return by an unworthy way of living to the old baseness. Remember who is your Head and to whose body you belong." These words are taken from the first of eight sermons St. Leo the Great gave on the Nativity of Our Lord. They richly deserve a place in the Christmas liturgy, coming from the pen of such a champion of Christ, true God and true man. In his sermons, in the leadership he gave to the Council of Chalcedon, in his vigorous war against the heresies of Nestorianism and Eutychianism, and in his famous letter known as "The Tome," St. Leo the Great established his unique role in Christology.

St. Leo sent the great letter which history has dubbed "The Tome" to St. Flavian, Bishop of Constantinople, in reference to the opinions of the archimandrite (Eastern abbot) Eutyches—which had been condemned in a synod held at Constantinople. The "Tome" is dated June 13, 449. Later, it was read to the more than 500 bishops assembled at the Council of Chalcedon, which was then meeting in its second session, October 10, 452. In the fifth and sixth sessions, the official definition of doctrine about Christ's natures and Person, largely based on St. Leo's "Tome," was presented and approved. Ever since, Catholic theology has followed this definition as the nucleus of its Christology.

The collection of St. Leo's letters numbers 173, of which about 140 are his own. "The Tome" is number 28 of this series. The selection used in the *Liturgy of The Hours* for the Solemnity of the Annunciation is taken from "The Tome." St. Leo's words describe the greatest moment in human history, that moment when God the Son took on our human nature:

> . . . Thus the Son of God enters this lowly world. He comes down from the throne of heaven, yet does not separate Himself from the Father's glory. He is born in a new condition, by a new birth. . . . He was born in a new condition, for, invisible in His own nature, He became visible in ours. Beyond our grasp, He chose to come within our grasp. Existing before time began, He began to exist *at a moment in time*. Lord of the universe, He hid His infinite glory, and took the nature of a servant. Incapable of suffering as God, He did not refuse to be a man, capable of suffering. Immortal, He chose to be subject to the laws of death. . . . He who is true God is also true man. There is no falsehood in this unity as long as the lowliness of man and the pre-eminence of God coexist in mutual relationship . . .

Another selection from "The Tome" describes these essential facts about Christ:

> He was born God from God, the Omnipotent from the Omnipotent, the Co-eternal from the Eternal, not coming later in time or inferior in power, not of unequal glory, not separate in essence. This same only-begotten Son of the eternal Father was truly born eternal of the Holy Spirit and the Virgin Mary. This birth in time in no way minimized His divine and eternal birth, nor did it add thereto. He sacrificed His entire self in order to redeem man (who had been deceived), to overcome death, and by His power to destroy the devil, who held sway over death. (Translation by Bro. Edmund Hunt, C.S.C., in *Fathers of the Church*, Vol. 34, NY, 1957).

"The Tome" has been called "the plain man's guide to the doctrine of the Incarnation." St. Leo expresses these sublime realities in a plain and unmistakable way. He was not an innovative, speculative theologian, but the exact and precise framer of traditional ideas. His interest was to put things in such a way that his flock could understand them. He thus presented the fruit of the studies of St. Cyril of Alexandria and others on the Incarnation in a lasting and easy-to-understand form.

In Letter 165 to the Emperor Leo, he sums up as well as could any modern theologian with the help of 15 centuries of Church history and theological refinements to support him, the whole substance of the doctrine on the Incarnation, as well as the position of those who opposed it.

Two enemies (the one shortly after the other) attacked the Catholic Faith, which is one and true; nothing can be added to or subtracted from it. The first of these to rise was Nestorius; then came Eutyches. They sought to introduce into God's Church two heresies, the one contrary to the other. As a result, both were rightly condemned by the advocates of truth, for the teachings of both men, false in different ways, were utterly foolish and blasphemous. Nestorius believed that the Blessed Virgin Mary was the mother of the man only and not of God; that is, in his opinion, the divine Person was different from the [supposed] human person. He did not think there was one Christ existing in the Word of God and the flesh, but taught that one was the son of man and the other the Son of God, each separate and distinct from the other. For this he was condemned. The truth is, that while that essence of the unchangeable Word remained (which is timeless and co-eternal with the Father and the Holy Spirit), the Word was made flesh in the womb of the Virgin in such a way that, by an ineffable mystery, through one conception and one birth the same Virgin and Handmaid was also the Mother of the Lord according to the reality of both natures . . . Eutyches is likewise crushed by the same condemnation. Wallowing about in the impious errors of old heretics, he picked out the third teaching of Apollinaris: that is, in denying the reality of the human flesh and soul, he stated that the whole of Our Lord Jesus Christ is of one nature, as if the very divinity of the Word had changed Itself into the flesh and soul.

Pope John XXIII in his encyclical quotes a passage from "The Tome" which shows the precision of St. Leo in speaking of the two natures and one Person in Christ.

The propriety of both natures remaining therefore integral, coming together in the single Person, human nothingness was assumed by Divine Majesty, weakness by power, mortality by eternity; and in order to satisfy the debt of our condition, the inviolable nature was united to a susceptible nature, in such a manner that, as was indeed needed for our salvation, the one and irreplaceable mediator between God and man, the man Jesus Christ, could indeed die according to one nature, but not according to the other. Therefore the Word, though assuming the complete and perfect nature of true man, was born true God, complete in His divine properties, complete also in ours.

Doctor of the Unity of the Church

In his encyclical *Aeterna Dei Sapientia* (1961), Pope John XXIII says, "St. Leo is celebrated above all as the Doctor of the unity of the Church." St. Leo's whole way of thinking and acting always tended to protect and strengthen unity. He was always bent on preserving the Church as one in teaching. For that reason he was prompt in stating the truth against any deviant teaching. Besides his chief work, that regarding the Incarnation, St. Leo the Great did much to combat Pelagianism and to make clear the teachings of St. Augustine on grace. Pelagianism, the heretical doctrine of Pelagius, a native of Britain, denied Original Sin, that death is due to Original Sin, that Baptism is necessary to blot out Original Sin (he said it was only a title for admission to the kingdom of Heaven), and that grace is necessary for salvation. As Pelagianism developed, it professed that grace is within the natural capacity of man. In *Letter* 2, a reply to a bishop concerning Pelagianism, St. Leo has a fine, epigrammatic sentence that expresses reams of theology: "Grace not actually given gratis is not grace at all."

St. Leo the Great vigorously combatted heresy in any form whatever. One of his first actions was against the Manicheans in Italy. He wrote against Priscillianism in Spain. Repeatedly St. Leo says that nothing can be added to or taken away from the Faith. "The integral and true Faith is a great bulwark to which nothing can be added or taken from by anyone."

St. Leo was also interested in an essential unity of liturgical practice in the Church. One interesting point in this connection is his effort to secure agreement on the proper day for the celebration of Easter. The astronomers of Alexandria and Rome differed in their methods of calculation. Although not convinced by mathematical proof, St. Leo gave in to those who upheld the Alexandrian system and admitted the celebration of Easter beyond April 21. He gave in on the basis of a concession to attain a unity of practice. Later mathematical calculations proved the Alexandrian system correct, and incidentally showed how St. Leo's wisdom and restraint triumphed over bad mathematics and the strong feelings and demands of the people in the West.

Flowing from St. Leo's love for unity was his constant appeal to the canons of the Council of Nicaea (325 A.D.). He himself by this appeal to these canons, by citing the decisions of preceding popes, and by his own far-sightedness in making decisions (keeping in mind that he spoke for the whole Church), had a lasting influence on the development of the Canon Law of the Church.

Papal Power Strongly Proclaimed

In particular it was Pope St. Leo's love for unity that led him to expound over and over the position of the Bishop of Rome as the successor of St. Peter and the visible head of the Universal Church. He would use the occasion of the anniversary of his consecration as Pope to emphasize his position as visible head of the Church. He tells the assembled bishops and faithful that

> St. Peter rejoices over your good feeling and welcomes your respect for the Lord's own institution as shown towards the partners of His honor, commending the well-ordered love of the whole Church which ever finds Peter in Peter's See, and from affection for so great a shepherd grows not lukewarm over even so inferior a successor as myself.

St. Leo the Great was a humble man, not a seeker of power for its own sake. His anniversary sermons run along the lines of Our Lady's *Magnificat*. He is unworthy, but at the same time God has done great things for him. If he asserted the power of the papacy and exercised it more vigorously than any before him, it was because he saw in it the divinely instituted bond of Catholic unity.

In commenting on the well-known text of St. Matthew (16:18)—"Thou art Peter; and upon this rock I will build my church, and the gates of hell shall not prevail against it"—St. Leo at times says that Christ placed St. Peter at the head of the Church as a reward for his faith and built the Church on that faith. More often, he identifies the foundation of the Church as St. Peter himself, "the Rock of the Catholic Faith, the surname of which Peter received from the Lord." (*Letter* 119). That St. Leo (who so strongly claimed and exercised the powers of a universal visible head of the Church) could use both interpretations shows that in his mind there is no opposition between them. As he says in *Sermon* 3: "For the solidity of that faith which was praised in the chief of the Apostles is perpetual: and as that remains which Peter believed in Christ, so that remains which Christ instituted in Peter."

In a passage that was quoted by Pope John XXIII, St. Leo says (*Sermon* 4):

> The Lord took care of Peter in a special way; He prayed for the faith of Peter in particular, almost as though the perseverance of the others would have been better guaranteed if the soul of their chief would not be overcome. In Peter, therefore, the strength of all is protected and the assistance of divine grace follows this order: the strength which was given to Peter through Christ is conferred on the other Apostles through Peter.

In the last of his anniversary sermons that is preserved, St. Leo the Great says:

> There is a further reason for our celebration, namely, the apostolic and episcopal dignity of the most blessed Peter, who does not cease to preside over his see and receives an abiding partnership with the eternal Priest. For the stability which the Rock himself was given by that Rock which is Christ, he conveyed also to his successors, and wheresoever any steadfastness is apparent, there without doubt is to be seen the strength of the shepherd. (*Sermon* 5).

Papal Power Strongly Used

Pope St. Leo's exercise of the papal power of jurisdiction is dramatized by his relations with another saint, St. Hilary, Bishop of Arles. St. Hilary, a holy and mortified man, but given somewhat to impulsive action, had summoned a synod which had deposed Celidonius, Bishop of Besancon. Celidonius came to Rome to appeal. St. Hilary also hastened to Rome, on foot and in the dead of winter. He lost his composure and protested too strongly before a Roman synod, which action did little to commend his side of the case. The appeal of Celidonius was sustained, and he was reinstated. About this same time, friends of Projectus, another bishop of France, came to protest that St. Hilary had consecrated a new bishop in his stead while he was sick. This brought up the question of whether or not the Bishop of Arles had the right to consecrate a successor for Projectus. This case too was decided against St. Hilary. In a letter to the bishops of Gaul (France), Pope Leo declared St. Hilary deposed from metropolitan jurisdiction and limited to just his own bishopric. (A metropolitan is an archbishop placed over other bishops and their dioceses in a certain region.) "It is but fair . . . he may now be kept by our command, in accordance with the clemency of the Apostolic See, to the priesthood of his own city alone."

In the beginning of this letter St. Leo speaks strongly of the charge given by Christ to Peter:

> . . . He has placed the principal charge on the blessed Peter, chief of the Apostles; and from him as from the Head, wishes His gifts to flow to all the body: so that anyone who dares to secede from Peter's solid Rock may understand that he has no part or lot in the divine mystery.

The error of St. Hilary had been an excess of zeal, which led him to place men from the monastic life in bishoprics, passing over canonical provisions for the election of bishops. He may have done this in ignorance of the extent of his own power at Arles, since that See had been granted some privileges of provincial jurisdiction. At any rate, he submitted to the papal decrees. The whole case supports the claim of special authority for the successor of St. Peter and witnessess the submission to that claim by the bishops of France.

St. Leo's power made itself felt much farther than just France. A second council met at Ephesus in 449 A.D. The papal legates were badly treated; the Council reinstated Eutyches and deposed St. Flavian as Bishop of Constantinople. St. Leo called the Council a den of thieves and rejected its decrees. History has kept the name he supplied, and it is known as the Robber Council of Ephesus. St. Leo also flatly rejected the 28th canon of the Council of Chalcedon, which raised the ecclesiastical powers of the See of Constantinople because of its growing civil importance. "Resolutions of bishops which are repugnant to the rules of the holy canons laid down at Nicaea, in cooperation with the loyalty of your faith," he wrote to the Empress Pulcheria, "we annul and cancel, with a decision of general application for the future, by the authority of blessed Peter the Apostle, since in all ecclesiastical questions we respect the laws which the Holy Ghost defined through the 318 [bishops at the Council of Nicaea], to be kept peaceably by all bishops." He also wrote a sharp letter of reproof to Anatolius, Bishop of Constantinople.

The two decades of St. Leo the Great's pontificate were years of upheaval in both Church and state. The distant rumblings of massive change could be heard through the clamor of present disputes. St. Leo kept pointing to the "rock of unity" on which the Church was founded. He kept reminding everybody that Peter lived in Peter's see.

Unity in Christ

St. Leo's love for unity proceeded from a deep spiritual well— his love for Christ and the conviction that the "saints" are united in Christ through the Church. *Sermon* 63 describes the unity of the Mystical Body of Christ.

> There is no doubt, therefore, dearly beloved, that man's nature has been received by the Son of God into such a union that, not only in that Man who is the first-begotten of all creatures, but also in all His saints, there is one and the self-same Christ, and as the Head cannot be separated from the members, so the members cannot be separated from the Head. For although it is not in this life, but in eternity that God is to be "all in all," yet even now He is the inseparable inhabitant of His temple, which is the Church, according as He Himself promised, saying, "Behold I am with you all days, even to the consummation of the world." (*Matt.* 28:20).

St. Leo the Great writes beautifully of Holy Communion:

> For naught else is brought about by the partaking of the Body and Blood of Christ than that we pass into that which we then take, and both in spirit and in body carry everywhere Him, in and with whom we were dead, buried and rose again.

Union with Christ in the Mystical Body and in the Sacraments should generate enough loyalty to overcome the obstacles generated by ignorance and weakness. St. Leo never hesitated to speak out, asserting the truth of doctrine and the demands of discipline according to established law. He acted strongly on behalf of doctrine and discipline, but he always used restraint and moderation with individuals. He gives us his own philosophy in a letter in which he chides Anastasius, Bishop of Thessalonica, for the misuse of power granted by delegation. First he quotes St. Paul (*1 Tim.* 5:1-2).

> Wherefore also it is that the blessed apostle Paul, in instructing Timothy upon the ruling of the Church, says: "Do not rebuke an elderly man, but exhort him as you would a father, and young men as brothers, elderly women as mothers, younger women as sisters, in all chastity." And if this moderation is due by the Apostle's precept to any and all of the lower members, how much more is it to be paid without offence to our brethren and fellow-bishops? That is, although men of priestly rank sometimes do things that are to be reprimanded, yet kindness may have more effect on those who are to be corrected than severity: exhortation than perturbation: love than power. But they who "seek their own interests, not those of Jesus Christ," easily depart from this law . . . The fact that we are obliged to speak thus, causes us no small grief.

In the life of St. Leo the Great there are many instances of his correcting bishops, some of whom were quite holy. We may think of St. Hilary of Arles. If we are inclined to be scandalized by all this, it is well to recall that holy people also make mistakes, have defects and sometimes sin. The saint is one who rises from mistakes and sins, and serves God despite defects. He is not born a saint, but grows into one. At some time before he dies, his whole being, with heroic virtue, is finally turned completely toward the love of God.

Just as there can and will be differences and problems within a family, which nonetheless do not sever but rather increase love, so within the Church problems arise. But if the true love of Christ and of one another is present, the bonds of union among the members are not broken, but strengthened. One of man's dearest privileges is to differ with vigor and without bitterness. He must also have the privilege of being forgiven after making mistakes. It is with these principles of love and with a realistic viewpoint of the humanness of Christ's Church as a background that Catholic unity can flourish.

St. Leo sternly rebuking, yet tenderly loving; St. Leo so devoted to Christ as the sole Mediator between God and man, and yet so devoted to Christ's plan for a supreme, visible authority in the Church, is worthily called "The Doctor of the Unity of the Church." In his life and in his words there is much to consider that can lead to this unity.

The last words we have from St. Leo close a letter of August, 460. He is speaking of mutual charity:

> . . . the same medicine must be applied to all wounds in all places, in order that the Lord's flock may be restored in all the churches through the zeal of the shepherds, and so that through concern for charity, all Christ's sheep may feel that they have one shepherd.

St. Leo's feast day is November 10 (April 11 in the 1962 calendar).

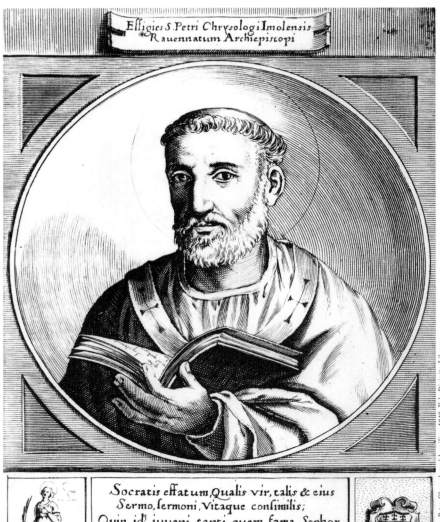

Effigies S. Petri Chryfologi Imolenfis
Rauennatum Archiepifcopi

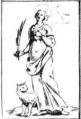

Socratis effatum, Qualis vir, talis & eius
Sermo, fermoni, Vitaque confimilis;
Quin id? iuueni, tanti quem fama Sopho꜓
Principis excierat, Fare, ait, vt uideam
In te vtrumq; cadit, mira benè note loquela
Antiftes, tibi funt aurea & Os, & Opus.

✠ Dominicus Mita Parochus Ecclefiæ S. Agnetis imprimj curauit .

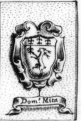

From a volume of *St. Peter Chrysologus' homilies,* 1643. Yale Divinity Library.

Saint Peter Chrysologus

13

SAINT PETER CHRYSOLOGUS
The Golden-Worded
c. 406-c. 450

"MAY our God deign to give me the grace of speaking and you the desire of hearing." (*Sermon* 96). With an interchange of pronouns, these words would make a fine prayer for the faithful as the priest walks to the pulpit. St. Peter Chrysologus, first archbishop and twenty-first bishop of Ravenna, Italy, used them at the end of a sermon. In a way, they sum up his life and achievements. He is commonly known as Chrysologus, which means "golden-worded." His baptismal name of Peter either goes before this title of honor or is often simply dropped.

History has left us this flattering title and little more to describe the life of St. Peter Chrysologus. Our knowledge of the facts of his life depends chiefly on a short biography and on what can be deduced from his own writings. The biography was not written until about 400 years after his death. It is one of a series by the Abbot Agnellus about the bishops of Ravenna (*Liber Pontificalis*), and is not considered entirely reliable.

The usual dates given for St. Peter's life are A.D. 406-450. He was born at Imola (formerly Forocornelio), 22 miles from Bologna, Italy. We do not know the names of Peter's parents nor anything about his family. In *Sermon* 165 he tells us of Cornelius, the Bishop of Imola, who had much to do with his training.

> He was a father to me. He begot me through the Gospel. Devout himself, he devoutly nourished me; holy himself, he trained me in the holy service. As a bishop, he brought me to the sacred altar and consecrated me.

Agnellus tells the famous story of how St. Peter Chrysologus became bishop. According to this, he was a deacon in the service of Bishop Cornelius, having charge of all his properties. When John (called Angelitis), Bishop of Ravenna died, the people and clergy chose a new bishop and sent him and a delegation to Rome to secure approval. Bishop Cornelius of Imola went along, accompanied by his deacon, Peter.

During the night before the delegation was to come before Pope Sixtus III, the Pope had a vision in which the Apostle Peter and St. Appolinaris, disciple of the Apostle for seven years at Antioch and founder of the Church at Ravenna, appeared to him, with Peter Chrysologus standing between them. St. Peter the Apostle told Sixtus: "See this man whom we have chosen and who stands between us. Consecrate him and no other." When the delegates from Ravenna presented themselves and the elected candidate, Sixtus said that he would ordain only the one he had seen, at which the group left quite confused and downcast.

The next day the Pope saw the group again and told them that somebody must be missing, as the one for whom he was looking was not among them. Sixtus had the same vision a second time. Still not seeing the chosen one upon the next visit by the delegation, Sixtus asked Cornelius to bring in all who were with him. As soon as he saw St. Peter Chrysologus, Sixtus went forward and saluted him, and told the assembly that this was the man who must be the new bishop of Ravenna. A great deal of argument and complaint arose. Then Sixtus finally related the story of his visions, and all were unanimous and enthusiastic in agreeing to accept the young deacon from a lesser see as their bishop. This was about 433 A.D. (The above story is condensed from the Latin of Agnellus.)

Ravenna at the time was the seat of government for the Western Roman Empire, which it remained until the eighth century. St. Peter Chrysologus became well acquainted with Galla Placidia, daughter of Theodosius the Great and Regent during the minority of her son, and he secured her help in constructing and artistically enriching various churches in Ravenna. In the apse of one of them which he consecrated, that of St. John the Evangelist, he was pictured with a long beard, celebrating Mass on board ship before the "Augusta," Galla Placidia.

Because of its imperial influence, the city is even today the richest treasure-house of ancient Christian art, noted in particular for its colorful and sparkling mosaics. Not even Rome can show as many examples of Church architecture from the fourth to the eighth centuries. It was in Ravenna that Dante spent his final years, composing most of *The Divine Comedy*, and it was here that he was first buried.

Toward the end of his life, St. Peter Chrysologus went back to his native city of Imola, and it was there that he died. He was buried in the church of the martyr St. Cassian. There also are kept the large gold chalice and silver paten which he had presented as a gift upon his return. Dominic Mita, parish priest at Imola, wrote a life of St. Peter Chrysologus in 1642 in which he relates that many people came to drink water poured from the paten, and were healed from the bites of rabid dogs and various fevers. They would come to venerate the remains of St. Peter Chrysologus and drink the water; often they took home water which had come into contact with the silver dish.

Chrysologus Neglected

Although Pope Benedict XIII named him a Doctor of the Church in 1729, St. Peter Chrysologus has received strangely scant notice in patrologies and in the history of theology. Some scholars tend to dismiss him as of very little importance. Another opinion says that Pope Leo the Great relied on him in formulating the renowned letter to Flavian—"Leo's Tome"—which was later accepted by the Council of Chalcedon as the basis of Christology. If this is so, then St. Peter Chrysologus had a large share in shaping our customary mode of speaking about Christ.

The most usual estimate of St. Peter Chrysologus is that he was primarily an orator who did not develop theology, but presented it in good, clear terms to the people. He spoke with unusual clarity on the Incarnation, the Blessed Virgin, St. Joseph, and the Mystical Body. His importance, in this same estimation, lies in his having been a good pastor to the people of Ravenna, a good teacher of morals and spiritual life.

It is well to remember several points that will have a bearing in guiding scholars to a more definite conclusion with regard to St. Peter Chrysologus' work. As Dominic Mita laments, it may be God's will that we know the lion only by a claw. St. Peter Chrysologus wrote many letters, commentaries, and sermons. But most of his writings have perished, some in the siege of Imola by Theodoric, others in the fire which destroyed the archbishop's library in Ravenna about the year 700.

Again, those writings which have survived need careful editing. Of St. Peter's works, all we have is a collection of 176 sermons, mostly short, and one letter. A few of the sermons are definitely not his, but in time, other writings of St. Peter

Chrysologus now listed in other collections may be identified as his.

The influence of St. Peter Chrysologus showed itself in a very direct way more than a thousand years after his death, when, in the period 1534-1761, 44 separate editions of his sermons were printed. Finally, the very fact that St. Peter Chrysologus has been admitted to the select circle of Doctors indicates that he has an importance for the Universal Church.

There is also some discussion about the title of Chrysologus, "The Golden-Worded" or "The Golden Speaker." It has been charged that the Latins invented the term so that they might have a champion with a title to correspond to that of St. John Chrysostom, the "golden-voiced" patriarch of Constantinople. The better explanation is that the name "Chrysologus" was given to St. Peter by the Greeks who resided at the imperial court at Ravenna. The memory of their own eloquent St. John Chrysostom was fresh, and when they heard the fervent outpouring from St. Peter, they noticed his sincerity and admired his well-balanced diction, and thus bestowed upon him the name of "Chrysologus." This explanation is given in the manuscript in the archives of the Capuchins in Bologna. (Cf. Mita in PL, v. 52, no. 36). The fact that St. Peter knew some Greek himself would have helped to make them more fond of him. The title "Chrysologus" is first met in the biography of St. Peter by the Abbot Agnellus (also called Andrew).

Cardinal Newman said that he preferred the Saints of the early Church and knew them better than later ones, just because with the early Saints he did not have to rely on biographies— these men spoke for themselves in their sermons and letters. "Words are the exponents of thoughts," Cardinal Newman said, "and a silent saint is the object of faith rather than of affection. If he speaks, then we have the original before us; if he is silent, we must put up with a copy, done with more or less skill according to the painter."

Almost one third of Chrysologus' sermons are at present available in English. (Vol. 17 of *The Fathers of the Church*). And for one who wants to ponder this part of the "lion's claw" there should emerge a living image. What we have left of Chrysologus' writings would constitute, in Cardinal Newman's opinion, a great deal of material for getting acquainted with him. As the Cardinal says of the Saints: "Some of them manifest themselves by their short sayings and their single words more graphically than if they had written a volume." We can still regret, however, that

Newman himself did not choose such excerpts from Chrysologus and weave them together to present a unified picture of the Saint's mind, character and teaching.

A Spiritual Guide

St. Peter Chrysologus was a real shepherd of the flock, who constantly turned to God for help and used all his own talent and energies to protect the sheep entrusted to him and guide them safely. He was very interested not only in helping them get to Heaven, but in having them reach the particular perfection of which their particular souls were capable.

> O man, beloved thus by God, return to God. Give your whole self to glorifying Him who for your sake humiliated His whole Self to bearing all His sufferings. Have confidence when you call Him Father whom you so lovingly accept, feel, and know as your Father.

St. Peter Chrysologus was not satisfied with half measures.

> Since you are named a Christian after Christ, you ask to have the privilege of having such a name glorified in your own case. For God's Name, which is holy by its nature and in itself, is in our case either glorified by our conduct or blasphemed among the Gentiles through our misdeeds. (*Sermon* 70).

The approach to God is by faith combined with humility:

> He who believes in God should not rashly try to fathom Him . . . The sun blacks out an imprudent gazing and . . . an unpermitted approach to God becomes a blinded one. He who desires to know God should observe moderation in his gazing. (*Sermon* 61).

In speaking of the virginal conception of Christ, St. Peter Chrysologus advises in a similar vein:

> Be reverently aware of the fact that God wishes to be born, because you offer an insult if you examine it too much. Grasp by faith that great mystery of the Lord's birth because without faith you cannot comprehend even the least of God's works.

In a phrase that must stun the rationalist's approach, St. Peter Chrysologus then asks: "What is so much according to reason as the fact that God can do whatever He has willed? He who cannot do what he wills is not God." (*Sermon* 141).

His Humble Reverence

As he approaches God with faith and humility, so does St. Peter Chrysologus approach men with reverence and humility. He is not a driver, but a quiet leader of men. Despite the vigor of his oratory, there is always a basic moderation in what he says. He advises fasting, but not overdoing it. The food for our souls which fasting is must be compounded "wisely and properly, lest something too salty or completely unsalted beget a fatal distaste for all nourishing food."

> Let the fast be one properly measured. And, as we received from tradition, let it be observed for the discipline of both the body and the soul. Surely, let not the one who is unable to fast start some innovation. Rather, let him acknowledge that it is through his personal weakness that he mitigates his fast, and let him redeem by alms-giving what he cannot fulfill by fasting. For the Lord does not require groans from him who has thus acquired the cries of the poor as pleadings for himself. (*Sermon* 166).

St. Peter Chrysologus gives us a fine insight into his reverent approach as he tells of the dilemma of St. Joseph when Mary was found with child of the Holy Spirit.

> "He was minded to put her away privately." This seems to be characteristic of a man in love rather than of a just man. [However,] justice does not exist without goodness, nor goodness without justice. If these virtues are separated, they vanish. Equity without goodness is savagery; justice without love is cruelty. Rightly, therefore, was Joseph just, because he was loving; he was loving because just. While he nourished his love, he was free from cruelty. While he kept his emotions under control, he preserved his judgment. (*Sermon* 145).

Then St. Peter Chrysologus makes the application for us and incidentally shows us further insight into his humble reverence.

We, too, brethren, whenever something troubles us, or some appearance deceives us, or the outward color of a transaction makes us unable to know its substance, let us restrain our judgment. Let us withhold punishment, refrain from condemnation, and tell the whole matter to God. Otherwise, while we perhaps easily impel an innocent man toward a penalty, we shall pronounce a sentence of condemnation upon ourselves. The Lord says, "With what judgment you judge, you shall be judged." But if we keep silent, the Lord will surely speak aloud." (as the Angel spoke to Joseph). (*Sermon* 145).

In a similar vein he tells us to do positive good to evildoers. (*Sermon* 38).

Therefore, brethren, he who wants to overcome vices should fight with the arms of love, not of rage. A wise man can readily see why endurance of injuries gives training toward a Christian way of living. Nevertheless, there are those who fail to understand that to do what follows is indeed a mark of strength, the summit of goodness, the pinnacle of piety, something characteristic of the divine outlook, rather than the human: not to resist the evil-doer, but to overcome evil with good; to bless the one who curses; to refrain from denying one who strikes you a chance to strike again; to give also your cloak to one who has taken your tunic, and thereby to give a gift to the one who has snatched booty; to add compliance for two more miles to one who forces you to go a mile; to do all this that willingness may take precedence over force, and love may overcome impiety, and that the very thing which your adversary forces may become the virtue of the patient man. Those examples teach us how a soldier of Christ is trained by injuries to the strength to practice virtues.

Centered on Christ

The spiritual direction of St. Peter Chrysologus centers on Christ. He emphasizes our adoption as sons of God. But he does not leave this as an empty, mystic phrase. In fact he warns against the idea of majesty and size, and spells out in plain, practical terms the virtues which he thinks most agreeably demonstrate our union with Christ, our supernatural adoption as sons, and our likeness to God. In his choice we can see, no doubt, the virtues he himself especially cherished and cultivated.

Let us who have been re-born to the likeness of Our Lord, (whom) God adopted as His sons—let us bear the image of our Creator in a perfect reproduction. Let it be a reproduction, not of that majesty in which He is unique, but of that innocence, simplicity, meekness, patience, humility, mercy, and peacefulness by which He deigned to become and to be one with us . . . May we desire Christ's poverty, which stores its everlasting riches in Heaven. May we preserve complete holiness of soul and body, that we may bear and enhance our Creator's image in ourselves in regard not to its size, but to our way of acting. (*Sermon* 117).

A modern doctoral study on the Incarnation in the sermons of St. Peter Chrysologus reports that

The just man who lives in Christ and in whom Christ lives is told of his great dignity by St. Peter in many beautiful passages. He becomes a consort, a partner, and a participant of the divine nature, and all this through Christ. No longer is his life to be limited by the bonds of earth, but its fullness is found rather in union with God. He is henceforth a partner of life, not death, and the fruit of his life now belongs to God, and not to the demands of flesh. (Robert H. McGlynn: *The Incarnation in the Sermons of St. Peter Chrysologus,* Mundelein, Illinois: St. Mary of the Lake Seminary, 1956, p. 134).

All of us receive our truest value from our union with Christ. The closer our union, the more do we share in His life and the more glory do we give to God. This basic thought brings St. Peter Chrysologus logically to the first one who was most closely and most uniquely united to Christ, His own Mother.

Let those come and hear who ask who He is whom Mary brought forth: "That which is begotten in her is of the Holy Spirit." Let those come and hear who have striven to becloud the clarity of the Latin tongue by a whirlwind of Greek, and have blasphemously called her *anthropotokos* ("mother of the human nature") and *Christotokos* ("Mother of Christ") in order to rob her of the title *Theotokos* ("Mother of God"). (*Sermon* 145).

Through the curse she incurred, Eve brought pains upon the wombs of women in childbirth. Now in this very matter of motherhood, Mary, through the blessing she received, rejoices, is honored, is exalted. Now, too, womankind has become truly the mother of those who live through grace, just as previously she

was the mother of those who by nature are subject to death
. . . It was by a soothing motion and holy affection that God
transformed the virgin into a Mother for Himself, and His handmaid into a parent. (*Sermon* 140).

Growth in Christ

The solidity of St. Peter's spiritual direction shows itself very
plainly in his ideas on spiritual growth. He knows that God
leads souls individually, that each has his own proper perfection. Therefore, he counsels much on attaining virtues; each person has to strive consciously to attain particular good habits.
But St. Peter Chrysologus never loses sight of the grand picture, that of a fully developed Mystical Body of Christ. Each
person should try to reach perfection, therefore, so that the full
beauty and glory of Christ may be reached. Christ is, of course,
already perfect as the Head of the Body. It is now up to the
members to strive for perfection, so that the Body may be perfect in all its parts. Nothing can be clearer than St. Peter
Chrysologus' own words on the subject:

> It is true that the individual members have, each one, their
> own function to perform. But they will fulfill these respective
> functions best if they are joined together and compacted and
> attain to the full beauty of the fully developed Body. This,
> therefore, is the difference between the glorious richness of a
> congregation and the presumptuous vanity of separation, which
> springs either from ignorance or negligence: that from the
> health and praiseworthiness of the entire body a beautiful
> unity arises, while from the separation of its members there
> springs base, deadly, and hideous ruin . . . The eye is precious
> for the healthy functioning of the members—but only if it
> remains in the body. Otherwise, when it fails the body, it also
> fails itself. (*Sermon* 132).

> Whoever he is who thinks that he is something, let him be
> instructed by such an example and remain in the Church, that
> he may be something. Otherwise, when he fails the Church, he
> soon terminates his own importance. If anyone desires a more
> extensive understanding of this, let him read the Apostle's trea-
> tise in which he speaks about the Body . . . Brethren, suppose
> that a man is evil to himself, and because of his shortcomings
> foolishly self-sufficient. Suppose that thus he seeks life outside
> the Church. He loses divine gifts, he spoils the outpouring of
> grace, he cheats himself of the benefits of charity. The bless-

ing of that unity will not await him. The Prophet testifies that that life is only in the Church: "Behold, how good and pleasant it is for brethren to dwell together in unity . . . For there the Lord hath commanded blessing and life forevermore." (*Sermon* 132).

In one of his seven sermons on the *Apostle's Creed*, St. Peter Chrysologus shows how deep his idea of unity really is.

The holy Catholic Church—yes, because neither are the members separated from the Head nor the spouse from her husband. But, by such a union, the Church becomes one spirit; she becomes all things, and God is in them all. Therefore he believes in God who acknowledges the holy Church as something united to God. (*Sermon* 57).

Need for Authority

St. Peter Chrysologus' final interest is always in uniting men to Christ. To be separated from Him is spiritual ruin. To keep unity with Christ, to prevent separation, St. Peter strongly endorses the need of a teaching authority:

When cautious physicians skillfully prepare a remedy of salutary juices against deadly diseases, and if the patient rashly takes it differently from the directions, or in an amount not conducive to healing, or with improper timing, that which was planned to bring health becomes a cause of danger. So too, if the hearer rashly tries to understand the word of God without the Teaching Authority, and learning, and the doctrine of the Faith, that which is the nutrition of life becomes an occasion of perdition. We must strive, brethren, that what has been divinely written for our progress may not turn out, through our lack of skill in hearing, to be something detrimental to our souls. (*Sermon* 156).

The only extant letter of St. Peter Chrysologus is a reply to Eutyches, who had written to St. Peter after he, Eutyches, had been condemned by the synod at Constantinople under Flavian for holding that in Christ there is only one nature. Eutyches, the archimandrite (or superior of a monastery in the East), was 70 years old and ill. St. Peter's reply is written in a kindly vein, and has a clear-cut reference to a Teaching Authority in the Church.

I have read your sad letter with deep grief and run through the details with a sympathetic regret corresponding to their sorrowful nature. For, just as peace among the churches, mutual harmony among priests, and the tranquility of the people cause us to rejoice with heavenly joy, so fraternal dissension afflicts and depresses us, especially when it arises from causes such as these . . . I have made these brief replies to your letter, dear Brother . . . However, we give you this exhortation in regard to everything, honorable Brother: obediently heed these matters which the most blessed Pope of the city of Rome has written, because blessed Peter, who lives and presides in his own see, proffers the truth of faith to those who seek it. For in accordance with our pursuit of peace and of faith, we cannot decide upon cases of faith without the harmonious agreement of the Bishop of Rome. May the Lord deign to preserve your love unharmed, very dear and honorable Son.

Oratorical Style

While some have criticized the style of St. Peter Chrysologus as labored and contrived, another estimation says that "no translation can adequately do justice to his concise, lapidary sentences." (R. Rios in *Clergy Review*, 1945, p. 312). His style is quite similar to that of Pope Leo the Great. It is easy to picture St. Peter Chrysologus spending many an hour composing his sermons, building up phrases, balancing them, framing antitheses. If there are a few labored phrases, there are many more of beauty and energy, often putting valuable truths in a way to be remembered.

You cannot easily forget such expressions as "the thief who stole paradise at the very time when he was hung upon the cross to pay the price for his brigandage." (*Sermon* 61). "The law of nature made Cain the firstborn son, but envious jealousy made him an only son." (*Sermon* 4). Of the sinful woman who bathed Christ's feet with her tears, St. Peter Chrysologus says: "Now the earth irrigates the heavens; even more the rain of human tears has leaped above the heavens, and all the way up to the Lord Himself." (*Sermon* 93). Slogan writers might envy St. Peter's way of giving advice on almsgiving: "Lest you lose by saving, gather in by giving out. O man, give to yourself by giving to the poor man. For you will yet possess what you leave to another." (*Sermon* 43). For laconic, wry humor combined with sober truth, we may consider this: "Although the heavenly region is very spacious, it does not admit the sinner."

The oratorical balance of St. Peter Chrysologus' thought and phrasing is illustrated all through the sermon on Mary Magdalen:

> She came to make satisfaction to God, not to please men. She came to provide a banquet of devotion, not of pleasure. She set a table of repentance, served courses of compunction and the bread of sorrow. She mixed the drink with tears in proper measure, and to the full delight of God she struck music from her heart and body. She produced the organ tones of her lamentations, played upon the zither by her long and rhythmical sighs and fitted her groans to the flute. (*Sermon* 93).

Chrysologus paints a colorful oratorical picture of the grief of the Apostles the night of the Resurrection before Christ appeared to them:

> At that time all the distress of the Lord's Passion had passed over to His disciples. The whole lance of sorrow was piercing not only to their sides, but their very hearts. Their hands and feet were held fast by the nails of the clinging grief. The bitter spirit of the Jews was then giving them vinegar and gall to drink. For them the sun had set and the day had waned. At that time severe temptation of thought was dashing them against the crags of infidelity to shipwreck their faith. Despair, which is worse than all evils and is in adversity always the last one to arrive, was already laying them out in sombre tombs. (*Sermon* 83).

Various Examples

One can pick up a short saying full of meaning or a paragraph that is graphic and clear on most of the pages of St. Peter Chrysologus. Consider: "He who thinks that he knows everything does not know himself." (*Sermon* 44). "The man who does not do what the Lord has commanded hopes without reason for what the Lord has promised." (*Sermon* 38).

Following are some sample paragraphs on forgiveness, envy, confidence in God, the ways of the devil, mildness, sin, adversity, the love of Christ.

> [*On forgiveness*:] "Forgive us our debts as we also forgive our debtors." By these words, O man, you have set the manner and measure of forgiveness to yourself. You ask the Lord to forgive

you exactly as much as you forgive to your fellow servant. Therefore, forgive the whole offense to the one who wrongs you if you wish to be liable to the Lord for nothing because of your own sins. For your own sake, be forgiving in the case of another man, if you wish to avoid the avenging sentence. (*Sermon* 70).

[*On envy:*] Envy is an ancient evil, the first sin, an old venom, the poison of the ages, a cause of death. In the beginning, this vice expelled the devil from Heaven and cast him down. This vice shut the first parent of our race out of Paradise. It kept this elder brother out of his father's house [brother of the Prodigal Son]. It armed the children of Abraham, the holy people, to work the murder of their Creator, the death of their Saviour. Envy is an interior foe. It does not batter the walls of the flesh or break down the encompassing armor of the members, but it plies its blows against the very citadel of the heart. Before the organs are aware, like a pirate it captures the soul, the master of the body, and leads it off as a prisoner. (*Sermon* 4).

[*Confidence in God:*] If God invites a man to work, and man comes burdened and anxious with a wallet, bread, and wages, how inhuman he believes God to be! That man approaches the work either as a tired or sluggish worker, or perhaps he cannot even approach! God promises abundant rewards, by His numerous signed bonds and His witnesses. He promises a generous reward. Do you think that, in a niggardly spirit, He will supply neither bread nor clothing? He granted you existence when you were not. Whatever you have, O man, He gave to you.

[*The ways of the devil:*] In guiding those entrusted to his care, St. Peter Chrysologus often warns of that enemy of mankind so commonly forgotten today, namely, the devil. On top of the growing crop of the Gospel, sown with the seed from Heaven, he sowed heretical cockle. Thus the Enemy caused a puzzling mixture, that he might make the sheaves of Faith bundles for Hell, that no wheat might get stored in the barns of Heaven. What more should I say? After he was himself changed from an angel into a devil, he hastened to use ingenuity, tricks, devices, and deceit to keep any creature from remaining secure in his own state.

"He sowed weeds among the wheat"—because the devil has become accustomed to sow of his own accord heresies among the faithful, sin among the saints, quarrels among the peaceful, deceptions among the simple, and wickedness among the innocent. He does this, not to acquire the weeds of cockle, but to destroy the wheat; not to capture the guilty ones, but to steal away the innocent. An enemy seeks the leader rather than a soldier. He does not besiege the dead, but attacks the living. Thus, the devil is not seeking to capture sinners whom he already has under his dominion, but is laboring thus to ensnare the just . . . The devil does not wish to possess a man, but to destroy him. Why? Because he does not wish, he does not dare, he does not allow the man to arrive at the Heaven from which the devil fell. (*Sermon* 96).

Chrysologus tells us how the devil tries to destroy beginnings.

The devil ever disturbs the first beginning of good; he tests the rudiments of the virtues, he hastens to destroy holy deeds in their first origins, well aware that he cannot overturn them once they are well-founded. (*Sermon* 11).

Again the devil plays his destructive game to the hilt. The devil's insatiable cruelty is what causes him to send his hirelings to the swine. Not content that men become criminal, he also makes them leaders in vice and teachers of crime. And once he has made them such, he does not let them get satisfied even with the food and fodder of the swine. Wanton men cannot find satiety; their passion cannot be satisfied; consequently, in their hunger they commit more vices still. (*Sermon* 2).

[*On mildness*:] He [God] wants us to smother anger when it is still only a spark. If it grows to the full flame of its fury, it does not get checked without bloodshed. Mildness overcomes anger, meekness extinguishes fury, goodness coaxes malice away, affection lays cruelty low, patience is the scourge of impatience, gentle words vanquish quarrelsomeness, and humility prostrates pride. Therefore he who wants to overcome vices should fight with the arms of love, not of rage. (*Sermon* 38).

[*On sins*:] Blessed is he who does not stand still on that way. He stands and loiters in that way who picks up burdens of sins, and arrives late like an overburdened traveler, and finds the heavenly mansion closed to him. (*Sermon* 44).

[*On adversity*:] Slaps are the beatings given to children, not to men. Hence it is that the infants of Christ are urged on by light commands, that when they are the men who live out the gospel, they may have the full strength to undertake its more serious precepts.

[*On the love of Christ*:] For the sake of His sheep, the Shepherd met the death which was threatening them. He did this that by a new arrangement He might, although captured Himself, capture the devil, the author of death; that although conquered Himself, He might conquer; that although slain Himself, He might punish; that by dying for His sheep, He might open the way for them to conquer death. (*Sermon* 40).

For our instruction the Lord often uses symbolic examples. He has always desired to be the Father of His servants and to be loved more than feared. He gave Himself as the Bread of life and poured His Blood into the cup of salvation. (*Sermon* 2).

Close to His Audiences

St. Peter Chrysologus watched his audience. "I observe that, as you listen, you are not experiencing fitting compassion nor deeming these matters our concern; rather, you are passing over them quickly with fleeting attention." (Sermon 2). He uses many examples from the world about us and from the events of daily living He speaks so often of physicians and medicine that we may perhaps assume that he had a special interest in these subjects because of ill health in his own life, or that he had an unusually tender heart for the sick. Chrysologus followed Christ, of whom he said: "He makes heavenly goods appear attractive through earthly examples. He uses beings of the present world to make us relish those of the future world. He represents invisible benefits by visible evidence. (*Sermon* 47).

We can easily feel how close St. Peter Chrysologus himself was to people by the way he describes Christ's closeness to us:

By the fact that He assumes human nature, acts the part of man, enters into the centuries, passes through the periods of life, teaches by word, works cures by His power, tells parables, gives examples, and manifests in Himself the burden of our emotions—by all this He reveals that He has an indescribable affection of human love. (*Sermon* 47).

The term "the burden of our emotions" seems to show the user to be a person of feeling, perhaps one who had to fight to keep his heart from overruling the dictates of cold intelligence. The piety of St. Peter Chrysologus had warmth. He did not reject the feelings as being an unsuitable partner for faith. In fact, he prayed for sensible devotion. "Let us beg, too, that the heat of that coal may penetrate all the way to our hearts. Thus we may draw from the great sweetness of this mystery, not only relish for our lips, but also complete satisfaction for our senses and minds." (*Sermon* 57).

His own strong feeling is quite evident in a very beautiful passage describing how the knowledge brought by faith strains for expression. It makes one sad over not being able to relate all that one feels and sees about God.

> As much as the flesh is limited, just that much are the lips too narrow for their spirit, and the tongue too short to explain its mind. A roaring fire is shut up in the flesh. It fills the veins with steam, inflames the inmost members, and seethes in the marrow. It always enkindles a man's whole interior, because he finds himself unable to express adequately with his mouth what he contemplates in the absorption of his mind. He cannot pour it out of his lips, adorn it with his language, and put it like steam into his whole speech. (*Sermon* 57).

St. Peter Chrysologus tried to speak to all who were in his audience.

> We should speak to the populace in popular fashion. The parish ought to be addressed by ordinary speech. Matters necessary to all men should be spoken about as men speak in general. Natural language is dear to simple souls and sweet to the learned. A teacher should speak words which will profit all. Therefore, today let the learned grant pardon for commonplace language. (*Sermon* 43)

It is possible that Chrysologus spoke more than once during the Mass, perhaps after both the Epistle and the Gospel. But he always showed sensitiveness to his listeners by his custom of giving short sermons. The average length for delivery would be about 15 minutes, and some of his sermons are much shorter. Many times he speaks of cutting off a discourse and continuing the same subject later. *Sermon* 1 ends with the words, "As you all desire, we shall investigate these matters in a later sermon." When being enticed "away from the customary brevity of our sermons, we preferred to cut our discourse in half lest it seem to start anew to such an extent as to overburden your patience to listen." (*Sermon* 36).

A True Shepherd

One critic says of St. Peter Chrysologus' sermons, "At times they carry us away with their pathos and the energy of their condensed diction." When we add up the impressions gathered from a perusal of his sermons, we see St. Peter Chrysologus as a man of great intensity and much compassion. The truths of Faith are so real and so full of meaning and value, his interest in the salvation of the people so deep, that his words at times seem to be bursting at the seams of his ability to express himself. He was himself sometimes affected by his sermons to such an extent that he was unable to continue them. His voice sometimes failed him, as when he grieved over the suffering Church, comparing her wounds to those of the woman suffering from a hemorrhage (*Sermon* 36); or he would shed tears, as when, on another occasion, he was speaking of the Passion of Christ. (*Sermon* 77).

St. Peter's sympathy for others made him a provider for the poor and for captives. His prayer to God for the sinner was for mercy, long-suffering and patience. He used to beg God to grant the erring one more chance. (Cf. Mita, No. 22).

According to St. Peter Chrysologus' first biographer, when he was near death he went to the Church of St. Cassian at Imola and prayed for a worthy successor.

> Send them, O Lord, a true shepherd who will gather the sheep, not by cruelly driving them to common ruin, but by calling them to the sheepfold of the Church . . . Send a shepherd, not one who strikes, but one who nourishes; not one who injures, but who defends; not one who spurns, but who seeks; not one who plunders, but who bestows . . . not a proud man, but a humble man; not a cruel man, but one who is meek. Protect them. They are Your people, the work of Your hands, Who art blessed forever. (*Agnellus*, Ch. 4).

In asking for these virtues in his successor, St. Peter Chrysologus gives us a good description of himself.

As stated earlier, St. Peter Chrysologus seems to be one Doctor of the Church who has been neglected by scholars, probably because he was chosen relatively late—by Benedict XIII in 1729—

to be among this illustrious group. This may be an indication that his work in his own time, and now, is for the common man. In fact, one of the things that strikes a person in reading St. Peter Chrysologus is how very common and down-to-earth he sounds. This could be a tribute to his influence in being copied (at first consciously and later unconsciously) by preachers through the centuries.

A selection of sermons and passages from his sermons could prove to be a popular and valuable book, one well suited for moral encouragement and spiritual guidance. As Fr. Ganss remarks, "In many passages, if the reader proceeds slowly while relishing each thought, he will discover that he is not so much reading a sermon as making mental prayer of contemplation." (Fr. George Ganss, S.J., *Peter Chrysologus*, Vol. 17, 1953, *Fathers of the Church* series).

If St. Peter Chrysologus were alive today, he might well be a popular speaker because of his mastery of words. He would also find acceptance because he had the universally loved quality of compassion for all men. And he would do much good because his soul was centered on Christ and because his mind arranged all truth in relation to Christ. He would be popular because he was not speculative, but practical in directing people along the path of virtue.

St. Peter Chrysologus was a lovable man, and for that he would be loved in any age. Our age would love him more because it is so interested in growth and advancement. One of the basic points he often made is that God wills the growth of each individual to higher spiritual perfection, rather than that the individual attempt to just slip into Heaven. He viewed this growth in its proper setting as a development of the Mystical Body of Christ. For this sweeping and universal view, St. Peter Chrysologus is deservedly honored as a Doctor of the Universal Church. He was a shepherd who tried to lead his flock to richer spiritual pastures. His feast day is July 30 (December 4 in the 1962 calendar).

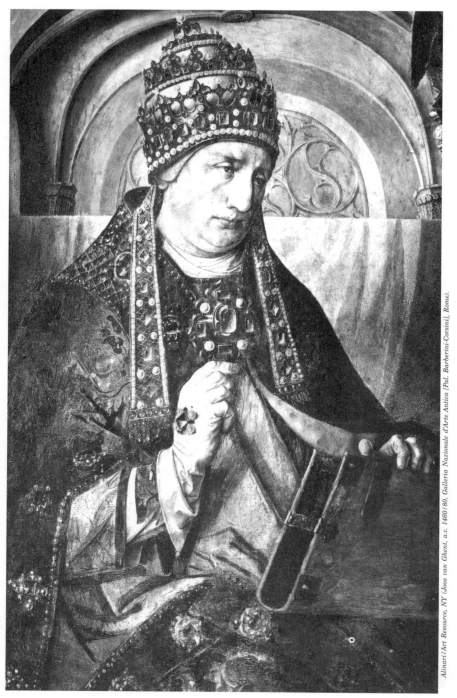

Alinari/Art Resource, NY (Joos van Ghent, a.c. 1460/80, Galleria Nazionale d'Arte Antica [Pal. Barberini-Corsini], Rome).

Pope Saint Gregory The Great

14

POPE ST. GREGORY THE GREAT

The Greatest of the Great

c. 540-604

IN a lonely rooming house in Rome a forgotten man died of starvation. When news of this came to the Pope, he felt so personally responsible and accused himself so deeply that he would not allow himself to say Mass for several days.

The incident gives us some insight into the mind and heart of that Pope—St. Gregory the Great, who reigned on the Chair of Peter from 590-604. He was a man of unusually deep humility plus a man with a profound sense of duty. He had a great ruler's ability to grasp worldwide problems and to deal with them without forgetting the smallest details close to home. He had a fully Christian heart, which made him his brother's keeper. Every day he invited 12 poor people to be guests at his table, and he was himself accustomed to pour the water with which they cleansed their hands. St. Gregory considered everybody to be his brother, especially the poor and the sinful.

Because he was a forceful and farsighted man, his influence had a broad, determining effect, not only upon the Church, but upon the growth of all medieval Europe. Historically, his was a tottering age, but he was the pillar on which it leaned. In his time, the city of Rome—which had been built to accommodate a million people—had been reduced to a relative ghost town of only 40,000. Rome was no longer the capital of the Empire. The real capital was Constantinople, established by the Emperor Constantine (who reigned from 306-337). The remains of the Western Roman Empire were weakly ruled by an exarch at Ravenna. St. Gregory, not by choice, but by the urgency of duty and love, rose to shape the channel of history in both the Church and the civil government.

Because St. Gregory the Great cared so much for each individual, his teachings have helped to form countless souls. His maxims have directed political rulers, bishops and priests. His words of advice have become a part of our Christian heritage.

All through his writings one can find thoughts that strike true to the human heart, sure evidence that he himself had an unusually good insight into that heart. For the throb of its over-elation and for the twinge or the stab of its sorrow, he had the remedy. He wrote to a friend who was grieving over criticism:

> Amid the words of flatterers and revilers we should always turn to our soul, and if we do not find there the good that is said of us, great sorrow should arise; and again, if we do not find there the evil that men speak of us, we should break forth into great joy. (*Epistle* 11, 2).

From a Saintly Family

St. Gregory was born in Rome about 540 A.D. of a renowned senatorial family whose exact name cannot be identified. We know that St. Gregory's father, Gordianus, held a civil post of some responsibility, and his mother, Sylvia, is venerated as a saint (November 3), as are two of his father's sisters, Tarsilla and Aemilia. He also had one brother, of whom nothing is known, not even his name. St. Gregory's childhood home was a spacious, palatial residence on the Coelian Hill, a site now occupied by the church and monastery of St. Gregory. Partial excavations indicate that the original palace, beneath this site, is still well-preserved.

Although Gregory received the best in liberal education of his day, the strongest influence on his mental development came from within his own deeply religious home. He was a thoughtful youth who liked to listen to the conversation of his elders. In later life, remembering this, he insisted repeatedly on the value of good surroundings for children. "For in truth," he says, "the words of those who bring up children will be as milk if they be good, but as deadly poison if they be evil." (*Epistle* 7, 23).

By about the age of 30, St. Gregory had attained the highest office in Rome. He was urban prefect and wielded more power in city government than does a modern mayor. At his father's death, he had also become one of Rome's richest men.

It must have caused quite a social stir when, still in his early thirties, he gave over his properties to found seven monasteries, and even more when he entered one of them himself. His own home became the Monastery of St. Andrew, and he placed himself there as a simple monk under a religious superior. A hospital was erected at the entrance to the monastery. Here it was quite a sight for the people to see their former prefect kneel at the feet of those whom he had formerly judged and perform humble services for them.

The fact that St. Gregory could make this change to the monastic life in his own familiar surroundings tells us much about the solidity of the piety and affection in which he had grown up. It also indicates how there dwelt within him at the same time the love of God, the spirit of prayer and penance, and a tender human love and concern for others. In St. Gregory the Great, detachment from the world never interfered with a warm attachment for friends. After many long years' absence he could write to his friend, St. Leander, Archbishop of Seville, "The image of thy countenance is impressed forever on my innermost heart." (*Epistle* 1, 41).

The few years he spent in strictly monastic life St. Gregory later recalled as the happiest of his life. When as Pope he was beset by many daily secular cares, he looked back and sighed for the peace of the monastery.

> My poor mind, distracted by the worry of business, reverts to old monastic days when passing events glided along far beneath it, while, soaring above the whirl of activity, it dwelt on things of God alone, and though still in the body, escaped from the bonds of flesh in contemplation, looking upon death, which almost all consider a penalty, as the entry into life and the crown of its labors . . . For now I am tossed on the waves of a mighty ocean and, like a vessel, my mind is dashed to and fro by the gusts of a violent storm; and when I recall my former life, looking back into the past, I sigh for the distant shore. And what is still worse, while I am borne on these high beating billows, I can scarcely get a glimpse of the harbor I have quitted. (Preface to *The Dialogues*).

John the Deacon, the ninth-century biographer of St. Gregory the Great, described his appearance minutely, referring to a picture on the wall of Gregory's Monastery of St. Andrew, which showed him and his parents. St. Gregory was of average height and of good proportion. He had a tawny, spare beard. His high forehead was topped by two sparse curls, which turned to the right. He was rather bald but had dark curly hair above the ears. His eyes had an open look and were touched with green. His nose was fairly long and slightly curved, his chin strong.

His hands were graceful, with slender fingers.

Deacon and Abbot

Though St. Gregory's life was hidden during his monastery years, his talents and reputation were remembered. Pope Benedict I (575-579) asked him to serve as a counselor and one of the seven deacons of the city. The next Pope, Pelagius II (579-590), chose St. Gregory to be his aprocrisarius (representative) at the court of the Roman Emperor in Constantinople. St. Gregory spent six years there, taking with him some monks, and in part was able to observe a monastic routine. It was at Constantinople that he did the basic work on his famous *Moralia* or *Morals on the Book of Job*, delivered as lectures to his monks. He felt a keen sense of failure because he could not obtain from the Emperor the troops that were asked for back in Italy. Yet for his own future career, his stay in Constantinople was invaluable, for he gained an insight into the workings of the imperial court, and he learned that if Italy were to be saved, vigorous independent action at home was necessary.

St. Gregory returned to Rome in 586 and was elected the abbot of the monastery he had founded. At this time there occurred the incident which he relates in the fourth book of his *Dialogues* and which in time gave rise to the custom of having Mass offered 30 consecutive days for a departed soul, still called a "Gregorian Mass." The incident illustrates very well, too, the balance of St. Gregory's severity and charity.

The "Gregorian Mass"

A certain monk named Justus, skilled in the art of medicine and who had often ministered to Gregory, fell sick. He knew that he was at death's door, and therefore told his brother Copiosus, who was attending him, that he had hidden three gold pieces. The money was found hidden among the medicines, and the fact was reported to St. Gregory. Wishing to benefit the erring Justus as well as all the monks, Gregory decided on a course that today seems quite severe—until, perhaps, we recall the case of Ananias and Saphira recounted in the *Acts of the Apostles* (Acts 5:1-11). All the brethren of the monastery were forbidden to visit Justus. When he called for them, none came, and it was pointed out to him why. Thus bemoaning and repenting his sin, he died. As further directed, his body was meanly buried in a dung heap apart from the other deceased of the monastery, and before the earth was put over him, the monks cast the three gold pieces onto his body, crying out, "Thy money go with thee to perdition!"

Thirty days after this, St. Gregory began to feel much compassion for poor Justus, and he summoned Pretiosus the prior, and told him sorrowfully:

> Our brother is a long time dead, and is suffering in fire: we ought to show some charity to him, and so far as we can to help him, that he may be released. Go therefore and see that the Holy Sacrifice is offered for him for 30 days, starting from today, and let not a single day pass by without the saving Host being immolated for his absolution.
>
> Engaged over other things [St. Gregory writes], we did not count the days as they passed, but one night the deceased monk appeared to his brother Copiosus in a vision. Upon seeing Justus, he questioned him, saying, "What is it, brother? How fare you?" Justus replied, "Up to this I have fared badly, but now, indeed, I am happy, for this day I am received into the Communion of Saints."

When Copiosus went to the monastery and reported this, they counted the days and found that it was exactly the 30th day since the Holy Sacrifice of the Mass had begun to be offered. (*Dialogues* 4, 55).

Almost a Missionary

Very likely it was at this time, too, that there occurred the event first recorded a century later by an unknown monk of Whitby. In telling the story, he speaks of English visitors; whereas, St. Bede makes them slaves.

Going through the Roman forum one day, St. Gregory saw three slaves for sale, their flaxen hair hanging down, their blue eyes glancing half-timidly, half-defiantly at the crowd. Struck by their beauty and grace, St. Gregory asked where they came from. Being informed that they were from Britain and were still pagan, St. Gregory exclaimed, "Ah, what a pity that the author of darkness owns such fair faces, and that, with such grace of outward form, they should lack inward grace!" Hearing that their nation was called Angles, St. Gregory exclaimed, "True, for they have angelic faces and should be co-heirs with the angels in Heaven. What is the name of the province whence they came?"

"Deira."

"Yes, *de ira*, snatched from ire and called to the mercy of Christ."

"Who is their king?"

"Alla."

"Alleluia," St. Gregory responded, "the praise of God must be sung in those parts." This story very likely has an historical basis, although it is dressed up in its details and wording. But it is nonetheless certainly true that St. Gregory had an intense interest in converting England.

In fact, he himself set out as head of a mission to England, having obtained the permission of a reluctant Pope Pelagius. The people of Rome were more reluctant still when they learned of his departure, and besieged the Pope's quarters with entreaties until he sent messengers to recall St. Gregory. Thus, Gregory returned to Rome and never himself became a missionary. But some years later, in 596, when St. Gregory was Pope, he sent the prior of his monastery on the Coelian hill, the tall and commanding St. Augustine of Canterbury (St. Austin), and a company of monks to England. Thus, the history of the Catholic Faith and the history of England itself point back to the obedience of a would-be missionary whose feet turned back, but whose zeal kept marching forward.

Strength in Weakness

In February of 590 Pope Pelagius II died of the plague. St. Gregory was quickly elected his successor, according to the custom, by the people and clergy of Rome, but the confirmation from the Emperor at Constantinople did not come until August. In the meantime, for the first part of this period, the plague had continued. In April St. Gregory organized a great procession to the Basilica of the Blessed Virgin. According to one ancient report, he himself carried a picture of Our Lady, painted by St. Luke, in the procession. According to a yet earlier report, when the procession came near the mausoleum of Hadrian, St. Gregory and all the people saw the Archangel Michael standing on its summit in the act of sheathing a flaming sword, symbolizing that the plague was over.

The crowning achievements of St. Gregory's life were to be

crowded into the relatively short period of his pontificate—590-604. His letters, of which there are more than 800, are collected into 14 volumes, one for each year of his pontificate. They testify to his minute interest in all the spiritual and temporal affairs of the Church. They testify to his strong conception of the supreme governing power of the successor of St. Peter. It was the great but humble Gregory who popularized the title "Servant of the Servants of God," which since the ninth century the Popes have reserved for themselves. But it was the forceful and systematic Pope Gregory who, by a strong exercise of his office, made the papacy more workably powerful and left in men's minds a more vivid and enduring image of its greatness.

St. Gregory had accepted the papacy very unwillingly. He had hidden himself and tried to escape it after his election. But once consecrated, he never tried to escape its responsibilities and burdens. A remarkable fact attesting to this is that he kept up his unflagging work in the midst of great pain and sickness. For he had suffered since his early days as a monk from stomach trouble, perhaps brought on by imprudent penitential eating habits. And in later years he had the gout.

Many times he rose from a sickbed to force himself heroically to go through several hours of Church services. His sicknesses, in addition to the extremely disorganized and weakened political conditions in Rome, undoubtedly helped to establish his conviction that the End of the World was near.

"Sometimes the pain is moderate, sometimes excessive, but it is never so moderate as to leave me, nor so excessive as to kill me. Hence it happens that I am daily in death, and daily snatched from death," St. Gregory wrote to Eulogius of Alexandria. (*Epistle* 10, 35). To another friend, Marinianus, Archbishop of Ravenna, he wrote, "At one time the pain of the gout tortures me, at another I know not what fire spreads itself over all my body, and sometimes it happens that at the same time the burning struggles with the pain, and body and mind seem to be leaving me." (*Epistle* 11, 32). But outwardly, St. Gregory's decisions continued to be clear-cut and his powers of mind undimmed.

His sickness never impeded his care for the Church, nor his interest in each person. To the same Marinianus he wrote,

I have made careful inquiries of each of the physicians here . . . They prescribe [for you] rest and silence above all things, and I am doubtful whether Your Fraternity can obtain them at your church. Therefore . . . Your Fraternity ought to come to me before the summertime, so that I may take your illness under my special care as far as I am able . . . As for myself, who seem near to death, if God should call me before you, it would be fitting for me to pass away in your arms. (*Epistle* 11, 33).

In his sickness St. Gregory always recognized the mercy of God.

But we, who are strenuously scourged, have a sign that we are not deserted, according to the testimony of Scripture, which says: "For whom the Lord loveth he chastiseth, and he scourgeth every son whom he receiveth." In these stripes of God we call to mind both His gifts and our losses by our guilt. Let us think how much good the Lord has done to us above our malice, and how much evil we have committed under His goodness. (*Epistle* 11, 30).

His *Pastoral Care*

One of the most influential of St. Gregory's writings was finished early in his pontificate. In fact, it explained why he had been so reluctant to accept his election as Pope. It was addressed to John, Archbishop of Ravenna, who had chided him for this. In English-speaking countries, it has always been known by its first words, *Pastoral Care*. The title that St. Gregory himself used, however, was *The Book of Pastoral Rule*. King Alfred in the ninth century, assisted by some of his clergy, translated it into English and ordered a copy to be given to every bishop in his realm. Charlemagne made its study an obligation for bishops of his territories. The custom grew up in France of putting a copy of *Pastoral Care* into the hands of bishops at their consecration.

It is a treatise which gives advice to all who rule others. In particular, it explains the high dignity and office of both the priest and bishop (those charged with the spiritual rule of others) and gives many suggestions on how the priest or bishop should live and how he should guide others. "The government of souls is the art of arts," St. Gregory writes, quoting his namesake, St. Gregory of Nazianzen, whose famous oration he follows to some extent.

For who does not realize that the wounds of the mind are more hidden than the internal wounds of the body? Yet, although those who have no knowledge of the powers of drugs shrink from giving themselves out as physicians of the flesh, people who are utterly ignorant of spiritual precepts are often not afraid of professing themselves to be physicians of the heart . . .

The principles contained in *Pastoral Care* have helped many who have guided others on the earthly as well as the spiritual plane. Of the four parts, Book III has been the most read. It gives directions on how to deal with 40 different classes of people: those who always succeed and those who always fail; the quarrelsome and the peaceable; the joyful and the sad, the humble and the haughty; the slothful and the hasty, and so on. Throughout, St. Gregory shows much insight into human nature.

He shows the same insight in another popular work commonly called the *Moralia*, or *Morals (Morals on the Book of Job)*. A modern writer describes the insight he displays in this book. "It seemed to me that my mind was laid open before me, all its thoughts read, the shifting, multifarious, discreditable ocean of its consciousness brought to light [and] described accurately." (Nicolete Gray, *The Month*, Vol. 17, pp. 364-375).

The same writer says of St. Gregory: "Of all the people whom I have 'met' he is the person who I feel was most completely conscious of himself and his actions. He was conscious of the whole world of his time in the same light to an extent which seems to me unique in history. It is this consciousness that is the peculiar quality of his sanctity."

St. Gregory the Great gained his deep insight into himself and others by prayer and meditation, by dealing with a multitude of men of all classes and by being always animated by a sincere love for them and an interest in their welfare. St. Gregory may have erred at times in making decisions, but the errors were not based on pettiness or prejudice. He has been especially criticized for leniency on a few occasions toward the rich and the powerful, notably with Venantius, an ex-monk, and with Phocas, the usurping Emperor. The common consensus, however, is that he succeeded to a remarkable extent in transferring his principles and advice into the many and varied decisions he made in dealing with those he ruled.

In dealing with others St. Gregory sought to make the proper combination of three different virtues which are rather difficult to describe by just one word in English. They were *rectitude*, or fidelity to law, joined to loyalty; *discretion*, "common sense" in the application of the law; and *suavity* or *"blandness,"* meaning the ability of the leader to apply the law in such a way that his subjects will still love him. (The words in Latin are *rectitudo, discretio,* and *blandimentum*.) In the combination of all these, of course, we can notice that the emphasis is on law, order and principle. History attests that St. Gregory was himself successful in blending the proper combination of these qualities, for he was a strong leader and yet was much loved.

The Pope's Death

No one has described the last hours of Pope St. Gregory, who had himself left us such beautiful descriptions of the deaths of St. Benedict and St. Scholastica. The Pope died on March 12, 604, and was buried the very same day in the Portico of St. Peter's Basilica.

The fickleness of the public is well illustrated by a temporary wave of revilement of his memory which took place shortly after St. Gregory's death. There was a famine at the time, and the report went out that no help could be given the people because Gregory had squandered the property of the Holy See. His friend, Peter the Deacon, who used to take dictation from St. Gregory, cleared his memory by relating the story of the dove, representing the Holy Ghost, who had assisted St. Gregory in his writing. On the basis of this story, the dove has become a special symbol of St. Gregory in art. The story of the temporary ill feeling against him seems to be based on fact, but the details are given in various forms.

Also, some controversy exists concerning the final resting place of St. Gregory's body and its various parts. Tradition favors St. Peter's Basilica in Rome, but some hold that it is now at Soissons in France. A number of places claim to have in their possession the head of St. Gregory, the cathedral at Sens apparently having the strongest claim. There are other lesser relics at various places. In Spain there was (and perhaps still is) a picture of the Blessed Virgin supposed to have been sent by St. Gregory to Leander of Seville. In the Church of St. Gregory at Rome is the marble table that is said to have been the one used for the entertaining of his poor guests.

Gregorian Chant

One historical opinion, dating from the beginning of the twentieth century, maintains that all we can say for sure of St. Gregory's liturgical work is that he introduced five reforms. (F. Homes Dudden [non-Catholic], *Gregory the Great: His Place in History and Thought*, 2 Vols. NY: Longmans, Green, 1905). These were the chanting of the *Alleluia* outside the Easter time, the transferring of the *Pater Noster* to its place at the end of the Canon of the Mass, and the addition of the words to the *Hanc Igitur* prayer of the Mass: "Order our days in Thy peace, and cause us to be saved from eternal damnation and to be numbered among the flock of Thy elect." In the matter of ceremony, St. Gregory forbade sub-deacons to wear the chasuble and limited deacons to the singing of the Gospel.

Later scholars lean more to the ancient tradition, which assigned to St. Gregory the entire groundwork of our liturgy in both Mass and Office. This refers not to the composition, but to the arrangement of the parts. Very likely St. Gregory composed eight of the hymns used in the Divine Office from his day until the post-Vatican II changes. (*Primo Dierum omnium et Nocte surgentes vigilemus omnes*, Sunday at Matins; *Ecce jam noctis tenuatur umbra*, Sunday at Lauds; *Lucis Creator optime*, Sunday at Vespers; *Clarum decus jeunii* in Lent at Matins; *Audi benigne Conditor*, at Vespers in Lent; *Magno salutis gaudio*, on Palm Sunday; and *Rex Christi factor omnium* in Passiontide). During the same period of time, there had been 68 Gregorian contributions to the *Roman Breviary*, which is the largest number from one person, after those of St. Augustine. (Strangely, no contribution to the Breviary has been taken from the famous *Pastoral Care*.)

The exact role that St. Gregory played in furthering liturgical music and the exact amount he contributed to it are hard to define. According to his biographer of the ninth century, John the Deacon, St. Gregory founded two schools of chant and himself listened to the boys practice and kept them in order with properly timed taps of a rod.

Of the eight modes ascribed to his name, *four* probably existed before his time, to which he added *four* subsidiary modes. Not very well known is the part St. Gregory played in the modern revival of Gregorian chant. Pope Leo XIII in 1891 held a Gregorian Congress to commemorate St. Gregory's fifteenth centenary, counting from the beginning of his pontificate. In 1904, Pope St. Pius X had another congress to commemorate the fifteenth centenary of his death. These meetings helped to start the modern revival of Church music, especially in stirring up the interest of those in high places.

John the Deacon has some rather uncomplimentary comments to make about the way Germanic and Gallic voices rendered St. Gregory's chant. "For Alpine bodies, deeply resounding in the thunder of their voices, are not readily accommodated to the sweetness of sustained modulation; for when the barbarous roughness of a bibulous throat strives to produce soft singing with inflections and accents, it casts their voices into a certain natural grating, like the confused sound of wagons coming down stairs, and instead of soothing the minds of hearers, rather provokes them to exasperation and clamorous interruption." (Quoted in Snow, O.S.B., *St. Gregory the Great: His Works and His Spirit*, 2nd ed., rev. by Huddleston, O.S.B., London: Burns Oates and Washbourne, 1924, p. 319). John's "confused sound of wagons coming downstairs" certainly provides a fine phrase for an exasperated choirmaster of any age or clime.

One study sums up St. Gregory's role in Church music thus: "The great work of Gregory was to organize, set in order, and fix." (Wyatt, *St. Gregory and the Gregorian Music*, London: Plainsong and Medieval Music Society, 1904, p. 25). Another study says, "The Office also owes its arrangement to the same Pope, according to a well-attested tradition. According to the tradition, Gregory did not compose the melodies of the Mass and Office, but either arranged them himself or had them arranged." (*Cecilia*, Vol. 85, p. 166). The same writer ventures an opinion: "Maybe the Gregorian form has remodeled the Ambrosian and is a clear abbreviation of it."

Mysticism and Monasticism

A favorite expression of St. Gregory the Great was "the chink of contemplation." He thought of God as boundless light. At times a shaft of this light floods the souls of those who have prepared themselves by getting rid of sin and attachment to it and who continue to occupy themselves in fruitful labors. In this life man cannot look directly at the divine essence, just as he cannot look directly at the bright sun. But occasionally, for those who are ready, the sunlight comes in through a chink and fills the room of the soul.

Two things are to be remarked. The filling of the soul with light is short and momentary. It passes swiftly. Secondly, the light, just like the sunlight which shows all the floating dust particles, shows the soul to be filled with numerous flaws and faults. That is why the mystic is always truly humble. He does not exaggerate, but fully means what he says about his own baseness. He has seen his flaws in the light of a moment's contemplation.

Especially important to remember is that in this life contemplation is only momentary. St. Gregory himself was much impressed by how short it is and how steadily and faithfully a person has to continue in a sinless life, filled with good works, in order for God to grant him another moment of contemplation. He insisted over and over on good works as a conditioning of oneself to receive again the boost of contemplation. This viewpoint is much more understandable than the more current idea that contemplation is a state which one enjoys for long periods. To remember that contemplation is momentary, that it should result in good works, that good works condition one for a new "boost," is also to realize that many people are called to it.

St. Gregory writes of the momentary nature of contemplation in his *Morals*:

> Not even in the sweetness of inward contemplation does the mind remain fixed for long, in that, being made to recoil by the very immensity of the light, it is called back to itself. And when it tastes the inward sweetness, it is on fire with love, it longs to mount above itself; yet it falls back in broken state to the darkness of its frailty. (*Morals* 5, 57).

Allied to St. Gregory's viewpoint that contemplation is a very brief dip into a subdued eternal Light is his strong emphasis on active work. He gave not only a strong but a deciding second to St. Benedict's proposition that monks must work. Work must be part of their everyday life. Contemplation was the fruit freely granted by God only after much tilling. The fervor and joy and love it stirred in the soul led to more readiness to continue in active work and to spend time in spiritual reading, study and prayer. Only the few, even among those devoted to the monastic and contemplative life, were called to spend their time completely apart from active work on behalf of other men.

It was St. Benedict who gave the direction, but St. Gregory who added the authority and force to this idea of the monastic life. In doing so, St. Gregory had an immeasurable influence in shaping monastic life as it developed in the West, and as it continues even to this day. He paved the way for the great work of the monks in preserving culture and in teaching. (Cassiodorus had the greatest single influence in turning the work of the monks to cultural pursuits in particular.)

By trying to further their work and make it fruitful for the Church, St. Gregory did much to define the relations of the monasteries with the bishops and clergy. The privileges (*privilegia*) which he granted became the basis of much of that part of Canon Law which defined and governed those ecclesiastical and monastic boundaries.

Tremendous Influence

The generosity, sympathy and charity of Pope St. Gregory the Great, his strong sense of social justice, would be admirable qualities in any man. But in him they have a special meaning and importance. It was his interest in the poor and the mistreated that made him interested in keeping and administering the patrimonies of St. Peter, i.e., the landed estates of the Church. He was also much interested in obtaining the cooperation and support of the civil government for the same reasons. By his own forceful pursuing of these purposes, he made the papacy a civil power, and he linked the Church and the state in an harmonious working relationship. He did not, strictly speaking, originate this arrangement. But he helped more than anyone else to establish it on a firm footing.

Historians may speculate whether St. Gregory's particular decisions were the best or even the only ones possible at the time. But it is quite possible that St. Gregory's course of action, humanly speaking, preserved the Church and allowed it to function as the preserver itself of culture and the fashioner of a new Europe.

The works of St. Gregory, if published today in condensed form, might prove to be popular once again. During the Middle Ages, St. Gregory was spoken of as "Gregory of the *Dialogue*." The common people in that world, in which life was quite hard, eagerly sought the evidence of God's providence in the marvels

St. Gregory related in his *Dialogue*. People still seek marvels, though the approach is more cautious.

Today, in an age deeply interested in the inner workings of a man's own mind, St. Gregory, who in his own terms described the inner man, should prove very readable for the average person. Moreover, people today, in an age again of unrest, are interested in finding a stable moral guide.

St. Gregory, using Scripture and appealing to unalterable Natural Law, giving rules of conduct in unadorned, clear phrases, could again come into vogue. "Learn the heart of God from the word of God," he advises. (*Epistle* 4, 31). Many who value the word of God would be willing to read him further. "My brothers, when you do good, remember always what you have previously done that was bad, so that, seriously considering your faults, you may not be too foolishly happy over your good actions." His words strike close to the heart.

> God . . . has not promised to His elect the pleasures of delight in this life, but the bitterness of tribulation; so that, as is done by medicine, through a bitter draught they may return to the enjoyment of eternal health . . . Consider, I beg you, where would there be room for patience if there were nothing to be endured? (*Letter to Theoctista*, sister of the Emperor).

To Andrew, a man of means, St. Gregory wrote:

> Our life is like a voyage. He who sails, though he stand, sit, or lie down, yet goes on, because he is led by the motion of the ship. So is it with us, whether sleeping or waking, whether silent or speaking, whether walking, whether willing or unwilling, through the moments of time we approach daily to the end. When the day of our end shall come, where will be all that we have amassed with such anxiety and such solicitude? Honor, therefore, or riches are not to be sought, for they pass away.

In giving direction to rulers, to bishops, priests, monks, to the average person, St. Gregory is at his best. He is a great spiritual guide, a great moralist and teacher of ethics.

St. Gregory's theology is not contained in formal treatises, but in his *Moralia*, his *Sermons* and *Letters*, and in *Pastoral Care*. The painstaking non-Catholic biographer of St. Gregory, F. Homes Dudden, says that "for a period of nearly four centuries the last word on theology rested with Gregory the Great." This was not because St. Gregory was necessarily an original thinker or a developer of dogma. It was rather because he summarized the teaching of St. Augustine and "re-stated his views in simple, unphilosophic form." He taught what other great Fathers and Doctors had taught before him, but he put things into clearer and more understandable form—for example, the doctrine on grace, on the Mass, on invoking Saints, on Purgatory.

Within St. Gregory's writings a person can find the strength and basic appeal which he garnered from Scripture, on which he relied so fully. He was not a man lost in non-essentials of any kind, nor in any kind of pedantry. By what he says of Holy Scripture we gain a good idea of his own cast of mind.

He says that Scripture

> is incomparably superior to every form of knowledge and science. It preaches the truth and calls to the heavenly fatherland; it turns the heart of the reader from earthly to heavenly desires; it exercises the strong by its obscurer sayings, and attracts the little ones by its simple language; it is neither so closed to view as to inspire fear, nor so open as to be despised, but familiarity with it removes distaste for it, and the more it is studied the more it is loved; it helps the reader's mind by simple words and raises it by heavenly meanings; it grows, if one may so speak, with the readers, for the ignorant find therein what they already know, and the learned find therein always something new. (Quoted in Dudden, p. 300, from Vol. II of *Morals*, 20, 1).

St. Gregory the Great is the fourth great Doctor of the West, following Sts. Ambrose, Jerome and Augustine. He is the last great Doctor of the ancient Church, and because of the firm mold which he gave to theology by selecting and summing up the preceding teachers, he is theology's link with medieval Scholasticism.

As a teacher of morals, as a molder of theology, as a Pope, St. Gregory is deservedly called "the Great." Some say that of the entire line of Popes, none deserves more to be named the greatest than does Pope St. Gregory the Great. His feast day is September 3 (March 12 in the 1962 calendar).

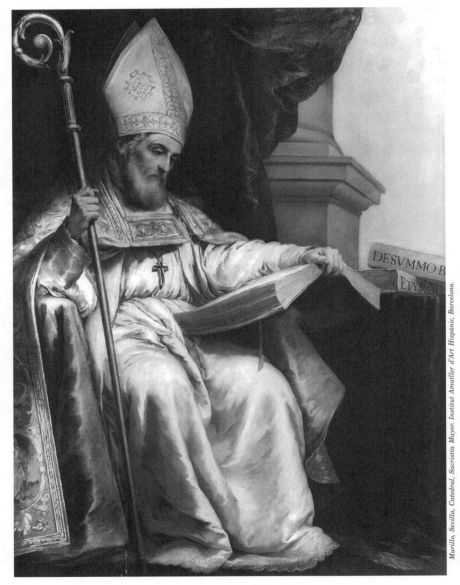

Murillo, Sevilla, Catedral, Sacristía Mayor. Institut Amatller d'Art Hispànic, Barcelona.

Saint Isidore of Seville

15

SAINT ISIDORE OF SEVILLE

Schoolmaster of the Middle Ages

c. 560-636

A WEARY and thirsty boy rested near the well. He had run away from the daily grind of prayer and study and scolding under his much older brother. Now he was observing the hollowed-out stones of the well. A woman who came to draw water followed his questioning gaze and explained that the hollow in the stone was caused by the constant dripping of water. As the lad kept thinking about the work that the patient drops of water could do, he decided that by patient day-to-day study he could acquire knowledge.

This story is told of St. Isidore of Seville, known as "The Schoolmaster of the Middle Ages," the compiler of all the secular and religious knowledge of his time. In a 1943 doctoral dissertation presented at the University of California, Larry Nepomuceno tells us: "His universal knowledge, the wonder of his contemporaries, was the fruit of a lifetime [of] study rather than the by-product of his youthful education. Isidore was truly the principal representative of Spanish culture, a great historian of note, and the most learned man of his time in all Spain." (Nepomuceno, dissertation: English translation of St. Isidore's *Historia Gothorum Waldalorum Sueborum*, with valuable introduction listing all materials used). The boy who found it hard to study is considered the last of the Latin Fathers of the Church. Montalembert calls him "the last learned man of the ancient world."

The *Etymologies*

It is seven years, if I am not mistaken, since I requested you to write the books of Origins. And in various ways you have frustrated me . . . with subtle delay explaining now that the books are not finished, now that they are not written, again that my letters have been lost; and with other such excuses

we have come to this day and remain with no answer to my
petition.

In this plaintive way a letter of St. Braulio, Bishop of Neocaesarea,
chided his friend St. Isidore for not fulfilling a request. He was
asking for something almost impossible to deliver, an encyclopedia, a summary of all knowledge. Yet in the last years of his
life, Braulio's friend obliged him, and all the students of medieval
Europe for centuries to come, by writing the *Origins* or
Etymologies, his most famous work—which proves that a friend
is sometimes needed to stir up even a voluminous writer like
St. Isidore of Seville.

Braulio divided the work into 20 books. Though it was never
entirely completed, its scope was such that Braulio could say of
it that it "contained about all that ought to be known." It is
aptly named, because St. Isidore bases so much on the derivation of words. The *Etymologies* covers, of course, not only religious topics but all kinds of secular subjects, such as war,
amusements, medicine, music, geography, building, garments,
ornaments, animals and many others.

What St. Isidore has to say of horses (Book 12, Ch. 4, 3) is
interesting.

> Horses have a high spirit; for they prance in the fields, they
> scent war, they are roused by the trumpet sound to battle, they
> are roused by the voice and urged to the race; they grieve when
> they are beaten, they are proud when they win a victory. Certain
> ones know the enemy in battle, so that they bite the foe. Some
> recall their own masters and forget obedience if their masters
> are changed; some allow none but their master to mount them;
> when their masters are slain or are dying, many shed tears.
> The horse is the only creature that weeps for man and feels
> the emotion of grief.

A Three-Bishop Family

Though St. Isidore was acknowledged as the leading scholar
of his age, even in his lifetime, no contemporary took the trouble to write his life. Contemporary sources, therefore, are but
short. Besides the nine letters of his own which are left to us,
there are four short notices: a passage in Leander's *Regula* or
rule, Bishop Braulio's introduction to Isidore's works, St.
Ildephonse's summary in his continuation of St. Isidore's *De*

Viris Illustribus ("About Illustrious Men") and a letter of the clerk (cleric), Redemptus, describing the Saint's death.

St. Isidore's family came from the province of Carthagena in Spain. Whether he was born there or in Seville is disputed. The year of his birth is not known exactly and is usually given as 560 A.D. His father's name was Severian (*sic*), and the mother's name is given either as Theodosia, Theodora, or Turtura. It is most probable that both his parents died when St. Isidore was very young, as his much older brother, Leander, took over his training and education.

Leander became Archbishop of Seville in 579, and is noted for his educational efforts, as well as his strenuous opposition to Arianism. Spain honors him as its chief preserver of the Catholic Faith, which it had received from apostolic times. Leander exerted a strong influence on the formation of the young Isidore. When Leander was sent into exile for opposing Arianism, he wrote to tell Isidore not to fear even death for the Faith. This indicates that there was danger for St. Isidore, even though his youth saved him from exile.

Another older brother, Fulgence, became the Bishop of Astigi. For his sister, Florentina, who was a nun, St. Isidore wrote a treatise on the Catholic Faith, marshalling many texts from the Old and New Testaments to answer the objections of the Jews. There has been some uncertainty about whether or not another sister, named Theodosia, actually belonged to the family. She married Leovigild, the King of the Goths, and became the mother of the famous martyr, Hermenegild. Very likely, the family of St. Isidore had been Catholic for at least several generations. Leander, Fulgence and Florentina are honored as Saints by the Church, as is St. Isidore.

Just what St. Isidore did between his years of formal schooling and his consecration as Archbishop of Seville, succeeding his brother Leander in about 600 A.D., is not definitely known. There is no positive proof that he was a monk. It seems more likely that he helped Leander as a priest and teacher. Very likely his own brother, Fulgence, was one of the consecrating bishops for Isidore. There is little doubt that St. Isidore went to Rome sometime during his episcopate and took part in a regional council assembled there. He was at several councils in Spain, and notably presided at the most important one, the Fourth Council of Toledo in 633. He did not preside as a figurehead, but actively influenced and shaped its decisions.

St. Isidore was a contemporary of Mohammed (c. 570-632), but stories about his meeting him and prophesying that Mohammed would be a scourge of the Church and of his driving Mohammed from Spain are false. Mohammed never went to Spain.

Death, Echo of Life

The generally accepted date of St. Isidore's death is April 4, 636. April 4 is also the date of his feast day. Since we do not have much personal data on St. Isidore's life but we do have a more detailed account of his death, we may learn something of the heart and mind of the Saint by considering the manner of his death.

When St. Isidore had a presentiment of approaching death, he set up a program of distributing his goods to the poor, and for six months spent much of his time in doing this. Attacked by a fever and unable to keep food in his stomach, he had himself taken to the Church of St. Vincent. The sorrow and sighing of the people, Redemptus says, would dissolve an iron heart into tears.

Inside the Basilica, the priests placed ashes on his head as a token of penance, and St. Isidore raised his hands and prayed humbly to God for forgiveness of his sins, which he said were more numerous than the sands of the sea. He had drunk iniquity as water and taken sin as milk.

> O Lord . . . You know that after I came unworthy to this holy church [to become Archbishop of Seville], unhappily as to a burden rather than to an honor, I have never stopped sinning nor laboring to commit iniquity . . . Be near and receive my prayer, and grant to me, a suppliant sinner, the pardon asked for.

He asked the people to pray for him so that his petition to God for forgiveness might be heard. Then he asked them for pardon.

> Forgive me, although unworthy, whatever wrong I have done against any of you. If I have shown contempt for anyone, if I have refused anyone the embrace of charity, if I have hurt anyone by advice or injured anyone by anger, forgive me, a petitioner and penitent.

After they had prayed for him, he exhorted them:

> Most reverend bishops of my Lord and all who are here, I ask and beg that you show charity to one another, not rendering evil for evil, nor give cause for complaint to the people; may the ancient enemy not find in you something to punish, nor may the raging wolf find one left by you to carry away; but rather, may the shepherd joyfully carry the lamb snatched from the mouth of the wolf on his shoulders, to this sheepfold.

Isidore then commanded that the rest of his goods be given to the poor, and sought to be kissed by all, saying:

> If you forgive from your heart all the wrong or evil things I have till now done to you, may the Almighty Creator dismiss all your sins, so that the water of the sacred font which the devout people are to receive today may be unto you for the remission of sins, and this kiss between me and you may remain as a testimony for the future.

St. Isidore was taken back from the church to his home and died on the fourth day.

An Astonishing Man

The charity of his giving and the deep humility of his begging pardon of God and man show a generous and sensitive soul. St. Isidore's death was not haphazard, but a studied exit to which he gave specific and exact attention.

St. Ildephonse says that those who heard St. Isidore were astonished at his eloquence. The word "astonished" sounds unusual at first, but when you picture a man of Isidore's vast mastery of facts and ability to arrange them, joined to the humility, frankness and directness he showed in his final dramatic hours, you can appreciate it. There is something unforgettable in picture of this dying bishop, the light of his age and the counselor of kings, his head covered with penitential ashes, begging pardon of all and counseling his clergy to have a special care for those sheep who are almost lost. There is something astonishing in the way he took hold of things as a true leader, and yet sought the testimony of a kiss of peace, remembering how he may have erred as a leader.

In the preface to his valuable *History of the Goths, Vandals and Sueves*, St. Isidore addressed his native country poetically:

> Of all the lands of the world from the West to the Indies, thou art the most beautiful, O sacred . . . Mother Spain! . . . Thou who art located in the most delightful zone of the world, art neither scorched by the summer sun's heat nor devastated by winter's cold, but enveloped by a temperate climate, nourished by gentle zephyrs . . .

Spain responded just 17 years after his death. For the Eighth Council of Toledo in 653 called him an eminent Doctor and the newest ornament of the Catholic Church. St. Isidore has remained the Great Doctor of the Spaniards. He is also recognized as a fashioner of the Spanish nationality. In 1936, under the gathering clouds of civil war, the thirteenth centenary of St. Isidore's death was observed throughout the Iberian peninsula. Pope Benedict XIV on April 25, 1722, named St. Isidore a Doctor of the Universal Church.

St. Isidore was first buried between Leander and Florentina in the cathedral at Seville. King Ferdinand the Catholic, shortly before the voyages of Columbus, recovered the relics from the Moors and transferred them to the Church of St. John the Baptist at Leon, where they remain to this day.

Moderate Rule for Monks

St. Isidore wrote a *Rule for Monks*, which Braulio says "he agreeably tempered for the use of his homeland and for the spirits of the weak." According to the canons in force in Spain at the time, a bishop had large share in directing monks; he could choose the abbot and correct violations of their rule. (St. Isidore's brother, Leander, also wrote a rule for nuns, requested by their sister, Florentina, and besides a homily, this rule is Leander's only extant work).

The *Rule for Monks* seems to be a good index to St. Isidore's own character and spirituality, bearing the impress of his personality more than his other encyclopedic writings. It is a rule of moderation, showing fine consideration for the needs of human nature. While the Rule is strict, a spirit of charity and prudence breathe through it. St. Isidore made careful provision for punishments for transgressions, but he never wanted any monk dismissed entirely, thinking he might lose his soul if he were sent away. Exclusion from the community was only to be temporary, even for grave, repeated faults.

When an applicant to monastic life first arrived, he should first serve outside the monastery for three months, administering to guests and the poor. Then he must put his intention of being a monk into writing. The abbot must not inquire whether the man be rich or poor, a slave or free. All in the monastery were to take their places according to the time of their coming. Those who had been rich should not despise those who had been poor, nor should the poor feel elated because their former rich neighbor was now equal to them in the monastery.

Whereas St. Isidore provides that the ailing should do less work, he knows that some healthy persons will feign illness. These should be borne with, for at times the sickness is not apparent to an outsider. If malingerers get away with doing less than their share, it is not a cause for anger but for sadness, since they are sick at heart or mind. While treating of the work of the monks, St. Isidore recalls the example of St. Joseph and says definitely that he was a "worker in iron" (*faber ferrarius*). (Ch. 5, n. 2).

At work the monks may sing, for if seculars can do their work and sing love songs, so can the monks do their work in such a way "that they always have the praise of God on their lips, and serve Him with their tongues by psalms and hymns." On this point St. Isidore shows freshness and insight and a singular freedom from an artificial approach to regulations.

In the summer months a rest period is allowed from noon to three o'clock. A departure from earlier rules allows meat on Sundays. There was, however, to be no murmuring about what was served at table, and there was to be just one meal a day, during which there was reading from Holy Scripture.

It would indeed have been difficult to fall asleep during Divine Office, since the rule called for a prostration after each psalm. But one who went through this strenuous routine should have little difficulty sleeping afterwards. After Compline the brethren were to bid each other good night before retiring.

One who needed food or drink between meals could obtain permission from the abbot, but must not eat or drink in front of others, lest they find it too hard to continue fasting. One caught eating ahead of time was to be punished. Only one monk, the hebdomader, was allowed to taste the food. Guests were to be given bread baked not by a monk but by a skilled layman. Some of these regulations show a kindly and deep insight into human nature that must have been tinged by a degree of humor.

St. Isidore's rule devotes one of its 24 chapters to the sick, and another to guests. "Those who are able to [work], let them thank God and work. Those who cannot work, let them make known their sickness and be treated more leniently." Guests were to be graciously received and housed. Their feet were to be washed and all humane treatment given them within the limits of prudent expense. Visiting monks were to receive most special consideration.

Provision was made for Mass to be offered for the deceased before burial and on the second day after Pentecost, "so that being made partakers of the blessed life, they may, having been purged, receive their bodies in the resurrection."

The historian Gibbon calls St. Isidore's rule "the mildest of the western monastic rules." In another work, the *Sentences* (Book 2,44), St. Isidore gives a bit of the thinking behind his moderate regulations.

> Weakness of the body also breaks the powers of the soul and makes the talent of the mind to grow feeble; nor can it accomplish anything good by its weakness. Enough of this. For whatever is done with moderation is salutary, but whatever is done immoderately is dangerous and turns to the opposite. It is proper, therefore, to be moderate and temperate in every work. For whatever is excessive is dangerous: just as water, if it bestows too much rain, not only has no use, but brings danger.

A Textbook Writer

St. Isidore was primarily a compiler. He has been criticized as being merely a copyist, which is not quite fair. He not only copied facts, but arranged them and summed them up. "Isidore's completeness of resume surpasses all writers of his own and immediately preceding periods. He goes back to the tradition of the Roman encyclopedists . . ." (Ernest Brehaut, Ph.D., *An Encyclopedist of the Dark Ages—Isidore of Seville*, Longmans Green, 1912). He worked on the guiding idea that the way to knowledge was through words, and that words were to be made clear by reference to their origin. St. Isidore had an unusual ability to define words, although the derivations at times, it has been pointed out, are more ingenious than factual.

"I have gathered together the writings of the Fathers like flowers from different meadows," St. Isidore says of his religious writings in general. The three books of *Sentences* make up a summary and systematic treatise on dogmatic and moral theology. Together they are "a manual of Christian faith and practice." (Mrs. Humphrey Ward, article on St. Isidore in *A Dictionary of Christian Biography*, Vol. 3, pp. 305-13, ed. Smith-Wace, 4 Vols., AMS Press, NY, 1967). The *Origins* or *Etymologies* contain in a condensed form almost all that St. Isidore has written elsewhere. Therefore, St. Isidore accomplished his purpose of making knowledge, both religious and secular, available in compact and handy form.

A scholar at the University of Chicago (C. Beeson in 1913) made a study and concluded that apparently the number of extant manuscripts of St. Isidore's works surpasses those of any other author. The conclusion is the more revealing since the study covers manuscripts only outside of Spain, and attests to the immense use and influence of St. Isidore's writings. There are at least 950 manuscripts of the *Etymologies* still extant. In medieval Europe, every library of Western Europe had this work as an indispensable source of information.

What St. Isidore had to say of astronomy, physics, medicine and similar subjects naturally contains much that today seems quaint.

> The body is made up of the four elements. For earth is in the flesh; air in the breath; moisture in the blood; fire in the vital heat. For it is by the spleen we laugh, by the bile we are angry, by the heart we are wise, by the liver we love." (*Etymologies*, Book 11, 127).

Music lovers should love St. Isidore, for he says that

> Without music there can be no perfect knowledge, for there is nothing without it. For even the universe itself is said to have been put together with a certain harmony of sounds, and the very heavens revolve under the guidance of harmony. Music rouses the emotions, it calls the senses to a different quality . . . For the enduring of labors, too, music comforts the mind, and singing lightens weariness in solitary tasks.

Master of Summary

St. Isidore says of his writing: "The student reads not my doctrines but re-reads the ancients . . . It is they who say what I teach, and my voice is merely their tongue." Nepomuceno comments about this. "True enough, he selected from various authors what seemed most suited to his thinking, but he adds a color of his own. He epitomized, revised, or omitted the superfluous, and injected remarks and phrases applicable to his own time and circumstances . . . in many cases, most of the passages flow from the affluence of his fertile mind, and are based upon the personal conviction of the writer . . ."

As a summarizer of the earlier Church Fathers, St. Isidore has special value for presenting the common doctrine of the Church. He makes a strong case for the need of authority in teaching. (Book 8, Ch. 3 of *Etymologies*).

> Heresy is so called in the Greek from "choosing," because forsooth each one chooses for himself what seems to him to be better, as the Peripatetic philosophers, the Academic, the Epicureans, and the Stoics, or as others who, following perverse belief, have of their own free will departed from the Church. And so heresy is named in the Greek from its meaning of "choice," since each at his own will chooses what he pleases to teach or believe. But we are not permitted to believe anything of our own will, nor to choose what someone has believed of his [own free will]. We have God's Apostles as authorities who did not themselves of their own will choose anything of what they should believe, but they faithfully transmitted to the nations the teaching received from Christ. And so, even if an angel from Heaven shall preach otherwise, he shall be called anathema.

After summarizing some Christian heresies, St. Isidore says,

> These heresies have arisen against the Catholic Faith and have been condemned beforehand by the Apostles and the holy Fathers, or by the Councils, and while they are not consistent with one another, being divided among many different errors, they still conspire with one assent against the Church of God. But whoever understands the Holy Scripture otherwise than as the sense of the Holy Spirit, by whom it was written, demands, though he withdraw not from the Church, he can still be called a heretic.

At the same time, St. Isidore is definitely opposed to forcing the Faith on anybody. "Faith should come by persuasion, not by extortion," he said.

St. Isidore provides us with valuable summaries like the following:

> It must be believed with complete faith that Mary, Mother of Christ [our] God, conceived as a virgin and brought forth as a virgin and remained a virgin after the birth. The blasphemy of Helvidius must not be acquiesced to, who said: she was a virgin before the birth, but not after the birth. (*Eccl. Dogmas*, Ch. 69).

> The Church was founded first by Peter in Antioch and there the name of Christians first arose through his preaching, as the Acts of the Apostles testify. (*Acts* 11:26). They are called Christian, the word being derived from Christ. The Church is called Catholic because established throughout the world, or because it is Catholic, that is, general in its doctrine for instructing man about things visible and invisible, heavenly and earthly. (*Eccl. Offices* 1, 1 & 3).

It would be hard to find a more succinct and clear summary of the first four Councils of the Church than the one given by St. Isidore. (Bk. 6, ch. 16 of *Books and Services of the Church*).

> Among the rest of the councils we know there are four venerable synods which embrace the whole Faith in its chief heads, like the four Gospels or the four rivers of Paradise. Of these the first, the Nicene synod of 318 bishops, was held when Constantine was emperor. In it the blasphemy of the Arian perfidy was condemned, which the same Arius gave utterance to concerning the inequality of the Holy Trinity. The same holy synod in the creed defined God the Son as consubstantial with God the Father. The second synod, of 150 Fathers, gathered at Constantinople under Theodosius the elder, and condemning Macedonius, who denied that the Holy Spirit was God, proved that the Holy Spirit was consubstantial with the Father and the Son, giving the form of the creed which the whole confession, Greek and Latin, preaches in the churches. The third synod, the first of Ephesus, of 200 bishops, was held under Theodosius II, and it condemned with a just anathema Nestorius, who asserted that there were two persons in Christ, and showed that the one person of the Lord Jesus Christ was immanent in the two natures. The fourth synod, of 630 priests, was held at

Chalcedon under Martianus, and it condemned by the unanimous vote of the Fathers, Eutyches, Abbot of Constantinople, who asserted that the nature of the Word of God and of flesh was one, and his defender, Dioscorus, Bishop of Alexandria, and Nestorius himself a second time, along with the remaining heretics, the same synod stating that Christ the Lord was so born of the Virgin that we confess in Him the substance both of the divine and of the human nature. These four are the principal synods, stating most fully the doctrine of faith; and whatever councils there are which the holy Fathers, full of the spirit of God, have ratified, after the authority of these four, they continue established in all strength.

Educational Influence

St. Isidore had a strong influence on education. "The influence which he exerted upon subsequent generations was felt far and wide and represented every existing branch of knowledge of the time. His organization of the field of science was widely accepted throughout the early medieval period. The many references to him by later scholars, the many manuscripts and successive editions of his works, even after the invention of printing, testify to the leading role he played in medieval civilization." (Nepomuceno).

Brehaut says that "there was contained in his writings . . . the embryo of something positive and progressive, namely, the organization of educational subjects that was to appear definitely in the medieval university and dominate education almost to the present day." His attitude was hospitable toward secular subjects, "unsurpassed in his own period and . . . never surpassed throughout the Middle Ages."

Braulio tells us that St. Isidore considered it his mission in life "to restore the monuments of the ancients, lest we lapse into barbarism." St. Isidore said that "ignorance nourishes vices and is the mother of all errors." St. Isidore, however, gave the first place to the study of theology, and especially to Holy Scripture.

By his strong insistence on learning for the clergy and his part in the Fourth Council of Toledo, which provided for the establishment of schools for their training, St. Isidore influenced the Church's program of seminary training. "The priest must be distinguished both by his learning and sanctity," St. Isidore says, "for learning without a good life makes one arrogant, and a good life without learning renders one useless."

Along with his brother Leander, St. Isidore, by his part in the councils of Spain, in which bishops and kings sat together, had a strong influence on Visigothic legislation. Historians in turn regard this legislation as having had a strong effect on the development of representative forms of government. St. Isidore's advice on framing a law is often quoted.

> The law should be honest, just, possible, according to the nature and custom of the country, suited to the time and place, useful and also clear, lest anyone by its obscurity should be deceived, written not for the benefit of any individual, but for the common good of the citizens.

St. Isidore "stood as it were on the line between two ages, with one foot in the Roman civilization of the past and the other in the Christian culture of the future. Thus he could view them both and discuss their mutual relations. The movement of his mind carried him, too, along the entire framework of the modern critical and scientific thought." (Nepomuceno, n. 11).

A Spiritual Guide

Just as St. Isidore culled the maxims of the Fathers, so can we gather a few of his thoughts for spiritual guidance. The following are taken here and there from his three books of *Sentences*, a systematic treatise on Christian doctrine and morals culled largely from St. Gregory's *Morals*.

> There are two kinds of martyrs, one in open suffering, the other in the hidden virtue of the spirit. For many, enduring the lyings-in-wait of the enemy and resisting all carnal desires, have become martyrs even in time of peace, because they have sacrificed themselves in their heart to the omnipotent God, and if they had lived in time of persecution, they could have been martyrs in reality.

> As art returns praise to the artist, so is the Creator of things praised by His creature . . . God makes known His beauty, which cannot be limited by the beauty of the limited creature, so that man may return to God along the path he went when turning from God, so that he who took himself from the form of the Creator through the love of the beauty of a creature, may again, through the grace of the creature, return to the beauty of God.

The Symbol of faith [Apostles' Creed] and the Lord's Prayer suffice for the whole law, allowing the little ones to capture the kingdom of Heaven. For the whole breadth of the Scriptures is contained in the same Lord's Prayer and the shortness of the Symbol.

"Compunction of heart is humility of mind with tears, rising from the recollection of sin and fear of the judgment." Compunction, St. Isidore says, has four elements: 1) remembrance of past sins, 2) anticipation of future punishments, 3) considering the space of this life as merely a journey, and 4) the desire of the supernal homeland.

> Everyone sinning is proud, in as far as by doing what is forbidden he has contempt of the divine law. . . . The way from pride often leads to abominable uncleanness of the flesh . . . for God often casts down the unseen pride of the mind by the manifest ruin of the flesh.

> Cupidity never knows how to be satisfied. The greedy man is always in need; the more he acquires, the more he seeks, and he is not only tortured by the desire of gaining, but by the fear of losing. . . . We are born poor into this life, and shall leave it poor. If we believe the goods of this life are perishable, why do we want them with so much love?

> The active life uses worldly things well, the contemplative life, renouncing the world, delights in living only for God. . . . Whoever first makes progress in the active life does well to ascend to the contemplative. Deservedly will he be sustained in that one who is found useful in the first. Whoever meddles with temporal glory or carnal concupiscence is prohibited from contemplation, so that placed in the work of actual life, he may be purged. In this life [meaning the active], all vices are to be rooted up by the exercising of good works, so that the person may pass with a sharp mind to the contemplation of God. And although converted, he wants immediately to rise to contemplation, he is however forced by reason to continue working first in the active life.

The Encyclopedist

Fr. Stephen McKenna, C.SS.R says of St. Isidore that he is "the first Christian writer who essayed a *Summa* or encyclopedia of human knowledge. In his books is found all the wisdom of antiquity, and it was he who preserved it and transmitted it to the Europe of the Middle Ages." (*Amer. Eccl. Rev.*, Oct., 1936). Cardinal Schuster has said: "The authority which he exercised throughout the Church in the early Middle Ages is beyond dispute, for the Venerable Bede and other writers of the Carolingian era are in great measure indebted to him for their ecclesiastical learning." (Quoted by R. Rios, *Clergy Review*, 25, 508).

Braulio says that St. Isidore was "more outstanding than anybody in sound doctrine and unsurpassed in works of charity." St. Isidore is especially remembered as the man of universal knowledge, the encyclopedist, the "first Christian who arranged for Christians the knowledge of antiquity."

And when we think of his charity and humility in his last illness, when we recall how he did not want any sinner to be lost, nor any monk to be dismissed, we may also recall St. Isidore as the man of universal charity. His feast day is April 4.

A Prayer to the Holy Spirit

The following is a 7th-century prayer of St. Isidore of Seville, composed for the Synod of Toledo and frequently used in General Councils of the Church, including Vatican Council II. (Oikoumene, Archdiocese of St. Louis, May, 1964).

O HOLY SPIRIT, Lord, we stand in Thy Presence aware of our sinfulness, but conscious that we have gathered together with special purpose in Thy name. Come to us and be with us. Be pleased to touch our hearts. Teach us what we must do, how we must proceed, and show us what we must accomplish, that by Thine aid, we may please Thee in all things. Be for us the only instigator and guide in our judgments, Thou Who alone with God the Father and His Son bear this ineffable name. May Thou Who lovest perfect equity not permit us to be disturbers of justice. Do not permit ignorance to turn us from what is right; do not permit unworthy motives to change our course, nor considerations of person or gain to corrupt us. Rather, join us to Thyself effectively with the gift of Thy grace. May we be one in Thee and not be deflected from truth. As we are presently gathered in Thy Name, so may we always join justice with religion that for the present time our convictions may not separate us from Thee, and in the future, we may attain an eternal reward for our deeds well done. Amen.

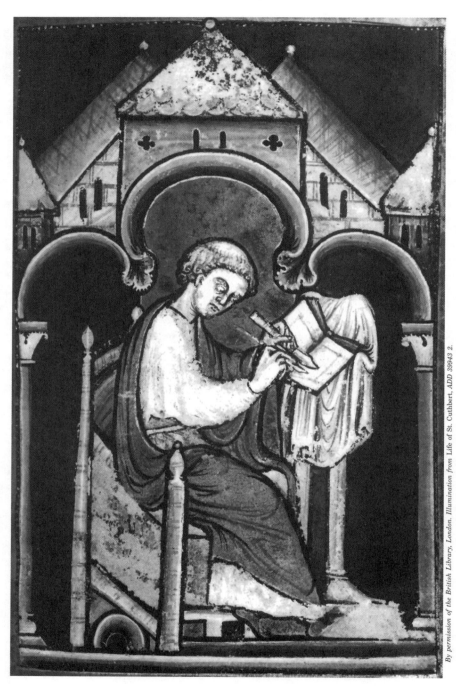

By permission of the British Library, London. Illumination from Life of St. Cuthbert, ADD 39943 2.

Saint Bede the Venerable

16

SAINT BEDE THE VENERABLE
Father of English History
c. 673-735

WHENEVER we mention a date in history or refer to the current year, we pay unconscious tribute to St. Bede. For he popularized the system of using "B.C." and "A.D." The system had been devised, he himself tells us, by Dionysius (Denis), an aged Roman abbot, starting with the Feast of the Annunciation in 527 A.D. But it lay unused for 200 long years until adopted by St. Bede in his works on Time and in his histories. The Cycle of Dionysius, using Christ as the centerpiece of history, then took root in England; it then went via English missionaries and teachers, and Bede's own works, to the Continent. Adoption by Charlemagne, and in the century following him by the Popes, brought it into universal use in the West.

The poet Dante places St. Bede in Paradise with another Doctor of the Church, St. Isidore of Seville. St. Bede does have much in common with the great Spanish Doctor, whose works he valued and used. For he had a universal interest and wrote voluminously about many subjects. He collected the treasures of knowledge that he might share them. He was a loving teacher, kind, quiet and devoted to bringing to others the lore of the ancient Church Fathers and the fruits of Scripture. In former times his name was a familiar one to English school children.

Usually he is spoken of as The Venerable Bede. This title comes from the Council of Aix-la-Chapelle in 835. The Fathers of this Council called him Venerable and an Admirable Doctor for Modern Times.

St. Bede describes himself as always "rejoicing to serve the Supreme Loving-Kindness." He made his mark on the pages of history, and he wrote about history. But he lived for eternity and wanted to help men reach a happy eternity. "Many a learned man," says the Venerable Bede, "will be found at last among the lost; and many a simple soul that has kept God's Commandments will shine among Apostles and Doctors." (*Op.* xi, 283.).

Father of English History

When St. Bede was about 59, he finished *The Ecclesiastical History of the English People*. It is considered his most important work and won him the title, "Father of English History." The *Ecclesiastical History* was very popular, and there are said to be 160 manuscript copies still in existence, at least two of which go back almost to his own time. One authority calls Venerable Bede "our greatest medieval historian." In the Catholic University of America library there is an edition of *The Ecclesiastical History* published in 1723 and bearing this complete title: *Ecclesiastical History of the English Nation from the Coming of Julius Caesar into this Island in the Sixtieth Year before the Incarnation of Christ till the Year of Our Lord 731*.

At the end of the fifth and final book, Bede gives a short summary of his own life. Outside of this short notice and a report on his death by a pupil named Cuthbert, practically no details concerning St. Bede are available. It may be said, however, that the simplicity and goodness, the zeal and humility and honesty of St. Bede show through his writings with unusual clarity.

Nothing whatever is known of his parents or family. At the age of seven he was brought by his relatives to the new monastery of St. Peter at Wearmouth, Northumbria, England. His birthplace was within the territory of the monastery. Monkton in County Durham is often pointed to as the exact place. The little Bede was given as an oblate boy into the care of the abbot, St. Benedict Biscop. (This early taking of a boy to the monastery was not unusual at the time, and was a common practice for some centuries to come.)

St. Bede would have many fellow oblates as companions. He would take his turn helping in the kitchen or barn, gathering eggs, or sometimes going with the monks who fished for their dinner in the nearby Wear River. But his chief interest was in prayer and study.

From his descriptions of the pictures in the Monastery Church of St. Peter, we can almost see him as a thoughtful lad, silently drinking in their story and meaning. There were

> likenesses of Blessed Mary Ever Virgin and of the twelve Apostles, also some figures from the Gospel story . . . from the Apocalypse so that . . . everyone who entered the church . . . wherever they turned their eyes, might have before them the amiable countenance of Christ and His saints . . . and with

watchful minds might revolve on the benefits of Our Lord's Incarnation, and having before their eyes the perils of the Last Judgment, might examine their hearts the more strictly on that account. (*Lives of the Abbots*, 6).

St. Benedict Biscop built a second monastery, one dedicated to St. Paul, five miles north of the one at Wearmouth. Both monasteries were under one abbot and were conducted as one. St. Bede says that they were "one single monastery built in two different places." To St. Paul's at Jarrow St. Bede went while still in his boyhood, and here he stayed for the rest of his life. Communication between Wearmouth and Jarrow was very free, so there were doubtless happy walks and visits back and forth.

In his nineteenth year, St. Bede was ordained a deacon by Bishop John of Beverly, and in his thirtieth year he was ordained a priest, in each instance at the express wish of the abbot. King Alfred's translation of St. Bede's History calls him a "Mass-priest." Besides offering the Holy Sacrifice, St. Bede exercised the office of preaching. His 50 authentic homilies that are preserved belong to the last part of his life, 730-735. Most of them would average about 20 minutes in speaking length. More than his earlier commentaries on the Gospels, they reveal St. Bede's own personality and the character of his spiritual direction.

St. Bede visited York and Lindisfarne. And he may have gone into neighboring villages to preach in the streets. One of the Franciscan-flavored stories connected with this work tells that in his later years St. Bede was blind. A boy who led him out to preach, took him one day, as a practical joke, to a lonely and stony place. St. Bede preached, thinking there were people about. When he finished, the stones cried out: "Amen, Venerable Bede!"

There is no reason for believing that St. Bede ever went to Rome or did any further traveling. His life passed within a very limited radius of about 50 miles. John A. Giles, who edited and translated some of St. Bede's works into English says, "It seems not a little surprising that one who had scarcely moved away from the place of his nativity, should so accurately describe those at a distance: and this quality in his writings, when considered with reference to the age in which he lived, is the more remarkable as there is but one other recorded in history who possessed it in equal perfection—the immortal Homer." (Cf. *Biographical Writings and Letters of Venerable Bede*, trans. from Latin by John A. Giles, incl. biography by Giles, London, 1845).

The Ecclesiastical History of the English People

The *Ecclesiastical History* includes many stories which have become famous, including many accounts of saints and miracles and of bodies of saintly persons being found incorrupt. It gives the well-known account of Drithelm's trip to the next world and the severe penances he then undertook for the rest of his life. When people asked why he was so hard on himself, Drithelm would answer, "I have seen it harder." Bede tells of the conversion of England by St. Augustine of Canterbury, recording correspondence between St. Augustine and Pope St. Gregory (who had sent Augustine to England) on various moral questions.

St. Bede devotes much space to the "Easter controversy" over determining the date of this feast each year. His description of the decisive moment at the council at Whitby in 664 is famous. King Oswiu was hearing out the two viewpoints on the date of Easter: the Roman one, supported by the priest Wilfrid, and the Irish one, supported by Bishop Colman. After much discussion Wilfrid quoted Our Lord's words giving St. Peter the keys to the Kingdom of Heaven. When Colman admitted that there was no comparable promise to back up his own position, King Oswiu said: "Then, I tell you, since he [St. Peter] is the doorkeeper, I will not contradict him; but I intend to obey his commands in everything to the best of my knowledge and ability; otherwise, when I come to the gates of the kingdom of heaven, there may be no one to open them because the one who, on your own showing, holds the keys has turned his back on me." (307). The decision of Rome had prevailed.

St. Bede relates another incident in which some heathens "with barbarian audacity" demanded to receive the Eucharist without first being cleansed by Baptism, which they claimed they did not need. The Bishop refused, and was forthwith expelled from the region.

St. Bede's story of the conversion of King Edwin and his retinue includes the words of one of Edwin's chief men comparing this present life to the brief moment in which a bird flew through their warm dining hall in winter: "So this life of man appears but for a moment; what follows or indeed what went before, we know not at all. If this new doctrine brings us more certain information, it seems right that we should accept it." (185). The pagan high priest Coifi admitted that the pagan religion was worthless, whereas the Christian religion offered life, salvation and eternal happiness. The King accepted the Gospel, renounced his idolatry and confessed his faith in Jesus Christ. Then he provided arms and a horse for Coifi, who mounted and set off to profane and destroy the pagan shrine.

He Always Read . . . Always Wrote

St. Bede summed up his own life in one sentence:

> All my life I spent in the same monastery, giving my whole attention to the study of the Holy Scriptures, and in the intervals between the hours of regular discipline, and the duties of singing in the church, I always took delight in learning, teaching and writing.

The old Benedictine breviary capsulized the life of St. Bede: "He always read, he always wrote, he always taught, he always prayed."

When as a little boy of seven, he was given into the charge of St. Benedict Biscop, he came under a very broadening and stirring influence. St. Benedict brought back stone masons to build the church and glaziers to put in colored windows. He had visited 17 different monasteries on the Continent, and he incorporated in his rules the best practices of each, following essentially the Benedictine scheme. He was determined to establish a model monastery in England. From St. Peter's in Rome he brought back John, the arch-chanter, to teach the proper chants. He was determined to have the best available manuscripts for the monastery library. His successor, Ceolfrid, continued to add to the collection of manuscripts. St. Bede describes Ceolfrid, who was his abbot until he reached the age of about 43, as of "acute intellect, bold in action, experienced in judgment, and zealous in religion." Trumberet, Irish and well-loved by his pupil, was St. Bede's teacher in theology.

Thus St. Bede had good men to guide him in his younger years. As his scholarship matured, he had the materials at hand for research. Monasteries in those days had guest-houses attached. St. Bede used the opportunities for fruitful exchange of facts and ideas with learned guests. When he was collecting information for his historical works, he left nothing undone to produce a thorough investigation. He shows an amazing scientific approach in gathering and classifying information, carefully distinguishing it as being direct evidence, secondhand, or hearsay.

In a letter to Bishop Acca, whom he greatly admired, St. Bede tells of his care in quoting.

> Since I do not want to be thought a thief in putting down as mine what is really theirs, I have decided to place the first letter of the name of each authority in the margin, against each passage taken from his writings. I beg and pray that these marks be copied from my original if at some future time my works shall be judged worthy of reproduction.

The marks of which St. Bede speaks gradually disappeared from the copies of his works, until it became very difficult to distinguish his own thoughts from those of his sources. Careful scholarly work in our day is restoring some of them.

It was also his diocesan bishop, Acca of Hexham, who once wrote to St. Bede asking him to hurry with his commentary on St. Luke. "I am sure that the Author of Light," he said, "will aid a student who works as hard as you do, night and day." In answering, St. Bede modestly demurred: "I do not really work 'night and day,' but it is quite true that I do toil hard to reach a right judgment on all that I read."

St. Bede wrote on music; he also wrote poems about poetry. Although he is best known today as a historian, four-fifths of his writing was in the field of Scripture commentary. His own contemporaries thought of him as a theologian. The statistics may vary, depending on how the summary is made, but we can count 39 works of St. Bede contained in 74 books.

The Venerable Bede had the enviable distinction of being Our Lady's homilist. The lessons for the Common of her feasts were his. The ninth lesson ended with this beautiful thought: "For the Mother of God was blessed indeed in that she gave flesh to the Word of God in time, but still more blessed in that she ever keeps that same Word in her love throughout eternity."

He Always Taught

St. Bede did not begin to write until about the time he was ordained a priest. His writing proceeded originally from his teaching at Jarrow, as he compiled manuals for his pupils. Then at the urging of Ceolfrid, and of Bishop Acca, "dearest and best-loved of all bishops on this earth," he wrote that he might teach a wider group of people. In a letter to Acca he explains that he wrote that he might abridge larger works and make the acquiring of knowledge easier for his countrymen. Much of his effort was spent in bringing to Englishmen in a simplified form the teachings of the four great western Doctors: Sts. Jerome, Ambrose, Augustine and Gregory.

The historian, J. R. Green, says of St. Bede:

> First among English scholars, first among English theologians, first among English historians, it is in the monk of Jarrow that English literature strikes its roots. In the six hundred scholars who gathered round him for instruction, he is the father of our national education.

Egbert, one of St. Bede's pupils, became the bishop of York and founded its famous school. It was Alcuin, a pupil of Egbert, who carried the torch of learning to the court of Charlemagne. They and hundreds of other missionaries and teachers owe much to the quiet scholar at Jarrow who centered in himself, and passed on in his writings, the sum of the day's knowledge.

St. Bede's style reflects the desire to teach. It is not ornate; words are used only to convey ideas and facts, not for show. The Latin flows readily. His works show a passion for truth and exactness. He admires and praises people in all classes of society, but points out evil when necessary. His aim is always to lead people to moral goodness, to help them praise and thank their Creator better.

It has often been pointed out that St. Bede is a specially valuable witness to early Church teaching and practice. He had a fine library of manuscripts; he labored to know the past; his whole effort was bent on teaching history and doctrine exactly. We can be sure St. Bede believed that the Church he was a part of, the Church whose teachings, practices and history he writes of, reached back to apostolic times.

A book was published at Antwerp in 1650 that counted up 49 items of belief and practice held by St. Bede which were at this time rejected by the new English Church. The book went through several editions, despite the fact that to be found with it meant imprisonment. Among the items listed as held by St. Bede were praying to the Blessed Virgin and the Saints, the use of holy water and holy oil, the hearing of Confessions—with absolution being given or deferred, the offering of the Mass, reservation of the Blessed Sacrament and praying for the dead. (Henry Martin

Gillette, *St. Bede the Venerable*, Burns & Oates, London, 1935, chap. 7). St. Bede also upheld the indissolubility of marriage.

He Still Teaches

St. Bede may possibly have been the first to use the word "Purgatory" as a noun. There is no doubt, however, about his doctrine, which was fully developed and expressed. In a homily he says, "But some . . . on account of various faults with which they departed from the body, are received by the flames of the fire of Purgatory (the purgatorial fire) to be severely chastised after death." Such souls may be detained till the Day of Judgment or may "certainly be freed from punishment sooner by the prayers, alms, fasting, tears and offering of the Saving Host by their friends among the faithful."

In his letter to Egbert, written in 732, St. Bede advises frequent Communion. The bishop should tell his people

how salutary it is for all classes of Christians to participate daily in the Body and Blood of Our Lord, as you well know is done by Christ's Church throughout Italy, Gaul, Africa, Greece, and all the countries of the East. Now this kind of religion and heavenly devotion, through the neglect of our teachers, has been so long discontinued among almost all the laity of our province that those who seem to be the most religious among them communicate in the Holy Mysteries only on the day of Our Lord's birth, the Epiphany and Easter, whilst there are innumerable boys and girls of innocent and chaste life, as well as young men and women, old men and old women, who without any scruple or debate are able to communicate in the Holy Mysteries on every Lord's Day, nay, on all the birthdays of the holy Apostles or martyrs, as you yourself have seen done in the Holy Roman and Apostolic Church.

After his death, Bede's homilies, written in clear and simple Latin, were often read in monastic chapels. His words still reach us after more than a millennium with the simplicity of a catechism of today.

St. Bede writes on the Mass:

He washes us day by day from our sins in His own Blood when the memory of this same blessed Passion is unfolded anew at the altar; when things created, bread and wine, are transferred into the Sacrament of His Body and Blood by the ineffable sanctifying of the Spirit. . . .

Pope Pius XI commemorated the twelfth centennial of St. Bede's death in a letter addressed to the English bishops and to the Benedictine Order on May 27, 1935. He spoke of the Saint's works giving witness to the Church.

> Those works testify most eloquently to the fact that the See of Rome is the centre and firm foundation of the universal Church; indeed, evidence of this may be found on nearly every page . . . It is our fervent hope that this solemn festivity may stimulate all Englishmen to unite together in faith and in action: that those who are already the children of the Catholic and Roman Church may cleave still more closely and more lovingly to the centre of Christian unity, and that those who are cut off from unity, may confidently and loyally return to the bosom of Mother Church.

What Pope Pius XI was thinking of is stated very clearly in one passage of St. Bede's Homily for the Feast of Sts. Peter and Paul.

> Blessed Peter in a special manner received the Keys of the Kingdom of Heaven and the headship of judiciary power, that all believers throughout the world might understand that all those who in any way separate themselves from the unity of this faith can neither be absolved from the bonds of their sins, nor enter the gate of the heavenly kingdom. (Quoted in *The Tablet*, p. 672, May 25, 1935).

He Always Prayed

In Anglo-Saxon the name *Bede or Baeda* means prayer. St. Bede certainly merited the name. For he was always primarily the monk, devoted to praising and thanking God. Nothing came before this. It was a part of himself from the time he entered the monastery.

When the yellow plague struck at Wearmouth and Jarrow in 685, only one boy and the Abbot Ceolfrid were left alive of all those at Jarrow who could chant the Office. With hardly any doubt this boy was Bede. With the monastery cut down so drastically, Ceolfrid held limited hours of prayer; but after a week, he could stand it no longer, and he chanted the Office with just the boy.

About 70 years after St. Bede's death, Alcuin, writing from France, reminded the monks at Jarrow of Bede's regularity in prayer:

> But, of a truth, angels often visit your holy places. Once, so men tell, blessed Bede, my master and your patron, said during his life at Jarrow: "I know that the angels are present when our monks chant their Office and meet in chapter. What if they did not find me among them? Would they have to say: Where is Bede? Why comes he not to the appointed prayers with his brethren?" (*Monumenta Germaniae Historica,* epp. IV, 284).

St. Bede's practice on those occasions when he was away from the monastery may be gathered from his comments on the text, "And Jesus entered into Jerusalem and into the Temple." (*Mark* 11:11).

> Whenever ye enter a village or a town or any other place in which there is a house of prayer consecrated to God, let us first go aside within it; and so, after we have commended ourselves to Him, then let us pass on to the business for which we have come.

St. Bede found it especially refreshing to pray Mary's hymn, the *Magnificat*, at the close of day.

> And so this good and wholesome practice has become customary in holy Church, that her hymn be sung every day by all at the chanting of Vespers, for the kindling of our devotion by the memory of the Lord Incarnate and the buttressing of our will to virtue by the remembrance of His Mother. Fitly, too, was this prescribed for the hour of Vespers, in order that the mind, tired by labors and distracted by divers problems, in dwelling awhile on the *Magnificat*, might be lifted from the day's pressing businesses and hurts to face the night in the reality of penitence and new resolve. (Giles, V, 305).

St. Bede rejoiced too that the pagan rites in February honoring the spirits of the dead had been replaced by a procession in honor of Mary at Candlemas Day. Priests and people, carrying candles, walked through the church and the streets as they chanted hymns. (*Bede of Jarrow*, by E. Duckett, p. 310).

The spirit of prayer breathes through the writings of St. Bede. He is always turned toward God. He closes *The Ecclesiastical History* with a formal prayer:

> And now, I beseech Thee, good Jesus, that to whom Thou has graciously granted sweetly to partake of the words of Thy wisdom and knowledge, Thou wilt also vouchsafe that he may some time or other come to Thee, the fountain of all wisdom, and always appear before Thy face, Who livest and reignest world without end. Amen.

Death the Echo

As a man lives, so usually does he die. Death is the echo of life, it has been said. In the death of St. Bede we see him doing what he had done all his life. Fr. Herbert Thurston, S.J. says that "the story of St. Bede's last hours is one of the most beautiful in history." It has been translated by Cardinal Newman, among others.

About two weeks before Easter, 735 A.D., St. Bede was much oppressed by shortness of breath; he rallied and continued his full schedule, giving his students' daily lectures and chanting the Divine Office. "And soon as he woke he was busy in his customary way, and he never ceased with uplifted hands giving thanks to God. I solemnly protest, never have I seen or heard of anyone who was so diligent in thanksgiving."

At this time St. Bede continued to take notes from St. Isidore and to translate the Gospel of St. John into the vernacular. Because of this circumstance, Bishop Lightfoot calls Bede's death the "opening scene of the long, glorious and eventful history of the English Bible." On the Wednesday before the Ascension, toward evening, the young man who had been taking dictation told Bede that there was a sentence to be completed. Bede told him to take his pen and write quickly. Shortly the young man, named Wilbert, said, "Now it is finished." St. Bede replied:

> "Good, you have said the truth, it is finished; take my head into your hands, for it is very pleasant for me to sit facing my old praying place and thus to call upon my Father." And so, on the floor of his cell he sang, "Glory be to the Father, Son and Holy Ghost," and just as he said "Holy Ghost," he breathed his

last and went to the realms above.

St. Bede was buried at Jarrow. In the eleventh century, his bones were taken away secretly to Durham and interred in the cathedral there with those of St. Cuthbert. Later, they were enclosed separately in a shrine of gold and silver. During the time of Henry VIII, St. Bede's tomb was despoiled. In 1831, bones were found buried in the ground beneath the site of the tomb. These relics are perhaps those of St. Bede. A large marble slab above them in the cathedral carries the famed epitaph: *Hac sunt in fossa Bedae Venerabilis ossa.* ("Here lie buried the bones of Venerable Bede.")

On November 13, 1899 Pope Leo XIII declared St. Bede a Doctor of the Church, and made official and universal the title of Saint. May 27 was set as his feast day.

"Candle of the Church"

To know St. Bede is to love him. He was sensitive, yet very humble. He was devoted to God and to his friends—to the service of all. As he taught in his commentary on St. Luke, we are called on to serve God first in adoration, and then in His children by charity of service. St. Bede's devotedness was joined to tender personal feeling. He missed Ceolfrid very keenly when the abbot left for Rome hoping to die there. Because of this parting Bede was even unable to work for a time.

On the afternoon of the day St. Bede died, he made a special point of giving away to priests of the monastery a few prized trinkets of his own. He also begged them urgently to offer Masses and prayers for him regularly, and they willingly promised to do so. St. Bede's eyesight was poor, and perhaps he was even blind in his later years, but he worked on in order to be of service. Regarding his writings he said, "I have made it my business for the use of me and mine." David Knowles, former history professor at Cambridge, says, "He appears as one with all the attraction of holiness, yet not showing what is unfamiliar or inimitable."

The mind of St. Bede ripened to maturity, quietly fed by the silent springs of prayer and reflection. It was not, like that of St. Augustine, fashioned after recoiling from the bitter cup of sin. Yet he knew human nature in depth, and he painted enduring pictures of the abbots whom he knew. Moreover, he understood the depravity and the weakness of men, as he described these so well in his letter to Bishop Egbert. He mastered the learning of the great Doctors and passed it on in simplified form. As St. Boniface, his fellow countryman, says, St. Bede was "the candle of the Church lighted by the Holy Spirit in the English lands."

We might allow a shaft of his light to help guide us in our personal spiritual life. The Venerable Bede says in his homily on St. Vedast,

> Let each of us, in whatever vocation he is placed, strive therein to work out his own salvation. The door of the heavenly kingdom is open to all; but the quality of men's merits will admit one man and reject another. How wretched must it be for a man to be shut from the glory of the Saints and to be consigned with the devil to eternal flames! . . . Let us throng frequently to the Church of Christ; let us diligently hear therein the word of God; and what we receive in the ear, let us retain in our hearts, that we may bear the fruit of good works in patience, and with brotherly love may each study to assist the other.

St. Bede's feast day is May 25 (May 27 in the 1962 calendar).

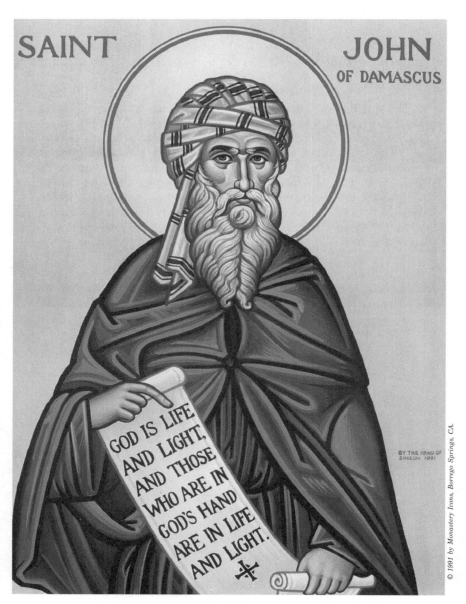

Saint John Damascene

17

SAINT JOHN DAMASCENE

Doctor of Christian Art
Doctor of the Assumption
c. 676-c. 749

WHENEVER we wear our favorite medal or look over the holy pictures we were so happy to have as children, we can thank St. John Damascene. We can thank him again when we look at the crucifixes on our walls, or when in church we see the stained-glass windows, the paintings on the walls, the statues in their niches. All these have nourished thought and devotion.

St. John Damascene is the outstanding champion of sacred images. As such he is also the champion of that article in the Creed which says, "I believe in the Communion of Saints."

We often recite the Creed trippingly. That precious summary of truths takes only a few moments to recite. Yet every article in it has been fought over, sometimes not just by verbal argument—by pens dipped in ink, but by swords that dripped blood. Those who would decry religion because of this must also logically look down on patriotism and love, which have also caused much spilling of blood. Men will always defend what they hold to be most precious.

Doctor of Christian Art

The Eastern Roman Emperor Leo III, the Isaurian (717-741), violently attacked a particular part of Catholic teaching on the Communion of Saints. In 726 A.D. he forbade all his subjects to keep any images, or icons, as the Greeks called them. He ordered the icons in the churches to be destroyed. A few years later, he threatened Pope Gregory II: "I will send an army to break your idols and to take you prisoner." Leo's son, Constantine V (741-775), continued the persecution. The monks were the strongest defenders of icons; many were martyred and many monasteries were burned down. The large church of the Blessed Mother in

Constantinople was stripped of its icons and repainted. People said it then looked like a bird cage or a fruit shop.

The periods of image-breaking or "iconoclasm" lasted 116 years, until the great triumphal procession when icons were carried through the streets of Constantinople on February 19, the First Sunday of Lent in 842 A.D.

Early in the controversy, about 729 A.D., St. John of Damascene (St. John of Damascus) wrote three apologias attacking the Emperor and defending the use of images. In these, he gave such a classical expression of the truths involved that nobody has ever had to improve upon it. He has supplied all the arguments from reason, from the past history of the Church, and from Sacred Scripture. If we wish to explain the use of statues, medals and holy pictures to ourselves or others, we need look no further.

St. John entered the conflict, not to win an argument, but the truth. "Conquest is not my object," he said. "I raise a hand which is fighting for the truth—a willing hand under divine guidance."

He felt strongly the implied charge by the image-breakers that the Church could have been wrong in the past to allow the use of images.

> It is disastrous to suppose that the Church does not know God as He is, that she degenerates into idolatry, for if she declines from perfection in a single iota, it is as an enduring mark on a comely face, destroying by its unsightliness the beauty of the whole. A small thing is not small when it leads to something great, nor indeed is it a thing of no matter to give up the ancient tradition of the Church held by our fore-fathers, whose conduct we should observe and whose faith we should imitate.

St. John Damascene said that the repeated commands given to the Jews not to make an image referred to the making of an image of the invisible God, lest they think He had a shape like a man or beast. Plus, they were very prone to idolatry. But, says St. John, "We have passed the stage of infancy and reached the perfection of manhood. We receive our habit of mind from God and know what may be imaged and what may not."

"Especially since the invisible God took on flesh," says St. John, "we may make images of Christ, who was visible, and picture Him in all His activities, His birth, baptism, transfiguration, His sufferings and resurrection." St. John also asks the pointed question why God, who forbids the making of images to adore, would also command the making of the Ark of the Covenant and the cherubim above the Ark if His previous prohibition were to be absolute. Many times St. John insists that we pay an altogether particular honor to God alone, called *latreia*.

St. John Damascene carries the argument forward. He shows why it is good to have images.

> We proclaim Him [God] also by our senses on all sides, and we sanctify the noblest sense, which is that of sight. The image is a memorial, just what words are to a listening ear. What a book is to those who can read, that an image is to those who cannot read. The image speaks to the sight as words to the ear; it brings us understanding. Hence, God ordered the Ark to be made of imperishable wood, and to be gilded outside and in, and the tablets to be put into it, and the staff and the golden urn containing the manna, for a remembrance of the past and a type of the future. Who can say these were not images and far sounding heralds? (1, 17).

Therefore, St. John Damascene sums up, "You see that the law and everything it ordained and all our own worship consist in the consecration of what is made by hands, leading us through matter to the invisible God." (2, 23).

Acts 6 and 7 of the seventh General Council name St. John Damascene, along with St. Germanus, Patriarch of Constantinople, and St. George of Cyprus as worthy of eternal memory for their defense of sacred images. The same three men had been singled out by the Council of the Iconoclasts held in 753 in the Palace of the Hieria near Constantinople, and anathematized. Constantine V further ordered St. John to be publicly cursed or anathematized once a year. It is not without good cause that St. John Damascene is called the "Doctor of Christian Art."

Golden-Flowing

A river flows through Damascus which the ancients called Chrysorrhoas, or the golden-flowing. This epithet has also been given to St. John Damascene, "who is called Chrysorrhoas because of the golden and shining grace of the Spirit which flowed in both his words and his manner of life." (*PG* 94, 507).

Not too much can be said with certainty regarding the details of St. John Damascene's life. He was born in Damascus of a good Christian family. His father, Sergius, was a tax collector for the Mohammedan Caliph of Damascus. St. John was also known by the surname of Mansur, after his grandfather, who had held a more important job under the Caliph. St. John Damascene succeeded his father as tax collector, but retired, perhaps before 715 A.D., to the Monastery of St. Sabbas, south of Jerusalem as one goes toward the Dead Sea. He was ordained a priest by John V, Patriarch of Jerusalem, before 726. His sermons on the Assumption of Our Lady indicate that he was called upon to preach for special occasions. "Suffer me now to revert again to her praises. This is in obedience to your orders, most excellent pastors, so dear to God." (*Sermon* 2).

But St. John Chrysorrhoas was primarily the monk, praying, leading an ascetical life, studying and writing. Accounts of his life give a great variety of dates for his birth and death. The traditional date for his birth is 676 A.D. He died sometime between 743 and 753; the most accepted date is December 4, 749. All the early sketches of his life say he attained a great age; one menology says he died at the age of 104. (*PG*, 94, 501).

He was buried at the Monastery of St. Sabbas, where his empty tomb can be seen today. His relics were transferred to Constantinople, very likely by the time of the 14th century. His feast day is December 4 (formerly March 27).

The original *Life* of St. John Damascene by John V, Patriarch of Jerusalem, tells the famous legend about the cutting off of his hand. By forging a letter, the story goes, the Emperor Leo III convinced the Caliph that St. John was plotting against him. Leo was smarting under the Damascene's strong defense of images. The Caliph, believing the Emperor, had St. John's hand cut off as a punishment. But St. John prayed to the Blessed Virgin, reminding her, "This hand often wrote hymns and canticles in praise of you, and many times offered the Sacred Body and Blood of your Son in your honor for the salvation of all sinners." (*PG*, 94, 500). He continued his prayer all night. Then Mary appeared to him and said, "Be comforted, my son, in the Lord. He can restore your hand who has made the whole man from nothing." Then she took the hand from where it had been hung in the monastery, and in a moment it was restored to his arm.

Another story from the same source illustrates St. John's undoubted obedience. When he first came to Mar Saba he was placed under the tutelage of an old and very strict monk. Now

St. John "had this one thing engraved in his mind, as on a tablet, that according to the counsel of Paul, whatever he did or was told to do, he would do without complaint." His master was one who knew how to test such a resolve to the limit. He told St. John to go to Damascus and sell baskets there, asking an unusually high price. So John went back to this city where he had been known and where he was held in a position of honor and, dressed in poor and dirty clothes, sang out his chant about the baskets, asking for the ridiculously high price. The onlookers laughed and scoffed. But finally somebody who had known him before recognized him, took pity on him and bought from the Saint at the asking price.

We can readily believe the biographer who relates that John tried to imitate the virtues of the Greek Fathers he studied. "He imitated the studiousness of one Father, the meekness of another, the restraint of another. . . " (*PG*, 94, 495). In later life St. John went through his writings and cut down whatever he judged superfluous or exuberant. A Protestant writer says that it was this same "brilliant fault" of exuberance which had earned him the name of Chrysorrhoas. (Smith-Wace).

The First Summa

In Eastern Christendom, St. John of Damascus has the stature which St. Thomas Aquinas enjoys in the West. He has summed up for them philosophy, doctrine and morals. His original work on morals is not extant, but it has come down to us in two shortened sections known as the *Sacred Parallels*. These are a collection of sayings for guidance in moral and ascetic living, taken from Scripture and the Fathers.

His work known as the *Fount of Knowledge* (also called *Fount of Wisdom*) is, however, a truly original synthesis of philosophy and dogma. It is St. John's greatest work. Its latest English translator says: "The *Fount of Knowledge* not only contains much that is original and a fresh viewpoint on many things, but is in itself something new. It is the first real *Summa Theologica*." (Frederick Chase, Jr., Vol. 37 in *Fathers of the Church* series, p. xxvi).

The *Fount of Knowledge* has three parts. The first is a manual of philosophy that provides a framework for the study of Christian doctrines. In writing these chapters, commonly known as the *Dialectica*, St. John proved himself to be a forerunner of scholasticism. He also gave us a first of such manuals and provided an aid in the understanding of Greek theology that is still of much importance. The second part of the *Fount of Knowledge* lists 103 heresies. St. John supplied only a few original definitions here. The third and most important part is known as the *Exact Exposition of the Orthodox Faith.* It has 100 chapters. It was translated into Latin at the request of Pope Eugene III. Its powerful influence on the West can be surmised from the large number of Latin manuscript copies still in existence. Peter the Lombard used it and may have owed much to it, and St. Thomas Aquinas quotes from it.

St. John Damascene is especially clear in writing about the Incarnation, and the greatest of those who wrote about Christ in later ages owe him a considerable debt. "The *Fount of Knowledge* as a whole remains a fitting monument and landmark to mark the close of the Patristic Age, of which it is one of the greatest single achievements." (F. Chase). St. John's words are precise and clear. Christ

> was in all things and above all things, and at the same time He was existing in the womb of the Holy Mother of God, but He was there by the operation of the Incarnation. And so He was made flesh and took from her the first fruits of our clay, a body animated by a rational and intellectual soul, so that the very Person of God the Word was accounted to the flesh . . . And so we confess that even after the Incarnation He is the one Son of God, and we confess that the same is the Son of Man, one Christ, one Lord, the only-begotten Son and Word of God, Jesus our Lord. And we venerate His two begettings— one from the Father before the ages and surpassing cause and reason and time and nature, and one in latter times for our own sake, after our own manner, and surpassing us. (Book 3, ch. 7).

It may be easier to appreciate St. John Damascene's comments on man.

> He made him a sort of miniature world within the larger one, another adoring angel, a compound, an eyewitness of the visible creation, an initiate of the invisible creation, lord of the things of earth, lorded over from on high, earthly and heavenly, passing and immortal, visible and spiritual, halfway between greatness and lowliness, at once spirit and flesh— spirit by grace and flesh by pride, the first that he might

endure and give glory to his Benefactor, and the second that he might suffer and by suffering be reminded and instructed not to glory in his greatness. He made him a living being to be governed here according to this present life, and then to be removed elsewhere, that is, to the world to come, and so to complete the mystery by becoming divine through reversion to God—this, however, not by being transformed into the divine substance, but by participation in the divine illumination. (Book 2, ch. 7).

Here is how St. John answers the knotty question concerning why God creates a man He knows will be lost.

Being comes first, and afterwards, being good or evil. However, had God kept from being made those who through His goodness were to have existence but who by their own choice were to become evil, then evil would have prevailed over the goodness of God. Thus, all things which God makes He makes good, but each one becomes good or evil by his own choice. (Book 4, ch. 21).

The *Exact Exposition of the Orthodox Faith* ends with a chapter on the resurrection of the body. St. John asks those who say this resurrection from the dust is impossible to consider how the body is formed in the first place from a little drop of seed that grows in the womb.

And so, with our souls again united to our bodies, which will have become incorrupt and put off corruption, we shall rise again and stand before the terrible judgment seat of Christ. And the devil and his demons, and his man, which is to say, the Antichrist, and the impious and sinners will be given over to the everlasting fire . . . And those who have done good will shine like the sun together with the Angels unto eternal life with our Lord Jesus Christ, ever seeing Him and being seen, enjoying the unending bliss which is from Him, and praising Him, together with the Father and the Holy Ghost, unto the endless ages of ages. Amen. (End of St. John's book).

A Writer of Hymns

The notice in the Menaion for December 4 asks: "What shall we call you, O holy one, John the Theologian or David singing his song: a cithara stirring the spirit or a pastoral flute, since

you sound so sweetly both to the ear and the mind?" (94, 507).
St. John Damascene's contribution to theology was great, but
his contribution to hymnody was also great. The problem posed
by the Menaion, if it had to be solved, would need a very tal-
ented balancer of merits. St. John wrote both words and music.
In the East, his work in music has been compared to that of St.
Gregory the Great in the West. But it requires more study before
it can be described in detail.

St. John's hymns, at least with regard to the words, are scattered throughout the Byzantine liturgy. Some accounts make
him responsible for all the Byzantine liturgical office from the
end of the Easter season till the following Lent. The best-known
English translations are his hymns on the Resurrection, Ascension
and All Saints. Rev. John Mason Neale, noted translator of Greek
and Latin hymns, calls St. John Damascene the greatest poet
of the Eastern Church. Following are a few samples, translated
by Neale.

Ode VII says of the Resurrection:

> We keep the festal of the death of death;
> Of Hell o'erthrown: the first fruits pure and bright,
> Of life eternal, and with joyous breath
> praise Him that won the victory by His might,
> Him Whom our Fathers still confest,
> God over all, forever blest.

Ode I for St. Thomas Sunday calls the Resurrection the "spring
of souls":

> 'Tis the spring of souls today;
> Christ hath burst His prison;
> And from three days sleep in death
> —As a sun, hath risen.
>
> All the winter of our sins,
> Long and dark, is flying
> From His light, to Whom we give
> Laud and praise undying.

Ode III for the same Sunday prays:

> On the rock of Thy commandments
> Fix me firmly, lest I slide:

With the glory of Thy presence
Cover me on every side;
Seeing none save Thee is holy,
God forever glorified.

For the Feast of All Saints a hymn attributed to St. John Damascene looks up from earthly labor to sigh after the glory of the Saints. It is known as "Those Eternal Bowers," from the first lines. Here is an excerpt:

While I do my duty
Struggling through the tide,
Whisper Thou of Beauty
On the other side!
Tell who will the story
Of our *now* distress:
Oh, the future glory!
Oh, the loveliness!

(Fr. Adrian Fortescue, renowned liturgist who lived 1874-1923, criticizes Neale's translations as being too free, and hindered by rhymes. He offers his own translation in *The Greek Fathers*.)

Doctor of the Assumption

On November 27, 1950, St. Peter's in Rome held a large crowd of more than 50,000. When Pope Pius XII raised his voice to give the blessing, he spoke the words in Greek. He was presiding at a Pontifical Divine Liturgy according to the Greek Byzantine Rite celebrated by the Patriarch of Antioch. The occasion commemorated the twelfth centenary of the death of St. John Damascene, the last of the Greek Fathers.

The whole setting pointed to his importance. He is a Saint and a Doctor of the Universal Church, proclaimed so by Leo XIII on August 19, 1890. His hymns and beautiful liturgical poetry are liberally used in the Byzantine Rite of the Catholic Church. Among the Orthodox, separated from Rome, he is looked upon as the leading theologian. So St. John Damascene stands as a powerful bond between East and West, just as Damascus, his birthplace, lies between East and West.

"In every attempt to bring about union between Rome and the East, the teaching of Damascene has served as a point of agreement, and should reunion eventually come, St. John

Damascene and the Lady of whom he sings will play an important part." This is the comment of Paul Palmer, S.J. in his book, *Mary in the Documents of the Church.* (p. 60).

Just a few weeks before the November 27 Mass in St. Peter's, Pope Pius XII had defined the dogma of the Assumption. The teaching of this truth as a dogma was new, but the truth itself was revered and ancient as a tradition. Pope Pius' definition only brought it into its final and sharpest focus. In *Munificentissimus Deus*, defining the dogma of the Assumption, the Pope called St. John Damascene "the interpreter of this tradition par excellence." He then quoted St. John:

> There was need that the body of her who in childbirth had preserved her virginity intact, be preserved incorrupt after death. There was need that she who had carried her Creator as a babe on her bosom, should linger lovingly in the dwelling of her God. There was need that the bride whom the Father had betrothed to Himself should live in the bridal chamber of Heaven, that she who had looked so closely upon her very own Son on the Cross, and who there felt in her heart the sword-pangs of sorrow which in bearing Him she had been spared, should look upon Him seated with His Father. There was need that God's Mother should enter into her Son's possessions, and as a Mother of God and hand-maid, be reverenced by all creation. (Par. 21).

The words are taken from the second of St. John's three homilies on the Assumption of Mary. From the opening words of the third sermon it seems that all three were preached on the same day at Mary's tomb in Jerusalem. The occasion was the Feast of the Assumption of Our Lady—also called her "Dormition" or "Falling Asleep."

The third sermon opens in this way:

> Lovers are wont to speak of what they love and to let their fancy run on it by day and night. Let no one, therefore, blame me if I add a third tribute to the Mother of God on her triumphant departure. I am not profiting her, but myself and you who are here present . . . She does not need our praise. It is we who need her glory . . .

St. John Damascene's words about the Blessed Mother overflow with love, humility and gratitude. You can feel the surging emotion and understand that the beautiful words do not satisfy his yearning to say something better and more fitting. "She is greater than all praise." In his "winter of poverty" he wants to "bring garlands to our Queen, and prepare a flower of oratory for the feast of praise." (*Sermon* 2).

Grateful, humble love can hardly speak more convincingly: "But what is sweeter than the Mother of my God? She has taken my mind captive and held my tongue in bondage. I think of her by day and night. She, the Mother of the Word, supplies my words." (*Sermon* 3).

St. John addresses Mary's empty tomb and asks:

> Where is the pure gold which apostolic hands confided to you? Where is the inexhaustible treasure? Where the precious receptacle of God? Where is the new book in which the incomprehensible Word of God is written without hands . . . Where is the life-giving fountain? Where is the sweet and loved body of God's Mother? (*Sermon* 2).

St. John concludes his third homily:

> Accept then my goodwill, which is greater than my capacity, and give us salvation. Heal our passions, cure our diseases, help us out of our difficulties, make our lives peaceful, send us the illumination of the Spirit. Inflame us with the desire of thy Son. Render us pleasing to Him, so that we may enjoy happiness with Him, seeing thee resplendent with thy Son's glory, rejoicing forever, keeping feast in the Church with those who worthily celebrate Him who worked our salvation through thee: Christ, the Son of God, and our God. To Him be glory and majesty, with the uncreated Father and the all-holy and life-giving Spirit, now and forever, through the endless ages of eternity. Amen.

Marian Theology and Devotion

St. John Damascene at various places in his writings shows a clear belief in Our Lady's Immaculate Conception. He explains in a sermon on Mary's nativity why she was born of a sterile mother. "Since the Virgin Mother of God was to be born of Anne, nature did not dare to precede the product of grace, but remained sterile until grace had produced its fruit." (PG, 96, 664). In the homilies on the Assumption, St. John is at pains to explain that

Mary, although not subject to death, died nonetheless. Death, of course, is the penalty for sin, and only one preserved even from Original Sin would be exempt.

> For how could she who brought life to all, be under the domination of death? But she obeys the law of her own Son and inherits this chastisement as a daughter of the first Adam, since her Son, who is the Life, did not refuse it. As the Mother of the Living God, she goes through death to Him. (*Sermon* 2).

In the East, Marian devotion probably reached its high point with St. John of Damascus. It would be easy, for example, to go through his sermons on the Dormition and from them alone make up a new litany of the Blessed Virgin Mary. She is the perennial source of true light, the treasury of life, the richness of grace, the cause of all our good. She is life-giving ambrosia, true happiness, a sea of grace, a fountain of healing, a fruitful tree, the lily of the field, the rose among thorns, the gladness of angels, the sweetness of patriarchs, refreshment of the weary. She is as shining as the dawn, beautiful as the moon, conspicuous as the sun; she is Queen, Virgin Mother of God, a rich treasure-house of the Godhead. Mary is the Saint of Saints, the spotless Virgin, most dear among women, all fair; her fragrance is sweeter than all ointment, the Ark of God. Over and over St. John Damascene calls her the Mother of God.

St. John was a man who sought wisdom humbly. He did not push himself. Only near the close of his life did he write his greatest work, the *Fount of Knowledge*, and that at the request of Cosmas, Bishop of Maiuma, once his fellow-monk.

St. John Damascene had a penetrating and exact mind that made him a great theologian; at the same time he had the fine feeling and beauty of expression that made him an outstanding poet. This combination of talents must have made him a superb orator. It is a pity that just nine of his sermons have come down to us, for they show his character so well and are truly golden-flowing.

But the point that seems most striking and endearing about St. John Damascene is his constant gratitude for being able to serve God and sing the praises of his Lady, the *Theotokos* or "God-bearer." Perhaps he expressed this best when he said: "We know that in celebrating her praises we pay off our debt, and that in so doing we are again debtors, so that the debt is ever beginning afresh."

St. John Damascene's feast day is December 4 (March 27 in the 1962 calendar).

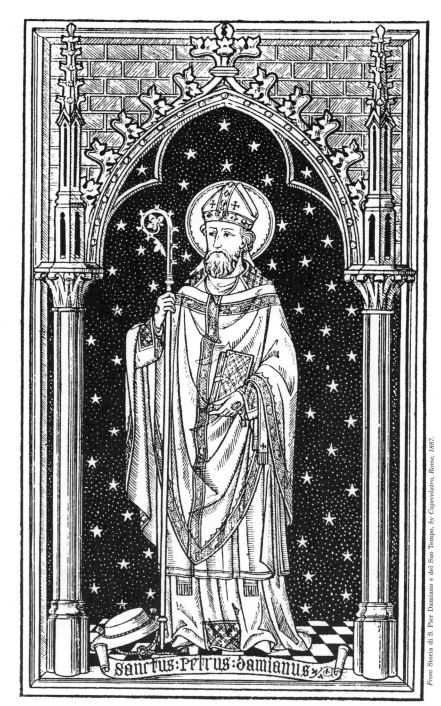

From Storia di S. Pier Damiano e del Suo Tempo, by Capecelatro, Rome, 1887.

sanctus Petrus damianus

Saint Peter Damian

18

SAINT PETER DAMIAN
Monitor of the Popes
c. 1007-1072

"FOR shame! We are already so big that the house can hardly hold us; and how sad the difference between this mob of heirs and the limited inheritance," an older son complained in Ravenna about 1007 A.D. when the youngest boy was born into an already large family. Nobody has noted the name of the complainant, but the unwelcome newcomer in due course left such a legacy of holiness and renowned teaching that in 1828 Pope Leo XII declared him a Doctor of the Church.

The fact that there was a complaint about an inheritance indicates that the family was not altogether poor. The youngest boy was baptized Peter and, when both parents had died, seems to have come under the successive charge of a sister and two brothers. The sister treated him well, but according to St. John of Lodi, St. Peter Damian's biographer, an older brother mistreated him quite severely. Later, another brother, named Damian, who was to become archpriest of Ravenna, took the boy under his care, and noticing his talent, secured for him the best of educations. It is assumed that St. Peter Damian added the name "Damian" to his own out of gratitude to his brother.

Two incidents related by St. John of Lodi show St. Peter's intensity of character. As a little boy he once found a coin and thought for some time about how he might most agreeably spend this unexpected treasure. When the idea suddenly occurred to him that he might have a Mass offered for his father, he dropped the visions of pleasure and gave the coin to a priest.

As a youth, he wore a hairshirt and did much fasting and praying. One night, being severely tempted to carnal pleasure, he arose and immersed himself in cold water until he could hardly move. Then he spent the remainder of the night reciting the whole *Psalter*.

St. Peter Damian helped the poor, often providing meals and serving them with his own hands. For some time he was a successful and acclaimed teacher, but in his late twenties he entered the monastic hermitage at Fonte Avellana. The location was the lower slope of an Apennine peak, about 15 miles northwest of Gubbio. Today the buildings are deserted.

The rest of St. Peter Damian's career could be summed up by saying that he loved and sought solitude, while others kept breaking into his quiet, seeking his talents and influence. The first evidence of others seeking him out was a request from another monastery to have him sent there to preach to and instruct the young monks.

In 1042, St. Peter became prior at Fonte Avellana, and the renown of the monastery grew. He introduced stricter practices and founded "daughter" monasteries, which he visited regularly. Much of his writing was aimed at helping the monks achieve perfection. He wrote the life of St. Romuald and other Saints, for instance, to hold them up for the monks as models of holiness. He can be considered as the founder of a reform based on the Benedictine rule.

St. Peter Damian's writing and example also had a strong influence on other monks not directly under his priorship. In particular, he corresponded often with Desiderius, Abbot of Monte Cassino. On the occasion of a visit there in 1061, he persuaded its monks to take up the use of the discipline. Later he wrote *On the Praise of Scourging* to encourage them to continue this practice. (No. 43, *Opuscula*).

A Papal Legate

St. Peter Damian has been called "The Monitor of the Popes." That they listened to him and valued his advice is well proved by the missions they entrusted to him as their legate. Their esteem is also attested by the pressure put upon him to be consecrated a bishop and receive the title of cardinal. This took place in Rome during November, 1057, under Stephen IX, when Peter Damian was made cardinal and bishop of the fading seaport of Ostia. The regard of the Popes for St. Peter Damian is also shown by the refusal of succeeding Pontiffs to heed his repeated appeals to be released from his duties and to become once again a simple monk. Pope Alexander II finally granted this in 1070, just two years before his death.

Before that date, he had been sent on three great missions. In 1059 he went to Milan and upheld the right of the Church of Rome to intervene in a dispute over clerical reform at Milan. From the human viewpoint, it was "a triumph of bold oratory backed by a great personality." (*Cambridge Medieval History*, Vol. 5, p. 42).

"What province of all the kingdoms of the earth," asked St. Peter Damian, "lies outside her [the Catholic Church's] authority? He who founded the Church of Rome on the rock of the newborn faith was He who gave to the keeper of the keys of life everlasting the rights of heavenly and earthly rule." (*PL* 145, 191).

In 1063 St. Peter Damian went to settle the dispute at Cluny between the monastery and the Bishop of Macon. He upheld the claim of Cluny to be free of episcopal visitation. In 1069 he made his third important trip as representative of the Pope. He travelled to Frankfurt and convinced the Emperor, Henry IV, that he should not divorce his wife, Bertha. It was a turning point in the Emperor's life. He became thereafter not only a good husband, but a good ruler. St. Peter Damian was so very convincing because, as he said, "I seek the favor of no one. I fear no one."

The Monastic Life and Contemplation

St. Peter Damian has been classified as a Camaldolese monk. However, he himself never spoke of anyone but St. Benedict as "our holy father." He admired St. Romuald, the Camaldolese founder and fellow native of Ravenna, but he considered himself and the monks at Fonte Avellana and other monasteries that he himself had started as belonging to the Benedictine family. In fact, he took pains to show that St. Benedict, like himself, had preferred the hermit's way of life to that of the monks. To St. Peter Damian the monastery was just a preparatory stage for the more perfect life of solitude as a hermit. It was a training ground. In the arrangements at Fonte Avellana, some of the brethren lived two by two in small cells near the central church. They came together for the Divine Office. But the more advanced might live at a little distance singly, and recite the Office alone, except on Sundays and feast days of major importance.

> To him who is aiming at the heights of perfection the monastery is a stage, not a dwelling place; a hostel, and not a home; not the end of his striving, but a resting-place on the

way . . . (*PL* 145, 537ff.). For indeed that is good, but this is better . . . It removes almost all the occasions of sin and directs us to an increase of those virtues which please God; so that it destroys the power of sinning and imposes by force of necessity perseverance in good works.

It is from St. Peter Damian's view on the eremitical versus the monastic life that we find a clue to his whole spiritual outlook. Man's aim in this life is to rise to the vision of God, that is, to be able to contemplate. "Holy men are even now able to look upon their Creator by the grace of contemplation." (*PL* 145, 537, ch. 8).

Once, in writing to Desiderius, he commiserates him on the troubles an abbot meets in attending to his duties, thus missing the sweetness of contemplation. He compares the vision of God in this life to a flying fish. It springs into the air and quickly falls back into the sea. So the soul by the wings of virtue springs into the heavenly air of contemplation, but soon must sink back into the sea of everyday life.

If we understand the prime importance St. Peter Damian gave to reaching these little flights into vision here on earth, we understand too the apparent scorn he had for secular learning and the emphasis he put on bodily penance.

Worldly learning can be a hindrance instead of a help to contemplation. "Who lights a lantern that he may see the sun, or candles that he may behold the glory of the stars?" asks St. Peter Damian. (*PL* 145, 701-2). He was not basically opposed to secular studies. He was opposed to monks getting involved in such studies to the neglect of the spiritual life. He himself was a master of Latin and a one-time teacher of secular subjects. He was anxious for his nephew Damian to receive a good liberal education. He asked the Frankish abbot to whom he had sent the boy to send him back wedded to the twin brides of the trivium (grammar, rhetoric and logic) and the quadrivium (arithmetic, music, geometry and astronomy).

Still, secular learning was at best only ancillary to theology. If he made fun of it at times, it was because of the false importance others gave it because they lacked his deeper vision.

What are the inventions of crazy poets to me? What do I care for the melodramatic inventions of pompous tragedians? Let the comedians put an end to the poisoned stream of scurrilities flowing from their noisy lips, and the satirists cease to

burden their audiences with bitter banquets of insidious slander. The Ciceronians shall not sway me with their smooth speech,
nor the followers of Demosthenes convince me by skilled argument or captious persuasion . . . Let the simplicity of Christ
instruct me, and the true humility of the wise loose me from
the chains of doubt . . . (Ch. 1 of *Book of Dominus Vobiscum*).

Penance and Contemplation

Penance was necessary to atone for sin, but it had a greater
purpose as a conditioner for the reception of the gift of vision.
Once this is seen, St. Peter Damian looks much less like his traditional image of one fighting only sin. He appears more like a
determined athlete, doggedly enduring long fasting, stilling the
errant appetites of the flesh, so that the spirit may taste the
sweetness of victory. Once tasted, once the soul gets a glimpse
of God, then the penance itself becomes much easier, and the
spiritual athlete rushes on toward new victory. To see St. Peter
Damian only as a preacher of penance is like looking at an athlete's rugged training program and forgetting about his noble
victories.

Thus, St. Peter Damian's emphasis on penance was not blind;
rather, his chief emphasis was on preparation for union with
God in prayer and in the ultimate refreshment given to man on
this earth, the gift of contemplation. He often spoke of contemplation as "rest":

> For our whole new way of life and our renunciation of the
> world has only one end, rest. But a man can only come to that
> state of rest if he stretches his sinews in many labors and striv-
> ings so that, when the clamor and disturbance is at an end,
> the soul may be lifted up by the grace of contemplation to
> search for the very face of God. (Ch. 8 of *On the Perfection of
> Monks*).

He advised, therefore, against immoderate vigils, but at the
same time he did want his monks to be thoroughly sleepy before
retiring.

> Sleep often on an empty stomach; let drowsiness lessen the
> thirst too that accompanies you to your bed. A moderate vigil
> is the cause of pure prayer, but an indiscreet and idle vigil pro-
> vides the material for talking; for when drooping eyelids and

yawning lips do not allow one to read or pray, it may be convenient to indulge in gossip. Therefore, retire late and rise more moderately for vigils. Let sleep precede the lying down and not the lying down the sleep. (*PL* 145,349).

It is also significant that St. Peter Damian allowed a siesta. "For it is indeed better to make a moderate concession to the flesh in sleeping and fervently to pray later the praises of God, rather than to spend the whole day sleepily yawning." He cautioned against excesses in scourging oneself; even his own monks were not bound to use the discipline, but only advised to.

A Pamphleteer and a Poet

Many of the shorter works of St. Peter Damian, known as *opuscula* ("little works"), were in the form of open letters to the Popes, cardinals, various bishops, abbots, and lay people. He wrote to all the Popes of his era: Gregory VI, Clement II, Benedict IX, Damasus II, St. Leo IX, Victor II, Stephen X, Nicholas II, Alexander II. He wrote often to Hildebrand, who became Pope Gregory VII shortly after St. Peter Damian's death. His writing to Cadalus, an anti-pope, is dramatic. He wrote especially to important lay leaders. The Empress Agnes was a favorite recipient of his letters.

In this manner St. Peter Damian exercised a deep influence on the Church. His remarks were always very much to the point. He is not so much the philosopher explaining principles at length, but rather the crusader giving practical advice. Today many of St. Peter's "little works" would well be called pamphlets.

Their titles explain the trend of his thoughts and efforts: "On Holy Simplicity, to be Placed Before Knowledge Puffing Up" (45); "On Bearing Correction With Equanimity" (46); "On the Perfect Formation of Monks" (49); "Against Sitting at Divine Office" (39); "On Refraining from Anger" (40); "On Patience in Bearing the Insults of the Wicked" (53); "About Miracles" (34); "True Happiness and Wisdom" (58); "About the Catholic Faith" (1); "About Contempt of the World" (12).

In the opusculum "About Chastity and the Means of Guarding It" (47), which is addressed to his nephew, St. Peter Damian recommends daily reception of Holy Communion:

. . . If I may speak so, in order that you may drive the rag-

ing beast from the field of your jurisdiction, try to be strengthened daily by receiving of the Body and Blood of the Lord. Let
the hidden enemy see your lips rubied by the Blood of Christ,
at which he will fear and flee in fear to his lair of darkness.
For that which you receive under the appearance of visible
bread and wine, he, willing or not, knows to be the Body and
Blood of the Lord. (*PL,* p. 712, no. 743, ch. 2).

Opusculum 3 uses a technique still favored by pamphleteers
today. It is in the form of a question-and-answer dialogue. The
dialogue is between a Christian and a Jew. The Jew proposes
the questions, and the Christian answers them.

Among St. Peter Damian's 225 poems, the best-known in
English is "A Hymn of Paradise." It begins:

> Unto the spring of purest life
> Aspires my withered heart,
> Yea, and my soul confined in flesh
> Employs both strength and art,
> Working, suing, struggling still
> From exile home to part.

The first two lines of the epitaph which he wrote for himself
are often quoted. (Op. 1, 1v, p. 162).

> What you are now, we once were;
> What we are now, you shall be.
> Do not put your faith in that
>   which you see is perishable.
> Let frivolous imaginings give way to sincere truth.
> Endless ages will follow passing time.
> Live mindful of death, so that you may live forever.
> Whatever is present will pass,
> And that which is enduring shall come . . .

The *opusculum* or "little work" on almsgiving (9) gives a piece
of advice that is very helpful in developing Christian perfection,
namely, that it is better to keep working on one virtue and try
to become a specialist in that one, than to try to master all the
virtues at once. For nobody can acquire all the virtues at one
time. But by trying to acquire just one, and that thoroughly, all
the others will be brought into play, for they will be needed to
help in acquiring the one emphasized.

In St. Peter Damian's writing you can see the truly mystic

soul, peering longingly through the veil of visible reality (always lumpy even for mystics) to the more solid and enduring, but presently invisible, reality beyond.

A Reformer

St. Peter Damian wrote to everybody, from the Pope and the Emperor on down, giving very pointed advice. Sometimes the recipients had requested his advice, sometimes not. To the cardinals as a group he wrote (*Letter* 51-52):

> In the ecclesiastical order, discipline is neglected almost everywhere; due reverence is not given to priests; canonical sanctions are trodden underfoot; and the work of God is done only for temporal gain. Where are robberies lacking, where thefts, where false oaths, where sinful allurements? Who fears sacrilege? In fact, who has a horror of even the most atrocious crimes?

St. Peter Damian's most influential works were two writings against the basic clerical abuses that weakened the Church in the eleventh century. They were the *Liber Gomorrhianus*, against clerical incontinence, and the *Liber Gratissimus*, against simony (the buying and selling of things sacred, especially offices, benefices, etc.). Simony was really the most basic evil, for the unworthy clerics who became priests or bishops by buying an office were not interested in the Church in the first place. They were interested in their own material well-being, and thus would make little or no effort to observe the Church canons on clerical celibacy.

The *Liber Gomorrhianus* was in the form of a letter to the Pope, St. Leo IX. It is so very frank in describing the evils of clerical incontinence that only an enemy of the Church or a man of much faith and holiness could have written it. The work made bitter enemies for St. Peter Damian—to such an extent that the Pope, who first welcomed it, later held a hushed attitude toward it. The book accomplished its purpose, though, of stirring up opposition to the abuses it outlined.

The *Liber Gratissimus* expressed the opinion that the ordinations of simoniacal candidates were valid, as also the Sacraments which they administered. St. Peter Damian, here and elsewhere, gave clear expression to this truth, which at the time was acridly debated and was finally settled only in the following century. St. Peter Damian is important, therefore, in the theology of ordination.

St. Peter Damian and Cardinal Humbert of Silva Candida were the forerunners of Church reform of these two abuses. However, they differed in their approach to the question of cooperation between the rulers of Church and state, St. Peter favoring more their mutual working together. He was perhaps inclined to allow privileges to the state because of his friendly relations with Emperor Henry IV. He also cared little for the practice of the Popes in maintaining and leading their own armies. Pope Gregory VII (Hildebrand) was indebted for his success as a reformer Pope to the work of Cardinal Humbert and St. Peter Damian. He owed much to their ideas and to the foundations they had laid for reform.

Modern in Devotions

It is quite possible that a thesis could be developed to show the influence of St. Peter Damian on St. Francis of Assisi, and through St. Francis and others, on modern monasticism and modern devotional thinking and practice. St. Francis was also seeking a workable combination of the monastic with the eremitic life. St. Peter Damian introduced fasting on Friday among his monks in memory of the Passion of Christ; St. Francis also put this into his rule. This was evidence of a whole trend of thought that wanted to make the Passion something re-lived and felt in a realistic, very personal way. St. Peter Damian's plea for scourging keeps recalling the suffering and humiliation of Christ receiving the lashes on His naked Flesh. St. Peter Damian asks repeatedly: "Why then should you not be willing to receive the same on your flesh?" Our modern use of the Stations of the Cross, promoted by St. Francis' followers, is one evidence of that trend. Use of the scourge in monastic life may be uncommon today, but we do indeed still recall the journey to Calvary in the form of the Stations of the Cross in our devotional practice.

St. Peter Damian tries to bring the Cross of Christ into the very fabric of the virtues, especially the most basic ones. He speaks of the Cross as representing faith, hope and charity. That part of the Cross which is planted in the earth is faith, which is the foundation of our religion. The top of the Cross, reaching out to Heaven, stands for hope. The twin arms of the Cross are the love of God and the love of neighbor. (*Epistle* 6, 22). The

Saint uses the Cross again to teach about the cardinal virtues: the right arm is prudence, the left temperance. The part reaching upward is justice, and that which bears adversity unshaken is planted solidly in the ground as fortitude. (*Epistle* 6, 22).

To Mary Especially

In his way of speaking of the Blessed Virgin Mary and in his practices in her honor, we can especially see St. Peter Damian's strong trend in the direction of modern Mariology. St. Peter Damian said, in speaking about Christmas, "There was a star in the sky, a star on the earth, the sun in the crib. The star in the sky was that which shone, the one on earth was the Virgin Mary, and the sun in the crib was Christ our Lord." *(Sermon* 1).

He returns to comparing Mary to a star in a sermon for the Feast of the Epiphany.

A star shines in the night, and the Virgin shines in the night of this world with an incomparable light so that it was said of her, "Thou alone hast destroyed all heresies throughout the whole world." (The votive Mass in honor of Mary, *Salve Sancte Parens.)* Such is our star, brethren, such is the Virgin Mary, "the Star of the Sea," and because she has left us an example, that we should follow her steps of such kind should our souls be.

His sermon for the Feast of the Annunciation (*Sermon* 11) begins on a note of fine joy.

Rejoice in the Lord, Brothers, because now there will be a word about that Lady who holds a very special, first place in our hearts. She is the one at whose name you humbly bow your body, at whose hours you reverently assist, whose memory you shower with feast days. She is the one who so delightfully makes sweet your affections, because great is the sweetness of herself. Sweeter than honey is her spirit, in which the sweet Lord rests with all His own sweetness. For when the Lord made all His works very good (*Genesis* 1), He made this one better, consecrating for Himself in her a golden couch on which He might find rest after the tumults of angels and men.

When St. Peter Damian spoke of the Blessed Virgin Mary, his words had a lyrical expression. His ending for the same sermon

(*Sermon* 11) shows this well:

> My Lord is sweet and my Lady is sweet, because He, my
> God, is merciful and she, my Lady, is the door of mercy. May
> she lead us as the mother to the Son, as the daughter to the
> Father, as the bride to the Groom, who is forever blessed, Amen.

Peter Damian had great confidence in Mary's intercession. He
relates a number of incidents to prove her powerful aid. It was
his custom when relating miracles or heavenly appearances to
say carefully just how sure he was of the facts, a rather unusual
scientific trait for his day. He tells, therefore, in relating one of
his stories of Mary's power, that he is not sure of the truth of
the facts but that he is sure of the truth of her powerful help,
which the story shows:

A cleric who had been guilty of many sins in his lifetime had
nevertheless kept up the practice of reciting the Office of the
Blessed Virgin and had confidence in her. As he lay dying, she
appeared to him and assured him that by God's mercy his sins
had been forgiven. St. Peter Damian concludes: "We know beyond
doubt that whoever says her daily office will find a helper and
patron in the Mother of his Judge in the day of need." (*Opusc.*
10, ch. 10).

In a small work addressed as a letter to Desiderius, Abbot of
Monte Cassino and later Pope, he tells the story of the Blessed
Virgin's appearing to a bishop and commanding him to restore
a benefice to an unworthy cleric who was in need. The unworthy cleric had the custom of daily reciting the Hail Mary in her
honor. (*Letter* 33). How much more can we expect, then, St. Peter
Damian asks, if we daily render the homage to her of all her
Hours. In the same letter he refers also to the custom of the
Saturday Mass in Mary's honor. "Therefore, the beautiful custom has also grown up in some churches of celebrating Mass in
her honor every Saturday unless a feast or a Lenten ferial day
hinders it."

His love for "the daughter of kings, but the mother of the
King of Kings" (*Sermon* 46, PL 144, 761) made St. Peter Damian
a promoter of Saturday as her special day. He made Saturday
devotion to Our Lady a custom among the monks of his own
congregation and helped to spread the custom in Italy. He was
not the originator of setting aside Saturday to honor Mary; the
roots of this devotion go back at least 200 years earlier. (Cf. L.

Gougaud, *Devotions et pratiques ascetiques du moyen age*, Paris, 1925, pp. 65-73).

St. Peter Damian gives the reason for choosing Saturday. "Saturday, which means rest, on which day we read that the Lord rested, is aptly enough dedicated to the most holy Virgin. Wisdom made her into a home for Himself (Itself) and rested in her as on a most holy couch through the mystery of assuming lowliness."

Clear in Explaining the Mystical Body

Before he was made a cardinal, St. Peter Damian wrote a little work that is still held in esteem by liturgical scholars. It is *The Book of the Dominus Vobiscum.* The propriety of using the plural form in praying the Office when alone had been questioned by some of the monks. St. Peter Damian addressed his answer to Pope Leo IX, seeking approval of what he had said. (Trans. in Patricia McNulty, *Selected Writings on the Spiritual Life*, Harper, NY, 1960). "Many of the brethren, followers of the eremitic [hermit's] life, have asked me whether, since they live alone in their cells, it is right for them to say 'The Lord be with you [plural]' . . . and the like." In making his reply, St. Peter Damian gives us a very clear and beautiful statement about the Mystical Body of Christ. Today, even with the intensive study of the past decades and the theological foundation of several centuries to help us, it would be hard to give a better explanation than St. Peter Damian's of the unity of Christians with Christ and with one another:

> Indeed the Church of Christ is united in all her parts by such a bond of love that her several members form a single body, and in each one the whole Church is mystically present; so that the whole Church universal may rightly be called the one bride of Christ, and on the other hand every single soul can, because of the mystical effect of the Sacrament, be regarded as the whole Church. (Ch. 5).

He uses an example to explain further this mysterious unity:

> Now just as the Greeks call man a microcosm, that is to say, a little world, because his body is composed of the same four elements as the universe itself, so each of the faithful is a little church, since without any violation of the mystery of

her inward unity, each man receives all the Sacraments of human redemption which are divinely given to the whole Church. (Ch. 10).

Where one part of the faithful prays the official prayers of the Church, there the whole Church prays:

> And so it is good that whatever action in the holy offices is performed by any one section of the faithful should be regarded as the common act of the whole Church, joined in the unity of faith and the love of charity. (Ch. 7).

The Holy Ghost is the cause of the Church's unity:

> For indeed, although holy Church is divided in the multiplicity of her members, yet she is fused into unity by the fire of the Holy Spirit; and so even if she seems, as far as her situation in the world is concerned, to be scattered, yet the mystery of her inward unity can never be marred in its integrity. "The charity of God is poured forth in our hearts, by the Holy Ghost, who is given to us." (*Rom.* 5:5). This Spirit . . . gives to holy Church which He fills, this power: that all her parts shall form a single whole, and that each part shall contain the whole. (Ch. 6).

Therefore, he concludes, it is indeed most proper that when praying alone the person should use the plural form of the particular prayers said in the Office of the day.

A Complex Man

St. Peter Damian signed himself "Peter the Sinner" or "Peter the Sinner-Monk" in his letters. His contemporaries thought of him, unless they were among his enemies, as the holiest man of the eleventh century.

Art shows him as a cardinal holding a knotted cord, recalling his promoting the practice of scourging oneself. The illustration is apt in more ways than one. St. Peter Damian was a man who used the lash against himself, and also the lash of biting correction against the evils of the day. He was not a man who minced his words.

The traditional historical picture of St. Peter Damian is stern and forbidding. He has been called "Old Jerome," a title that would compare him to the fierce fighter and strong rebuker, the great Doctor of the fourth century. St. Peter Damian is pictured as an extremist, seeing sin everywhere, asking for impossible penances, belittling the body and everything in this world.

But he was actually a realist, and his sternness comes from looking stern reality in the face. His age was an age of grave abuses. He was a reformer and an eminent forerunner of other reformers. The age is named after his reforming friend, Hildebrand, later Pope Gregory VII, whom he called a "holy Satan."

St. Peter Damian was a realist too, as all saints are, because he saw the world as it truly is, a place not to rest in, but wherein to work out one's salvation. As he said,

> It is absurd and disgraceful that we should show the same care and precision in human affairs that we devote to the things of God and of the spirit. (*Opusc.* 58, ch. 3).

Those who pay such a saying only lip service will naturally fail to understand the man who honored this truth with his best energies and talents.

Pope Paul VI said that we can study only one part of reality at a time; it is so complex. The same can be said of most people, and especially of those great personalities like St. Peter Damian, who are very complex. History likes to use a bright spotlight, but in doing so, it narrows its range and may light up only one part of a man. Distance in time may help to enlarge it, as eventually more careful study reveals the whole person. In the case of St. Peter Damian, some of this study has been done and more needs to be done. Very little of his work, e.g., has been translated into English, and there is no English biography. But there *is* continuing work in English on his spirituality.

A careful look at St. Peter Damian shows that the traditional historical picture is one-sided. He was himself many-faceted. He was stern, but basically a man of tender feeling. He urged scourging, but forbade excess in its use. He demanded much from his monks, but also he left much to their free choice. He preached penance, yet the motive behind it was to find rest and sweetness in closer union with God.

A Simple Soul

One author explains that St. Peter Damian was a great mystic, and as such so genuinely interested in helping others that he had to be practical and specific and insistent in telling them what to do. We might consider him an awful busybody if we forget that he told others what to do because he loved them. Before God, St. Peter Damian was essentially a very simple soul, for all his thought and effort centered on Christ and on cooperating with His Passion in order to win Heaven. Before men, St. Peter Damian appeared complex, because people could not see the unifying love of God which made a tenderhearted man so stern.

"It is robust common sense and discretion which mark his actions in spite of his blunt talk and occasional violence of manner." This is the opinion of one modern reviewer. (*Downside*, Vol. 77). And Pope Alexander II called him his "eye and the immovable foundation of the Apostolic See." (*PL* 145, 13).

St. Peter Damian was one who stood firmly by the principles which he held. Yet he was also personally quite susceptible to feeling shown against him. This can be noticed in his letters. He complains that Hildebrand (*Epistle* 8, bk. 8) has not sent him one word. He endures a "painful confusion" at the jokes and levity, the tales at his expense, admitted by Hildebrand in company, which are so pleasing to his enemies. "But why should I go on with this writing which I am not sure you will even read? Certainly there is none in the flesh to whom I would more willingly write, if you would deign to give it your attention." In this letter he says too: "I return to you the bishopric which you bestowed," giving a strong indication that Hildebrand had been instrumental in having him made a bishop.

The extravagance of St. Peter Damian's statements, in the setting of continued friendliness, shows the closeness of the friendship between himself and Hildebrand. It was Hildebrand that Peter Damian described, again with the license of friendship, as "the flattering tyrant who showed pity with the love of a Nero, caressed by boxing the ears, stroked with an eagle's talons."

A suffering author's poignant plea sounds in Damian's complaint to Hildebrand and Stephen about the loss of a book. (*Letter* 6, bk. 2). It had been taken by the Pope. "He has taken our book, which I have plucked from the poverty of my own poor little talent with much labor and which I embraced with the arms of a mother's sweetness as an only son."

St. Peter Damian's campaign for penance and for reform proceeded from a real love of God and the Church, bolstered by the passionate feelings of a very sensitive man. He felt strongly and acted strongly, but there is always something measured in his attitudes.

St. Peter Damian's advice to the priors of monasteries may help to explain his driving attitude toward penance, as well as his own cast of mind. The Saint states that the prior should represent strict justice and never deviate from any rule. Let the abbot represent mercy. His kindness will show up all the more against the sternness of the prior. We may suspect that the scourges St. Peter Damian recommended often inflicted a wound on his own basically tender heart.

In a wider sense he wanted each man to be his own prior, to be strict with himself and let the mercy of God shine forth in an outpouring of special graces. For this reason St. Peter Damian is not likely to be popular in our age because it insists on each man's showing mercy to himself and tends to forget justice, or at least to push it off to a hazy and uncertain future. Devotion to St. Peter Damian might help modern man to realize that one who preaches penance and justice does not necessarily forget mercy.

St. Peter Damian's feast day is February 21 (February 23 in the 1962 calendar).

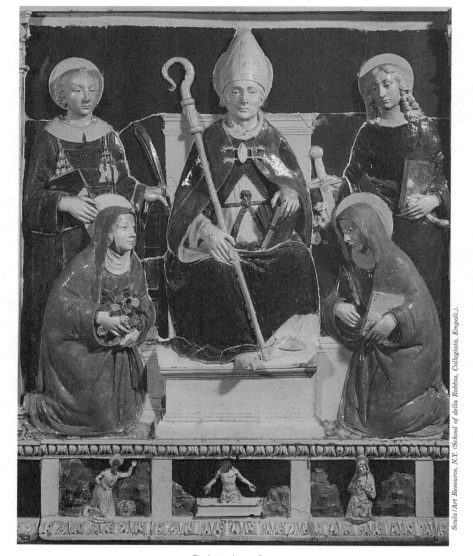

Saint Anselm

19

SAINT ANSELM
Father of Scholasticism
Defender of the Rights of the Church
1033-1109

S T. ANSELM is usually recalled as a profound and original
thinker and the first great Doctor of the Middle Ages. He
made pioneer contributions to the development of philosophy
and theology and paved the way for men like St. Thomas Aquinas
and Duns Scotus.

Yet when you read his biography by Eadmer, his fellow monk,
pupil and secretary, when you sample some of his more than
475 extant letters, it is not St. Anselm's learning that impresses
most. It is rather his lovableness and his profound and tender
spirituality. He was a man who loved God with mystical intensity and loved men with true and touching affection. He speaks
often and with simplicity of this unaffected love.

"May I seek Thee, O Lord, by my desires—may I desire none
but Thee in all my quest! May I find Thee by loving Thee, and
may I love Thee when found." (Eadmer in *St. Anselm, Archbishop
of Canterbury*, London: Sands & Co., 1911). He speaks thus to
Our Lord: "Thou hast given the honey its sweetness, and sweeter
than honey art Thou. Thou hast given all the spices their perfume, and Thy perfume, O Jesus, is above all spices, sweet and
grateful [pleasing]."

Writing to the monks at Bec, he tells of his love for those
with whom he had lived as a monk and an abbot, and he explains
how new attachments do not lessen his old affection.

> But true affection does not love its former friends less, even
> if it be unable to show itself outwardly when it is extended to
> a greater number; just as neither does it fear to be less loved
> by the earlier, if they be true friends, when it obtains the affec-
> tion of a greater number. (*Cur Deus Homo*, 148).

Another time, he tells of his tears while dictating.

> Even now in this very address which I am making to you
> by dictation, tears which my eyes cannot restrain are my wit-
> nesses, as also sobs bursting from my throat and choking it up
> as they overflow from the groaning of my heart, interrupting
> the writer by delaying the words from my mouth. (*Cur Deus
> Homo*, Trans. John Grant, Edinburgh, 1909, 140).

Again, to the monks at Bec he wrote of re-reading their letter.

> I have read in your letter your most affectionate and tender
> love for him whom you love and who loves you; I have read it
> often, and again and again the depths of my heart have been
> deeply and tenderly moved by the contemplation of your love,
> and tears flowed down my cheeks. (*Cur Deus Homo*, 151).

Tears might be a sign of weakness, but not in a man who
withstood kings and fought for justice; they might be a sign of
the mere emotionalism of one unable to face facts, but not in
one whose penetrating intellect wrestled with the most perplexing questions concerning God and man. In him their salt is
the sweetness of strength.

Boyhood in Italy

Pope St. Pius X issued *Communium Rerum*, an encyclical on
the occasion of his own golden jubilee as a priest and the 800th
anniversary of the death of St. Anselm (April 21, 1909). He sums
up St. Anselm's career very neatly.

> It is a pleasure for Us to be able to exhort you to fix your
> eyes on this luminary of doctrine and sanctity, who, rising here
> in Italy, shone for over thirty years upon France, for more than
> fifteen years upon England, and finally upon the whole Church,
> as a tower of strength and beauty.

St. Anselm was born around 1033 in Aosta, Italy, cathedral
city in a valley of the western Alps. His mother, Ermenburga,
was related to the lords of the region; his father, Gandulph, had
come from Lombardy. Just one younger sister, Richera, completed
the family.

Shy and imaginative, St. Anselm's soul responded to his gentle and spiritual mother, who spoke of God as of a kind and good
King. Eadmer relates the story of how the boy dreamed one

night that he had ascended the nearby mountain and found the King. He spoke with Him and finally was fed with bread of dazzling whiteness. When he awoke, the impression was so strong that he was convinced he had been in Heaven. Even in later years St. Anselm spoke of this event.

Another boyhood impression that remained deeply imbedded in his memory was his ill-treatment at the hands of a tutor who drove him beyond endurance. St. Anselm had to return to his own home, either with or close to a nervous breakdown. Ever after he had a special understanding for the problems of the young. Years later, an abbot complained to St. Anselm about the schoolboys at his monastery: "They are utterly perverse and incorrigible . . . In every way we constrain them to obedience, and they will not improve." In reply, St. Anselm gave the example of a tree that is always tied up.

> Would it be anything but a mass of tangled and misshapen boughs? . . . Yet that is just the way you deal with your boys. You plant them in the garden of the Church that they may grow up and bear fruit to God. And then you cramp them so heavily with threats of terrors and blows that they are utterly prevented from making use of any freedom. Depressed in this unwise way, their minds gather all kinds of evil thoughts and become entangled as if with thorns . . . Why are you so harsh with these boys? Are they not human beings? Are they not of the same human nature as you are? . . . You must lift them up and help them in every way with fatherly kindness and gentle treatment . . . Every soul requires its suitable food . . . The weak and tender in God's service need milk, the milk of babes, gentleness from others, kindness, mercy, cheerful encouragement, loving forbearance. (Joseph Clayton, *St. Anselm: A Critical Biography*, Bruce, Milwaukee, 1933, pp. 34-35).

St. Anselm's early wish to enter a monastery was blocked by his father, who had ambitions for him to be at least a bishop. After a while, St. Anselm's fervor cooled, and he no longer had any desire to be a monk; even his love for study left him, and his interest centered in the sports and current events of Aosta. Ermenburga died in 1056, and differences arose between St. Anselm and his strong-willed father.

A Monk in France

At the age of 23, St. Anselm left home and traveled for three years. The fame of the great teacher, Lanfranc, drew him to the abbey of Bec in Normandy. At 26 he settled down there to study. But before long, he went to Lanfranc with a vocational question. He did not know whether to be a hermit, a monk, or a layman living in the world who would help the needy. Lanfranc took the brilliant student to Maurille, Archbishop of Rouen, on whose advice St. Anselm entered the monastery at Bec.

Three years later, he was made prior by the saintly founder, Herlwin. In 1078 when Herlwin died, the monks unanimously chose St. Anselm as their abbot. The scene of their pleading with him to accept and his refusal is memorable. After several days' delay and repeated denials of his fitness, St. Anselm fell on his knees before the hundred monks and then lay prostrate to beg them not to make him abbot. Caught by surprise, they did not know at first what to do; then, replying in turn, they lay prostrate before him. In the end his conscience made him accept.

St. Anselm spent the largest span of his adult life as a monk, i.e., more than 30 years. This is the life he loved, a prayerful, quiet life, where the soul felt the closeness of God, where the days passed in fruitful teaching and study. Even the office of abbot St. Anselm considered a distraction and a burden, especially since it often took him on journeys and brought with it the care of many scattered properties.

Archbishop of Canterbury

It was while on a visit to England to help reorganize a monastery that St. Anselm was chosen Archbishop of Canterbury. He objected that he was 60 years old, that he was incapable and that he owed allegiance to the Duke of Normandy.

St. Anselm first came to England to be at the bedside of King William Rufus ("The Red"), just as he, Rufus, had gone earlier to his own dying father, William the Conqueror. Rufus promised St. Anselm to stop confiscating Church lands and interfering with and usurping the powers of bishops. He thought himself to be dying. Moreover, the King agreed with the bishops that an appointment must be made for the archbishopric of Canterbury; this see had been vacant since Lanfranc's death three years before and its rents had been seized by the Crown.

St. Anselm was selected, and the scene of his being chosen as abbot was repeated. This time, those beseeching him, the bishops, went down on their knees first, at the behest of the King. Then St. Anselm in turn fell on his knees before them. In irritation, the bishops arose, forced a crozier into his hands and carried him into the church. This was in the spring of 1093. Further discussions and formalities delayed his consecration until December 4, 1093.

The more than 15 years of St. Anselm's episcopate were years of struggle with William Rufus, who had recovered from his illness, and later with his brother, Henry I. The repentance of William the Red had lasted only as long as his sickness. The bishops who had so strongly urged St. Anselm to become Archbishop of Canterbury were usually weak and leaned to the side of the King.

While the details of those long years of struggle—over lay investiture, the paying of homage to a secular ruler, and the recognition of the Pope as the pre-eminent ruler throughout the Church—are complex, they amount to a fight for the freedom of the Church. In upholding his rights as Bishop and the principles claimed by the Church, St. Anselm was forced to spend two three-year periods in exile away from England, first under William Rufus and then under Henry I. It was during the first of these that he attended the Lateran Council and wrote his greatest work, *Cur Deus Homo* ("Why God Became Man"). This is considered to be "the most able if not the most comprehensive work on the mystery of redemption in all Christian literature." Emphasizing the demands of God's justice, it undercut the old idea that exaggerated the role of the devil in making Christ's coming necessary. It laid the foundations for future thinking in Christology.

The final settlement between the Bishop and the Crown is called by Monsignor Mann "a satisfactory compromise—the source of spiritual jurisdiction was elsewhere than in the crown." Hilaire Belloc saw it as a victory for the lay power. Beyond all doubt St. Anselm made clear the principles he upheld concerning the freedom of the Church. Their practical application at the time of the Council of London on August 3, 1107 settled the problems of the time. Whether for long-range effects St. Anselm should have driven a harder bargain, or whether he could have, is naturally difficult to establish. Pope St. Pius X speaks approvingly and at length of St. Anselm's part in fighting for the rights of the Church. He said that he could not express his own feelings better than by quoting the energetic words of St. Anselm himself: "In this world, God loves nothing more than the liberty of His Church."

Defender of the Apostolic See

The Encyclical introduces St. Anselm as "Doctor Anselm of Aosta, most vigorous exponent of the Catholic truth and defender of the rights of the Church, first as monk and abbot in France, and later as Archbishop of Canterbury and Primate in England." Later, Pope St. Pius X mentions that St. Anselm illustrated in his life most strikingly the zeal of a good prelate and his fear of the evils that beset the souls under him. But in the grief he felt at seeing himself culpably abandoned by many, even including his brethren in the episcopate, his one great comfort was his trust in God and in the Apostolic See.

The Pope also quotes one of St. Anselm's letters in reference to bad princes.

> Disdaining obedience to the decrees of the Apostolic See made for the defence of Religion, they surely convict themselves of disobedience to the Apostle Peter whose place he holds, nay, to Christ who recommended His Church to Peter . . . because they who refuse to be subject to the law of God are surely reputed the enemies of God.

At the Council of Rockingham St. Anselm placed himself squarely against almost all the bishops of England in resisting the demands of King William Rufus. St. Anselm addressed the assembled bishops in church:

> From Him do I seek guidance. It was He who said to Blessed Peter, "Thou art Peter, and upon this rock do I build My Church." He said to all the Apostles, "Who hears you, hears Me" and "Who touches you, touches the apple of My eye." As we know He said these words to Blessed Peter, and through him to the other Apostles, so we hold that these things are meant first and foremost for the Vicar of St. Peter, and through him for the bishops who fill the place of the Apostles—they are not addressed to emperor or king, to duke or count. (Eadmer, Sands, pp. 172-173).

What our duty of submission and obedience to our earthly princes is, that same Angel of Great Counsel teaches us, saying, "Render to Caesar the things that are Caesar's and to God the things that are God's" . . . Wherefore, hear ye. In those things that are of God, I shall obey the Vicar of Blessed Peter, and in matters which touch my earthly sovereign's rightful dignity, I shall give him all the counsel and help in my power.

In 1097, when trying to leave England to take his case to Pope Urban II, St. Anselm told William Rufus: "He who forswears Blessed Peter, forswears Christ, who placed him as prince over His Church. When, therefore, O King, I have denied Christ, I shall pay to your court whatever fine it may impose for the sin committed in so swearing."

In a letter to Pope Paschal II, St. Anselm wrote: "I do not fear exile, or poverty, or torture, or death; for being strong in God, my heart is ready to bear all these for obedience to the Apostolic See and the liberty of my mother, the Church of Christ." (2, 39).

Father of Scholasticism

Writing in the *Dublin Review*, April, 1943, the Benedictine scholar R. Rios says of St. Anselm: "His position as a Doctor of the Church is unique, for it was he who closed the patristic period and opened the age of the Schoolmen with the golden key of his theological speculation . . . his was a giant mind. His treatises make it evident that he was possessed of a keen intellect, that he was a profound as well as an original thinker."

St. Pius X, in the encyclical mentioned, calls St. Anselm the precursor of the schoolmen, the scholastic philosophers/theologians whose work was to flower in the twelfth and thirteenth centuries.

It may well be said that Anselm was raised up by God to point out by his example, his words and his writings, the safe road, to unseal for the common good the spring of Christian wisdom and to be the guide and rule of those Catholic teachers who, after him, taught "the sacred letters by the method of the school," and he thus came rightly to be esteemed and celebrated as their precursor. Not indeed that the Doctor of Aosta reached all at once the heights of theological and philosophical speculation, or the reputation of the two supreme masters, Thomas and Bonaventure. The later fruits of the wisdom of these last did not ripen but with time and the collaboration of many doctors.

Even more to the point, St. Pius X says:

> Yet Anselm accomplished far more than he ever expected or than others expected of him. He secured a position in which his merits were not dimmed by the glory of those that came after him, not even of the great Thomas, even when the latter declined to accept all his conclusions and treated more clearly and accurately questions already treated by him. To Anselm belongs the distinction of having opened the road to speculation, of removing the doubts of the timid, the dangers of the incautious, and the injuries done by the quarrelsome and the sophistical, "the heretical dialecticians" of his time, as he rightly calls them, in whom reason was the slave of the imagination and of vanity.

Whereas Scholasticism is hard to define precisely, it can be called a system of philosophy whose essential aim is to give a philosophical basis and a system to the teachings of religion. T. J. Motherway says that "St. Anselm was, however, the first to institute systematically philosophic discussion of the teachings of the Church. He was the first to take the truths of Revelation as a starting point and with reason alone to go out in search of the principles and truths which would lead him back as far as possible to the doctrines from which he had started." (*Modern Schoolman*, 15, 79-83). Motherway calls St. Anselm's *Monologion* the "first complete theodicy ever produced."

The "Ontological Argument"

After St. Anselm had written his *Monologion*, he composed another book, the *Proslogion* ("Discourse"), which was originally called *Faith Seeking Understanding*. It was the result of his own seeking for one single argument for God's existence—one that would require no other proof except itself. He lost both sleep and appetite in mulling over the problem, and just about the time he was ready to give up, the flash of discovery suddenly illuminated his mind. To him the whole proof had become crystal clear. But great thinkers who have examined his "proof" differ over this famous "ontological argument" of St. Anselm. Duns Scotus and Alexander of Hales accepted it. St. Bonaventure praised it, but St. Thomas rejected it. This difference of weighty opinion makes it a point of special interest for those who like to think things through on their own.

The flash that St. Anselm saw was the necessity for existence to be a part of the idea of God as a Being "than which nothing greater can be imagined." Many could agree with him that God was that Being above all others, above whom nothing could be imagined. But as the monk Gaunilon objected (and others agreed) in "The Case for the Fool," how could a person know that the highest thing thinkable existed? St. Anselm's answer for that was that if it did not exist, it was not the highest thing thinkable, for the highest thing thinkable that did exist must be higher. In short, the mind demands a supreme being, and existence must belong to the essence of the Being that is demanded. Otherwise, it would not be supreme.

Faith and Reason—Not Faith versus Reason

Whether this particular argument is valid or not, St. Anselm's whole system and its underlying principles are especially valuable for settling many modern problems. St. Anselm knew that truth is one, that there can be no conflict between faith and reason. His plan was to use reason to better understand the truths of faith.

But St. Anselm's starting point for philosophizing was faith. His approach is especially good for our age, which tends to overemphasize the role of reason. In the ordinary affairs of life, we would be helpless if we had to understand everything first. We must act on human faith to use a radio, electricity, an airplane, medicine, etc. So also is a person helpless supernaturally unless he starts with supernatural faith. Reason can and should be used to the highest degree, but when it comes to religion, reason is helpless unless it joins and acts with a faith that is already active, dynamic.

At the end of Chapter One of the *Proslogion*, St. Anselm gives a summation of his approach:

> . . . I long to understand in some degree Thy truth, which my heart believes and loves. For I do not seek to understand that I may believe, but I believe in order to understand. For this I also believe, that unless I believed, I should not understand.

Completely Human

One of St. Anselm's special talents was to be able to fall asleep at a moment's notice. When he was engaged in a law trial, as happened in fulfilling his duties as abbot, he seemed to pay little attention to the arguments of opponents. Often he napped while they vehemently pleaded their cause. But when his turn to speak came, he set forth the truth of the case so clearly that an observer might have thought the other person had been napping.

To a former pupil named Maurice, St. Anselm confided that he had been remiss in teaching grammar. "You know that it was always tiresome to me to teach boys grammar, so that I did it much less than would have been useful for you. I know that under me you went back in parsing."

When asking the prior at Canterbury for a copyist, St. Anselm's charity was not above specifying one who wrote well. "I beg of you to cause to be written out for me the book *Cur Deus Homo* in one volume, for I want to send it to the lord pope, and I would ask that someone who writes clearly and distinctly may transcribe them." This innocent request brings up the picture of the gentle abbot exercising patience on the many occasions when the writing was not clear and distinct.

To his nephew Anselm, son of his only sister, the Saint confides a special love and tells of worries over the young man's progress.

> Since of all my relations it is for thee that I feel the most special love, I long for thy improvement in the sight of God and before everyone . . . Study carefully . . . spend no time in idleness. Strive most to acquire a thorough knowledge of grammar by declining and parsing, by dictation; and practice reading prose, rather than verse. Above all keep guard over thy behavior and thine actions before men, and over thy heart before God, so that when, God permitting, I see thee, I may rejoice in thy progress and thou be glad in my joy.

One day a hare pursued by dogs ran toward St. Anselm. He reined in his horse to protect the hare and rebuked the page boys who were urging on the dogs. Then he called off the dogs, and the hare scampered to safety.

Another time he saw a boy with a bird on a string. The boy allowed some slack, and the bird flew off, only to be stopped abruptly by the string and hauled back in. "I wish the string would break so that it could fly away," St. Anselm said. This happened almost as soon as he had said the words. The Saint then took advantage of the occasion to tell his companions that the devil also used men's passions to ensnare them, and that unless God helped, and men made a great effort to break the cord, they would not be free.

Completely Spiritual

If it is human to err and divine to forgive, St. Anselm showed himself completely devoted to the divine by ready forgiveness. When he was first made prior, some in the monastery objected because he was young and had been there just three years. In particular, there was one monk named Osbern who went out of his way to be mean and difficult. The young prior set himself to win him by gentleness, granting him ready dispensations and privileges. His warmth and love gradually brought Osbern around, and then the prior, having won his confidence, led him back to stricter observance for the good of his soul. When Osbern grew sick, St. Anselm watched at his bed day and night. When Osbern died, St. Anselm could not forget him. He wrote of "dear, dead Osbern" and asked for prayers. "Wherever Osbern is, his soul and mine are one . . . do not forget the soul of my dear Osbern; and if I seem too troublesome, forget me and remember him."

The same can be said of St. Anselm's treatment of King William Rufus. The King caused him untold grief by harming the Church; not only that, but Rufus often insulted Anselm and reviled him personally. Yet when in the end William Rufus, having gone out to hunt, was found stiff and cold with an arrow through his heart, St. Anselm was the chief mourner. He wept and grieved for him, especially because he had not received the Sacraments.

The loving, spiritual and refined nature of St. Anselm drew hearts to him. Wherever he went, men were attracted to him whose face was "not that of a man, but of an angel." (Eadmer, Sands, p. 203). When he traveled incognito in Italy, men came to ask his blessing after seeing him. He was tall and slim, though in later years a bit stooped. Those who came into contact with St. Anselm could feel the depth of a nature in close contact with God and a character at once firm and gentle.

His glowing piety and sensitive, spiritual nature are shown in his writings, even those that are philosophical. He is ever seeking God. The first chapter of the *Proslogion* makes in itself a touching prayer, springing from the depths of man's littleness, yearning to understand something of God.

> Pity our toilings and strivings toward Thee, since we can do nothing without Thee. Thou dost invite us; do Thou help us ... Lord, in hunger I began to seek Thee; I beseech Thee that I may not cease to hunger for Thee. In hunger I have come to Thee; let me not go unfed. I have come in poverty to the Rich, in misery to the Compassionate; let me not return empty and despised . . . Teach me to seek Thee, and reveal Thyself to me when I seek Thee, for I cannot seek Thee except Thou teach me, nor find Thee except Thou reveal Thyself. Let me seek Thee in longing, let me long for Thee in seeking; let me find Thee in love and love Thee in finding . . .

His prayers and meditations, beautiful and flowing in style— as are all his writings—reveal the sweetness of his soul even more. Some of them have been translated into English by Cardinal Manning. (Most of those in the PL [*Patrologia Latina*] collection are not, however, considered genuine.)

At the Monastery of St. Mary at Bec, the monks, though Benedictines, wore white in honor of the Blessed Virgin Mary. St. Anselm's writings reveal the purest affection and the highest esteem for her. Although he did not write about Mary in formal treatises, he deserves to be called a great Marian Doctor. For he set forth the tradition about her with clarity and force, showing the divine maternity to be the foundation of all Our Lady's privileges. "Nothing is equal to Mary; nothing except God is greater than Mary," St. Anselm said.

St. Anselm did not, strictly speaking, profess the doctrine of the Immaculate Conception (which had not yet been defined as a dogma by the Church), but he formulated the principle which later thinkers used in developing the proofs for the doctrine. "It was becoming that the Virgin should shine with that purity than which none greater under God can be thought of." Anselm never made the final application because of the absolute nature of his ideas concerning the transmission of Original Sin by human generation.

The Feast of the Immaculate Conception was celebrated even before St. Anselm's time in England; it had already been suppressed at the time of the Norman conquest. St. Anselm's nephew of the same name helped to restore it.

If the doctrine of Mary as the Mediatrix of All Graces is defined, the name of St. Anselm will be prominent in that regard. He upheld the truth of her universal mediatorship both in the meriting and the distribution of grace.

We have a familiar legacy of St. Anselm's Marian devotion in the hymn, "Daily, Daily Sing to Mary." It is a translation of the first part of his hymn of praise called the *Mariale* (defended by Ragey as authentic).

He Has Exalted the Lowly

Pope St. Pius X speaks of St. Anselm's force and gentleness, his singleness of purpose and his humility. He quotes approvingly some words of St. Anselm regarding the need for a humble approach to the study of divine things.

> For there are some who, immediately they have begun to grow the horns of an overweening knowledge—not knowing that when a person thinks he knows something, he does not yet know in what manner he should know it—before they have grown spiritual wings through firmness in the Faith, are wont to rise presumptuously to the highest questions of the Faith. Thus it happens that while . . . against all rules they endeavor to rise prematurely by their intelligence, their lack of intelligence brings them down to manifold errors.

Once a friend, not agreeing with what St. Anselm wrote, added a paragraph of refutation on the original document before sending it back. (This was not a mere note of criticism, but was written on the finished product.) St. Anselm was not angry, and when the book was to be copied over, he left the paragraph in, adding another to clarify the point.

St. Pius X throws light on St. Anselm's humility in all his writings.

> Anselm himself, with that great modesty so characteristic of the truly wise, and with all his learning and perspicacity, never published any writings except such as were called forth by circumstances, or when compelled thereto by some authority, and in those he did publish, he protests that "if there is anything that calls for correction, he does not refuse the correction."

St. Anselm's life was dotted with miracles—which he completely disclaimed. A nobleman suffering from leprosy prayed and gave many alms, asking for a cure. In a vision one night he was told to go to the Abbot of Bec and ask to be allowed to drink the water used to wash his fingers during Mass. St. Anselm was embarrassed and at first refused—until his kindness succumbed to the nobleman's entreaties. The man served his Mass quite early at a side altar, drank the water, and was cured.

Another time, when men came rushing to save a house from fire, they were met by the lady of the house, who told them not to fear, since Archbishop Anselm was staying there. His companions, Gundulf and Baldwin, hearing this, asked St. Anselm to do something, as the fire from neighboring houses was perilously close. They asked him to go out and make the Sign of the Cross. This he refused to do, but he did go out lest he be burnt alive. The two companions seized his hand and raised it in a Sign of the Cross; the flames quickly subsided, leaving the neighboring house half burnt.

When St. Anselm was staying in exile near Lyons, many reported themselves cured of fever by eating bread left over from his table. At Macon the people begged him to pray that their four-month drought might end. Before he left the city, the rain came, refreshing the parched soil.

Near Schiavi in Italy, where he wrote *Cur Deus Homo*, he picked an unlikely spot to dig at, in answer to a lay brother's request for help in getting a good well. But on the third day of digging, an abundant supply of water sprang out of the rocky ground. The water has never failed to this day, and is still pointed out as "St. Anselm's Well."

St. Anselm died as the morning of April 21, 1109, was breaking. It was Wednesday in Holy Week. The monks at Canterbury had laid him on the ground, according to monastic custom, on sackcloth and ashes.

He is buried in the Cathedral of Canterbury in the chapel originally dedicated to Sts. Peter and Paul, which is now called St. Anselm's Chapel. After almost 400 years, he was canonized in 1494 by Alexander VI and declared a Doctor of the Church by Pope Clement XI in 1720.

In 1791, the abbey at Bec was suppressed; the church and chapter house were destroyed. In 1948 the Benedictines returned to Bec, and in 1959, they held a congress there commemorating the ninth centenary of St. Anselm's coming to Bec. (*Tablet*, July 25, 1959).

St. Anselm was Archbishop of Canterbury, a speculative and original thinker, and the pioneer of Scholasticism. But he was most truly a monk, a man seeking God in prayer and meditation. It is fitting that the monks have returned to the monastery of Herlwin, of Lanfranc, and of Anselm.

There is no great popular cult of St. Anselm, though few, even among the Saints, can match his lovableness. Perhaps St. Anselm still prefers, even in Heaven, to observe the hidden life. His feast day is April 21.

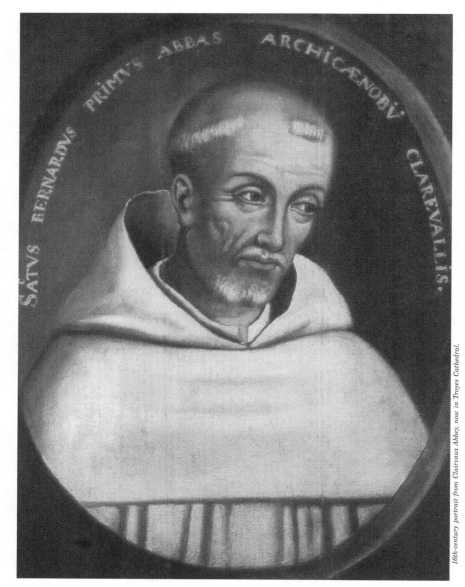

16th-century portrait from Clairvaux Abbey, now in Troyes Cathedral.

Saint Bernard of Clairvaux

20

SAINT BERNARD OF CLAIRVAUX

The Mellifluous Doctor
Oracle of the Twelfth Century
Thaumaturgus of the West
Arbiter of Christendom
The Last of the Fathers
c. 1090-1153

"WE all take to ourselves St. Paul's injunction to St. Timothy, 'Use a little wine [for thy stomach's sake].' Only somehow we do not lay enough stress on that word, 'a little.'" St. Bernard was complaining about monks who had suddenly discovered that they possessed weak stomachs and needed the agreeable medicinal help suggested by the Great Apostle. In the phrase of George Bernard Shaw, St. Bernard's character sketches, which were aimed at monastic reform, "dissolved the Middle Ages in a roar of merriment."

The holy Abbot of Clairvaux was not trying to be funny. But the foibles of human nature tend to appear comical when caught assuming a dignified pose. And St. Bernard had a habit of sending a direct, searching beam of truth on whatever subject he explored. It might be theology, philosophy, asceticism, political affairs, or an everyday problem. His intuitive grasp of a subject and his flowing but punchy style make it hard to miss the point.

Users of costly apparel and cosmetics might not agree with St. Bernard's advice to Sophia, but would find it difficult to frame an equally pungent rebuttal:

> Silk and purple and the ruby dyes applied to the skin exhibit their own loveliness but impart it not. Surely a beauty which is put on with a garment, and laid aside with it, belongs to the clothes and not to the wearer. Do not emulate the evil-minded, who painfully seek artificial attractions because they are conscious they have none of their own. Deem it unworthy to borrow comeliness from the skins of little beasts and the

281

toil of caterpillars. Be content with your own. Oh, how lovely the bloom with which the jewel of true modesty tints a virgin's cheek! . . . Self-discipline gives a graceful dignity all its own to a maiden's deportment and countenance. It bends the neck, smooths the brows, represses the contortions of laughter, assuages anger . . .

The Gallic Bee

A little book by Theophilus Reynauld which appeared in 1508 entitled *The Gallic Bee* was the first to call St. Bernard "The Mellifluous Doctor." This has been his most common description ever since, and it was used as the title of the encyclical letter of Pope Pius XII commemorating the eighth centenary of his death, May 24, 1953. During the Middle Ages a common epithet for St. Bernard was *Theodidaktos*, which is Greek for "Taught by God."

St. Bernard is aptly called "mellifluous," not only because of his flowing, elegant Latin, but more so because of his sweetness of spirit. His words rise as the fragrant aroma of an incense burning in a heart on fire with the Holy Spirit. His words are honey-flowing because, as a diligent bee, he has extracted the sweet essence from Scripture and the Fathers and refined it in loving meditation. What he says is a synthesis of Scripture (which he is said to have known by heart) and the ancient writers, yet it is not old or copied, but rather new because he has made it completely his own.

He has also colored it with the rich and varied tints of the beauty he so much loved in nature. St. Bernard used to sit with the Scriptures open on his lap, read a while, then look out over the Burgundian landscape and reflect. He meditated too when he took his place with the other monks in the fields.

Characteristic of his intensity of spirit was the way he went about this manual labor. He was so awkward at first with the scythe that his superiors had to make him work apart from the others, lest they suffer injury. So he practiced in private, and before long he could take his place with the best swingers of the curved blade.

"The Gallic Bee" could also sting. But St. Bernard's stings were always either to turn people away from spiritual danger, to stir them to pursue good, or to chase them away from harming the Church. Those he chided usually understood that even his painful stings proceeded from love—that they hurt only in order to cure. In his direct and forceful way, he went to the heart of the problem like a doctor lancing an abscess.

Writing to a nun who had for a time lived unworthily of her vows, he says:

> While you were trying to live as one of the world under the habit and name of religion, you alone had rejected God by your own will. But you found that you were not able to do what you stupidly thought you could: the world rejected you, but not you the world. So while you turned away from God, the world turned away from you, and you fell, as the saying goes, between two stools. You did not live for God, because you did not wish to, nor for the world, because you were not able to. You were dead both to God and to the world, to the former willingly and to the latter unwillingly. This is what is apt to happen to those who make vows and do not keep them, who according to their profession are one thing and in their heart another . . . Why did you feign by the veil on your head a gravity that your impudent glances belied? The veil you wore covered a haughty brow; under the outward guise of modesty, you carried a saucy tongue in your head . . . (*Letter* 114).

St. Bernard called Arnold of Brescia "this scorpion with the dove's head." Arnold was a seditionist who led a model ascetical life, but preached that all goods should be taken away from the Church and given to the laity. In St. Bernard's description, "Arnold of Brescia is a man who neither eats nor drinks, but like the devil he thirsts only after the blood of souls."

The Saint wrote to King Louis VII of France:

> You have not listened to words of peace nor kept your own compacts nor hearkened to wise counsel: but I know not under what judgment of God you have so perverted everything as to count shame honor, and honor shame; you have been afraid of what was safe and have despised what ought to be feared; you have loved those who hated you and have held in hatred those who desired to love you . . . In the murders of men, the burning of dwellings, the destruction of churches, the scattering of the poor, you take part with the robbers and ruffians, according to the word of the prophet: "when you saw a thief, you ran in company with him, and took your portion with adulterers," as if you had not strength enough in yourself to do evil. (*Letter* 223).

This rebuke served in good part to effect the reconciliation of the King and the Count of Champagne, with whom he was warring.

Writing to Pope Innocent II (1124-1130), St. Bernard said, "I speak faithfully because I love truly . . . Whoever are criminal or quarrelsome among either people or clergy, with monks outcast from their monasteries, rush to you; and returning, they boast, with passionate gestures, that they have found protectors where they should have found punishers . . ."

For Pope Blessed Eugene III (1144-1145) he wrote in his treatise *Concerning Meditation*,

> Brush aside the deceit of the fugitive honor, despise the glitter of painted pomp, and think of thyself simply as naked, even as thou camest from thy mother's womb! Art thou ornamented with badges, shining with jewels, brilliant in silks, crowned with plumes, stuffed out with golden and silver embroideries? If thou shalt expel from contemplation all these things, so swiftly passing and soon utterly to vanish like the morning mists, there will appear to thee a man naked, poor, needy, miserable, grieving because he is a man, blushing at his nakedness, deploring his birth; a man born to labor, not to honor; born of a woman, and so under condemnation; living only a little while, and therefore full of fear; replete with miseries, and weeping because of them. (ii, 9).

The Famous Debate with Abelard

The story of his dealings with the brilliant Peter Abelard has been at times cited as an illustration of a ruthless streak in St. Bernard's character. But there was nothing whatever ruthless about St. Bernard; he was always essentially lovable and loving, but the gesture of truth sometimes has to be not a pointing finger, but a mailed fist. It was Abelard who entered the ring and set himself up for the knock-down.

The ideas of Abelard set down in two books called *The Theology of Peter Abelard* were dangerous to the faith of his followers and especially to the faith of the common people. Naturally the zeal of a man so devoted to the Faith as St. Bernard was aroused. He called Abelard's theology "fool-ology" and his reasoning "raving." But when St. Bernard was called to refute Abelard, he spoke to him at first only in private, hoping to win him over to the proper, more traditional expression of theology. Later he wrote letters asking the Pope and various cardinals to do something to avert the danger to souls posed by Peter Abelard.

But Abelard issued a challenge to Bernard to meet him in public debate, where the odds would be on Abelard's side. He was a renowned rhetorician and debator. As a young man he had already crushed and humiliated his teacher, William of Champeaux, in a public debate. He was not only brilliant, but trained in logic and debate. St. Bernard was more of a philosopher of the intuitive type; therefore, he was not anxious to meet Abelard in debate. He feared that it would harm the cause of True Religion if he were made to look bad by a man of such brilliance. To his archbishop, who wanted St. Bernard to engage in the debate, he wrote: "Where all flee before his face, why should he pick me out for single combat: I am but a child, and he a man of war from his youth."

There was, however, no choice but for St. Bernard to accept the debate. To refuse would in itself look like a defeat. So he went to the synod at Sens, where the debate was to be held in the cathedral. The King was there; so too many high churchmen, priests and religious, as also many of the simply interested and curious. Enormous excitement was in the air as the time for the debate between the two foremost men of the age approached. Yet the outcome would be indeed strange.

St. Bernard walked slowly past the gathered crowd, his eyes downcast. Abelard walked with head held high, proud and disdainful. St. Bernard opened the case by merely calling on Abelard to retract the passages now to be read by the clerk. The clerk had barely begun to read when Abelard cried out for him to stop; he wanted to appeal the case to Rome. So the encounter came to an end like a boxing match before round one could even begin. But St. Bernard pursued the case and Abelard was condemned. Later Peter Abelard met St. Bernard and was reconciled to him, and he wrote an official apology, retracting his errors. Later too, he explained to friends that at the synod, "his memory failed him, his understanding faltered, and he lost his presence of mind." (IER, May 62).

From a Saintly Family

St. Bernard, the third son in a family of six boys and one girl, had been born in 1090 (or 1091) at Fountaines les Dijon, his father's castle near Dijon in the Burgundy province of France.

Both his father, Tescelin, and his mother, Aleth (or Elizabeth), belonged to the nobility and were strongly Catholic. Aleth was a woman totally devoted to God. Besides caring for her own family, she spent much time helping the sick and the poor, and in praying.

According to her custom she always had the priests of the neighborhood in for a meal on the feast of St. Ambrose. Although feverish and having a presentiment of being near death, she did this as usual when Bernard was about 19. The guests left the table at her request to gather at her bedside and pray the litany for the dying. At the words: "By Thy Cross and Passion, deliver her, O Lord," she lifted her hand to trace a cross, and died at that moment, her hand remaining upheld.

Aleth's example had a strong influence on St. Bernard and saved him, shortly after her death, from an inclination to follow a worldly career. Hesitating over what path in life to choose, St. Bernard seemed to hear her voice and to see her pointing out the cloister to him. Perhaps she did the same for others in the family, for it would probably have required even more than Bernard's winning personality to induce his uncle and four of his brothers to accompany him to the religious life. Later, his father, his youngest brother and his sister, Humbeline, also entered the monastic life.

When St. Bernard appeared at Citeaux, the original and founding Cistercian abbey, to ask admittance, he brought with him 31 companions. Three years later, at the age of 25 and not yet ordained a priest, he was sent as abbot to make a new foundation at Clairvaux, to which abbey his name would ever after be associated.

The chosen spot was then called Valley of Wormwood. It was dark and desolate. The monks felled many trees to make a clearing, and they put up simple monastic buildings and went about their daily routine of penance and prayer with extreme simplicity. As orderly fields appeared under their toiling hands and as the atmosphere of peace and prayer settled over the countryside, the name of the place was changed to Clairvaux, which means "Valley of Light."

A Charming Personality

Before St. Bernard's death he would be in charge of more than 700 monks at this monastery, and Clairvaux itself would have sent out monks to found 68 other monasteries, these in turn making new foundations, until the total number came to 160 at the time of his death. The charm of St. Bernard and the power of his holiness were obviously at work.

Very remarkable in the life of St. Bernard were his many accomplishments, despite frail health. Throughout his monastic years, his stomach could tolerate little food other than moistened bread. For long periods he could hardly retain anything. In his early days at Clairvaux, after about 18 months there, St. Bernard had been ordered by the local bishop and the Cistercian chapter to live apart from the community, to try to restore his health. William of St. Thierry, one of the three principal biographers of the original *Life*, came to visit him in the little hut set apart for him from the monastery. St. Bernard lived here for about a year. There was nothing done for him that could have cured him, but he recovered anyway, perhaps being cured by the Blessed Virgin. St. Bernard mitigated somewhat the extreme rigor that had broken his health and grew in prudence and sympathy, although throughout his life he remained very penitential, hardly eating or sleeping. Yet his works were prodigious, and his burning spirit seemed to energize and almost to look through his frail body.

In his younger years, St. Bernard was described as having beauty of face and charm of manner. He was of average height, always slim, and as he grew older, became very thin. His eyes are described as "dove-like." His hair was light in color and his beard reddish, gradually mingling with white. His countenance had a peculiar brightness. Those who saw him felt the presence of a rare charm and the glow of the Spirit which filled him.

When he preached the Second Crusade in the French language to the Germans, they were moved to tears, for though they had not yet heard the words of the translators, they nonetheless understood St. Bernard. Many times men at first said no to his suggestion that they enter the monastery, but soon, under his influence, they would change their minds. He seemed to be able to accept a candidate with the worst possible background and yet fashion him into a good monk. Once, he saved a criminal from the hangman and took him to the novitiate. He seized the rope, already around the neck of the criminal, saying: "Give him to me, and I will put him to death with my own hands." He insisted before the presiding Count that he would see to it that the man expiated his offenses by a daily, constant death to self. The criminal became a monk and lived a holy life for some 30 years.

A Man of Strong Friendships

St. Bernard's friendships were strong and affectionate. To William of St. Thierry he apologized because he had not answered his letters: "Are you worried because I have not yet once answered your many letters to me? How could I possibly suppose your mature wisdom would be satisfied with my ignorant scribbling? . . . Although I love you less than I should, yet I love you as much as I can according to the power that has been given me . . ."

St. Bernard wrote to comfort a couple whose son had left them to come to the monastery. "You are not losing him; on the contrary, through him you are gaining many sons. All of us at Clairvaux . . . will receive him as a brother and you as our parents . . . I will be for him both a mother and a father, both a brother and a sister . . ." (*Letter* 110).

St. Bernard once wrote to Pope Innocent II: "If things always went wrong, no one could endure it; if they always went well, anyone would become arrogant."

A most poignant example of St. Bernard's affectionate nature is set forth in the letter traditionally placed first in the long list of some 469 pieces of his extant correspondence. (Translation by Fr. Bruno Scott James, Regnery, 1953). He writes to Robert, a young cousin (often referred to as a nephew because of the difference in ages) who had left Clairvaux to join the Benedictines at Cluny.

> Long enough, perhaps too long, have I waited, dearest Robert, for the Lord that He might deign to touch your soul and mine through yours, moving you to salutary regrets for your error and me to joy for your deliverance. But seeing myself still disappointed of my hope, I can no longer hide my sorrow, restrain my anxiety, or dissemble my grief . . . I will forget old injuries . . . Unhappy man that I am who have not you by me, who cannot see you, who am obliged to live without you for whom to die would be to live, and to live without whom is no better than death! So I do not ask why you left me. I only grieve that you do not return; I do not blame your going away; I only blame your not coming back . . . No doubt it may have been my fault that you left. I was too severe with a sensitive youth; I was

too hard on a tender stripling. Hence your grumbles against me (as I remember) while you were here; hence your ceaseless complaints about me even now that I am absent. The fault of this will not be laid at your door. I might perhaps excuse myself by saying that only in this way could the passions of youth have been curbed and that, at first, a strict way of life must be hard on a raw youth . . . Now that I am become gentle, return to me from whom you fled when fierce. My severity frightened you away; let my tenderness draw you back . . .

The long letter ends with a warning that "at the Last Judgment you will incur a greater penalty on account of this letter of mine if, when you have read it, you do not take its lesson to heart." The letter shows the heart of St. Bernard, always tender and loving, yet strong enough to direct with much severity one who is held in unusually strong affection.

St. Bernard's letters show a man who played on a full diapason of the emotions. Strong indignation and anger contrast with praise, approval and affection. Light-heartedness and joy mingle with grief and sorrow. Fr. Bruno Scott James, who translated his letters, says in his Introduction to them that if we are surprised at St. Bernard's emotions, we have perhaps forgotten that to be a man of God, it is first necessary to be a man. St. Bernard, he says, was a *whole* man *just because* he was a holy man.

St. Bernard's brother Gerard became his closest companion, helping him to govern the monastery and traveling with him on his trips. When Gerard fell sick while he and Bernard were at Viterbo, St. Bernard turned to God and pleaded that he would not die away from home. "Wait, O Lord, until our return. Then Thou shalt take him if Thou wilt, and I will utter no complaint." Gerard recovered and returned to Clairvaux, but did not live long afterward. Grief at Gerard's death cut deeply into St. Bernard's soul. He controlled his tears at the funeral, but when he spoke to the monks later, preaching on the *Canticle of Canticles*, he had to break off and explain to them how he felt:

> The sharpness of my grief paralyzes my will, and my very heart fails me . . . I was weak in body and he sustained me, downcast in spirit and he encouraged, slow and negligent and he spurred me on . . . Nothing escaped his sagacity in the matter of buildings or drainage, or the art of husbandry . . . He was my Gerard, truly mine! My brother by blood, my son by

profession, my father for his care of me . . . My words are laden
with grief, but not with murmuring. Righteous art Thou, O
Lord, and Thy judgments upright! Thou gavest Gerard! Thou
hast taken him away! And if we mourn because he is taken,
we forget not that he was given.

St. Bernard's lively mind and ready sympathy led him at times
to show the quite human trait of a delightful sense of humor.
Once, when he had cured a possessed man, he brushed aside
the admiration caused by this by explaining, "It were small wonder that the devil suffered defeat; for with such a helpmate as
I, God could not fail. Besides, we were two against one."

Geoffrey of Clairvaux, another of the three early biographers
of St. Bernard—who became a secretary and traveling companion in 1140 after the death of Gerard—made the first collection
of his letters. He had great insight into St. Bernard's character,
and he summed up his impressions of him by saying that St.
Bernard was strong in will, sometimes headstrong, swift in decision, subtle in resource and undismayed in his work by long
years of intermittent ill-health.

The Thaumaturgus of the West

One of the titles often applied to Bernard was "Thaumaturgus
(miracle-worker) of the West." Cardinal Baronius (1538-1607),
chronicler of the Saints and possibly the Church's all-time greatest historian, estimates that St. Bernard worked more miracles
in his lifetime than any other saint whose miracles are recorded.
During his travels in Germany, when he preached the Second
Crusade, dozens of miracles were often recorded for a single day.
The blind, the lame, the insane, the possessed were cured, sometimes when St. Bernard blessed them, sometimes when they
touched his garments. The *Liber Miraculorum*, which records
his miracles, tells of more than 100 people raised from the dead.
But the miracles and the praise and enthusiasm of the people
never affected his serene humility. He used to say that it seemed
to him, when he was received with tumultuous welcome, that
the people were really honoring someone else. He felt more like
himself back in the fields or at the monastery at Clairvaux.

St. Bernard distinguished between his reputation and his actual
life. The people had come to believe him holy, he said, so God
was willing to help them pursue His own holiness through these

signs. "Signs of this kind," St. Bernard argued, "do not contemplate the holiness of the one, but the salvation of the many."

When St. Bernard was dying, the Archbishop of Treves came to tell of civil war between the people of Metz and the nobles. Two thousand people had already been killed. Unable to eat or sleep and swollen with dropsy, St. Bernard triumphed over his weakened body by the flame of his indomitable spirit and arose from his bed to travel to Metz. Once there, he spent a whole day going about among the burghers, urging them to peace. The nobles, on the other hand, at first refused to see him, but they later sent a delegation to him at night. When he cured a palsied woman in their sight, he won them over completely and peace was restored. St. Bernard returned home to his monastery and to his sickbed, getting up only to drag himself daily to the altar to offer Mass.

By making a weak, sick body obey the force of a commanding will, St. Bernard only displayed with emphasis what he had actually done all his life. In answering a plea to help settle a civil strife and successfully restore peace, he was repeating what he had done time and again throughout his life, namely, bringing aid, solace, peace or a true understanding of the Faith wherever it was needed and wherever he could be of assistance.

The Arbiter of Christendom

There was no cause too lowly nor one too great for St. Bernard to aid. In his last days he wrote to the Count of Champagne on behalf of a poor man whose pigs had been stolen: "I had much rather that my own pigs had been stolen, and I require them at your hand." As the man's suzerain, the Count would simply have to take up the matter and bring the thief to justice, as his duty called him to do.

In a time of famine, the monastery at Clairvaux gave out tokens to 3,000 people. The holders of these tokens were entitled to receive free meals at the monastery for the duration of the famine. Eyes were ever turning to Clairvaux and its holy abbot. Men were willing to listen to one so wise and so holy. And when, at times, they were not willing, his mere presence made them change their minds. The story of his encounter with William, Duke of Aquitaine, who was of violent, terrible strength and uncontrollable, vicious temper, illustrates the persuasive power of St. Bernard's presence alone, as well as his fearlessness.

St. Bernard's first meeting with this man produced no lasting results. Four years later, after further fruitless discussion,
St. Bernard was celebrating Mass as the terrible Count, who by
this time was excommunicated, took his place at the door. After
consecrating the Host, St. Bernard placed It on the paten and
walked toward William, his eyes flashing. He spoke with tremendous authority:

> We have besought you, and you have spurned us. This united
> multitude of the servants of God, meeting you elsewhere, has
> entreated you, and you have despised them. Behold, here comes
> to you the Virgin's Son, the Head and Lord of the Church which
> you persecute! Your Judge is here at whose Name every knee
> shall bow, of things in Heaven and things on earth and things
> under the earth. Your Judge is here, into whose hands your
> soul is to pass. Will you spurn Him also? Will you despise Him,
> as you have despised His servants?

The Count fell to the floor and, when raised by his men, could
not stand, but fell again. St. Bernard then told him to stand up,
to give the Bishop of Poitiers (whom he had cast out of his diocese) the kiss of peace and to restore to him his rights. Without
a word this warrior obliged, despite a waiting army standing
by. This time his repentance continued, and his spirit, which few
had challenged and none had conquered, was completely subdued to the end of his life.

St. Bernard actually achieved a much greater general influence in the Church at large by refusing the many bishoprics
that were offered him than he would have possessed had he
accepted one of them. Langres, Chalons, Rheims, Genoa, Pisa,
Milan, all had asked, and he had turned down all of them. In
the case of Milan, his sense of humor had helped. A delegation
of the clergy and people came to carry him off bodily to be their
archbishop. He told them to wait till the morrow, at which time
he would mount his horse. "If he shall bear me beyond the walls,
I shall hold myself free from all engagement. If he remain within
your gates, I shall be your archbishop." Many gathered to witness the scene the next day. St. Bernard mounted and galloped
off so suddenly that he was soon beyond pursuit.

Confidant of Popes

The most famous instance of St. Bernard's power of arbitration came with the Papal Schism, which began in 1130. Called to the French Council at Etampes, St. Bernard stood for Innocent II and held Anacletus II to be an antipope. A year later, after traveling with Pope Innocent II as his adviser and trying everywhere to establish his claim, St. Bernard wrote: "Nor have I labored in vain. The Kings of Germany, France, England, Scotland, Spain, and Jerusalem, with all the clergy and people, adhere to the Lord Innocent like sons to a father." St. Bernard continued to spend much of his time during the seven years of the schism traveling with and working for the Pope. It was, in fact, chiefly the weight of St. Bernard thrown fully onto the side of Pope Innocent II that kept Catholicism from a deeper, more lasting schism.

In 1145 a former monk of Clairvaux was elected Pope as Eugene III. St. Bernard frequently advised him and admonished him as a spiritual son.

From the beginning of the schism in 1130 until his death in 1153, St. Bernard was really the most influential man in the Church, not excepting even the Popes, a truth emphasized by the fact that they often called upon him and leaned on him for support. In the words of Henry Cardinal Manning, "There is, perhaps, in the annals of the Church no more remarkable instance of the power of an individual over the men of his age than in St. Bernard." (Preface to *Life and Times of St. Bernard* by M. L'Abbe Ratisbonne.)

Preacher of the Second Crusade

It was at the command of Pope Eugene III, after the plea of the French king had failed, that St. Bernard went forth as preacher of the Second Crusade. He opened his campaign at Vezelai le Rideau in France, King Louis VII standing at his side. The enthusiasm was so great that the King could say nothing, and St. Bernard could not properly expound all his ideas. The demand for crusade crosses was instant. At Pentecost a council at Chartres elected St. Bernard commander-in-chief, to march at the head of the soldiers. He appealed to the Pope against this choice and was relieved of such a duty. Instead, the Pope sent him to Germany to preach the Crusade there.

His progress in Germany was like that of any of the greatest apostles of history: crowds flocked to him wherever he went. There were conversions and miracles. The journey through the cities and towns was as much a missionary event as a stirring call to the Crusade. St. Bernard was at this time at the height of his renown.

But with the failure of the Crusade, he became the scapegoat. He was blamed for its failure, accused of misleading men by his preaching and his miracles. France especially had never before had so many widows and orphans. Many men, including some close to St. Bernard, thought that any insult hurled at him was acceptable. At this time, too, Nicholas, a monk of Clairvaux and secretary to St. Bernard, caused him anguish by writing letters under his name and recommending unworthy men to positions of honor. When exposed, he turned against St. Bernard and did all he could to besmirch his reputation.

St. Bernard bore the humiliation and ingratitude in silence. It was, as he acknowledged, the immorality within the crusading armies—leading to excesses, factions and reverses—which had led to their misfortunes, defeats and disintegration. These things were not his doing. St. Bernard called this time of his life the "season of disgrace." It was not until after the reaction of a more reasonable opinion had set in that St. Bernard wrote an apology to the Pope. This was after a year. He pointed out that he had acted under obedience and for the glory of God. Moses and other prophets had done the same in ancient times, and yet the people, by their sins, had often brought defeat upon themselves. St. Bernard said he was glad that the slanders and blame were directed at himself and not at God.

(Portugal, incidentally, saved at this time by Crusaders from the on-marching Moslems, declared itself a fief of Clairvaux.)

His Influence on Piety

Despite his tremendous activities, St. Bernard was nonetheless one of the world's great contemplatives. In fact, his activities in the affairs of his time were so successful just because he was primarily a man of silence and prayer.

St. Bernard wrote or spoke chiefly for the occasion at hand. He actually wrote only a few treatises, such as, *On the Necessity of Loving God* and *The Degrees of Humility*. His *Life of St. Malachy* was a lone and stellar effort at biography. Most of his teachings are set down in his sermons. A group of 86 of these on the *Canticle of Canticles* is considered by many to be his greatest work. St. Bernard was not a systematic writer, but in what he did set down there can be discovered a body of very systematic teachings.

St. Bernard had an influence on the development of many of our modern, popular devotions. Devotion to the Sacred Heart, the Holy Name, the Blessed Virgin, to St. Joseph and to the Guardian Angels, all owe a great debt to St. Bernard. Sometimes he has been taken to task by modern critics for being responsible for a trend of piety away from the liturgy, a trend toward becoming too individualistic. Even if such were true—that there could possibly be too much individual piety in the Church— Catholics have always regarded the Holy Sacrifice of the Mass as the center of their prayer life. And even presuming, for the sake of argument, that such a charge were true, it would be not a result but a corruption of the unction and sweetness of St. Bernard's teachings. His system centered on devotion to the Sacred Humanity of Christ and the love of God. As "a restorer and promoter" of the Cistercian Order, in the phrase of Pope Pius XII, he was dedicated to a strict renewal of the liturgical life of the primitive Benedictine rule. (The Cistercians are a development from the Benedictine Order and are often referred to as "the White Benedictines.")

During the Middle Ages no writer except St. Augustine was read more than St. Bernard. There have been about 500 editions of his works published. It has been claimed that the *Imitation of Christ*, printed more than any other Catholic book except the Bible, is in substance contained in the works of St. Bernard. And St. Bernard's influence can be seen in the formation of the spirituality of St. Francis of Assisi, with its strong and loving emphasis on the humanity of Christ. St. John of the Cross, St. Alphonsus Liguori, St. Francis de Sales and, in fact, practically every spiritual writer since the twelfth century owes a great debt to St. Bernard of Clairvaux.

He also wrote a treatise on meditation for Pope Eugene III called *De Consideratione*. A later pope, St. Pius V, had part of this book read to him daily while he dined. The book influenced St. Ignatius and his famous *Spiritual Exercises*. In fact, St. Bernard's treatise had a large influence on the development of the practice of meditating.

The history of the hymns attributed to St. Bernard is hard

to trace. Some of our very well-known hymns, such as the *Jesu, dulcis memoria* and the prayer known as "The Memorare" seem quite certainly to have come from his sermons. St. Bernard's passage on the Holy Name (from *Sermon* 15 on the *Canticle of Canticles*) is much quoted and appears in the encyclical of Pope Pius XII.

> . . . If thou writest, thy composition has no charms for me unless I read there the name of Jesus. If thou disputest or conversest, I find no pleasure in thy words unless I hear there the name of Jesus. Jesus is honey in the mouth, melody in the ear, a cry of joy in the heart. Yet not only is that name light and food. It is also medicine. Is any amongst you sad? Let the name of Jesus enter his heart; let it leap thence to his lips; and lo, the light that radiates from that name shall scatter every cloud and restore tranquillity! Has someone sinned, and is he, moreover, abandoning hope, rushing in desperation toward the snare of death? Let him but invoke this life-giving name, and straightaway he shall experience a renewal of courage . . . Whoever, when trembling with terror in the presence of danger, has not immediately felt his spirits revive and his fears departing as soon as he called upon this name of power . . . There is nothing so efficacious as the name of Jesus for restraining the violence of anger, repressing the swelling of pride, healing the smarting wound of envy.

"Mary's Faithful Bernard"

St. Bernard's sermons on the Blessed Virgin amount to nothing less than a complete Mariology. His famous letter to the canons of Lyons concerning the feast of her Conception has been at times interpreted as evidence that he did not believe in the Immaculate Conception. But Fr. Bruno James, translator of the letter into English, said there is no evidence that St. Bernard used the term "conception" in the sense used in the definition of the dogma in 1854. But in the course of this letter St. Bernard makes a clear summary of the teaching about Mary.

> Let us honor her for the purity of her body, the holiness of her life. Let us marvel at her fruitful virginity, and venerate her divine Son. Let us extol her freedom from concupiscence in conceiving and from all pain in bearing. Let us proclaim her to be reverenced by the Angels, desired by the nations, foretold by the patriarchs and prophets, chosen out of all and pre-

ferred before all. Let us magnify her as the channel of grace, the mediatrix of salvation, the restorer of the ages, and as exalted above the choirs of angels to the very heights of Heaven. All this the Church sings in her praise and tells me too to sing. What I have received from the Church I firmly cling to and confidently pass on to others; but, I confess, I am chary of admitting anything that I have not received from her. Certainly the Church has taught me to keep that day with the greatest veneration on which, when she was taken up from this evil world, she brought a festival of great joy to Heaven.

St. Bernard was an eloquent witness to the Blessed Virgin Mary's Assumption and her position as "Mediatrix of Graces." So well and clearly did he express the traditional doctrines about Mary, so well did he express his love for her, that one can hardly speak of Mary without borrowing from St. Bernard. The poet Dante places St. Bernard in Paradise as the supreme panegyrist of Mary. He calls him "Mary's faithful Bernard."

Pope Pius XII quotes at length in his encyclical a great passage of St. Bernard on Mary, "Star of the Sea." Of this passage he says that "there is perhaps none more beautiful, more impassioned, more apt to excite love for her, more useful for stirring devotion and inspiring imitation of her virtuous example." The passage is then quoted as follows:

"Mary". . . is interpreted to mean "Star of the Sea" and admirably suits the Virgin Mother. There is indeed a wonderful appropriateness in this comparison of her to a star, because as a star sends out its rays without detriment to itself, so did the Virgin bring forth her Child without injury to her integrity. And as the ray emitted does not diminish the brightness of the star, so neither did the Child born of her tarnish the beauty of Mary's virginity. She is therefore that glorious star which, according to prophecy, arose out of Jacob, whose ray illumines the entire earth, whose splendor shines out conspicuously in Heaven and reaches even unto Hell . . . She, I say, is that resplendent and radiant star placed as a necessary beacon above life's great and spacious sea, glittering with merits, luminous with examples for our imitation. Oh, whosoever thou art that perceivest thyself during this mortal existence to be rather floating in the treacherous waters, at the mercy of the winds and the waves, than walking secure on the stable earth, turn not away thine eyes from the splendor of this guiding star, unless thou wishest to be submerged by the tempest! When the storms of temptation burst upon thee, when thou seest thyself driven upon the rocks of tribulation, look up at the Star—call upon Mary. When buffeted by the billows of pride or ambition or hatred or jealousy, look up at the Star—call upon Mary. Should anger or avarice or carnal desires violently assail the little vessel of thy soul, look up at the Star—call upon Mary. If, troubled on account of the heinousness of thy sins, confounded at the filthy state of thy conscience, and terrified at the thought of the awful judgment to come, thou art beginning to sink into the bottomless gulf of sadness and to be absorbed in the abyss of despair, oh, then think of Mary! In dangers, in doubts, in difficulties, think of Mary—call upon Mary. Let not her name depart from thy lips; never suffer it to leave thy heart. And that thou mayest more surely obtain the assistance of her prayer, neglect not to walk in her footsteps. With her for a guide, thou shalt never go astray; whilst invoking her, thou shalt never lose heart; so long as she is in thy mind, thou art safe from deception; whilst she holds thy hand, thou canst not fall; under her protection, thou hast nothing to fear; if she walks before thee, thou shalt not grow weary; if she shows thee favor, thou shalt reach the goal. (Homily II on *Missus Est*).

His Love for God and for Man

The tolling of bells sounded sorrowfully over the countryside around Clairvaux on the morning of August 20, 1153. If they were heard in Heaven, it would have been as a paean of joy. For they announced the death of St. Bernard. His last words sum up the theme of his life.

The monks had gathered around, begging him to stay with them. Accustomed to wonders from him, they trusted that he could obtain from God the favor of longer life. He had answered, "I know not to which I ought to yield, the love of my children, which urges me to stay here; or the love of my God, which draws me to Him." Love of God and of man had been the theme of St. Bernard's life.

Called "The Last of the Fathers, and surely not unequal to the first," because of his learning and influence, he is also in the tradition of those untrammeled spirits of the early Church who could feel and express to the fullest both joy and sorrow. "I say it boldly, I cannot be separated throughout eternity from one whom I have so loved," St. Bernard had written when one of his friends, the Abbot Suger, was dying. The following inscription from one edition of St. Bernard's works gives a good summary of his life and work: "Who, bearing a heart of universal love, called against his will from the cloister, never ceased to defend, ardently, patiently, and humbly, the one and immaculate Church."

In 1830, Pope Pius VIII declared St. Bernard to be a Doctor of the Church. But the title had already been applied to him unofficially ever since his death. At the time of St. Bernard's canonization in 1174, Alexander III assigned the Gospel used for Doctors to his feast day Mass: "You are the salt of the earth . . ." (*Matt.* 5:13).

St. Bernard had said that when he thought of God's judgments too long, he grew fearful, and if he thought too long of God's mercy, he grew lax. "And this experience has taught me to sing not alone the mercies of the Lord, and not alone His judgments, but judgment and mercy united in one embrace." (*Life of St. Bernard*, Sands & Co., 1916, p. 232).

St. Bernard contained in himself qualities of forcefulness and zeal, gentleness and sweetness, qualities that, taken together in one person, might confuse those who look at only one aspect of his character. Greater minds and spirits than ours, people closer to the truth of the unity of God—with its baffling paradoxes— have a wider vision of life and a wider scope of action as a result. The unity of their personality is there, even if not readily apparent. In St. Bernard the unifying force that directed his thinking and his action was a consuming, heartfelt love for God. "The reason for loving God is God Himself. The measure is to love Him beyond measure." (*On the Necessity of Loving God*, 1, 1).

St. Bernard's feast day is August 20.

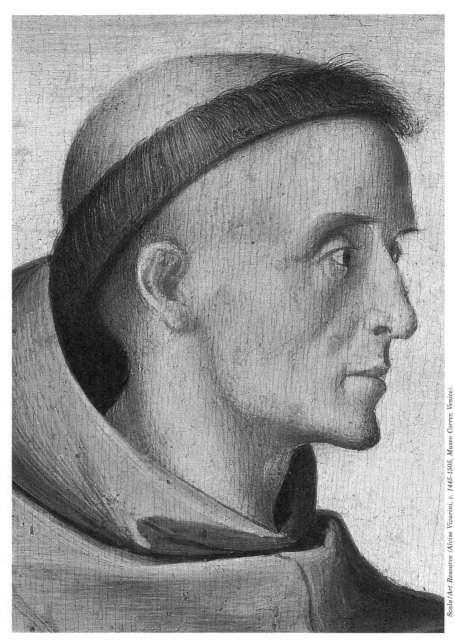

Saint Anthony of Padua

21

SAINT ANTHONY OF PADUA

Doctor of the Gospel

Hammer of Heretics

Ark of Both Covenants

1195-1231

CANDLES that pilgrims brought to his tomb were so large that it took 16 men to carry them, relates the writer of the earliest life of St. Anthony of Padua. The candles are not so large today, but the numbers of them that burn throughout the world to honor and petition this Saint are still fantastic.

Considering such popularity, it is remarkable that there are few biographies in print in English about St. Anthony of Padua, and one of these (Clasen's) was originally written in German. (Sophonius Clasen, O.F.M., *St. Anthony: Doctor of the Gospel*, Chicago: Franciscan Herald Press, 1961). Among Catholics there seems to be a happy indifference to the facts of his life and to his special dignity as a Doctor of the Church. Simple and good people, and children too, who might quake and stutter when talking to a man with a scholastic degree, turn easily to this Doctor of the Universal Church and say, "St. Anthony of Padua, please look around; something is lost and must be found."

Exult, Happy Portugal

The apostolic letter of Pope Pius XII of January 16, 1946, which declared St. Anthony of Padua a Doctor of the Church, begins with an invitation: "Exult, happy Portugal, rejoice, happy Padua; for you have given birth for earth and Heaven to a shining star, a man who has illuminated and still dazzles with a radiant light the whole earth, not only by holiness of life and fame of miracles, but by the splendor of his celestial teaching."

It was in Lisbon in 1195 in the shadow of the cathedral that Anthony was born. He was the first child of parents of noble stock and "still in the first flower of youth." The young couple gave their boy the name of Ferdinand. According to an account written in 1317 by a Friar Minor, his father's name was Martin and his mother's was Mary. A sister is also mentioned, and the account may have been written by Anthony's nephew, her son. We know nothing in explicit detail about Ferdinand's boyhood.

Ferdinand's mother dedicated him to the Blessed Virgin, and nurtured in him a deep devotion to the Mother of God and a faith that treasured the grace of Baptism. At the age of 15, feeling the tug of adolescent temptation, he decided that if he were to carry this treasure unsullied through life, he should enter religion.

He joined the Augustinian Canons located at St. Vincent's outside the city walls. At the age of 17, he asked to be transferred to the monastery of Holy Cross at Coimbra. Here he would be away from the interruptions to study and prayer occasioned by the visits of his home town relatives and friends.

Ferdinand spent the next nine years as an Augustinian canon at Coimbra, then the chief city of Portugal and a center of learning. He applied himself assiduously to his studies and made such progress as to amaze his teachers and fellow religious. His memory was so remarkable that he retained almost all he studied, whether of Scripture or the Church Fathers. His 11 years as an Augustinian were chiefly quiet and peaceful, although political evil and intrigue were casting a disturbing shadow within the cloister at the latter end of Ferdinand's stay at Coimbra.

Wanted to Be a Martyr

On January 16, 1220, five Friars Minor were put to death in Morocco. The remains of these first martyrs of the Order were brought to Portugal and given to the Augustinians of Holy Cross at Coimbra. Ferdinand, the young guestmaster of the monastery, shared the general awe and enthusiasm. In him was born the desire to join them in martyrdom. Ferdinand asked some of the begging friars who came to the monastery to see if it could be arranged for him to join their order, the Friars Minor, so that he could go to Morocco. Receiving the reluctant consent of his Superior and fellow monks (the monastery had the privilege of a requirement that anyone leaving must ask each one), Ferdinand left to be clothed in the habit of the Friars Minor, or Franciscans, as they are more commonly called. He asked for the name of

Anthony, patron of their chapel. At this time, no novitiate was required among the friars. This was in the summer of 1220, and the new Anthony was 25 years of age.

There remained to him just 11 more short years of life, which he was to spend as a Franciscan. He received permission to go to Morocco, where no glorious martyrdom awaited him—nor any fruitful work either. Rather he fell terribly and ingloriously sick, and after a long siege of illness, he decided to return to Portugal. But adverse winds drove the ship off course, and it brought him instead to Sicily.

Perhaps St. Anthony may have wanted to ask the question that so many tearful faces have since phrased before his statue: "Why all these troubles?" God certainly did not seem to be in a hurry to have St. Anthony begin his active work.

A Preacher Discovered

At Messina, he joined other friars to go to the Chapter of the Order, held in 1221 at the chapel of the Portiuncula near Assisi. When it was over, the unknown Anthony was left unassigned. Nobody had asked for him. So he requested Gratian, the provincial of Romagna, to take him along to northern Italy. There Gratian granted his request to live in the little hermitage at Monte Paolo near Forli and Bologna. One of the friars had a place in a nearby cave in which to retire and to pray. St. Anthony asked him for permission to use it, and he often spent the day there in fasting and prayer.

Pursuing his love for solitude and prayer, St. Anthony did not at first help the other friars in the household tasks. Then, noticing this defect, he first humbly asked permission and then took his turn at sweeping, cleaning and scouring.

In 1222 St. Anthony went to Forli, and it was at this time that he was most likely ordained, along with a few other Franciscans and some Dominicans. Afterwards, when the group gathered for a meal in the Dominican monastery refectory, the suggestion was made that instead of the usual table reading, a friar deliver a speech. Between the lines we might conjecture that this was a not too subtle invitation by the minister provincial, aimed at putting the new priests on the spot and having at the same time a little innocent fun. All declined the unsought honor. Then the superior chose St. Anthony.

As Anthony spoke, all present began to realize that the simple friar was a man of profound knowledge and filled with the Holy Spirit. When he had finished, perhaps the food was cold, but the hearts of the amazed listeners were warm. There was no doubt about what assignment would be given to St. Anthony now. He was quickly appointed preacher to northern Italy. And after two years there, he went on to France (1224-1227), then returning to spend the last years of his short life in Italy.

During his first tour of preaching in Italy, St. Francis himself appointed St. Anthony lector of theology. As such, he is, in the words of Pope Pius XII, "The first of all lectors in the Seraphic Franciscan Order." Teaching the young friars, going about preaching to the faithful, and correcting those who were teaching false doctrines made up his days. He combined the life of a teacher with that of a preacher.

St. Anthony also held administrative posts of local and regional scope: Guardian and Custos in France and Provincial in Italy. He was released from the office of Minister Provincial of Romagna at his own request a year before he died.

Doctor of the Gospel

St. Francis of Assisi had said that his friars should live after the manner of the Holy Gospel. He really wanted no other rule. It is fitting, then, that St. Anthony, the first theologian of the Order, should be known as "the Doctor of the Gospel." In his apostolic letter of January 16, 1946, Pope Pius XII said: "It is because Anthony so very often uses thoughts and examples taken from the Gospel that he clearly shows himself worthy and deserving with full right the title, Doctor of the Gospel."

St. Anthony's sermons are the only undisputed evidence of his teachings. (No autographs remain to us.) They are divided into "Sermons on the Feasts," "Sunday Sermons" and "Sermons in Praise of the Blessed Virgin Mary." In the 1905 edition by Anthony Mary Locatelli, the sermons with accompanying notes cover more than 900 pages. Shortly before his death, St. Anthony of Padua had in mind to write a book for the whole Christian people, but he never had the opportunity to do this book. Had he written it, we might have not only a valuable guide of Christian perfection, but a better index of St. Anthony's popular style than appears in the sermons. The sermons we have were not the sermons he actually gave, but were prepared near the end of his life, chiefly perhaps as a guide for other preachers.

At the end of his Sunday Sermons, St. Anthony gives thanks, as he also heaves a sigh of relief for coming to "the long-desired end of this work." "Well then, dearest brothers, I the least of all, your brother and your servant, have in some fashion composed this work of the Gospels of the year's cycle, for your consolation, the edification of the faithful and the remission of my sins . . ."

In the prologue to his work, St. Anthony says that for the honoring of God and the bettering of souls he was fashioning a chariot in which, with Elias, the soul might fly to Heaven. "And note, that as there are four wheels on a chariot, so this work rests on four materials: the Sunday Gospels, the stories of the Old Testament as read in the Church, the Introit, and the Epistles of the Sunday Masses . . ." He uses these elements, interweaving them, to point out doctrinal and moral truths, and to raise the soul to closer union with God.

Locatelli, in his introductory letter addressed to Pope Leo XIII, says: "There is hardly a doctrine which Anthony did not defend or eruditely explain by solid arguments and reasons in his books." (XIV). He singles out for special mention St. Anthony's defense of the Real Presence of Christ in the Eucharist, the Assumption of Mary, her Immaculate Conception, and the infallibility of the Pope.

In his apostolic letter, Pope Pius XII says:

> If anyone attentively considers the sermons of the Paduan, Anthony will stand forth as a most skilled master of the Scriptures, an outstanding theologian in examining doctrine, an excellent doctor and master in treating of ascetical and mystical things.

The primitive writer calls Anthony a "pen of the Holy Spirit." Pope Gregory, who requested St. Anthony to preach before him, called him an "ark of the covenant." As the original Ark contained the Scriptures, so did St. Anthony possess them in himself. His wonderful versatility in making a mosaic of Scripture texts to prove a point or to draw an analogy rested in part on his memory. He knew both Testaments by heart. He knew the Bible in two ways: first, by study, whereby he had committed the Scriptures to memory and sought out their meaning; and second, by the light of the Holy Spirit, which he had merited by his prayerful and penitential life.

The variety and extent of St. Anthony's use of scriptural texts, especially in the allegorical and spiritual sense of the passages, is so profuse that the reader may grow weary since he does not have before him the living preacher to explain them. Undoubtedly, the full explanation of the points, as given to a live congregation, is missing. Some commentators have suggested that parts of St. Anthony's sermons as we have them are quite sketchy.

St. Anthony quotes St. Augustine more than any other Father, 54 times in all. He also quotes St. Gregory the Great 48 times and St. Bernard 35 times. His life and training as an Augustinian, too, shaped his mind along the lines of the great African Father's philosophy. In God's providence, the minds of St. Augustine and the heart of St. Francis met in St. Anthony, the first lector of the Friars Minor, and St. Anthony in turn had an enduring formative influence in creating the particular flavor of Franciscan thinking. It is a thinking that is always tinged by the mystical, and yet approaches truth in a fully human way, allowing some room for intuition and even emotion, and veering away from the coldly abstract and disembodied approach.

St. Anthony prepared his written sermons in Latin. When he spoke, he used the language of the people of the territory, Portuguese, Italian, or French, as they existed in their developing stages at the time. The spirit of St. Anthony's sermons can be gathered from the prayers he used to end them. A note of joy and hope sounds as he often concludes with the word "Alleluia." (A translation of these prayers concluding his sermons would be quite valuable.) The prayer he composed for himself to recite before his sermons also reveals his approach.

Light of the World, Infinite God, Father Eternal, Giver of Wisdom and Knowledge, most Holy and Ineffable Dispenser of spiritual grace, Who hast known all things from the beginning, Who hast made darkness and light, guide my hand and touch my lips that they may be like a sharp sword to set forth Thy truth. Make my tongue, O Lord, like a swift arrow to declare Thy marvelous works.

Send forth, O God, Thy Holy Spirit into my heart that I may perceive, into my mind that I may remember, into my soul that I may meditate. Inspire me to speak with piety, holiness, tenderness and mercy. Teach, guide, and direct my thoughts and senses from beginning to end. May Thy grace help and correct me, and may I be strengthened now with wisdom from on high, for Thine infinite mercy's sake. Amen.

Elsewhere, St. Anthony tells us what a sermon should be like.

> The sermon must be true, not false, without frivolous jest-
> ing or highsounding words, and it must call men to weep and
> do penance. Just as a thorn draws blood when it pierces the
> skin, and a nail that is driven through the hand will cause
> great suffering, so should the words of the wise man, like a
> thorn, pierce the heart of the sinner and draw forth the blood
> of his tears, and cause him to have sorrow over his past sins
> and fear of the punishment of Hell. The sermon, moreover, must
> be sincere, which means that the preacher may not deny by
> his actions what he says in words, for the whole force of his
> eloquence is lost when his word is not helped by his deed.
> Lastly, it must direct its hearers to correction in such a way
> that, having heard the sermon, they will change their lives for
> the better. (Clasen, p. 70).

Very valuable for understanding the mind and the character
of St. Anthony are the words of his dear friend, the learned
Augustinian abbot, Thomas Gallus. (It was to him that St.
Anthony appeared in a dream shortly after his death and said,
"I have left the ass [i.e., his body] at Padua and am returning
to my home.")
Gallus said of St. Anthony:

> Often love can enter where mere natural knowledge is
> excluded. We read of some holy bishops that they were but
> poorly versed in the natural sciences, and yet they had the gift
> of readily understanding mystical theology. Having left all nat-
> ural knowledge behind, their purified souls ascended, as it were,
> to the very heavens, even to the most Blessed Trinity. This very
> thing I myself, as a close friend, have been able to observe in
> the holy Brother Anthony, of the Friars Minor. Though he was
> not well-read in the natural sciences, he had a pure spirit and
> a burning heart and was a man on fire for God. All this enabled
> him easily to understand with all his heart all the riches and
> depths of mystical theology. Therefore, I may well apply to him
> the words which Sacred Scripture says of John the Baptist:
> "He was a lamp, burning and shining. Because his heart was
> burning with love for God, he was a shining example also to
> men." (Quoted in Clasen, p. 54).

Devotion to Mary

Pope Pius XI in his apostolic letter of March 1, 1931, *Antoniana solemnia*, commemorating the seventh centenary of the death of St. Anthony, singles out his virtue of purity.

> Among the gifts of sanctity with which by every effort he adorned his soul, the beauty particularly of his perfect chastity shines forth. On account of this virtue he was regarded by all with the greatest admiration as a very angel in human form. St. Anthony acquired this virtue, however, not without enduring temptations and the sting of the flesh, which, as we all know, arise from a nature fallen through Original Sin . . . Yet he so steadfastly and diligently resisted this law that, by keeping in check and overcoming the passions of lust and the disorderly forces of nature, he preserved immaculate the snow-white flower of chastity.

Art pays tribute to this victory of St. Anthony by showing him holding a lily, the symbol of purity. St. Anthony was able to preserve chastity and in fact to keep from all mortal sins through his tender devotion to the Blessed Virgin. Dedicated to her as an infant by his mother, he found, as he tells us, that

> Our Lady's name is a strong tower. To her the sinner has recourse, and there finds security and salvation. O sweet name, which gives the sinner strength and blessed hope. We pray you, Our Lady, Star of the Sea, shine upon us in our distress on the sea of life, and lead us to safe harbor and the ineffable joys of eternity.

St. Anthony's sermons on Mary give evidence of his profound thought about her place in God's plans. He speaks strongly of her role in giving all graces. He says that she is the "door of graces." He speaks affectionately of her as a "beautiful rainbow," the "sign of God's agreement" that peace has been made with mankind.

Pope Pius XII, defining on November 1, 1950 the dogma of the Assumption of Our Lady, singles out St. Anthony from among the writers of his time.

> Among the holy writers who at that same time employed statements and various images and analogies of Sacred Scripture to illustrate and to confirm the doctrine of the Assumption,

which was piously believed, the Evangelical Doctor, St. Anthony of Padua holds a special place. On the feast day of the Assumption, while explaining the prophet's words, "will glorify the place of my feet," he states it as certain that the divine Redeemer had bedecked with supreme glory His most beloved Mother, from whom He had received human flesh. He asserts that "You have here a clear statement that the Blessed Virgin has been assumed in her body, where was the place of the Lord's feet." Hence it is that the Holy Psalmist writes: "Arise, O Lord, into Thy resting place, Thou and the ark which Thou hast sanctified."

And he asserts that, just as Jesus Christ has risen from the death over which He triumphed and has ascended to the right hand of the Father, so likewise the ark of His sanctification "has risen up, since on this day the Virgin Mother has been taken up to her heavenly dwelling."

A Plainspoken Man

We are so accustomed to seeing St. Anthony on a pedestal that it is difficult to think of him as a man. We are so accustomed to thinking of him as a miracle worker, a helper in need, that everything else about him fades into obscurity. It is somewhat like thinking of a person only as a ball player, as a doctor, or as a teacher. He is "good St. Anthony," better loved than a close friend, yet keeping his personal struggles and thoughts in impenetrable solitude.

Near the close of his life St. Anthony went to spend some time on the mountain of LaVerna, where St. Francis had received the stigmata. This was part of his pattern of life. Like St. Francis, he was fond of going off to dwell in a lonely cave or cell. St. Anthony was most of all a prayerful, contemplative soul, seeking God and wanting to be hidden. It seems that even now, despite his worldwide following, he has succeeded in hiding himself in the impersonality and obscurity of fame.

He wrote of the soul's hidden secrets:

> The secret of the heart is like a veil that must hang between us and our neighbor, so that he cannot look behind that veil. It should be enough for him to see the lamps which we carry ready in our hands and which will give him light. For Jesus alone is our High Priest. All hearts are open to Him, and He

sees everything despite that curtain, for He searches the heart
and its deepest thoughts.

St. Anthony was fearless and plainspoken to the point of blunt-
ness. Invited by Simon de Sully, Archbishop of Bourges in France,
to preach to a national council, St. Anthony turned to the Prelate
during the sermon and addressed him: "And now I have something to say to you who wear the mitre." Then he proceeded to
point out some faults of the Archbishop that hindered reform.

Julian von Speier, who wrote an Office of St. Anthony, said
in its lessons:

> Overflowing with sound doctrine, to every man he awarded
> the pound of justice that was his due. Gentle and simple alike
> he pierced with the javelin of plain speech. For this saint, who
> in former days had thirsted for the chalice of suffering with
> such a greedy heart, was not to be deterred by the lofty estate
> of any man, nor yet by the fear of death, but with admirable
> courage resisted the tyranny of princes. And indeed with such
> severity did he rebuke certain reprehensible potentates that
> some other preachers who were present, aye, and famous preach-
> ers, too, trembled at the intrepid constancy of the man, and
> suffused with shame and confusion, hid their glowing faces in
> their handkerchiefs or their sleeves and wished they were any-
> where else rather than where they were.

His sermons against the Cathari, those "apostles of earnestness," the Patarines and Albigensians, earned him the title,
"Hammer of Heretics." Yet his force came from logic and indis-
putable supremacy in the knowledge of Scripture—it did not come
from stinging attacks. And in his sermons for regular congregations, Anthony practically avoids mention of heretics. His title,
"Hammer of Heretics," can, in fact, be misleading if taken as a
clue to his character. Pope Pius XI places it in the correct light:

> And though with the sublime force and incisiveness of his
> eloquence he attacked every form of heresy and immorality,
> nevertheless, he displayed a most fatherly spirit towards all
> men: the unenlightened seeking the light of the Gospel; the
> straying souls searching for the right road; the prodigal chil-
> dren desiring the pardon and embrace of their heavenly Father.

A Very Sensitive Man

At the same time and more notably, if possible, St. Anthony was sensitive to the feelings of others; he was very sensitive to the external conditions and circumstances of his own life. His compassion for the suffering and unfortunate has linked his name to the first bankruptcy law of Padua, March 15, 1231. It reads:

> . . . At the request of the venerable friar (and holy confessor), Anthony of the Order of Friars Minor, it was established and ordained that henceforth no one was to be held in prison for any pecuniary debt or debts, whether past, present or future, if he shall have agreed to relinquish his possessions. . . .

After Easter of 1231, in poor health and near exhaustion, St. Anthony went to Verona to confront personally the tyrant Ezzelino and to intercede for the release of certain prisoners. This brave act of compassion could have led to his death. It ended in mere failure. More than the working of miracles, it helps us to understand God's ways with men to know that St. Anthony was unsuccessful in this mission. Holiness does not march down a rosy path of constant success. Men who have helped open the doors of Heaven for many of their fellowmen still face the closed doors of prejudice and find the doors of ill will slammed in their faces. St. Anthony's failure with Ezzelino came after his final and brilliantly successful season of Lenten preaching.

The facts of St. Anthony's life point to a man who had the sensitivity of a perfectionist. Even after he was a renowned preacher, he continued his studies. One story relates his distress at not having his notes to look over before a sermon. The eager crowds were seeking the great man, and the great man was seeking a notebook. In the prologue to his written sermons, he tells us plainly that he added some examples taken from physics and other sciences, just to make the word of God more palatable and more profitable. He says, "The fastidious taste of readers and hearers of our time has become so delicate that if they do not find an elegant, rich and elaborate style, with a sense of novelty, they are displeased with what they read, and they despise what they hear."

In our age St. Anthony might easily be classified as change-able and an unlikely candidate for the religious life. He was highly sensitive to his surroundings. Twice as an Augustinian he asked for release from a vow of stability, once on leaving St. Vincent's and again on leaving Holy Cross. For his first assignment as a Friar Minor he asked to be sent to Monte Paolo, and once there, he asked a particular friar for permission to use his private, secluded cave. Near the end of his life, he had a little cell made in a walnut tree. This was near the friary at Camposampiero. St. Anthony spent his days in his leafy dwelling, while nearby two companions occupied little huts provided, as was his own, by his nobleman friend, Tiso.

When he first joined the Friars Minor, he asked to change his name from Ferdinand to Anthony, although at the time there was no custom of taking a new name upon entering religion. Very likely his motive was to remain hidden from the entanglements occasioned by visits and requests of friends.

St. Anthony joined the Franciscans in the hope of martyrdom as a missionary. The desire for martyrdom abstractly viewed is simply an expression of the highest form of love, one which seeks immolation. In an individual, however, there can be a wider meaning and a more complex motivation. Many who love God in a perfect way do not specifically want martyrdom. In St. Anthony the desire for martyrdom could well have been the seeking of a solution to the problem of attaining perfection. A man very aware of the inroads of external distractions on the quiet of the soul, St. Anthony seems to have been anxious to find the ideal surroundings for personal peace and the fullest serving of God; perhaps, fearful of forces within himself that might destroy grace, he may have seen in early martyrdom the perfect solution. In martyrdom he would be able say the perfect "I love You" to God, which perhaps he never quite felt able to speak perfectly in the din of a workaday world, even a monastic workaday world.

Denied martyrdom, it may be that St. Anthony saw a new light and found in the Franciscan way of life and its greater allowances for individual expression the answer to his quest. At least there is no indication that he tried to return to Morocco. Or could St. Anthony at that time have seen himself in a new light and discovered that the desire for martyrdom was in reality a highly dignified form of escape from the Will of God for him?

You cannot tell much about the complexities of St. Anthony's personality from his pictures. The oldest picture of him, which is probably by Giotto and is in the Basilica of St. Anthony of Padua, shows him as short and slightly stout. The nose is classically straight, its angle not much different from that of the forehead. The mouth is small and ruby, the face is shaven. Another very ancient picture—from the thirteenth century—shows him with a beard. His eyes are very steady, but have an inscrutable look.

The Wonder-Worker

Most of the wonders performed by St. Anthony, as far as actual, undisputed miracles are concerned, were worked after his death. At his canonization, less than a year after his death, an official list of 46 miracles was approved by the Holy See. Of these, only one had occurred during his lifetime. The rest had been granted to people who invoked him after his death. The one which was worked while he was alive, the cure of Paduana, a four-year-old girl not able to walk, does not fully answer the current requirements of the Church for classification as a miracle, for the cure occurred gradually.

The author of the *Dialogue Legend* lists these 46 miracles and says:

> Of the many and great tokens of holiness attributed to Anthony far and wide by common report I will say nothing, but with no faltering tongue will I proclaim the wonders worked at Padua after his decease, for these, after a most searching scrutiny undertaken by the venerable Bishop of Padua and the Prior of the Dominicans and the Prior of the Benedictines of the same city, commissioned thereto by the Pope, were approved by the Holy See.

The appearance of St. Francis hovering in the air and blessing the friars while St. Anthony preached to the chapter at Arles in 1224 is authentic. St. Francis came to show approval of St. Anthony, whom he used to refer to as "my bishop." So also the statement of St Anthony just before his death is authentic. He said, "I see my Lord," for evidently Christ had appeared to him at this time.

St. Anthony fell sick and had to stay for some time in a Benedictine monastery. The monk who nursed him in his sickness told St. Anthony of his violent temptations against purity. Fasting and prayer had not lessened them. St. Anthony told him to put on his habit (i.e., Anthony's) for a minute. After this, the monk was freed from the severity of these temptations.

The story of the Infant Jesus appearing to St. Anthony has been disputed and has been placed at various locations, as have other events in his life. The representation of this incident in art first appears in 1439; the same is true of written accounts of the story. Pope Pius XII, however, in his apostolic letter of 1946, has this to say:

> For frequently, while he stood alone in his quiet cell praying, Anthony, with eyes and mind sweetly fixed on Heaven, behold: the Infant Jesus suddenly in shining radiance embraces the neck of the young Franciscan with tender arms and, smiling gently, heaps childlike caresses on the Saint; and he, rapt from his senses, made from man into an angel, now "feeds among the lilies" [*Cant.* 2:16] with the angels and with the Lamb.

Two famous incidents have been placed at Rimini in northern Italy by writers of a later date than the primitive authors, John Rigaldus in 1317, and *Liber Miraculorum*, after 1367. These are the stories of the conversion of Bonillo and the preaching to the fishes. Bonillo was a heretic in France who refused to believe in the Real Presence of Jesus Christ in the Holy Eucharist. St. Anthony made an agreement with him: If, after Bonillo withheld food from his donkey for three days, the donkey would kneel in adoration before the Blessed Sacrament, rather than first partake of hay that would be offered him, Bonillo would agree to believe in the Real Presence. Bonillo brought the fasting donkey, and behold, the donkey knelt before the Blessed Sacrament being carried by St. Anthony rather than eat the hay presented to it.

These and other stories bear dramatic witness to what can be rhetorically called the great continuing miracle of St. Anthony's preaching. Many times shops were closed and business ceased when he preached his long sermons. As many as 30,000 gathered to hear him preach in the open fields when the churches no longer could hold the crowds. Women came with scissors to snip away pieces of his habit for relics.

Many of the stories about St. Anthony concern miracles worked to cure not pain, but embarrassment. Representative of these is the story of the woman who, in her excitement at having St. Anthony as a guest, forgot to turn off the tap on the wine barrel. Then one of St. Anthony's companions broke the only glass. When St. Anthony prayed, the glass was made whole, and it was found that the wine barrel was still full.

Perhaps because St. Anthony was himself sensitive to little things—was bothered or helped a great deal by the atmosphere of his own surroundings—he wanted to help others. It seems that from Heaven he continues to be a compassionate helper in the many small problems of life that are so important at the time to the individual who implores his aid.

Spiritual Director

St. Anthony was a spiritual director of immense influence. By his preaching and his work as a confessor, he brought many thousands to live a full Christian life. He was, in the words of Pope Pius XI, a "herald of divine truth" for farmers, merchants, soldiers and artisans. "And indeed, having heard him, they returned to their tasks with the firm resolution henceforth to lead better lives." (*Apostolic Letter*).

Pope John XXIII, in a letter of January 16, 1963 concerning the centenary of the translation of the remains of St. Anthony of Padua, remarked on the aptness of commemorating the Saint during the Second Vatican Council, which aimed at spiritual renewal. For St. Anthony, by his pastoral work, implemented the decrees of the Fourth Council of the Lateran. ". . . His actual pastoral work harmonized with the salutary decrees of that council."

St. Anthony said of Confession:

> Truly, it is the gate of Heaven, the gate of Paradise, since it leads the penitent to God, that he may kneel and kiss the foot of the all-merciful Lord, then be lifted up to kiss the hand of our gracious God, and finally be embraced by our loving Father and received to the kiss of His mouth.

He would have nothing of a rattled, mechanical Confession. In fact, he wanted, like a good doctor of souls, not just an idea of the present ailment of the soul, but a history of past ailments. Therefore, he recommended that when a penitent first approach a new confessor, he make a General Confession. "I give you sound and salutary counsel and very necessary to your soul, that as often as you go to a new confessor, you confess as though you have never gone to Confession before . . ."

His particular words of advice in the confessional would be long remembered by the individual penitent. Most of this is, of course, recorded only by the angels. One reported instance tells of a group of 12 robbers who were converted by hearing St. Anthony's preaching. The writer later became a friar. When they went to Confession, he told each one in turn: "This, maybe, is your last chance; if you return to your vomit, I foresee that a terrible punishment will overtake you; but if only you will strive to walk in the footsteps of our dear Lord, I promise you in His name the happiness of Heaven."

St. Anthony preached often on the evil of loving money.

> Earthly riches are like the reed; its roots are sunk in the swamp, and its exterior is fair to behold, but inside it is hollow. If a man lean on such a reed, it will snap off and pierce his soul and his soul will be carried off to Hell.

He preached hardly a sermon without mentioning the mercy of God. He often set before the people the picture of heavenly joy, in order to spur their efforts and their hope. Once he explained how there would be no jealousy in Heaven, even though the splendor of one would differ from that of another.

> . . . I shall rejoice over your well-being as though it were my own, and you will rejoice over mine as though it were yours. To use an example: see, we are standing together and I have a rose in my hand. The rose is mine, and yet you no less than I rejoice in its beauty and its perfume. So shall it be in eternal life: my glory shall be your consolation and exultation, and yours shall be mine.

Dispute over a Peacemaker

During the Lent of 1231, St. Anthony had preached daily in and around Padua, and he had heard the Confessions of the many people who had resorted to that Sacrament as a result. The people of this city loved him, and he loved them in a special way, although he spent less than two years there, and that at the very end of his life. Wearied by this hard Lent and saddened by his unsuccessful visit to Ezzelino, St. Anthony went to Camposampiero, about one mile north of Padua. Here he had the little cell in the tree.

During this Lent in which he had expended such tremendous effort, he should really have been resting, because for some time he had had dropsy, caused most likely by a weakened heart. One night at the beginning of that Lent, St. Anthony had not been able to get his breath. He spoke of it as the devil trying to choke him. Praying to the Blessed Mother, whom he invoked in all his needs, he obtained relief, and his cell was bathed in light.

On June 13, 1231, which was a Friday, St. Anthony felt suddenly weak while at table with the friars for the noon meal. He asked to be taken to Padua to the Friary of Holy Mary. So he was put into an ox cart and the journey to Padua began. Nearing the city, however, they met a friar coming to visit St. Anthony, who suggested that they go to Arcella, to the friars' house there at the convent of the Poor Clares.

Having arrived there, St. Anthony had another attack, which left him momentarily shaken and fearful. But his spirit rallied to conquer this sudden feeling of insecurity; he went to Confession and then sang happily and clearly the hymn to the Blessed Virgin: *O gloriosa Domina*.

> O glorious Lady, fairest Queen,
> Exalted high in Heav'n above!
> The Great Creator, Mighty Lord
> Was nursed with mother's love.
> What sinful Eve has lost for us,
> By thy dear Son thou didst restore.
> The Gate of Heaven thou hast been made,
> That we may entrance find and weep no more.
> Through thee the Saviour came to us
> To be our guiding light and King.
> To Christ, our Life, of Virgin born,
> Ye ransomed peoples praises sing.
> O Mother dear, of grace divine,
> God's mercy for us sinners plead,
> Protect us from the enemy,
> In life's last hour to Heaven lead.

Shortly afterwards, his faithful servant Ruggiero, noticing his shining eyes, asked him: "Do you see anything?"

"I see my Lord," St. Anthony replied. He was anointed and joined in the penitential Psalms, and shortly after this, he died. He was just 36.

In life St. Anthony had always been a peacemaker. But his

death was the occasion for a dispute between Padua, on the one hand, and Arcella and suburban Capo di Ponte across the river, on the other, as to which place would claim his body. While the squabble lasted, his burial was delayed for almost a week. The destruction of a bridge of barges, hastily built to take his body across the river to Padua, brought both sides out under actual arms. At this point the Poor Clares, seeing what their original request to have the body of St. Anthony had stirred up, asked for his remains to be taken away.

In 1263 the body was transferred to the new Basilica of St. Anthony in Padua. Another Doctor of the Church, St. Bonaventure, was present at the time. When he saw the remains, which consisted of the bones with the tongue still incorrupt, St. Bonaventure exclaimed: "O blessed tongue, you have always praised the Lord and led others to praise Him! Now we can clearly see how great indeed have been your merits before God." Writing in 1931, Edyth H. Brown said that the tongue of St. Anthony, once soft and ruddy, had become brittle and discolored, "a dark pod in a reliquary shaped like a monstrance." (*Catholic World*, 113, 311-320).

Today, the Franciscan Conventuals are the custodians of St. Anthony's remains. At his tomb in the great basilica dedicated to him in Padua, people come to pray, most often preferring to go to the rear of the tomb. Here they can get closer to the tomb and pray with one hand held against it. At Arcella a tomb has been built over St. Anthony's death cell.

Thus both at Padua and all over the world, the prayers to St. Anthony continue, offered up to ask for the intercession of the Saint who cares so much about so many of the minor desires of mankind. Aside from St. Therese of Lisieux, there is no Doctor of the Church more prayed to than St. Anthony.

St. Anthony of Padua's feast day is June 13.

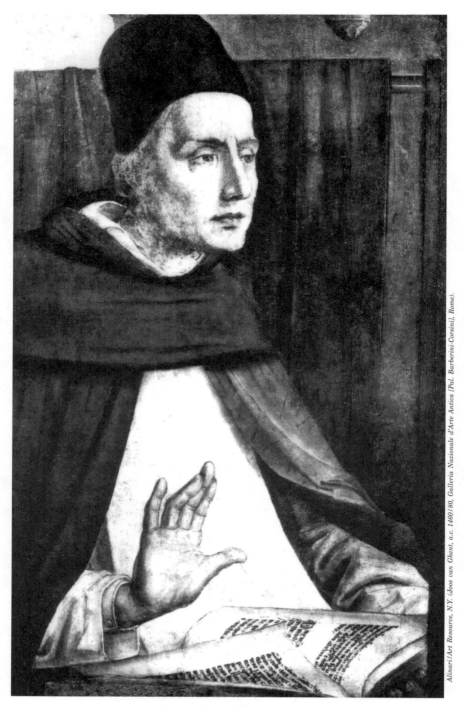

Saint Albert The Great

Alinari/Art Resource, N.Y. (Joos van Ghent, a.c. 1460/80, Galleria Nazionale d'Arte Antica (Pal. Barberini-Corsini), Rome).

22

SAINT ALBERT THE GREAT

(Albertus Magnus)
The Universal Doctor
c. 1206-1280

THERE is only one man in all history who is called "The Great" because of his scholarship. To a contemporary he was "the wonder and miracle of our age." Seven centuries later, Pope Pius XI said in his decretal (decree), *In Thesauris Sapientiae* (1931): "Albert is exactly the saint whose example should inspire this modern age, so ardently seeking for peace and so full of hope for its scientific discoveries." (*Decretal* in *Dominicana*, Washington, DC, Vol. 17, p. 350).

St. Albert, from his heavenly eminence, can appreciate exactly the task of scientific research. He did a great deal of it himself, not only in one subject, but in the whole field of science, which today is divided into so many specialties. St. Albert's specialty was no less than "everything created." He wrote on botany, mineralogy, astronomy, physics, chemistry, anthropology, cosmography, and other subjects. "No single science escaped his attention." (*Decretal,* p. 344).

St. Albert knew and wrote about 114 species of birds, 113 quadrupeds, 139 aquatic animals, 61 serpents and 49 worms. He was the first to mention the weasel and the arctic bear, the first to speak intelligently about the reproductive functions of birds. He was the first man in 1,500 years to study the physiology of plants. He had clear ideas about grafting. He described bees, ants, spiders, eels, salmon—and their habits.

At a time when the practice was forbidden by law, St. Albert dissected animals. He knew as much as or more than the doctors and dentists of his day about medicine, surgery and dentistry. He had a great fund of knowledge about herbal remedies. He wrote of eugenics. Overzealous admirers, especially his pupil, Thomas of Cantimpre, who gathered popular legends to glorify him, helped to cast an uncomplimentary historical shadow over

St. Albert's name as having been a practicer of magic.

St. Albert was a special expert on horses and their diseases. He can in fact be called both the father of veterinary medicine and the patron of veterinarians. He disposed of many popular legends, such as the one that the pelican feeds her young with her own blood, or that a rooster before dying lays one egg, from which a serpent hatches. Once Albert had a man lowered by a rope over a cliff to observe an eagle sitting on several eggs, in order to obtain proof of the falsity of the common belief that all the eagle's eggs except one are destroyed.

St. Albert knew that gunpowder could be made from sulphur, saltpeter and charcoal. He conducted chemical experiments and held the possibility of something that has only lately been accomplished, namely, that synthetic metals equal to some natural ones could be made. At a time when the shadows on the moon were thought to be reflections of the mountains and seas of the earth, St. Albert stated correctly that these were configurations on her own surface.

Patron of Scientists

In Seville, Spain, today there is preserved a set of St. Albert's writings which belonged to and were annotated by Christopher Columbus. Following Aristotle's lead, St. Albert taught that the world was a sphere. It was a fellow-Dominican, Diego Deza, confessor to Queen Isabella, who took up the case for Columbus with the Queen. St. Albert's writings also influenced another Dominican, George Anthony Vespucci, whose nephew, Amerigo Vespucci, gave his name to the New World.

On December 16, 1941, Pope Pius XII designated St. Albert the Great as patron of all who engage in scientific studies. As such, he is the special Saint for researchers, technologists, and all who engage professionally in any of the sciences, as well as of those who study science.

The title of the Pope's letter, "To God through the Knowledge of Nature," indicates why St. Albert was so chosen. Many people are puffed up, the letter said, "with a hollow science of words." But St. Albert has taught us "by his example how we should rather mount from the things of earth to the things above." The Pope's trend of thought in choosing St. Albert for this role is summed up in a text of St. Paul which the Pope uses in his letter and repeats in a letter of March 7, 1942 to the Dominican

Master General: "For the invisible things of him, from the creation of the world, are clearly seen, being understood by the things that are made; his eternal power also, and divinity." (*Rom.* 1:20).

The letter to the Dominican Master General, Martin Gillet, spells out the reason plainly.

> It is for this reason especially, beloved son, that we decided to select and constitute him Patron of Scientists: in order that the students of the natural sciences, bearing in mind that he had been given to them as their guide, might follow his footsteps and not cling too tightly to the investigation of the fragile things of this life, nor forget that their souls are meant for immortality, but use created things as rungs in a ladder that will elevate them to understand heavenly things and take supreme delight in them. May they discern the presence of God in all the forces of nature and, in meditation and veneration, admire the incorruptible rays of His splendor. May they see the beauty of God in the sweet and fragile loveliness of flowers; in the swelling waves of the sea may they reverence His power; and may they adore and revere His creative and eternal wisdom, not only in the harmonious and wondrous march of the stars, which obey the Supreme Will throughout the boundless spaces of the heavens, but also in the hiding-places of that tiny world which is known only to the eye of the microscope.

St. Albert's method was far ahead of his age. Had others taken it up consistently, the timetable of scientific advances would have been moved ahead by centuries. Things being discovered today could have been discovered before the American Revolution. "The aim of the natural sciences," St. Albert said, "is not simply to accept the statements of others, that is, what is narrated by people, but to investigate for ourselves the causes that are at work in nature."

Sometimes St. Albert relates what Aristotle or some other writer has said and then adds, "I have not been able to observe this." He passed on the information for what it might be worth, but considered himself bound to qualify it in this way. In his *Summa Theologiae,* written near the end of his life, he devotes a chapter to the "Errors of Aristotle," his favorite writer. (The *Summa* of St. Albert the Great follows Alexander of Hales.)

"He who believes Aristotle to be a god ought to believe that he never made a mistake. But whoever thinks him to have been a man must admit that he was as liable to make mistakes as the rest of us." (*Summa*, Ia, q. 62, a. 1).

Over and over again St. Albert asks for proof by experiment. "I have tested this." "I have proved this is not true." "I and my associates have experienced." "We have shown it to be false by experiment." "But this has not been sufficiently proved by a certain experiment." Writing about whales, he remarks: "We pass over what the ancients have written on this topic because their statements do not agree with experience."

St. Albert was against multiplying miracles as explanations of natural events. Medieval man thought of the Creator as hiding "just behind the outer crust of things" and controlling them. (*St. Albert the Great*, by Thomas Schwertner, O.P., Bruce, 1932, p. 243). In his work on *The Heavens and the Earth*, St. Albert says:

> In studying nature, we have not to inquire how God the Creator may, as He freely wills, use His creatures to work miracles and thereby show forth His power; we have rather to inquire what nature with its immanent causes can naturally bring to pass.

In St. Albert's manifold scientific treatises there are indeed conclusions that today we would consider crude. Yet what could be expected without the use of the many precise instruments of research now so common, or without the benefit of the hundreds of discoveries made since his day?

St. Albert made no single discovery of great importance, such as Newton did with the law of gravity. What he did accomplish was to provide an encyclopedia of all past scientific knowledge, which in many instances was corrected by personal experiments. But most of all, he is important because he gave such a strong impetus to the use of the scientific method, the way of modern experimentation. He rejected *a priori* reasoning in science (i.e., reasoning from pre-accepted principles). Everything had to be proved. To St. Albert, the ancient authorities were worthwhile only when their positions were backed by proof.

As a scientist and a Saint, St. Albert the Great proves there is no conflict between faith and reason, between holiness and learning. Pope Pius XI says of him:

> Like St. Jerome, Albert, as it were with powerful voice, declares and proves in his wonderful writings that science worthy of the name, and faith and a life lived according to the

principles of faith, can and indeed should all flourish together in men, because supernatural faith is the crown and perfection of science. It is not true, as modern atheists assert, that the Christian life and the pursuit of Christian perfection destroy the human spirit, weaken the will, impede civil activity, and rob men's minds of their native nobility; on the contrary, grace perfects nature, develops, improves and ennobles it. (*Decretal*, p. 351).

The Thirteenth-Century Man

St. Albert's long life corresponds roughly with the thirteenth century. Most likely he was born in 1206. (But it could also have been in 1193.) The place was Lauingen on the Danube, 26 miles northwest of Augsburg, Bavaria. His parents were of the lower nobility, in the service of the Emperor. The family name was Bollstadt. He may have had other brothers and sisters, for it is known that one brother, Henry, also entered the Dominican Order. Among the familiar titles by which people referred to St. Albert during his lifetime, were Albert the German, Albert of Cologne, Albert von Bollstadt, Albert the Teuton, Albert the Theologian. Since 1343, when the title appeared in a book by John of Vitry, history has always called him "Albertus Magnus," which is the Latin for Albert the Great.

As a young man St. Albert accompanied his uncle to Padua, where he pursued his studies. Because of his endless interest in learning things, he made an ideal student. He also liked to hunt and fish and to explore the countryside, observing all the activities of nature. He enjoyed telling about his findings and answering the questions of his young companions.

At Padua he heard the renowned Dominican preacher, Blessed Jordan of Saxony, and felt drawn to become a Dominican. However, his uncle made him promise not to go to the Dominican church for a certain period of time; after this St. Albert still hesitated, because he feared he might enter the Order and then leave. One day Blessed Jordan answered his doubts in a sermon, stating that the devil deceived the unwary by suggesting to them that they could not persevere. St. Albert, it seems, also had difficulties concerning his ability to submit his intellectual life to a religious superior. In accepting and in living the vocation of the religious life, St. Albert entrusted himself to the guidance and help of the Blessed Virgin Mary. He entered the Dominican Order most likely in 1229, probably at Padua, and spent the days of his novitiate probably at Bologna, where St. Dominic had died and where his body was venerated.

There is no record of the date of St. Albert's ordination to the priesthood, but it would have been about 1233. He soon thereafter went to Cologne as a teacher. It was here that he spent most of the rest of his life, though not in one continuous sequence. He also taught at other schools of his Order—at Hildesheim, Freiburg, Strasbourg and Ratisbon. For several years he taught at the University of Paris, leaving that city on June 27, 1248 to return to Cologne.

From his early teaching days at Cologne has come the story which most people associate with his name. In his classroom was a quiet young pupil, half German, half Sicilian, who had been dubbed "the dumb Sicilian Ox" by his classmates because he said so little. One day this pupil was forced to talk, defending a thesis he had written. He deftly answered a barrage of questions by a teacher who certainly knew how to think them up. It was then that that teacher, who was St. Albert the Great, declared: "You call him 'the Dumb Ox,' but one day the bellowing of this Ox will resound throughout the world." It is said that before long St. Albert had the pupil, St. Thomas Aquinas, placed in a cell near his own in the monastery and that he often chose him as a walking companion.

In 1254, St. Albert was elected the Prior Provincial of the German Province of the Dominican Order, which also included Austria, Switzerland, Holland, the Benelux countries, Latvia and part of Poland. He traveled by foot over this vast stretch, visiting the 40 houses of his province, which contained about a thousand friars.

Sometime between March 1 and March 29, 1260, St. Albert was consecrated a bishop at Cologne. On March 29 he stole into Ratisbon in order to avoid a noisy reception, and the next day, Tuesday of Holy Week, he was installed as Bishop of that city.

As a bishop, St. Albert continued to walk on his visitations about his diocese, and this wearing old shoes. All through life he was a great walker, and his pace was so swift that he was often goodnaturedly teased about it. Some, who looked down upon this mode of travel by a high ecclesiastic, were not so goodnatured, and gave him the nickname, "Boots the Bishop."

St. Albert resigned from his bishopric, and the resignation was accepted by Pope Urban IV in a letter of May 11, 1262. The records show that St. Albert continued to ordain priests, especially for the Dominican Order, that he acted as bishop conse-crator and that he also blessed churches, chapels and altars in various places throughout his career.

The year following his resignation, he was made papal nun-cio to northern Europe and given the task of preaching the Crusade launched by Urban IV. Despite his great zeal, ability and efforts, St. Albert was not successful in stirring up any enthusiasm among the people. Most of his later years St. Albert spent as a teacher at Cologne, but as in earlier life, we often find him acting as a legate of the Pope or being called in by warring factions to settle disputes, which were mostly political.

Philosopher and Theologian

When we read the list of St. Albert's works in the field of sci-ence, we could easily conclude that here was the literary work of a lifetime. But science, of course, was just a part of his inter-est and work. There is a popular adage about St. Albert which runs: "He was great in magic, greater in philosophy, greatest in theology." "Magic" here would mean science. It has also been said that St. Albert was a scientist by temperament, a philoso-pher by deliberate choice and a theologian by mood.

His exact place as a philosopher has never been fully defined. His great contribution in general has been summed up in one word: Aristotle. More than anyone else, he made Aristotle accept-able in Christian circles. At a time when Aristotle was either condemned outright or looked upon with suspicion, he worked to present the whole of his works with the parts dangerous to Christian principles properly explained. He gave the world the most complete and comprehensive exposition of Aristotle, and he introduced St. Thomas Aquinas to him.

St. Albert's importance as a thinker can be shown to be based on the fourfold purpose for which he studied Aristotle: 1) he wanted to make all of Aristotle's doctrines available; 2) he made a paraphrase of Aristotle; 3) he added many digressions, show-ing where he (Albert) differed from Aristotle; 4) he gathered into one handy collection all the elements necessary for the devel-opment of scholastic philosophy, though he did not weld it together himself.

His work may be described as "mining the ore." Others, espe-cially St. Thomas Aquinas, would refine the metal. St. Albert was the founding father of Christian Aristotelianism.

St. Albert's importance to theology lies in his bringing to its study the systematic use of reason. If his contribution to philosophy can be summed up under one word, "Aristotle," so his contribution to theology can be summed up either in the same way or by the one word, "reason."

> By Albert's efforts, the whole of philosophy, and in particular the Aristotelian philosophy, was adopted to serve—under the light of Revelation—as a sound and fit instrument for the Christian theologian. (*Decretal*, p. 346).

More than ever before, St. Albert introduced the reasoning process in explaining the truths of doctrine and morals. He said: "Whatever is known by two ways instead of one is better grasped; hence, what is known by faith and reason is better understood than that which is known only by faith." (*Summa*, Part I of the 3rd treatise).

One way in which his reasoning process showed itself was in the more critical presentation of the thoughts of earlier writers. St. Albert shows unusual ability in getting to the point. His Dominican biographer, Schwertner, says: "He selects with sure instinct the skeleton thought and cuts away ruthlessly the literary flesh."

St. Albert was appreciative of how the thinking of earlier theologians had clarified Catholic teaching. He therefore pointed out that there is a certain development of doctrine. Indeed, the doctrine itself does not change, but succeeding generations build on the insights of earlier generations, and the individual truth becomes better understood and its meaning and beauty become more apparent. St. Albert laid down norms that should govern the fruitful and true development of dogma.

Again, in line with his emphasis on reason, St. Albert brought into the explanation of doctrine many more examples from other fields than did other writers. Incidentally, this must have made his classes very interesting. But it left its mark on theology, making that subject less formal and linked more to daily modes of speech.

St. Albert had an especially far-reaching effect on moral theology because of his explaining and giving reasons for the norms it proclaimed. He helped moral theology along to its present status as an independent branch of theology. As it exists today, it consists very largely of using the reasoning process to apply moral principles to the practical conditions of life to decide what is right and what is wrong, morally speaking.

St. Albert covered new ground in exploring the exact nature of responsible acts and showing how bodily and mental health affected the degree of responsibility, and sometimes even destroyed it. Moralists and confessors today are paying increased attention to this aspect of morality.

Since St. Albert had so much to do in arranging the wedding of reason and faith, he has in some quarters incurred blame for the rationalistic rebellion of theology in later centuries. By introducing the works of Aristotle, he "introduced into Western Europe for the first time a body of positivistic knowledge modeled on the sciences of the Greeks." (*Encyclopedia of the Social Sciences,* Macmillan, 1937, p. 14).

Pope Pius XI saw only good in St. Albert's influence on theology. He said in the *Decretal* of Canonization (p. 347):

> It would be an endless task to recount all that Albert has done for the increase of theological science. Indeed, it was to theology that the whole trend of his mind was inevitably directed. The authority he had acquired in philosophy grew and increased, for, as we have said, he used philosophy and the scholastic method as a kind of implement for the explanation of theology. In fact, he is regarded as the author of the method of theology which has come down in the Church to our own time as the safe and sound norm and rule for clerical studies.

Secretary of the Blessed Virgin

An early biographer of St. Albert the Great, Rudolph of Nijmegen (1488), called him the "secretary and panegyrist of the Blessed Virgin Mary." Albert was so devoted to the holy Mother of God, Rudolph says,

> that he could not conceal her praises, and he, moreover, appended to all his works something in praise of his beloved Lady, or closed his studies with a song to her glory. He composed many sequences in honor of the glorious Virgin which are as remarkable for their depth of meaning as for their harmony and interior spirit. In the convent garden and elsewhere he delighted to sing them with intense sweetness, devotion, and enthusiasm. His sighs and tears would often interrupt his song, and thus disclose his fervor, love, and ardent piety. (*Sch.* 161-2).

Pope Pius XI said that "he was in all things wholly devoted to God, and he was especially remarkable for his tender devotion to Our Lady." (*Decretal*, p. 340).

In Volume I of St. Albert's works (edition of A. Borgnet, 1889), there is a metric eulogy:

> Albert was the philosopher of Mary;
> Thomas was the theologian of the Word.
> The one wrote well of the Son,
> And the other of the Mother.
> Now both were great indeed,
> But one was pupil and the other master.

St. Albert's sermons about the Blessed Virgin Mary in their German and German dialect versions were cut up and used as bookmarks or put on the walls of homes as mottos. In addition to nourishing piety, St. Albert's presentation of the Blessed Mother as the highest ideal of womanhood helped to stir the spirit of true chivalry and soften the manners of a rough age.

St. Albert quotes *Ecclesiasticus* 24:29-31 to give the background reasons for his writing about the Blessed Virgin. Then he explains:

> It is in hope of these promised riches that we undertake this work; otherwise, we should be too much exalted above our narrowness of mind and knowledge . . . It is from her that we expect the happy completion and reward of our task. It is she who guides our wills, who determines us to write and who knows our intentions . . . We are desirous only to render ourselves useful through these unpretending pages, to simple and untaught people like ourselves . . . (This is at the beginning of his *Mariale*, or "230 Questions concerning the Blessed Virgin.")

The questions center on the text of St. Luke: ". . . the angel Gabriel was sent. . ." (*Luke* 1:26). St. Albert gives reasons both for and against his own conclusions. The questions are very interesting, and the answers are often intriguing. The work shows exact and detailed thought, and proves to us that we take many beliefs about the Blessed Virgin Mary for granted, and never think at all of others.

Question 3 asks: "In what form did the angel appear?" The opinion of St. Bede is given, that he appeared as a serpent; then is explored the opinion that he appeared as a dove, representing simplicity, in opposition to the serpent's duplicity. St. Albert then explains his own conclusion, that the Angel appeared in human form.

Question 4 then asks: "In what sex did the angel appear?" Perhaps it seems more fitting that a woman should appear to a woman, a virgin to a virgin. But St. Albert thinks that the Angel appeared as a man because in all previous visits by Angels with reference to the coming of Christ, they had appeared as men. Then too, "The feminine sex is not so much illuminating as a subject of illumination, according to what the Apostle says: 'But I would have you know that the head of every man is Christ, and the head of the woman is the man, and the head of Christ is God.'" (*1 Cor*. 11:3).

Question 5 concludes, following Denis the pseudo-areopagite, that the Angel appeared in the form of a young man, since youth signifies something new and the perfection of vital power.

Question 7 inquires what time of day it was when the Angel appeared. It should perhaps be morning, since the day of grace was beginning; it should perhaps be noon, because then the sun is at its height; noon is the hour in which Christ suffered, and the hour in which the birth of St. John the Baptist, the forerunner, was announced. It should perhaps be evening, because "God sent his Son in the fullness of time." (*Gal*. 4:4). St. Albert again follows Denis, saying that the time was the morning, since the time should express the properties of the one announced. The coming of Christ was the rising of the True Sun over the earth.

Other questions ask such things as where the appearance took place, what Mary was doing at the time (praying or working), and how old she was at the time. On this last, which is Question 14, St. Albert concludes that she was at the height of her maturity in body and in growth of grace. This, he explains, would place her between the ages of 25 and 31. In other questions, St. Albert takes up the subject of Our Lady's beauty, her size and her appearance. All these are treated ingeniously, and as usual, the reasons for the opposite viewpoint are listed and explained.

St. Albert concludes the series of questions on Our Lady's appearance with this description: "And so, the Blessed Virgin was in color of skin ruddy white; her hair and eyes were temperately dark, as also we believe her beloved Son, most beautiful of the sons of men, was in color."

Did Mary know music? Did she receive Baptism, Confirmation, the Holy Eucharist? Did she go to Confession, and if so, to whom? Did she have the power of Holy Orders? The 230 questions of this work run to 317 pages of double-column quarto.

One interesting note is that St. Albert would not want to call Our Lady what she is so often termed today, a "second Eve." He said she should not be called Eve, because her role is in every way the opposite to that of Eve.

We must be like Mary in order to praise her, says St. Albert. Then we will praise her wisely.

> Wisely, in such a manner that he who praises may resemble him who is praised, and that this praise may be the faithful expression of the heart. How indeed can the voluptuous praise the Virgin? How can the proud man praise her who was humble? How can the cursed praise her who was loaded with heavenly blessings? (Schwertner, p. 163).

St. Albert was a great promoter of a practice which had a resurgence after the Marian year of 1954, the erection of shrines in Our Lady's honor along the roads and in homes. He wrote more extensively of Mary than any man of his period. His systematic treatment of the Blessed Virgin is unique even among the great writers of the Church. He provided a reservoir from which many great preachers have drawn to nourish their own devotion and that of the people. Like those of a true lover, St. Albert's thoughts must have kept returning to Mary. Otherwise, he could never have written in such detail and with so much feeling.

The Heart of a Scholar

As we would expect of a man whose passion was truth, St. Albert had a strict sense of justice. He showed this at times in his clear, unequivocal way of pointing out truths that hurt certain individuals.

> As a preacher he weighed all in the balance of justice and distributed to each one according to his needs, whether he preached to the rich or to the poor. He struck everyone with the arrow of truth. (Humbert de Romanis, fifth Dominican Master General).

As a bishop he stirred up violent opposition by his criticisms of the nobility who pampered themselves and oppressed the poor. A pioneer in pointing out the influence of bodily and mental weakness on responsibility, St. Albert still said of sins of impurity: "They who seek to excuse their faults by saying that such acts are conformable to nature should be taught that they are, on the contrary, opposed to it." (Schwertner, p. 67).

When St. Albert was provincial, he imposed penances on priors who came to the chapters in a carriage or on horseback (which was hardly the way to insure re-election). Fasting on bread and water and eating this fare while kneeling in the middle of the refectory before the community were some of the penances he imposed. When first elected provincial, he showed his strictness with regard to poverty by ordering the body of a lay brother on whom money had been found at death to be dug up and cast into the common sewer. As a confessor he once gave a penance that lasted seven years.

Yet St. Albert's outstanding characteristic was magnanimity. An early biographer says of him: "He had an eye for the good, an intellect for the noble, and an enthusiasm for the great." Despite the severity he showed in the interest of justice and truth, he was noted as a sympathetic and understanding confessor. He was a favorite confessor for lay people as well as for nuns. His door was never barred to anyone who came to confess or to ask counsel.

St. Albert found the task of dispensing justice very trying. As a bishop he used to retire to a villa to write and pray when the pressure of his office grew too great. Perhaps his retiring from his diocese stemmed from the same cause.

> Nothing is more easy, he wrote, than to lead inferiors with mildness and humility as far as circumstances permit. But when the irruption of evil constrains one to act seriously and with severity, the pastoral office becomes to a bishop, as of old to Moses, an insupportable burden, especially when he is unwilling to tolerate and protect evil-doers, as certain prelates are wont to do in these times. (Schwertner, p. 117, quoting from the *Commentary on the Gospel of St. Luke*).

In his old age, St. Albert's tenderness of heart showed itself when, as it is said, he wept whenever he heard the name of Thomas Aquinas, who had preceded him in death. And the many references to childhood and home scattered throughout his works show a man who had had a happy childhood and loved the simple joys of home.

St. Albert was genial and good-natured; he was winsome and an animated conversationalist. He loved to talk to others. This and his vast interest in all creation, plus his ability to present his thoughts clearly, made him a born teacher. Students from all over Europe flocked to his classes.

St. Albert's drive to serve God most fully, his love for neighbor that urged service, and the impelling inquisitiveness of his mind made him really deserving of that overworked word, "busy." "He was incessantly occupied, either in reading, writing, dictating, preaching or hearing Confessions. He never allowed his mind to repose where there was a question of divine works. . ." (Humbert de Romanis). Every day he prayed the entire *Psalter* slowly and thoughtfully. Today this would be considered by many people to be a good day's work. When too weary to work, or too sad, St. Albert sought the "solace of movement," walking back and forth, or perhaps going on one of his many journeys.

Writing within 30 years after St. Albert's death, an author described him as "the great Albert, great in his knowledge, small in his person." Albert was small to medium in size, but had broad shoulders, as his relics show and historians attest. His chin was small enough to be a notable characteristic. He was a man of great endurance, who needed little sleep and could work or travel for long periods beyond what the ordinary person could do. He was never known to complain of ill health, yet in 1932 when his relics were examined, a doctor gave the opinion that St. Albert had been a lifelong victim of chronic rheumatism.

The Soul of a Scholar

St. Albert's writings did not proceed from a merely cold, scientific spirit, but from a soul seeking union with God. He wrote many prayers, one, for instance, for each Sunday of the year, based on the Epistle and Gospel read for that particular Sunday. For the Fourth Sunday after Pentecost, the prayer reads:

O Lord Jesus Christ, Who seekest those who stray and receivest them when returning, make me approach Thee through the frequent hearing of Thy word, lest I sin against my neighbor by the blindness of human judgment, through the austerity of false justice, through comparing his inferior status, through too much trust in my merits or through ignorance of the divine judgment . . . Help me to search diligently each corner of conscience lest the flesh dominate the spirit. (*Vol.* 13, Paris ed.).

St. Albert considered the proper fear of death to be a grace.

For many neglect the fruits of good works on this account, that they think they will live long, but the Lord coming by graces, strikes them with the fear of death, so that they may more fervently sow on earth what they will reap in Heaven. (3rd of Advent, Vol. 13).

Besides his outstanding devotion to the Blessed Virgin Mary, St. Albert had an intense devotion to the Holy Eucharist. Speaking of God's goodness in giving us the Eucharist, St. Albert says: "In His sweetness God thinks sweetly of us. He can think of nothing sweeter or better than that God should be in us in His divinity and humanity as a spiritual food, which nourishes our life and brings to perfection our union with Himself." (*On Euch.*, Dist. 1, 2).

St. Albert wrote large works on the Mass and the Holy Eucharist. His *Sacrifice of the Mass* runs to 165 quarto pages, and his work on the Eucharist runs to 243 pages. Of his 32 sermons on the Holy Eucharist, Schwertner says: "No preacher could read them and be quite the same ever again." Of the work on the Mass the same biographer says: "Each sentence is written in starlight and the eternal tears of love." Pope Pius XI speaks of St. Albert's "incomparable work on 'The Blessed Sacrament of the Altar.'"

The great Dominican mystics Meister Eckhart, Bl. Henry Suso and John Tauler, were strongly influenced by St. Albert's works. The writings of the latter two especially had a strong influence on the language and literature of Germany.

St. Albert composed an office of St. Joseph, which remains lost but which had a great influence on devotion to St. Joseph in the Eastern Churches.

Pope Pius XI in his decretal letter of equipollent canonization says that St. Albert's mystical writings "show that he was favored by the Holy Ghost with the grace of infused contemplation." (*Decretal*, p. 348). He says of St. Albert's scriptural works in particular and of all his theological works that they make the soul want to cling to Christ. "We readily discern in them the holy man discoursing of holy things." (*Decretal*, p. 347).

Twenty Million Words

"You knew all that was knowable" was part of a saying addressed to St. Albert after his death. Nobody knows for sure the exact number of his writings. At present a critical edition of his works is being made at Cologne, five volumes having been finished by 1960. The edition of his works made at Paris in 1889-1899 contains some writings certainly not his, yet there are many more not included in that edition which *are* his. We can safely say that St. Albert wrote some 20,000,000 words. The Paris edition runs to 38 quarto volumes, which would make double that number of books in the usual size printed today. We might compare St. Albert's literary output to that of the indefatigable writer, Cardinal Newman, whose printed works run to 39 volumes (of smaller size than usual today, or sextodecimo).

St. Albert had a full life as a preacher, a teacher, an administrator and an arbiter of peace. Yet all his activities were as nothing, as Pope Pius XI says, in comparison with his written works. They range over the whole field of human knowledge. A list of the titles alone serves to illustrate the extent of St. Albert's knowledge. It is little wonder, then, that his title in his own lifetime and today is "The Universal Doctor."

It was the vastness of his work, as well as its clarity and value, that made men pick him out from all the great scholars of his time and name him "The Great." His field of knowledge was universal. Pope Pius XI says:

> He was a conspicuously great man in his own age and is still great in our day; by his pre-eminent qualities as a teacher and his surpassing skill in so many departments of knowledge, he has won the special title of "The Great."

In all the many writings of St. Albert, as we might expect, some things are not treated with finality, or arranged in the best order. Yet throughout his writings, clarity is an outstanding characteristic. They remain "the most colossal encyclopedia ever undertaken and carried through by a single individual." The most authoritative biography of Albert himself is that by Heribert Scheeben, *Albertus Magnus* (Bonn am Rhein, 1932).

Death and Glory

In 1274 St. Albert was at the Second Council of Lyons, but his part in it is not clearly known. In 1277 he journeyed to Paris to defend the works of his pupil, St. Thomas Aquinas, from imminent condemnation by Stephen Tempier, Archbishop of Paris.

Toward the end of his life, St. Albert's memory and his intellectual powers began to fail, probably due to a stroke. But he was able to pray and to move about to the end, although the once swift pace had slowed to a shuffle.

St. Albert died sitting in a large wooden chair in his cell, clothed in the Dominican habit. The friars were there and sang the *Salve Regina*. Its strains were in his ears and its greeting must have been in his soul when he went forth from earthly life to meet his Queen. His death occurred the evening of Friday, November 15, 1280. There were tears and grief in Cologne as men passed the news to one another: "Friar Albert is dead."

According to a story not contradicted by his confessor, Gottfried of Duisbert, St. Albert appeared to him one night shortly after death and told him: "Because in my lifetime I drew many persons out of the darkness of ignorance to the light of truth and the knowledge of God, the Lord has accorded to my prayers the deliverance of 6,000 souls from the flames of Purgatory." (Schwertner, p. 325).

Many people came to visit St. Albert's tomb, and many miracles were reported there. On a wrought-iron fence around the tomb was this inscription in Latin:

Prince of thought, in art, in science skilled,
Cask of Wisdom's waters, truth distilled,
Plato's better, master need he own
No mortal sage but Solomon alone;
Here in deathless fame, great Albert lies;
To Thee, O Christ, grant that his spirit rise.
Five days had passed since Martin's festal morn,
Twelve hundred years since Christ was born,
When, seeking Thee, O God, with every breath,
He found and made a jubilee of death.
Turn back, all ye that read this craven scroll,
And pray eternal rest unto his soul.

St. Albert's relics are now at the church of St. Andrew in Cologne. St. Albert was not beatified or canonized by the usual processes, but "equivalently." Innocent VIII granted the Dominicans at Cologne and Ratisbon the faculty to celebrate his feast and erect altars in his honor. This permission in 1484 was equivalent to beatification and entitled Albert to be called Blessed Albert. Pope Pius XI used the expression "equipollent canonization" in his decree of December 16, 1931, "In the Treasures of Wisdom." (*In Thesauris Sapientiae*). This decree established the feast of St. Albert the Great on November 15 and declared him a Doctor of the Universal Church.

From November 9 to 15 an Albertine Week had been held in Rome. Scholars from all over the world had lectured on different aspects of Albert's work. On the closing day of the three-day Canonization celebration, 30,000 people gathered at Cologne Cathedral. At the Triduum held at Oxford around Pentecost of 1932, speakers included the well-known Bede Jarrett, the Dominican General Vincent McNabb, the Abbot Vonier, Adrian English and Ronald Knox. In the United States there were special observances on the first anniversary of the Canonization, November 15, 1932.

St. Albert's life was a search for truth in all branches of knowledge. All who seek scientific truth today will, if they seek it humbly and lead an innocent life, find that the microscope and the telescope reveal only the wonderful works of God. The path of truth must lead to the Creator of all things, the God of truth.

St. Albert feared not that the truths of science could contradict those of faith. His practice of introducing the best of pagan philosophy into theology was something he was to call "snatching a weapon from the enemy's hands." And thus, "He used the ancient philosophy to support and defend revealed truth." (*Decretal*, p. 345). We could do no better in summing up the accomplishments of St. Albert and their meaning for us today than to use the words of two popes of the twentieth century.

Pope Pius XI describes his accomplishments:

> Albert had an insatiable thirst for truth, a patient, tireless energy of inquiring into natural phenomena, a vivid imagination joined to a tenacious memory, a sane esteem for the established wisdom of the past. Above all, his was a religious mind, ready to perceive the matchless wisdom of God shining out through all creation. His was the spirit of the psalmist who invites all the elements of the world to sound forth the praises of the Creator. (*Decretal*, p. 345).

Pope Pius XII illuminates the meaning of St. Albert for us today by a prayer:

> May St. Albert, who in his own very difficult times proved by his wonderful work that science and Faith can flourish harmoniously in men, through his powerful intercession with God, arouse the hearts and minds of those who devote themselves to the sciences, to a peaceful and orderly use of the natural forces, the laws of which, divinely established, they investigate and seek after.

St. Albert the Great's feast day is November 15.

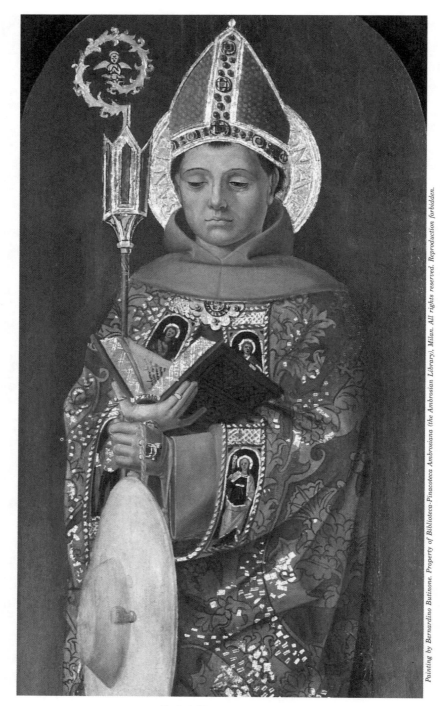

Saint Bonaventure

23

SAINT BONAVENTURE
The Seraphic Doctor
c. 1221-1274

"CAN one who has no book-learning love God as much as one who does?" This question was put by Giles, one of the primitive followers of St. Francis of Assisi and at the time venerable with age. The man who answered it was the Father General of the Order, St. Bonaventure, one of the most learned men of history.

"An old woman can possibly love God more than a master in theology," replied St. Bonaventure, who had given a strong impetus to study in the Franciscan Order—a fact which Giles, favoring simplicity and piety, could not accept nor understand. He feared learning because it might destroy simplicity and piety and puff up with pride those who acquired it. Giles then went to the edge of his garden and called out for any who might be listening: "Hear this, all of you: an old woman who never has learned anything and cannot read, can love God more than Brother Bonaventure!"

Giles knew that the Father General had not changed his mind about the value of learning. Giles was simply dramatizing the question by gleefully blowing to the winds the straw of a seeming victory over St. Bonaventure.

Yet in the substance of this little exchange we have the key to the character and the thinking of St. Bonaventure. With him the love of God always came first and last. Because St. Bonaventure gave the primacy to love, he could answer as he did. But he could never slight learning, for to him, to learn meant simply to explore creation, which contained the traces and images of God. Learning, properly guided by love, must lead to greater love of God.

St. Bonaventure held that love of God must be a love based on faith. Those who are capable of using their minds should do so to the fullest possible extent, in order to explore and understand the material world, the soul of man, and the Scriptures.

Those who are not capable of using their minds are better off not to try to exceed their powers, lest they fall into confusion. Still, they are already in possession of the highest truths through their love based on faith. Those who learn more formally should have as the final fruit of their study the love of God.

The ancient chronicle says of St. Bonaventure: "He made every truth a prayer to God and a praise of God." George Boas, professor of philosophy at Johns Hopkins University, says that St. Bonaventure makes observational science the fulfillment of a religious obligation. This is evident in the Saint's treatise, *The Soul's Journey to God*. Boas says that, without too much exaggeration, it can be maintained that "the impetus to the study of the natural world through empirical methods came from the Franciscans." (Boas, trans. and intro., *The Mind's Road to God*, Liberal Arts Press, NY, 1953, p. xix).

St. Francis of Assisi feared the errors that often came from learning. He feared learning which could extinguish the spirit of piety. Experience shows that the learned often stray the furthest from God; even among the good who are learned, there is the danger of cold, intellectual appraisal replacing warm piety and simplicity. Yet St. Francis himself was a student of the open book of Creation. Everything spoke to him of God.

St. Bonaventure, who came to such an opposite conclusion regarding formal study, did so just because he so thoroughly appreciated St. Francis' viewpoint. He had to reconcile in himself the complete following of Francis and the insistent demands of an inquiring mind. His system was the answer. In it he was able to reconcile the demand for the values of St. Francis and the undeniable practical necessity for formal study. The title of one of his works indicates his trend of thought: *The Reduction of All Things to Theology*. All branches of study should lead to God.

A Mother's Vow

St. Bonaventure was born in Bagnorea near Viterbo, Italy around 1221. (Early sources differ regarding the year; it may have been 1217 or 1218.) The family name was Fidanza, and Bonaventure's parents, John and Ritella, had their son christened John. But he was usually called Bonaventure, meaning "good coming," for some reason not clearly known. Some have said that the name was given him by St. Francis. But there is no proof that St. Francis, who died in 1226, ever knew of him.

As a boy, however, St. Bonaventure was cured of a serious illness by St. Francis. He tells of it himself in the prologue to his *Life of St. Francis*, giving as one of the reasons for writing: "The devotion which I am bound to bear to this our holy Father, by whose merits and invocation I was (as I well remember), while yet a child, delivered from the jaws of death." Bonaventure's mother had made a vow to St. Francis, asking for her boy's recovery.

No life of St. Bonaventure was written by any of his contemporaries, so details on his youth in particular are scarce. It seems that one of his Franciscan brethren, John Giles Zamorra, wrote a life; but it has either been destroyed, hopelessly lost, or it is waiting in some unknown archive for discovery.

St. Bonaventure most likely entered the Friars Minor in 1238 and came to Paris a few years later, probably in 1242, according to some writers (*Latin Life*). Others say that he was in Paris first and entered the Order there in 1243-44 (cf. *Cord* 7, 299). One of his teachers was the renowned Alexander of Hales, known as the Father of Scholastic Theology, whom he always held in much esteem and veneration and whom he followed in his writings. St. Bonaventure was in a center which at that time has been called "the oven where the intellectual bread of the whole world was baking." (*Cord* 7, 298).

We do not know when or where St. Bonaventure was ordained a priest. In 1248 he began to lecture at the University of Paris on the *Book of Sentences* of Peter the Lombard. His *Commentary on the Sentences*, written during these years of teaching, can be considered his greatest work, though it is not his most original. Its four large books cover all of scholastic theology. At the conclusion of Volume 3, he tells us:

> Everywhere I have tried to follow the common opinion as the safer course. Where I could not determine which was the common opinion, I chose that which seemed to me preferable. (Quoted by Ludger Wegemer, O.F.M., *Franciscan Studies*, Vol. II, July 1924, p. 16).

Second Founder

When he was just 36, St. Bonaventure was chosen to be the General of the Franciscan Order. He held this position until shortly before his death 17 years later. As ninth General of the

Friars Minor he solved problems both within and without the Order that were perplexing and even threatening to its very existence. His work in framing legislation, in visiting the provinces; his writing in defense of evangelical poverty, his writings explaining the Rule and expounding Christian perfection, have guided and molded the Franciscans ever since. It can also be said that his philosophy and mystical theology have stamped themselves on the Franciscan mentality.

St. Bonaventure said that St. Francis had a threefold ideal: to be a complete imitator of Christ in His virtues, to cling completely to God through prayer and contemplation, and to work for souls. St. Bonaventure embraced this ideal wholeheartedly in his own life. Men were willing to follow him because he was not only learned, but also holy.

As St. Francis had left it, and without further interpretation, the Rule could effectively have guided only a small body of saintly and dedicated men. St. Bonaventure built up the intellectual and juridical framework in the Order that would insure the preservation and the active application of St. Francis' ideal in a large body of men. St. Francis is remembered today, and St. Bonaventure is largely forgotten; but had it not been for St. Bonaventure, the master builder, the house of St. Francis might have been shaken to the ground.

In the Bull *Ite et vos* (p. 34, Wegemer), Pope Leo X said, "Under the leadership of St. Bonaventure, God-fearing men have in the third hour, with the help of the Blessed Trinity, re-established the walls of the vineyard which in all places threatened to crumble." Pope Sixtus IV had already said of St. Bonaventure in the Bull of Canonization: "Of all who came after St. Francis, he is the one who did most" for the Order.

St. Bonaventure was a kind but forceful administrator. In his first official letter to the Franciscan Order (April 23, 1257), he outlined his program:

> Drive out the buyers and sellers from the heavenly Father's house. Awaken in all the Brethren a desire for devout prayer. Limit the reception of candidates; for this statute I will have strictly observed. Root out these evil ways, though it be hard. The sublimity of your profession demands it; the calamities confronting us demand it; St. Francis himself, the Blood of Jesus Christ, and God demand it. (*Cord* 7, 303).
>
> Should I learn from the [ecclesiastical inspection] visitors, whom I desire to pay especial attention to these matters, that

my directions have been obeyed, I shall give thanks to God and to you. But if it should be otherwise, which God forbid, you may rest assured that my conscience will not permit me to allow the matter to pass unnoticed. Though it is not my intention to forge new chains for you, yet must I, in compliance with the dictates of my conscience, aim at the extirpation of abuses.

The Angelus

In the second and sixth of the General Chapters of the Order, those at Pisa in 1263 and at Assisi in 1269, over which St. Bonaventure presided, strong direction was given to devotion to the Blessed Virgin. At Pisa one provision asked the friars to exhort the people to salute the Blessed Virgin several times when they heard the bell rung at Compline. The reason given was that a good opinion held this hour to be the one in which the Angel had saluted Mary. This custom appears to be the start of the saying of the *Angelus*. (Other Marian provisions were legislated at the same time.)

The statute was renewed in the Chapter of 1269, and it was also decreed (or the decree was renewed—there is a dispute) that Mass be sung each Saturday in honor of the Blessed Virgin and a sermon given in her honor. These regulations embodied the tender devotion of St. Francis and St. Bonaventure for the Blessed Virgin.

St. Bonaventure relied much on Mary and often spoke of her in his sermons. (IX, 633-721 has his complete sermons on Mary.) He quotes at length from St. Bernard's beautiful passages on the Blessed Virgin, especially those dealing with placing confidence in her. St. Bonaventure himself says:

Let us go to the Virgin with great confidence, and we will tranquilly find her in our necessities. Therefore this tabernacle is rightly to be honored, and to this tabernacle flight should be made, in which the Lord rested so familiarly, so that the Blessed Virgin herself could say truly and literally, "Who made me rested in my tabernacle." (Fourth sermon on Annunciation, IX, 673).

The Saint compares Mary to the fount which irrigates thorns. The thorns, he says, are sinners.

For many who were thorns have been made—because of their confidence in the Blessed Virgin—trees of election. The sinner is never so thorn-choked that he may not become a healthy tree, if he goes to her. (Sermon IX, 697).

St. Bonaventure cannot find words to express his admiration for the Mother of God. (IX, 693).

Beloved, the excelling sublimity of the Virgin so transcends human capacity that words do not suffice to explain it; and therefore the Holy Spirit, who filled her with the charisms of the virtues, the Holy Spirit Himself speaking through the prophets and other doctors of Holy Scripture, praises her in many ways, not only by express words, but also by figures and metaphors.

In finding an apt use for passages of the Bible, in bringing together a multitude of texts that illustrate a point, St. Bonaventure shows remarkable command of Scripture and fertility of thought. No matter what his topic, he was endlessly imaginative in making a Scriptural mosaic to illustrate his point. He was also one of the great preachers of his time and one who found acceptance before all types of audiences, from popes and kings to the most common people.

St. Bonaventure wrote a treatise for the guidance of preachers. An early edition of this work carries the title *The Art of Preaching by the Seraphic Doctor, St. Bonaventure, in which the keys of the Scriptures are given for the task of making sermons.*

He shows an acute awareness of the need for preparing differently according to the audience that will hear his sermon. "The material must be divided one way when preaching to the clergy, another way when preaching to the people, because by the one it is grasped more keenly and by the other more slowly." A detailed demonstration is given on how to handle the same subject for different groups. (IX, 9, no. 4).

Fashioner of Unity

St. Bonaventure, who was so successful in maintaining unity in the Franciscan Order, also displayed an unusual power to inspire unity in larger contexts. Alexander of Hales had said of him: "Adam did not seem to have sinned in Bonaventure." The historian of the Second Council of Lyons (1274) wrote: "This grace the Lord had given him, that whosoever looked upon him was forthwith irresistibly drawn to love him." (X, 67). He was well-proportioned, and his countenance was angelic and grave, yet ever cheerful. It has been said that within his person he exemplified his own dictum that "a spiritual joy is the greatest sign of divine grace dwelling in a soul." (*Month*, 21, 183-82).

The respect he commanded was so great that the cardinals of the Church, not being able for two years to settle on a successor to the papacy, took his advice. At the time, St. Bonaventure had come to Rome from Paris. His counsel helped the cardinals quickly to settle on one of the six proposed candidates, Theobald Placentinus, Apostolic Legate to Syria. This was September 1, 1271. It took until the following March 27, 1272 for him to be crowned Pope Gregory X. (He is now known as Blessed Gregory X.)

In 1265 St. Bonaventure had excused himself from an appointment to be Archbishop of York, England. At that time Pope Clement IV had written to him:

> We have striven by every means in our power to find a worthy man, one devoted to the Apostolic See and suited to the wants of the aforesaid Church and zealous for the peace and welfare of the Kingdom—a man conspicuous for learning, remarkable for foresight—a man whom the Lord might love, in whose goodness He might dwell—a man whose good deeds render him worthy of imitation, by whom the Catholic flock, as by a shining light, may be led to salvation. Seeking for such a one, we have fixed our choice on thee—our mind has rested on thee with entire satisfaction. For we behold in thee religious fervor, candor of life, irreproachable conduct, renowned learning, prudent foresight, serious gravity. We see that thou hast so long and so laudably presided over thine Order and fulfilled so faithfully the office of Minister General—exercising it prudently and profitably for the welfare of the Order, striving to live innocently under regular observance, showing thyself peaceful and lovable to all.

It might seem impossible to resist such a letter from the Pope. St. Bonaventure was a humble man, but the reasons he gave the Holy Father, which he no doubt held as valid himself, were hardly based essentially on humility. It can be pointed out that St. Bonaventure was still much occupied with the affairs of the Franciscan Order, and that the office offered to him was one of extreme difficulty. Nor was his health robust.

But Pope Gregory X gave St. Bonaventure no choice. "We prescribe and command . . . that you acquiesce without urging any difficulty. We also command that you hasten to our presence without any tardiness or delay." (X, 64). St. Bonaventure was created a cardinal in the Spring of 1273. In November at Lyons, the Pope consecrated him a bishop, appointing him Archbishop of Albano and consecrating at the same time the Dominican, Peter of Tarantaise.

A universal tradition relates a charming circumstance connected with St. Bonaventure's receiving the red hat. He was in a friary near Florence, busying himself in the kitchen, cleaning the utensils, when the papal legates arrived. He continued with his work, even commanding perhaps that the red galero offered him be hung temporarily on a tree. When he had finished he commented: "We have finished the work of the Friar Minor and will find this [new work] more burdensome; believe me, Brothers, these things are salutary and healthful, but the work that goes with great dignities is burdensome and dangerous." Then he received the legates graciously and accepted the red hat. We can be sure that even as he accepted this high dignity St. Bonaventure recalled the truth he had pointed out to others on another occasion: "Just as waters crowd into the valleys, so the graces of the Holy Spirit fill the humble." (*Holiness of Life*, transl. by L. Costello, O.F.M. of *De Perfectione Vitae ad Sorores*, B. Herder, 1923, p. 18).

Also in 1273, St. Bonaventure was named Papal Legate to the Council of Lyons, which was the fourteenth Ecumenical Council of the Church. He had a large share in shaping the agenda of the Council and in conducting meetings of bishops and theologians. The Pope himself presided at the general sessions.

At this council a reunion, though destined to be temporary, was effected with the schismatic Greek Church on May 18, 1274. St. Bonaventure preached to the Council on the nature of religious unity, using as his text *Baruch* 5:5. "Arise, O Jerusalem, and stand on high: and look about towards the east, and behold thy children gathered together from the rising to the setting sun . . ." The occasion of this address was the second session of the Council; the Franciscans, who had been sent as delegates to the Greeks, had returned and brought news that rejoiced the Holy Father: The people were willing to submit to the Pope and thus end the Great Eastern Schism. The Holy Father then called all the prelates to the chief church at Lyons. (X, 66).

St. Bonaventure preached to the Council again on June 29 after the Eastern Church delegates had arrived. Then the Creed was sung in both Latin and in Greek; the much-disputed term *Filioque* —"and from the Son"—was repeated three times. St. Bonaventure, the leading light of the Council, whom the Greeks had affectionately named "Eutyches," stood with the Eastern delegates to the Council, weeping copious tears of joy.

St. Bonaventure took part in the fourth session on July 6, when the reunion with the Greeks was formally made.

A Mass from Every Priest

Just a week later, while the Council was still in session, St. Bonaventure died. It was on a Sunday morning, July 15, 1274. We do not know the exact cause of death nor the circumstances. The heavy burdens of his work at the Council may have hastened or actually brought it on. He was just 53.

Peter of Tarantaise, who would be the next Pope as Innocent V (now Bl. Innocent V), celebrated the funeral Mass and preached, using the text: "I grieve over thee, my brother, Jonathan." Pope Gregory X and the prelates of the Council attended; many of them wept openly as they followed the body to the grave. On July 16, the Holy Father ordered every priest and bishop in the world to offer a Mass for the repose of the soul of St. Bonaventure.

The famous story of how St. Bonaventure received Holy Communion miraculously is sometimes placed as happening on his deathbed, but it is more reliably related as occurring at an earlier date, between the Franciscan Chapters of 1266 and 1269. According to the story, St. Bonaventure did not celebrate Mass for some days, judging himself unworthy of receiving the Body of Christ. While he was assisting at Mass one day during this period, a particle of the Host came—not by the hand of the priest, but by divine command—into St. Bonaventure's mouth. (X, 59).

St. Bonaventure was buried in the church of the Friars Minor in Lyons. In 1434, when the remains were transferred to the new church of St. Francis in the same city, his head, hair, tongue, lips and teeth were found incorrupt. But in May, 1562, Huguenots sought and burned his relics, excepting some which had been separated and taken to other places, and the head, which had been in Lyons but hidden in a separate place. At the time the guardian of the monastery was killed and thrown into the river for his part in trying to protect the relics. During the French Revolution, the monastery and church of the Friars Minor were destroyed. The head had been hidden at this time also, but if it still exists, the place had not been found as late as 1902.

St. Bonaventure was canonized on the octave of Easter, April 14, 1482 by Pope Sixtus IV. The Bull of Canonization assigned him the office of a pontiff and doctor. Pope Sixtus V more solemnly and formally declared St. Bonaventure a Doctor of the Universal Church on March 14, 1587 and made July 14 his feast day. It had previously been the second Sunday of July. His feast is July 15 in the revised Church calendar.

In his Bull *Triumphantis Jerusalem* Pope Sixtus V said that he was approving and renewing what Pope Sixtus IV had already done, and that

> Bonaventure, by right assigned to and numbered among the holy Doctors by the same Sixtus IV, we by these presents decree and declare by apostolic authority is to be held and honored among the principal and foremost who excelled in the teaching of theology. (X, 72).

Prince of Mystics

St. Bonaventure does not speak of mysticism, but of union with God. Yet all his works can truly be said to be permeated with mysticism. His works bearing directly on the subject, however, are short compared to the remainder of his works. *The Triple Way* is a compendium of his mystical theology in particular, just as the *Breviloquium* is a compendium of theology in general. His *Soliloquium* is a compilation of the ascetical and mystical teaching of the Fathers. *The Journey of the Soul to God*, written on Mt. Alverno, where St. Francis had received the stigmata, explains philosophically the whole process of spiritual progress.

Besides treatises concerning points of the Franciscan Rule, St. Bonaventure wrote one for superiors, one for sisters, and one for people in general. *Concerning the Six Wings of the Seraph* counsels religious superiors. It was at one time printed and spread throughout the Society of Jesus (the Jesuits) by their famous Father General, Aquaviva. *Perfection of Life for Sisters* was written by St. Bonaventure for the Poor Clares and was addressed to Isabella, sister of King St. Louis of France. Its approach and content are suitable for anybody to read with profit. *The Wood of Life* is a series of meditations on the life of Christ and is also suitable for all. (Cf. Wegemer, p. 21).

B. Herder Book Co. published *Perfection of Life for Sisters* under the title of *Holiness of Life* and *The Six Wings* as *Virtues of a Religious Superior*, the latter translated by S. Mollitor, O.F.M. and the former by Lawrence Costello, O.F.M. Thomas Baker of London has published in English *Three Principal Questions* and *Memorabilia*, translated by D. Devas. St. Anthony Guild Press of Paterson, New Jersey published selected works of St. Bonaventure in English, of which *Breviloquium* is Volume II. And finally, Franciscan Herald Press of Chicago (now Franciscan Press at Quincy College, Quincy, Illinois) published St. Bonaventure's complete works in five volumes, with an introduction by Etienne Gilson.

Pope Leo XIII (1878-1903) said of St. Bonaventure: "Having scaled the difficult heights of speculation, he treats of mystical theology with such perfection that in the common opinion of the most learned he is easily the most distinguished." (*Of Mystics Understood, or Facile Princeps*, Wegemer, p. 21). Fr. James, O.F.M. Cap., the renowned Irish writer, said that St. Bonaventure was "God-intoxicated," and that as

> a man himself filled with the knowledge of God, he wished to awaken Christians to their God and to lead them in the paths of peace to the heights of mental transports and unheard of things.

St. Bonaventure's whole thinking and character have been summed up as a conscious turning to the presence of God as the sunflower turns to the sun. The presence of God is the basis of his philosophy, his mystical theology and his directing of practical affairs.

In St. Bonaventure's teaching, the road to contemplation is the road to peace. As the soul advances, it comes more and more to peace. St. Bonaventure's emphasis is on the quiet pursuit of knowledge and love of God. Purification by mortifications and by trials is necessary, but these things are not to be looked upon as one single stage in the spiritual life, but rather, taken all together, they constitute various stages or steps along the path to God, and to some degree, fit into one continuous whole. In

the beginning of advancement, more mortification may be necessary than later on. St. Bonaventure himself was not an ascetic
by the standards of his day. He believed in sufficient food and
drink and sleep, and he took them. In fact, there was some
reproach cast at him for this, and he feared that his moderation would be used as an excuse for laxity by others, as it was
in truth. St. Bonaventure's mortification lay not so much in penitential practices as in the orderly discipline of the exterior
senses and the interior affections. If these went awry, then the
mind could not think of God, nor could the heart seek Him.
Therefore, he cautions that the hands, the eyes and ears must
be occupied in work or in study, and the body kept in subjec-
tion by fasting. But the fasting he meant was for those days
moderate. (Cf. Sermon *De Modo Vivendi*, IX, 722-724).

The beginning of the path to peace lies in strong desire. The
person who achieves the peace of Christ and possibly mystical
contemplation begins by strongly wanting to achieve them.

> No man is in any way disposed for divine contemplations,
> which lead to mental transports and unheard-of things, unless
> he be, like the prophet Daniel, a "man of desires." In two ways
> are such desires enkindled in us: through the cry of prayer
> that ascends from anguish of heart, and by the splendor of high
> thought, which turns the eyes of the mind directly and intently
> upon the rays of divine light. (Prologue to *Itinerarium*, no. 3).

The true nature of desire is beautifully explained:

> Desire, again, is something chiefly directed towards that which
> most deeply moves it. But desire is most keenly aroused by
> that which is most deeply loved, and happiness is what all men
> most urgently seek. Happiness, however, is possible only by the
> possession of the Highest and Ultimate End. It follows that
> nothing is really desired by man except it be the Supreme Good,
> either as an installment of it and as leading to it, or else as
> bearing some resemblance to it. Such is the attraction of the
> Supreme Good that nothing can be loved by the creature with-
> out desiring It, but the creature is deceived and errs when he
> accepts an effigy and an appearance for the truth. Behold then,
> how near is the human soul to God. Its various activities of
> memory, intellect and will point to God: memory, which is a
> reflection of His eternity, intellect, which postulates His truth,
> and the power of choice, which leads to Him as the Supreme
> Good. (*Itinerarium,* no. 3, 4).

The final stage, which is the last part of "active contemplation" or the height to which the soul can actively reach, consists in the love of Christ crucified. "The road to final peace is none other than the most fervent love of the Crucified which so transformed Paul, when caught up to the third Heaven, that he could say (*2 Cor.* 12:2): '*With Christ I am nailed to the cross; I live, now not I, but Christ in me.*'" (Prologue to *Itinerarium*, no. 3).

All Are Called to Contemplation

St. Bonaventure teaches that God calls, not just a few people, but all, to contemplation. His invitation is general, but a person has to work diligently—through prayer and meditation, through the combatting of sin, the control of disorderly inclinations—to be ready to receive this gift.

St. Bonaventure emphasizes the sweetness of contemplation and the attractiveness of God, rather than the darkness of mind and soul that are preparatory stages to contemplation. With St. Bonaventure the way to advance spiritually is continually to keep progressing by degrees in the knowledge of God. Mortification is chiefly necessary to help this progress. When a person has reached the highest step possible to human effort aided by ordinary grace, then it is fitting that God reward him at times by taking over his faculties and giving him a deeper glimpse of knowledge, one that is beyond human effort, and which is properly called "contemplation" in the passive sense.

In short, by *working* at the spiritual life, man reaches a high degree of active contemplation. Then at a certain point, God takes over to give him a temporary but more exalted vision, one that on his own man could not achieve.

St. John of the Cross, known as a teacher of mystical theology, made the works of St. Bonaventure mandatory study in the Carmelite novitiate. He followed St. Bonaventure in teaching that contemplation is not just for the very few, still less something to be dreaded. All should aim at the highest union with God possible on earth, but we must know that it comes only at a price. Both Saints teach that few people reach passive contemplation because so few are willing to make the necessary sacrifices that are included in the preliminary steps for spiritual advancement.

St. John also follows St. Bonaventure in warning against the occasional "concomitants" of contemplation, such as visions, revelations and levitations. Contemplation should be desired and worked for, but these extraordinary phenomena are not to be desired, but rather distrusted and feared. (Cf. *Month,* v. 21, article by Anselma Brennell).

St. Bonaventure gives a warning against trying to rush ahead on the way of holiness too rapidly and without guidance.

> . . . It is of little or no avail to look in the mirror of creation unless the mirror of our minds be cleaned and polished. First then, O man of God, thou must exercise thyself in holy compunction, experiencing the prick of conscience, before thou may raise thine eyes to the rays of divine Wisdom reflected in her mirror, lest haply [perchance], from gazing on these rays, thou fall into a deeper pit of darkness. (Prologue to *Itinerarium,* no. 4).

Just before this, however, St. Bonaventure has invited the readers of his *Journey of the Soul to God* to read only if they are properly disposed.

> To these, therefore, who are disposed by divine grace, the pious and humble, the contrite and devout, to those who are anointed with the oil of divine gladness, to the lovers of divine Wisdom and to those inflamed with the desire thereof, and who wish to go apart in order to taste and magnify and appreciate God, I offer the following speculations . . .

A Guide in Devotion

One reason why St. Bonaventure may be misinterpreted, or at least considered difficult in his philosophy, is that he is a spiritual pragmatist. He was most interested in having men turn to God. As a consequence, he swings easily from the examination of a truth in a speculative way to using it as a means of raising a soul immediately to God. "Bonaventure's whole philosophy is built about the immediacy of God as a central postulate." (*Modern Schoolman,* May, 1938, p. 87).

Yet St. Bonaventure, who can be so deep and difficult to learned philosophers and theologians, has written so plainly and simply about prayer and virtues that he can be understood easily by the average person.

He is a good, practical guide for devotional purposes. One of his earliest titles was "The Devout Doctor." This is suggested by the way in which the sparks and flames of love constantly shoot through his writings. When he was a young religious, a chronicler wrote of him: "As in wisdom, so in the grace of prayer did he continually grow. He converted every truth into a prayer and repeated it incessantly in ejaculations." (Wegemer, p. 12).

St. Bonaventure, for instance, tells us: "You cannot understand the words of Paul unless you have the spirit of Paul." Prayer and a good life are necessary to attain the full perception of truth. You must be truly devout in order to reach Christian wisdom.

St. Bonaventure gives us an insight into his own way of life and an example of how simply he can put things when he states a rule for spiritual progress:

> No one can serve God perfectly who does not try energetically to break the bonds of the world and rise above all earthly cares. We must never permit our heart to be disturbed by any created thing. Cares manifold and unduly sought distract the spirit, disturb interior peace, bring the phantasy into disorder, and cause many a sorrow. Hence we will cast off the pressing burden of every earthly love and without delay or hindrance hasten to Him who invites us, in whom our souls find bountiful refreshment and that perfect peace which surpasses all understanding (Wegemer, p. 12 and taken either from *Regula Novitiorum* or the letter containing *Memoralia* VIII, 494; the *Latin Life* says that this letter is most valuable for giving us an insight into St. Bonaventure's soul.)

What he has to say of charity is unmistakably plain.

> Charity is a virtue of such power that it can both close the gates of Hell and open wide the portals of eternal bliss. Charity provides the hope of salvation and alone renders us lovable in God's sight . . . (*Holiness of Life*, p. 83). If your love for anything does not conduce to greater love for God, you do not yet love Him with your whole heart. If for love of anything dear to you, you neglect to give Christ those things which are His by right, again, I say, you do not love Him with your whole heart. (*Holiness of Life,* p. 86).

How happy will a person be in Heaven? In the same treatise, St. Bonaventure clearly gives the answer:

What measure men put to their love of God here will be the
measure of their rejoicing with God in Heaven. Therefore, love
God intensely here and your rejoicing will be intense hereafter.
Continue to grow in the love of God here, and afterwards in
Heaven you will possess the fullness of eternal joy. (*Holiness
of Life*, p. 98).

How can you make a perfect prayer? St. Bonaventure says
that there are three requisites: 1) You must ponder your helplessness because of past sins, present weaknesses and constant
need of God's grace in the future. 2) You should be thankful for
forgiveness, for your Baptism, for the sufferings and death of
Christ. 3) You must, in the act of prayer, occupy yourself with
and think of nothing else but what you are doing.

It ill becomes a man to speak to God with his lips while in
heart and mind he is far away from God. To pray half-heart-
edly, giving, say, half one's attention to what one is doing and
the remaining half to some business matter or other, is no
prayer at all. Prayers made in such a way as this never reach
the ear of God. (*Holiness of Life,* pp. 52-53).

The Seraphic Doctor

The title by which St. Bonaventure is most readily known was
given him while he was still alive. And it is apt for several reasons. His thought is entwined with love; it quickly springs to
seraphic or angelic heights. As a teacher, he gives intellectual
expression to the life of the Seraphic Saint, St. Francis of Assisi.
St. Francis pursued a way of life that kept reaching out to God
with the fullness of an ardent nature, the sternness and intensity of a logic that looked at things reduced to ultimate simplicity, and the color of a rich emotion. Everything spoke to St.
Francis of God because its very nature is made by Him.
Everything pointed to the Sacred Humanity of Christ, and in
return the Sacred Humanity shed its glow on everything.

St. Bonaventure saw all created things as flowing in a necessary way from God: not that creation is or was necessary, but
creation, once decided upon, had to mirror the perfections of
God. Each part of creation according to its dignity is either a
shadow, a trace, an image or a similitude of God.

Since in Christ all the stages of creation are contained as in
a perfect examplar, there is no true knowledge, understanding

or wisdom if He is left out. "In Christ are contained all the treasures of wisdom and knowledge of the hidden God, and He is the medium for all knowledge." (Cf. *Modern Schoolman*, Note 35, May, 1938).

To St. Bonaventure Christ is therefore necessary for any full philosophy. There is no such thing as a philosophy based completely on reason. Faith has to enter in and present Christ as the Supreme Exemplar of all creation. If you leave out this centerpiece of creation, then not only would theology be empty, but philosophy would be weakest where it should be strongest. St. Bonaventure's philosophy rests squarely on faith and on reason.

St. Bonaventure was by no means opposed to the arts. He has, however, said that you cannot judge them rightly unless you look at them in the light of higher values. St. Bonaventure therefore turns to the Incarnate Word "as the touchstone at which to measure the human enterprise." (*Franciscan Studies*, 19, 1-12).

The great value of this system is that learning can proceed in the spirit of devotion. In this way, there is less chance for reason to drop into the pitfalls of rationalism, to run to the extremes of empty intellectualism. The proud spirit of man is kept more humble as it learns by tasting "in the darkness of faith" as well as by seeing in the light of reason.

"Taste and see that the Lord is sweet." This is the invitation of St. Bonaventure to all who would delve into the secrets of the universe. You can taste "in the darkness of faith" and come to a surer knowledge than by seeing in the light of reason. When it comes to ultimate, important truths, you cannot judge by reason any more surely than you can tell whether an object is sweet or bitter by looking at it. You must taste it.

St. Bonaventure "made every truth a prayer to God and a praise of God." He has been called "the totally religious soul." "Multifarious, infinitely diverse and subtly shaded, his thought is but an ever-active charity, whose whole movement strives toward objects which escape our view or toward unknown aspects of those things we do in part perceive." (Etienne Gilson, Preface to *The Works of St. Bonaventure*).

Sometimes we read in the lives of holy people that they had a knowledge of natural science and of human nature that amazed learned men. The usual assumption is that this knowledge was preternaturally infused. Perhaps this knowledge was not so much infused as naturally developed from using the system of

St. Bonaventure, letting faith and reason work together.

It has been said that St. Bonaventure rejected Aristotelianism. It may be more true to say that he used it as part of his eclectic system. He used it as far as he could, and then passed beyond it. He could see no sense in riding in the buggy of pure philosophy when he had the strong chariot of Christian wisdom to carry him faster and further forward—a wisdom already refined through centuries of thought. To St. Bonaventure, philosophy is good as far as it goes, but it is too obscure on the most important questions.

St. Bonaventure has been placed on an equal footing with St. Thomas Aquinas by two different Popes. Yet he has not found general acceptance even among Catholic philosophers. Compared to St. Thomas, he remains practically unknown as a philosopher. In the future this may be different.

> What the Seraphic Doctor's ultimate ranking as a Christian philosopher is to be, must be left to a generation which will again experience the speculative and pragmatic necessity of Christ as the center of philosophy. (*Modern Schoolman,* May, 1938, p. 87).

"The oft-repeated phrase is well-known: 'Thomas is the Christian Aristotle; Bonaventure, the second Augustine.' But this difference must not be stressed, for the two complement each other in an admirable way: Thomas is the angel of the schools, Bonaventure the master of the practical life; Thomas enlightens the intellect, Bonaventure elevates the heart. Sixtus V justly places both side by side, and grants Bonaventure the same ecclesiastical honors as Pius V granted Thomas. 'They are,' he says, 'the two olive trees and the two shining lights in the house of God, who by the plenitude of their love and the light of their erudition illumine the entire Church. By the special providence of God, they are similar to two stars appearing at the same time. During their earthly pilgrimage they were intimately united by the bond of a true friendship and by the intercourse of holy labors. With equal step did both hasten toward their heavenly fatherland, that both might at the same time enter the joys of Heaven." (Ludger Wegemer in *Franciscan Studies*, Vol. 2, p. 19).

The Whole Man

It is not easy to summarize a man of such talents as St. Bonaventure. He was a great organizer, a great handler of men, one of the supreme theologians and philosophers of Christianity. He was known for moderation, but he drove relentlessly to his goals. He loved solitude, but traveled extensively. He was a renowned preacher. It may be said of him that he was a whole man, whose mind and heart clearly interpreted the things of both time and eternity.

A few sidelights on his personality can be seen in his remarks about study and books.

St. Bonaventure's rules for study given in his *Discourses on the Hexaemeron*, written near the end of his life, show something of his own approach. Study must be orderly and persevering. There should be a pleasure in study properly pursued, and study must remain within proper bounds. To attempt a learning beyond our talents is not good.

Defending the right of the friars not to lend books, St. Bonaventure gave reasons which showed how observant and practical he was—and indicated too a sense of humor.

> . . . Those who are most importunate in asking for them are the slowest to return them; books return torn and dirty; he to whom they are lent, lends them to another without your permission, and this other sometimes to a third, and this third not knowing by now who owns the book is not in a position to take it back; sometimes, again, he to whom a book is lent leaves the place and is then too far away to bring it back; and if he manages to find someone to bring it back for him, this someone wants to read it before giving it back, or lends it, and ends up by denying that he ever had it; finally, if a book is lent to one man, others are angry that it is not lent to them too, so that one is forced to do without it oneself while waiting for it to come back dirty, or be lost altogether. (*The Works of St. Bonaventure*, Franciscan Institute, St. Bon. U., St. Bon., NY, 1955, VIII, 371).

There are not many anecdotes about St. Bonaventure. Salimbene tells one that attests to his humility and need for and reliance upon a friendship.

> Brother Mark was my special friend, and to such a degree did he love Brother Bonaventure that he would frequently burst

into tears on recalling (after our father's death) the learning and the heavenly graces that had crowned his life. When Brother Bonaventure, the Minister General, was about to preach to the clergy, this same Brother Mark would say to him: "You are indeed a hireling," or "On former occasions you have preached without knowing precisely what you were talking about. I sincerely hope you are not going to do that now." Brother Mark acted thus to incite the General to more painstaking efforts. His deprecation was merely affected and in no way genuine, for Mark reported all the sermons of his master and treasured them greatly. Brother Bonaventure rejoiced at his friend's reproaches, and that for five reasons. First, because he was of a kind-hearted and long-suffering disposition; second, because thus he could imitate his blessed Father [St.] Francis; third, because it showed how loyally Mark was devoted to him; fourth, because it afforded him the means of avoiding vainglory; fifth, because it incited him to more careful preparation. (Cited in *Cord,* 7, 309).

That St. Bonaventure sometimes had to accept the barbs of criticism coming from much less kindly disposed people can be seen in a satirical stanza against himself and two other Franciscan members of the Second Council of Lyons. This Council suppressed new mendicant orders, excepting Franciscans and Dominicans.

> Bonaventure, Rouen, and Tripolitane
> Dispense papal laws and unmindful remain
> Of their Order which scorns all honors as vain.

The other two were the Archbishop of Rouen and the Bishop of Tripolis.

One of the greatest admirers of St. Bonaventure was John Gerson (1363-1429), Chancellor of the University of Paris. He says of the *Breviloquium* and the *Journey of the Soul to God*: "For more than 30 years I have studied them, and yet I must confess that I am just beginning to enjoy them." He also said that the scholastics who were devoid of piety neglected the writings of St. Bonaventure, "although no teaching is more sublime, more divine, more salutary, more pleasing."

Faith, Reason and St. Bonaventure Today

Our age has gone far in the direction of rationalism. Faith has grown less and less in importance. Maybe that is why the philosophy of St. Bonaventure is currently stirring a renewed interest. (Cf. *Franciscan Studies*, 19, 209-26). St. Bonaventure may tend to grow more important in the next decades. In literature, the emphasis on reason alone has led to intellectualism and sensuality—as a rebellion against the inadequate answers of reason with regard to man's destiny—to over-simplicity and functionalism in architecture, to abstractions in art. In many modern buildings, the mind, stretching always for the infinite, feels hemmed in. There are no mysterious curves, no intricate patterns. Straight lines and bald simplicity stare back with the aspect of coldness and incompleteness. There are no interesting corners or nooks hinting at unknown treasures beyond. Reason claims to be and indeed wants to be complete, though it is not. It pretends to have all the answers, though it does not. Men of this cast of thought put their thinking into literature, art and architecture; and intellectualism, sensuality, over-simplification and functionalism are the result.

In modern thought, the mind is fractured. The light that falls on the arts and sciences is not white, as it should be, but is separated into different colors—red, yellow, purple, orange. Thus, some people say all things are red, others say they are yellow or purple or orange. The blend that allows for clear vision is too complex for them to consider. Therefore, thought is dissected, and as a result, reality itself is dissected, to the detriment of wholesome thinking. Relativism and subjectivism take over. Experts abound in many sciences, men who use their minds to the limit within the boundaries of their own science. They often arrive at some very good conclusions. But at other times, especially in arriving at conclusions relating to man's nature, or involving man's conduct and destiny, they succeed only in distorting the truth. But falsehood is dressed in such an appealing garb these days and camouflaged by so much learned verbiage, that its crooked finger, which actually points to confusion and destruction, is eagerly followed today by many unsuspecting people.

St. Francis feared learning that might extinguish fervor. Since his day, learning in the empirical sciences has run wild, extinguishing not only fervor, but reason as well. When the present trend of overemphasis on reason has run man into further destruction, to predicaments that are no longer tolerable, then the philosophy of St. Bonaventure might well be sought for the answers to the modern problem of reason acting without the guidance of faith.

The rights of reason and its power for good are best served when its limitations are known. "I will not serve" sent the devil to destruction. That man who wants to live only by reason, and who shouts, "I will not serve under the leadership of faith," will also plunge to destruction, both here and hereafter.

Reason gets furthest when, like a child, it walks beside faith. Faith can see over the mountains and across the precipices. If reason leads, the child may get into trouble—to its own sorrow. The abundance of life for individuals and the fullness of the age of man for society will come only through Christ—both in the natural, human realm, as well as in the supernatural and divine. He is the Supreme Exemplar for understanding all problems, and for solving them. The philosophy of St. Bonaventure recognizes this. For him, everything is built upon Christ.

St. Bonaventure's feast day is July 15 (July 14 in the 1962 calendar).

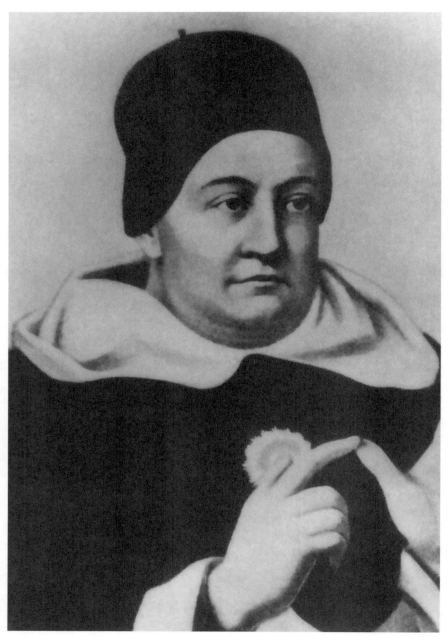

Saint Thomas Aquinas

24

SAINT THOMAS AQUINAS

The Angelic Doctor
The Common Doctor
c. 1225-1274

MANY Catholics, if asked, would say that they know nothing by heart in Latin. Yet, when the fragrant incense rises at Benediction of the Blessed Sacrament, they will quickly join in the familiar words of the *O Salutaris* and the *Tantum Ergo*. These words begin the concluding stanzas of two longer hymns, the *Verbum Supernum* and the *Pange Lingua*. Pope Pius XI has said that the Church "will always use" these hymns of St. Thomas Aquinas, "in which there breathes at once the highest warmth of the pleading soul and which contain an unequalled enunciation of the apostolic doctrine on the august Sacrament." *(Studiorum Ducem)*.

According to the traditional historical view, St. Thomas wrote these Eucharistic hymns, together with the *Sacris Solemniis* and the Mass sequence, *Lauda Sion*, for the Feast of Corpus Christi. Pope Urban IV had commissioned him to compose the Office and Mass for this feast, which was about to be extended to the universal Church in 1264. Fr. Reginald Coffey, O.P., a biographer of St. Thomas Aquinas, says that it was St. Thomas himself who asked for the universal observance of this feast; he did this on the occasion of refusing the cardinal's hat. These great Eucharistic hymns, along with the famous *Adoro Te*, which is also ascribed to him, are St. Thomas' only extant poetic works.

Despite his towering intellect, St. Thomas was not a man who sought for novelty in the way he framed his ideas. Rather, he simply saw deeply into the essence of the truth and thus stated it in such a way that no one could improve on it in the future.

The magnificent hymns on the Eucharist truly live up to this characteristic and ability of St. Thomas Aquinas. They use ideas and truths already thoroughly known, and even some expressions already a part of existing hymns. But the end is a finely chiseled, unbeatable product, a masterpiece, blending precise thought, solid doctrine and rare beauty.

The story told by Denis the Carthusian in this regard is very interesting and highly complimentary of St. Thomas Aquinas. He relates that St. Bonaventure too was commissioned by Pope Urban IV to compose a Mass and Office for the Feast of Corpus Christi, but when St. Bonaventure read the work of St. Thomas, he quietly tore up his own.

What Is God?

St. Thomas Aquinas was born in 1225 or 1226. A room in the castle of Roccasecca is still pointed out as his birthplace. The castle and nearby Aquino, from which the family took its name, are situated about midway between Rome and Naples. The chief branch of the family, the Counts of Acerra, had their palace in the town of Aquino. Thomas d'Aquino became known in later neo-classical Latin as Thomas Aquinas. St. Thomas was the youngest boy in a large family. His father, Landulph, was a knight of noble lineage and Lombard descent. His mother, Theodora, was a noblewoman from Naples and was of Norman descent. There were at least three older brothers, Aimo, Ronald, and Landulph; and four sisters, Marotta, Theodora, Mary and one whose name is not known. When St. Thomas was an infant, the little sister whose name is unknown was killed by lightning while he slept nearby in the same room of the castle.

The boys in the family were warriors, and St. Thomas grew up amid the pageantry of the age and the din of clashing arms. The eldest sister, Marotta, became an abbess. Ronald was later executed as a prisoner of war, a victim of the Emperor's wrath for having sided with the Pope in a political dispute. Not to be misleading, it should be said that the Aquino family usually had been on the other side, fighting against the armies of the Pope in his role as a temporal sovereign. This, of course, meant nothing with regard to their loyalty to the Church. They were staunch Catholics. At the age of five St. Thomas was sent to be educated by the Benedictines at Monte Cassino. He was offered by his parents as an oblate, the motives of which action might well have been a mixture of piety and ambition. They hoped, not without solid basis, that he would one day be the abbot. One of his early questions at this stage in his life was "What is God?" The probing mind of the future intellectual giant was already at work.

It could well have happened that St. Thomas would have spent his entire life at Monte Cassino. But political disturbances suggested that he be taken from the monks and sent to Naples to pursue his studies. He was then in his early teens. The particulars and the dates for this and many of the events in St. Thomas' life are uncertain.

About the end of his teens, after having given evidence of unusual and precocious talent in studies, he entered the Order of St. Dominic at Naples.

His choice of this newly founded, mendicant (begging) Order met severe opposition from his family. It is not known whether his father, Landulph, was alive at this time or not. His mother actively tried to break his will, even pursuing him to Rome. And St. Thomas was literally captured by his brothers and imprisoned in the family castle. His sisters, Marotta and Theodora, who for perhaps two years attended him and probably tried to weaken his resolve, were converted to his viewpoint after a time.

The most dramatic episode of his imprisonment, recounted by most biographers of the life of St. Thomas, came when his brothers sent a temptress to his quarters. As soon as St. Thomas saw that the girl's intention was to seduce him, he ran to the fireplace, seized a burning stick and, brandishing it, chased her from the room with it. Then he traced a cross on the wall with the charred wood.

When he fell asleep soon afterward, he dreamed that two Angels came and girded him about the waist with a cord, saying: "On God's behalf we gird you with the girdle of chastity, a girdle which no attack will ever destroy." It is often said that henceforth he had no temptations against purity. The words of the Angels would seem to indicate rather that he would be victorious over all such attacks. His faithful companion and confessor, Reginald of Priverno (Piperno), who heard his general Confession on his deathbed, testified later that St. Thomas had remained as innocent as a child throughout his life.

"The Dumb Ox"

When his family finally released him, St. Thomas returned to Naples, and from there was transferred to Rome. But he soon went by way of Paris to Cologne, where he was to study under St. Albert the Great, Albertus Magnus, from 1248 to 1252. He was perhaps ordained at Cologne, but the date and place are not known for certain.

The large, quiet young man from Italy was dubbed "the Dumb Ox" by fellow students at Cologne. He was so quiet and non-committal that another student offered to coach him. But when this student faltered in giving an explanation, St. Thomas continued in such a way that the student asked that the coaching roles be reversed. How was his brilliance finally revealed? Perhaps this student broke a promise not to say anything; perhaps St. Thomas dropped a sheet of notes which St. Albert found and was impressed by; perhaps it was just through a routine part of his participation in the academics of the school. At any rate, St. Thomas was called on to defend a thesis. His brilliance in presenting his thesis and answering objections to it called forth the famous remark of St. Albert the Great: "You call him 'the Dumb Ox,' but one day the bellowing of this Ox will resound throughout the world."

Through the influence of St. Albert the Great and despite the original refusal of the Master General of the Dominicans, St. Thomas was sent to Paris to study and to teach. In his early years there, he composed a masterful commentary on the *Four Books of Sentences* of Peter Lombard, and in his later years at Paris, the treatise *Concerning Truth*. Among other works of this period, he wrote a defense of the mendicant orders, for there was strong and bitter opposition to professors from the mendicant orders at the university. It took a Papal Bull by Alexander IV on October 23, 1256 to have St. Thomas and St. Bonaventure admitted to full membership on the university faculty.

St. Thomas left Paris for Italy in 1259 and was made a preacher general of the Dominican Order the following year. This position required his presence at the chapters of the Dominican province based in Rome.

From 1261 to 1265 he was also attached to the curia of Pope Urban IV as theologian and teacher. The papal court moved from place to place, so that St. Thomas, at this period of his life, had to do a good deal of traveling. His writings, however, continued uninterrupted. He finished the *Summa contra Gentiles* (the "Summa against the Gentiles") and wrote extensive Scriptural commentaries.

"Thomas, You Have Written Well of Me."

In 1269, he returned to Paris, where he resumed teaching at the University of Paris. St. Thomas, now at the height of his powers, poured forth his energy in a truly amazing amount of writing. Besides scriptural and philosophical commentaries and opuscula, he produced the bulk of his most famous work, the *Summa Theologiae* (known in English as the *Summa Theologica*), or "the Summary of Theology." This period of a little more than three years was the most productive literary period of his entire life.

St. Thomas was recalled to Italy in 1272. The general chapter of the Order and the chapter of the Roman province took place in Florence that year. As preacher-general, St. Thomas had the right to take part in the provincial chapter, not the general chapter. He was appointed by the provincial chapter to found a *studium generale*. To Fr. Thomas d'Aquino was entrusted the *studium generale* of theology, both with regard to where it would be and as regards who and how many would be sent there to study. (*St. Thomas Aquinas*, by Angelus Walz, O.P., trans. Sebastian Bullough, O.P., Newman Press, 1951, p. 140). St. Thomas chose Naples. It was there that he would work on the last part of the *Summa Theologica*, which he never quite completed.

On the way to Naples, both he and his faithful companion, Reginald of Priverno, fell sick at the castle of Molara. St. Thomas recovered, but Reginald continued with a high fever. Therefore, St. Thomas took a relic of St. Agnes which he had always worn and gave it to Reginald, telling him to recommend himself to the virgin martyr. Reginald was cured immediately. In gratitude, St. Thomas arranged a special celebration and banquet during the following year to honor St. Agnes on her feast day at the Dominican *studium generale* in Naples. This celebration was to become an annual affair.

It was at Naples, in this last period of his life, that the episode occurred of St. Thomas speaking with the crucifix. The evidence was given by Brother Dominic, sacristan of the priory at Naples, who had witnessed the scene. St. Thomas customarily came there before matins to pray alone before the crucifix. On one occasion, Our Lord spoke to St. Thomas from the Cross: "Thomas, you have written well of Me; what reward do you ask of your labor?" The reply was, "None other, Lord, but Thyself."

On December 6, 1273, St. Thomas "underwent a wonderful

transformation" while offering Mass. "After this Mass, he never wrote or dictated anything; in fact, he lay down the instruments of writing, being at the third part of the *Summa*, in the tract on Penance." (Walz, p. 139, quoting Neap. Proc., n. 79).

His friend Reginald was concerned and asked why Thomas had given up this great work which he had been doing "for God's glory and the instruction of the world." This repeated question brought the reply, "I cannot go on." Later he offered a fuller explanation: "Because all that I have written seems to me like so much straw compared with what I have seen and what has been revealed to me."

The ecstasy during this Mass may have taken place at Naples or at the castle of San Severino, residence of St. Thomas' sister, Theodora. But we can see a twofold meaning in St. Thomas' laying aside his pen. His new understanding and knowledge made the tortuous ways of human words seem hardly capable of leading the mind to an adequate idea of the truth about God and His creation. Perhaps, too, the disease which was soon to take St. Thomas' life was already sapping vital energy and preventing him from rising to the new challenge of providing expression for his increased depth of perception.

My Rest For Ever and Ever

After a stay at his sister's castle, St. Thomas proceeded on his way to the Council of Lyons, to which he had been summoned. In an accident, perhaps caused by absentmindedness, he hit his head quite violently against a fallen tree. Further along the way, he stopped at the castle of his niece at Maenza. She was the Lady Frances, wife of the Count of Ceccano. But finding that his condition was getting worse, he asked to be taken to the nearby Cistercian Monastery of Fossanuova.

"If the Lord is coming for me, I had better be found in a religious house than in a castle." (Walz, p. 164). After greeting the monks, St. Thomas went to visit the Blessed Sacrament. On entering the cloister he was heard to quote aloud the words of Psalm 131:14: "This is my rest for ever and ever: here will I dwell, for I have chosen it."

Wishing to show his gratitude for the great care that was given him, and in answer to the request of some of the monks, he gave them from his deathbed a short commentary on the *Canticle of Canticles*, which is not listed among his works. He received Viaticum on March 5, kneeling on the floor beside his bed. Present were the community of Cistercians, some fellow Dominicans and some Friars Minor. The Bull of Canonization records the beautiful words of St. Thomas when he received Our Lord:

> I receive Thee, redeeming Prince of my soul. Out of love for Thee have I studied, watched through many nights, and exerted myself: Thee did I preach and teach. I have never said aught against Thee. Nor do I persist stubbornly in my views. If I have ever expressed myself erroneously on this Sacrament, I submit to the judgment of the Holy Roman Church, in the obedience of which I now part from this world. (*St. Thomas Aquinas—His Personality and Thought*, by Martin Grabmann, trans. Virgil Michel, O.S.B., Longmans, Green, NY, 1928, p. 15).

St. Thomas received Extreme Unction on March 6 and died early Wednesday morning, March 7, 1274. The soul of the great yet humble Thomas went forth to the reward of the Beatific Vision. In the hushed death room the nearly blind sub-prior touched the still warm body, and immediately received back his sight. About a hundred witnesses were present when this happened.

From the University of Paris came a letter asking for the body of its most famous teacher. (Did it come from the faculty of theology or the faculty of arts, now headed by Siger of Brabant, once the greatest foe of St. Thomas?)

> It were surely in the highest degree improper and unworthy that any town or place other than Paris, the most noble city of all in studies, should guard the bones of him whose youth was nourished, fostered and educated here at Paris, which then received from him in return the inexpressible benefit of his teaching.

St. Thomas was buried originally at Fossanuova, where late in 1274 the monks noticed a strong fragrance coming from his tomb. In 1368 the relics were taken to Toulouse, to the Dominican Church. Since the French Revolution, they have been in the Church of St. Sernin (or Saturninus) in Toulouse, France.

St. Thomas was canonized by Pope John XXII on July 18, 1323. On April 11, 1567 Pope Pius V declared him a Doctor of the Church.

How to Become a Saint?

During St. Thomas' final visit with his sister Theodora, she asked him how to become a saint. His answer was, "Will it." To another question, "What is the most desirable thing in life?" he replied, "A good death."

Today, with his immense reputation for learning, it is easy to forget that St. Thomas Aquinas was first of all a man of holiness. His strong will, shown early in life by his tenacious clinging to a Dominican vocation, was always turned firmly toward God. His teaching and writing were not carried out just to satisfy his demanding, inquiring mind. His work proceeded from holy obedience and from an intense will to make better known those truths that would lead men to know, love and serve their Creator. His writings were not coldly planned, but issued like great sparks from the white heat of the controversies and problems of his time. They were his best effort to combat error, to avert damage to the Church.

He poured forth his energies in response to requests or assignments from the Pope or others, or to the need he himself saw at hand. For instance, at the request of Pope Urban IV, he wrote over a period of several years his discourse *Against the Errors of the Greeks*, to provide an argument that might help to end the Great Schism. His *Summa Contra Gentiles* "is a solid body of reasoned theology against the teachings of Islam." It has been said that it "saved European civilization." (*Irish Ecclesiastical Record* 95, 39-44). Without a doubt, it proved a most valuable textbook for missionaries in Mohammedan countries.

His greatest and best-known work, *The Summa Theologica*, was his response to the need for a summary of theology. It may seem odd to think of this monumental work as being designed for beginners. But that was St. Thomas' intention, as expressed in his prologue to the work:

> Since the teacher of Catholic truth must instruct not only the advanced but also the beginners, according to the word of St. Paul (*1 Cor.* 3:1-2), "As to little ones in Christ, I fed you with milk, not with solid food . . ." so the purpose and intent of this work is to treat those things that pertain to the Christian religion in a manner suitable to the instruction of beginners. For we have observed that beginners are greatly impeded by the writings of various authors, partly because of the multiplication of useless questions, articles and arguments; partly

because the knowledge necessary for beginners is not presented in orderly fashion, but in a manner dictated by the explanations of books or by the demands of disputations; and partly because the frequent repetition of the same matter causes disgust and confusion to the audience. In trying, therefore, to avoid these and similar things, we shall, with confidence in the divine help, try to present the contents of sacred doctrine as briefly and clearly as the matter allows.

St. Thomas, who fought for and is remembered for his emphasis on the place of reason in theology, relied primarily on the guiding hand of divine love. He wrote in his commentary on the Gospel of St. John: "For just as a lamp is not able to illuminate unless a fire is enkindled, so also the spiritual lamp does not illuminate unless he first burn and be inflamed with the fire of charity. Hence, ardor precedes illumination, for a knowledge of truth is bestowed by the ardor of charity." (Quoted in Grabmann, *Int. Life*, p. 30).

Real understanding of important, fundamental truth must come from divine love. Love for neighbor will then lead to the communication of this knowledge to him. "For just as it is better to illuminate than to shine," says St. Thomas, "so it is greater to pass on the fruits of contemplation to others than just to contemplate." (Walz, p. 172, from *Summa* II, II, 186, 6).

William of Tocco, relying on information given by St. Thomas' close associate, Reginald of Priverno, relates:

> Thomas did not acquire his knowledge by natural ingenuity, but rather through the revelation and infusion of the Holy Spirit, for he never began to write without previous prayer and tears. Whenever a doubt arose, he had recourse to prayer. After shedding many tears, he would return to his work, now enlightened and instructed. (Grabmann, p. 12).

Pope Leo XIII (*Aeterni Patris*, August 4, 1879, *On the Study of Scholastic Philosophy*) quotes *James* 1:5:

> If any of you want wisdom, let him ask of God, who giveth to all men abundantly, and upbraideth not: and it shall be given him. Then he continues: Therefore, in this also let us follow the example of the Angelic Doctor, who never gave himself to reading or writing without first begging the blessing of God; who modestly confessed that whatever he knew he had acquired not so much by his own study and labor as by the divine gift.

Pope Pius XI (in *Studiorum Ducem*) quotes the comment of St. Thomas indicating that knowledge of the truth is connected with a good life. "First life rather than doctrine: for the life leads to the 'knowledge of the truth.'" Pope Pius XI tells us that St. Thomas, in order to obtain the light of the Holy Spirit,

> often abstained from all food, spent whole nights in watching and prayer; repeatedly impelled by piety, he placed his head against the tabernacle of the august Sacrament, and he turned his eyes searchingly to the image of Jesus crucified; as he confessed to his friend, St. Bonaventure, whatever he learned he had learned chiefly from that book. (311-12).

In this encyclical Pope Pius XI mentions three specific occasions on which St. Thomas fasted and prayed to obtain light from above in his study and writing. This emphasis is worth noting because St. Thomas was a large, heavy man—"fat," if you will—and it is easy to imagine that he was a big eater. But his custom was actually to eat only twice a day, and sometimes just once. He was often so lost in thought that the plate could be taken away and he would not notice it. He had little concern for either food or clothes, and he did not take much sleep.

The only instance recorded of his asking for special food was at a time when he had no appetite. This was shortly before his death, when he had turned aside for a few days' rest at the castle of his niece at Maenza. At her urging him to select some particular food he might relish, he admitted that he might enjoy fresh herring. They were not obtainable in that district, but remarkably, it happened that when a passing fish vendor was asked, he did have a few fresh herring.

The best-known instance of St. Thomas' power of concentration is related by William of Tocco. St. Thomas and the prior of St. James, the Dominican house at Paris, were guests of King St. Louis IX at a banquet. The pleasant hubbub of the royal meal faded into the background for St. Thomas as his mind turned on a problem connected with his current writing. Suddenly the table clattered as he brought down his hand decisively, exclaiming: "*That* is the argument that will settle the Manichees!" The prior was mortified and the guests were startled. The King, however, had the ideal reaction: he summoned secretaries to take down St. Thomas' thoughts while the trend of the argument was still fresh in the mind of his abstracted guest.

The Angelic Doctor

It was common for St. Thomas to shed tears. The Bull of Canonization testifies that he shed abundant tears during prayer. He customarily offered Mass and then attended another while making his thanksgiving. He often broke out in tears during these Masses. They reveal a tender heart and a soul often touched by the nearness of God. The quiet overflow of tears, showing his goodness and emotion, as with so many of the great Saints and mystics, symbolized and were a release for the overflow of the soul. Tears may not always be evident or abundant with good people, but many even today, as in all ages, when they turn to God in the intimate communication of what is deepest in their souls—of their longing for Him, of their sorrow for their sins and their suffering friends—will pray with eyes brimming with tears.

There are reports of instances when St. Thomas was seen raised a few feet above the ground while praying. Reports tell of his having been visited by the Blessed Virgin Mary, and by Sts. Peter and Paul. He was likewise favored several times by an appearance of, or communication from, one of his family members or friends who had died. His sister Marotta appeared after her death and asked him for a number of Masses, that she might be freed from Purgatory. She answered a question about their brother, Ronald, saying that he was already in Heaven. Later, in another appearance to Thomas, she repeated that Ronald was in Heaven, but that Landulph, another brother, was detained in Purgatory.

Pope Pius XI lists chastity, humility and wisdom as the most characteristic virtues of St. Thomas. "If we are looking for the signs of holiness in him that are most properly his own, the one that strikes us first of all is that virtue by which Thomas seems like the Angels; we cite his chastity . . ." (*Stud. Duc.*) Later, Pope Pius XI says that "If Thomas had fallen from chastity, even when in extreme danger, it is very likely that the Church would never have had her angelic doctor." This is so because, as Scripture tells us, "For wisdom will not enter into a malicious soul, nor dwell in a body subject to sin." (*Wisdom* 1:4).

The title, "Angelic Doctor," dates from the fifteenth century; Pope St. Pius V used it officially in declaring St. Thomas Aquinas a Doctor of the Church. The reason had to do both with the innocence of his life and the greatness and sublimity of his intellect.

Pope Pius XI recommends the promotion of the Angelic Warfare, a society for the preservation of chastity among youth, founded under the patronage of St. Thomas. It had its inspiration in the incident of the Angels girding him after his victory over temptation. In order that members may more easily be won to enter the society, Pope Pius XI allowed the substitution of wearing a medal for the use of a cincture or cord. On one side of the medal is the image of St. Thomas being girded by the Angels, and on the other side the image of the Queen of the Rosary. (*Studiorum Ducem*).

Humble and Lovable

John Peckham, the Franciscan scholar, opposed some of St. Thomas' views. This he did on one occasion in public, and rather violently, perhaps at one of the sessions where the *Quodlibetes* (questions freely introduced by listeners) were allowed. He testified later that St. Thomas remained calm and mild in his replies, and he spoke of him as the "Humble Doctor."

St. Thomas was completely imperturbable in argument, speaking in a low, pleasant voice. His interest was always in coming to the truth, and having the other person see it. Therefore, rather than shout, he tried to see the other person's viewpoint, knowing that only by starting there could the other person be led gradually, by force of logic, to the position St. Thomas considered to be true.

Once a young friar, about to make a trip into town, was told by the prior to choose as a companion the first friar he met. St. Thomas was stopping at Bologna at the time and was pacing back and forth in deep thought. The young friar, not knowing him, told him that he was supposed to take as a companion the first brother he met. St. Thomas went without demur. But he had trouble keeping up with the young man and apologized for his slowness. When the young friar finally found out that he had chosen a famous professor, he in turn apologized. To some people nearby who complimented him for his humility, St. Thomas replied: "In obedience religious life is made perfect."

Thomas was no "disembodied intellect." Rather, he was a man of tender compassion, of affection for friends and family, of composure and mildness, of endless accommodation to others. Wisdom, charity and peace are listed as the special characteristics of his interior life by the renowned Thomistic scholar Martin Grabmann.

However, Grabmann says that "the works of Thomas furnish the chief basis for a delineation of his erudite personality, and they are written in such a rigorous matter-of-fact and impersonal manner that only an extended and profound study of them will reveal something of the personal character of their author." (Grabmann, p. 29).

There is little in all of St. Thomas' works that can be considered personal, hardly any evidence of a personal like or dislike. Occasionally, at the beginning of a work, he gives the reason for this particular composition, or he has a dedication. He addresses his *Compendium of Theology* to "Brother Reginald, most dear of companions."

St. Thomas left no correspondence, unless writings such as his very last, addressed to the Abbot Bernard of Monte Cassino, be considered as such. These are smaller works and are replies to particular questions. He shows a great charity in replying, although busy: "Although I have been busy with many things, nevertheless, lest I should fail the request of your charity, I took care to answer you as soon as the opportunity permitted." (*Resp. de VI articulis ad lectorum Bisuntinum*). "Although I have been very busy, I have put aside for a time the things that I should do and have decided to answer individually the questions which you proposed. . ." He also asks for prayers at the end of such replies to questions.

A Tireless Worker

Because St. Thomas sought wisdom in prayer, it must not be thought that he neglected the natural means of learning. He was a hard worker. In one treatise (*On Lots*) he tells us that he is using his vacation time to formulate the present answer. In another work, which was written in reply to the Duchess of Brabant, he remarks about "the many labors connected with the profession of teaching."

Much can be learned about St. Thomas from a reply he wrote concerning the method of study. (*Epistola de modo studendi*, of uncertain date). It is addressed to a friar John, a novice.

> Since you have asked me in Christ, dear John, to tell you how you must study for the attainment of a treasury of knowledge, I shall mention the following points of advice. Prefer to arrive at knowledge over small streamlets, and do not plunge

immediately into the ocean (of wisdom), since progress must go from the easier to the more difficult. This is my admonition and your instruction. I exhort you to be chary of speech, and to go into the conversation room sparingly. Take great heed of the purity of your conscience. Never cease the practice of prayer. Love to be diligent in your cell, if you would be led to the wine cellar of wisdom. Be ever loving toward all. Do not bother yourself about the doings of others. Nor be too familiar with anyone, since too great familiarity breeds contempt and easily leads away from study. Do not engage in the doings and conversations of the worldly. Above all, shun roaming about outside the monastery. Do not fail to walk in the footsteps of the saintly and the good. Do not consider from whom you hear anything, but impress upon your memory everything good that is said. Make an effort to understand thoroughly whatever you read and hear. In all doubts seek to penetrate to the truth. Try always to store away as much as possible in the chambers of your mind. What is too far above you, do not now strive after. If you follow these directions, you will produce useful blossoms and fruits in the vineyard of the Lord of Hosts, as long as you live. If you do all this, you will attain what you desire. Farewell. (Quoted in Grabmann, p. 51).

As a result of constant application, St. Thomas perfected his thinking. Scholars notice many individual instances of how he corrected and revised and enlarged upon earlier statements. His *Summa Theologica*, written after age 45, for example, shows much progress over the *Commentary on the Sentences*, written before he was 30.

In St. Thomas Aquinas' time, professors were not hemmed in by the clock; rather, they taught during the period between hours of the Office. So a lecture could run two to three hours. St. Thomas' daily routine can be briefly summarized. When he was not lecturing, studying or writing, he was praying. His usual exercise was a brisk walking back and forth. He aptly fits the description given by Cardinal Bessarion, who said that St. Thomas was "the most learned of the Saints, and the most saintly of the learned."

It must not be thought that St. Thomas was forever abstracted and absent-minded. His writing shows much insight into the feelings and thoughts of others. As a preacher, he could move people to tears. The second part of the *Summa*, on morals, shows a masterful knowledge of human behavior and psychology, an awareness of circumstances and problems that affect responsibility.

St. Thomas could be genial and a welcome guest to people interested in mundane affairs, who were completely out of the range of his own metaphysical thinking. On his many travels, he rubbed elbows with all sorts of people. As a good teacher, he had intimate contact with the minds of his pupils. His reputation was that of one who was kindly and lovable. Fra Angelico, a fellow Dominican of the following century, painted him as a man of charm and amiability.

His Style and Penmanship

There is no extant authentic portrait of St. Thomas Aquinas. According to Tocco, he was "heavily built, tall and upright, as befitted his upright spirit; his countenance was of wheaten hue, bespeaking the fineness of his fiber; his head was large, for his mighty intellect required a mighty brain; he was also slightly bald." (Grabmann, p. 116). He had great physical strength.

St. Thomas' style is precise and transparently clear. But it is also austere, because he brings in no personal comments and very seldom names any individual. It is likely that most modern readers would find a first reading of St. Thomas to be boring. His words move against error like a deliberate, invincible army; they march in stately harmony with the unfurled banner of truth; there is no cavorting, no verbal handsprings. With study and rereading, the style of St. Thomas should grip the reader's mind and imagination.

St. Thomas never tried to say things in a novel way; he tried only to state the truth with complete clarity. Therefore, the light touch, the startling figure of speech that captivates most readers is missing from his work. Pure, forceful thought and the drive of a clear mind relentlessly pursuing truth are distinctively present in his writing. But it takes a real student or the careful reader who has some familiarity with the problems St. Thomas is discussing to appreciate such writing.

Only a very few of St. Thomas' works are preserved in his own handwriting. His handwriting was so bad that even his close friend, Reginald, could barely read it, if he could at all. In part, no doubt, the difficulty lies with Thomas' intricate, personal system of shorthand. Practically all we do have of St. Thomas' own personal handwriting belongs to his earlier years. There is no trace of any autograph from the later years. The first modern scholar to make a serious study of St. Thomas' autographs, Pietro Antonio Vcelli (1816-1880), is said to have lost his eyesight as a result. A later work by Père Dondaine on St. Thomas and his secretaries concludes, "The fact that St. Thomas dictated most of his works cannot now fail to be taken into account."

St. Thomas on Our Lady

St. Thomas did not compose an extended treatise on the Blessed Virgin Mary nor leave us a systematic Mariology. His brief and beautiful *Exposition of the Hail Mary* is his most properly mariological work. Here and in other places he treats of her Assumption, virginity and queenship. Fr. Urban Mullaney, O.P., (*AER*, 123) says that St. Thomas makes a valuable contribution to the study of Our Lady's position and privileges because he reduces their derivation to one basic principle: She is the Mother of the Divine Redeemer, and in St. Thomas' view this is the single and simple basis from which all thinking about her derives.

In referring to the Blessed Virgin, St. Thomas usually uses a word that indicates this trend of thought. He employs the word that in the Latin so perfectly balances the term, "Lord." Christ is "Lord," or *Dominus*, and Mary is "Lady," or *Domina*. It seems that in all his writings he uses the expression "our Mother" only once.

There is, however, nothing cold about St. Thomas' devotion to Our Lady. In a prayer he composed he calls her "my sweetest Lady." Preaching during Holy Week, at the Church of St. Mary Major in Rome, he spoke of her sorrow in such a way as to move the people to tears. On Easter, when he spoke of her joy at Christ's Resurrection, a visible wave of joy swept through the congregation.

Of Mary's care for sinners St. Thomas said:

> She is endowed with this great privilege, that all sinners, all evil-doers who wholeheartedly hasten to her are saved . . . and all prayers which are poured forth to her are heard . . . Come, let us go confidently to this temple of grace, that we may find mercy.

Pope Pius XI recommends that all the faithful "follow the example of the piety of the Angelic Doctor toward the august Queen of Heaven, whose angelic salutation he used so often."

His Gradually Rising Fame

It may be shocking to note that not all St. Thomas' contemporaries thought well of him. Three years to the day after his death, some of St. Thomas' teachings were condemned by Archbishop Tempier of Paris. They were included in a list of 219 condemned propositions. Eleven days later, the Dominican Archbishop Edward Kilwardby of Canterbury listed these and other Thomistic doctrines as dangerous. He did this through the masters of Oxford. These condemnations resulted from the work of St. Thomas' personal foes and others who wanted to link his name with Averroist Aristotelianism. In his old age St. Albert the Great had hastened to Paris to defend the works of his most famous pupil. If his words had no immediate effect in Paris, they did influence the acceptance of St. Thomas' works in his own Order. The Dominican Order in its General Chapters of 1278, 1279, 1286, 1309 and 1313 passed resolutions that made the teachings of "the Ven. Bro. Thomas" official for the Order. The Paris condemnation was lifted only in 1325, a year and a half after St. Thomas' canonization.

Today, the stature of St. Thomas Aquinas as a theologian has been summed up in the statement that he was "probably the greatest theological master of Christianity, and his thought dominated Catholic teaching for seven centuries after his death. . . . In him the Middle Ages reached its full flowering and Christianity received its most towering and influential intellect." (John Delaney, *Dictionary of Saints*, Doubleday, NY, 1980.) The only other "nominee" for the title of the greatest mind in Christendom would be St. Augustine.

Although St. Thomas Aquinas has reached an eminence attained by no other in the Church, this rise to fame was not immediate. It was not until 1480 that the *Summa Theologica* replaced the *Sentences of Peter Lombard* as the text at the University of Pavia. Other universities followed. The first commentator on St. Thomas was Cardinal Cajetan. "From Cajetan's pen flowed the rebirth of St. Thomas." Cajetan knew the *Summa* so well that he could quote most of it by heart.

One writer, Frank Sullivan, has said that "It is doubtful whether until recently he was ever fully understood, but even in the midst of opposition, he stood out in the minds of men who knew him as a rock on which they might build, though they knew not its scientific composition, as a bridge, which though it did not turn aside the violent current of opinion, was nevertheless useful in getting across the swirling confusion." (*Modern Schoolman*, 18).

Grabmann, a giant of the neo-scholastic revival, said that "It is evident that the Thomistic philosophy had to overcome numerous difficulties before it could arrive at a position of leadership in the Dominican Order, and still more so, in the learned circles outside the latter." (Grabmann, p. 59).

"Go to Thomas"

Of all the Doctors of the Church, none has received higher praise nor more support from the Popes than St. Thomas Aquinas. At least 66 popes have expressed approval of his teachings. Pope Pius XI said that the documents of the Apostolic See about St. Thomas are "innumerable." Pope Leo XIII in his encyclical on scholastic philosophy called St. Thomas "this incomparable man." He called, moreover, for a renewal of the study of St. Thomas.

> While, therefore, We hold that every word of wisdom, every useful thing by whomsoever discovered or planned ought to be received with a willing and grateful mind, We exhort you, Venerable Brethren, in all earnestness to restore the golden wisdom of St. Thomas, and to spread it far and wide for the defense and beauty of the Catholic faith, for the good of society, and for the advantage of all the sciences. (Par. 56).

The following year, again on August 4, Pope Leo declared St. Thomas Aquinas to be the Patron of all Universities and Schools. The apostolic letter, countersigned by Cardinal Mertel, is said to have been written by the Holy Father himself.

Pope Pius XI, in an apostolic letter to Cardinal Cajetan Bisloti, singled out St. Thomas as the one to be followed by teachers of philosophy and theology, not only in method, but also in doctrine. (August 11, 1922). The following year, June 29, 1923, he issued the encyclical *Studiorum Ducem*. This was on the occasion of the sixth centennial of the Canonization of St. Thomas. Pope Pius XI renewed his declaration that St. Thomas should be the supreme guide of studies in seminaries and universities, and explained at length the reasons for this. The prayer so often used by St. Thomas, "O Ineffable Creator," was enriched by the Pope with an indulgence of seven years and seven quarantines (periods of 40 days).

It was near the end of his encyclical that Pope Pius XI remarked:

As it was once said to the Egyptians . . . "Go to Joseph," from whom an abundance of food would be supplied to them for nourishing the body, so now to those seeking the truth We say, "Go to Thomas," that they may request, for the everlasting life of their souls, the food of sound doctrine with which he overflows. (*Studiorum Ducem, Acta Apostolicae Sedis,* Vol. XV, no. 7, pp. 309-326).

What may well be the only free day from school provided for by any Pope is also mentioned. "And in order from now on to observe the feast of St. Thomas in a manner befitting the patron of all Catholic schools, we wish that day to be free for students . . ." (A better introduction to Thomism could hardly be imagined if youthful minds are to be favorably impressed and influenced.)

Pope Pius XI expresses a preference for St. Thomas' original scholastic title of "Common Doctor." He says that the title, "Common Doctor," is most apt because the Church has made his doctrine her own.

Pope John XXII, who canonized St. Thomas in 1323, made a statement that is hard to surpass: "He illuminated the Church more than all the Doctors; in his books a man will advance more in one year, than in the teaching of the others for a lifetime."

St. Thomas never personally attended any General Council of the Church. He died en route to the Second Council of Lyons (1274). But he has been present at all the Councils since then, as Pope Leo XIII observes. (*Encycl.,* 1879). This was especially true of the Council of Trent (1545-1563).

But the chief and special glory of Thomas, one which he has shared with none of the Catholic Doctors, is that the Fathers of Trent made it part of the order of the conclave to lay upon the altar, together with the code of [sic] Sacred Scripture and the decrees of the Supreme Pontiffs, the *Summa* of Thomas Aquinas whence to seek counsel, reason, and inspiration.

Pope Pius XII, in an address to the faculty and students of the Roman Athenaeum Angelicum, on January 14, 1958, singled out St. Thomas' commentaries on Scripture for special praise.

In the opinion of men of the finest judgment, the commentaries that St. Thomas wrote on the books of the Old and New Testaments, and especially on the Epistles of St. Paul the Apostle, reflect such authority, such a keen insight and such diligence that they can be counted among his greatest theological works and are considered in the nature of a biblical complement to these works, one to be held in the highest esteem. (*The Pope Speaks*, 1958, p. 93).

Pope Pius XII also asked his audience this question: "What above all did St. Thomas teach?" He answered his own question:

> This much is abundantly manifest: by his words and by the example of his life, he taught . . . that the greatest obedience, the greatest reverence was owed to the authority of the Catholic Church. This full observance of obedience toward the authority of the Church had its roots in the fact that St. Thomas was thoroughly convinced that the living, infallible Magisterium of the Church was the immediate and universal rule of Catholic truth.

Pope John XXIII dwelt on the title of St. Thomas as the "Common Doctor" (address to the Fifth International Thomistic Congress, September 16, 1960).

> His teaching was, more than any other, fully in keeping with the truths that God has revealed, with the writings of the Holy Fathers, and with the principles of right reason, and therefore Holy Church has adopted it as her own, and has given the name of common or universal teacher to its author. (*TPS*, 1960, p. 325).

Pope John XXIII wanted to see the "treasure unearthed," meaning that Thomistic teachings should "reach a much wider public in a language and form perfectly suited to the spirit and temper of our times." (*TPS*, 1960, p. 327). Not to leave out a personal note, Pope John XXIII recalled that he was linked to St. Thomas by the fact that his predecessor of the same name in the papacy, Pope John XXII, had canonized St. Thomas. He also confessed that he himself had been "quite attached from the earliest years of our priesthood" to Thomistic studies.

The 1917 Code of Canon Law mentioned St. Thomas twice. Canon 589, 1 said: "Religious instructed in the lower disciplines should diligently study philosophy for at least two years, and sacred theology for at least four, adhering to the doctrine of St. Thomas according to the norm of Canon 1366, 2."

Canon 1366, 2 provided that "professors should by all means conduct the study of philosophy and theology and the formation of students in these disciplines according to the method, teaching, and principles of the Angelic Doctor, and hold these as sacred." In the apostolic constitution of May 24, 1931, *Deus Scientiarum*, Pope Pius XI repeated in strong terms that St. Thomas' doctrine should be studied.

The 1983 Code states: "Lectures are to be given in dogmatic theology based always on the written word of God and on sacred Tradition; through them the students are to learn to penetrate more deeply into the mysteries of salvation, with St. Thomas in particular as their teacher." (Canon. 252, §3).

Ordinarily we may think of St. Thomas Aquinas as proficient chiefly in dogma or philosophy. But Pius XI says that he is also unusually proficient in morals and mysticism as well, and in fact, in all fields. If one wishes to know thoroughly the principles of ascetical and mystical theology, Pope Pius XI says, "it behooves him to approach first of all the Angelic Doctor." (320).

A Synthesis of Faith and Reason

St. Thomas Aquinas lived in an age in which theological opinions clashed to an unusual degree. It was his life's work and no doubt his conscientious burden to take the elements of truth from both sides in the various arguments and fashion a coherent whole. In his system, he combined elements that apparently differed as much as black and white. His black and white Dominican habit has been used as a symbol of this fact.

"The whole basis of his thought is this: If it is wrong to give up the Faith for the sake of reason, it is also wrong to give up reason for the sake of faith." (CD, June, 1944, p. 54, G. McVann). This is so because truth is one. In the thirteenth century, as now, some held that this life alone is worth living. Others held very strongly that the next life alone is worth living. By taking the reasoning of Aristotle, correcting it where necessary and combining it properly with the truths taught by faith, St. Thomas arrived at a viewpoint which included all of life, both here and hereafter. He said that both lives are worth living.

> Clearly distinguishing, as is fitting, reason from faith, while happily associating the one with the other, he both preserved the rights and had regard for the dignity of each; so much so, indeed, that reason, borne on the wings of Thomas to its human height, can scarcely rise higher, while faith could scarcely expect

more and stronger aids from reason than those which she has already obtained through Thomas. (*Aeterni Patris*, par. 49).

St. Thomas Aquinas had a high respect for the authority and wisdom of the Fathers of the Church. Pope Leo XIII quotes Cajetan, who said that St. Thomas, because "he most venerated the ancient Doctors of the Church, in a certain way seems to have inherited the intellect of all." (Par. 48). A year later Pope Leo XIII wrote, "His doctrine is so great indeed that like a sea it contains all the wisdom flowing down from earlier writers." (August 4, 1880). At the same time, St. Thomas freely and respectfully differed from the earlier writers on individual points.

As he said, "In accepting or rejecting opinions, a man must not be influenced by love or hatred of him who proffers the opinions, but only by the certainty of the truth." (Quoted in Grabmann, p. 35). The life of St. Thomas was a constant seeking after truth. "The study of philosophy is not to know what men have thought, but what the truth of things is in itself." (*De coelo et mundo*, lect. 22).

> Nothing may be asserted as true that is opposed to the truth of faith, to revealed dogma. But neither is it permissible to take whatever we hold to be true and present it as an article of faith. For the truth of our faith becomes a matter of ridicule among the infidels if any Catholic, not gifted with the necessary scientific learning, presents as a dogma what scientific scrutiny shows to be false. (Cf. Grabmann, p. 37).

St. Thomas said that "faith is a certain beginning in us of eternal life." Faith is absolutely necessary for the knowledge of mysteries; and even for those things which can be known by reason, faith is necessary for a sure acceptance. (Pope Pius XI, AAS, Vol. xv, p. 318). Vatican Council I quotes St. Thomas on this. Yet reason prepares the way for faith so that a man "would not believe unless he saw that the truths should be believed." (Pope Pius XI quoting St. Thomas' *Summa Theologica* II, II, Q.1, a.4).

A Cathedral of Love

Angelus Walz, O.P. summarized St. Thomas' work: "Aquinas' greatest achievement in the world of thought was the synthesis of Augustine and Aristotle."

Those who have studied St. Thomas deeply (e.g., Josef Pieper) hesitate to call Thomism a system. A system usually makes everything fit into convenient mental packages. St. Thomas rather took the items of truth, one by one, and built them, as has often been said, into a towering edifice, a great cathedral. Just as glass and stone and wood combine in the building to make a whole, so do the differing elements of truth combine in the mind of St. Thomas Aquinas into a unified structure of truth.

Pope Pius XI indicates a good way of looking at Thomas Aquinas: he is much like his own *Summa* (*AAS*, Vol. XV, p. 312), which revolves around and stems from God as the First Cause and Last End of all creatures.

There was a great unity in St. Thomas' life; everything was ordered toward the pursuit of truth. This is why Thomas drove himself so relentlessly, why he turned aside from honors and positions. He refused the abbacy of Monte Cassino, offered to him through the maneuvering of his family. He begged off the cardinalate offered by Urban IV. He was never even a local superior of the Dominicans. When his friend Reginald suggested that he might bring glory on the Order by accepting a cardinalate, he replied: "I can be of much more use to the Order as I am." St. Thomas, great champion of order as representing God's plan, ordered his own life in such a way as to use his talents to the greatest extent.

But for St. Thomas, who was forever looking for the underlying reasons for things, there was a deeper underlying reason for this making of himself a master seeker of truth. The driving force was the love of God. As he himself said: "Charity properly makes a man turn toward God, uniting him in affection to God, so that a man does not live for himself but for God." (Pope Pius XI quoting S.T. II, II, Q. XVII, a. 6, ad 3). For St. Thomas, the way to live for God was the pursuit of truth. The reason he pursued truth was first of all because he loved God. Therefore, St. Thomas was a great thinker because he was first a great lover. And the result of studying him should be, not only growth in the knowledge of God, but in the love of God as well. This does not happen when reason only is brought to this study. But it does happen when St. Thomas is studied with faith and reason. Those who use St. Thomas, overemphasizing reason, will be led to formalism and dry intellectualism. Those who use his works, bringing to them his own combination of faith and reason, may attain, as he did, a synthesis of knowledge and wisdom, of logical understanding and penetrating vision of the sublime truths.

St. Thomas' feast day is January 28 (March 7 in the 1962 calendar).

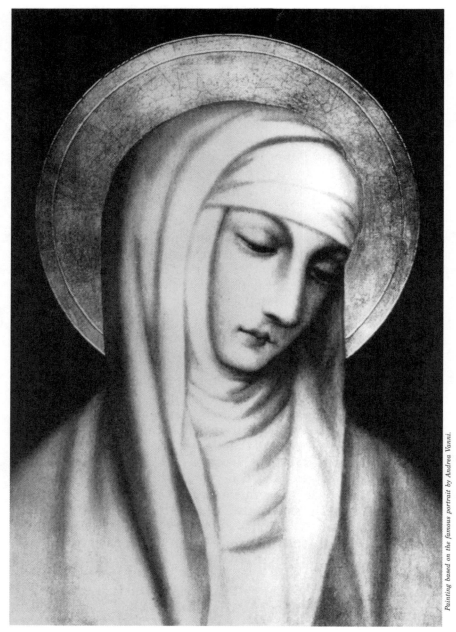

Painting based on the famous portrait by Andrea Vanni.

Saint Catherine of Siena

25

SAINT CATHERINE OF SIENA

The Seraphic Virgin
Mystic of the Incarnate Word
Mystic of the Mystical Body of Christ
1347-1380

JUST before the big city gates closed for the night, a rather frightened little girl of six ran all the way up the hill to Siena, Italy. Her decision to be a hermit had weakened at the sound of the bell for Vespers, which brought very near the thought of night outside the city walls and the worry of anxious parents. Giacomo Benincasa, the mild-mannered cloth-dyer, and his wife, Lapa, simple and devoted and of well-volumed voice, would worry greatly about little Catherine, the baby of the family.

Catherine's twin, Giovanna, had died at birth. They were the 23rd and 24th of 25 children. There was possibly another Giovanna, the 25th child of the family, who died young. The names of eight of the children who grew to maturity are known: Benincasa, Bartolo, Stephen and Sandro, Nicoluccia, Magdalen, Bonaventura and Lisa.

St. Catherine was born on Annunciation Day, March 25, 1347, which in that year was also Palm Sunday. By the time she was weaned, Siena had lost 80,000 people in the Black Death, which was sweeping over Europe. Overgrown fields and empty houses were grim reminders to those who were left and to those of the new generation. During a later plague St. Catherine worked heroically, comforting, caring for and even curing the sick. It was then that she met Blessed Raymond of Capua, who became her greatest confidante, her confessor and ultimately her biographer.

Everybody's Joy

The baby of the Benincasa family was everybody's joy. Happy, sprightly, with a merry laugh and swift of foot, she was often "borrowed" for a day or so by friends and relatives. Some called her Euphrosyne, the name of one of the graces of ancient mythology signifying joy, and also of a saint. Bl. Raymond of Capua thinks she invented the name for herself. Little Catherine had one thing in common with the Saint of that name, a childish wish to disguise herself as a man so as to enter a community of friars. She was captivated by the Dominicans. She used to watch in awe as the Dominican priests walked by and then she would dart out to kiss the pavement their feet had just touched.

Catherine continued to play the hermit at home, finding quiet corners in the big house at Fontebranda, Siena, in which to pray and to think. She was a natural leader of other children, and they joined her in this childlike piety. They also joined her sometimes when she went up the stairs pausing on each step for a Hail Mary. It is true to say that St. Catherine as a child was the same as other children; it is also true that she was different. She was different in her intensity and fullness of spirit, different in the natural gifts bestowed upon her by God, and different too in the extraordinary favors He gave her. These latter became manifest very early.

Jesus, Her Teacher

At the age of six, St. Catherine was returning home one day with her brother, Stephen, when she looked toward the Church of the Dominicans. Above it she saw a vision of Jesus Christ seated on a throne, clothed in priestly garments and wearing the papal tiara. Smiling upon Catherine, He blessed her in the usual manner of a priest. Stephen, who had gone on ahead, lost in his own thoughts, now returned and tugged at his sister's arm. She looked away from the vision, and then burst into tears. For when she looked back, the vision had vanished.

The pattern of St. Catherine's future is more or less contained in capsule form in this vision. For Jesus Himself was to lead her. He was to be her teacher. He was always tender with her. As she told Bl. Raymond of Capua:

> No one ever taught me what was needed in the path of salvation; but my most beloved Bridegroom, our Lord and Master Jesus Christ has taught me Himself, either by interior impulses, or in appearing to me and speaking to me, as I am now speaking to you.

In Jesus she also saw the Church, the priestly ministry and especially the Pope.

Catherine's vision at age six had a great effect upon her. Because of it, St. Catherine felt the need to do something special, to give herself more to Christ. Therefore, at the age of seven, she promised herself to Him, through Mary, by giving herself over to a life of chastity. She understood at least that this meant the complete giving of herself to the one she loved, to Jesus who had smiled upon her and had blessed her.

St. Catherine's great Teacher led her first along the quiet, hidden path of self-knowledge and humility, the way of detachment; then He brought her forth by degrees to wider and wider fields of activity and influence.

In the following St. Catherine's life story, we can conveniently divide it into three periods. The period of her hiddenness lasted until the end of her teens. During the final three years of this period, from age 16 to 19, she led a hermit's life in her own home.

After this, she entered again into family life, and also spent a great deal of time helping the poor and sick around Siena. In the third and last period of her short life, from age 25 to 33, her circle of influence grew until it embraced the Catholic world of her day. She counselled, she spoke, she wrote letters, both to the great and to the small. She went to Pisa, to Florence, to Avignon and to Rome. She died there, the most influential and celebrated woman of her time and one of the most extraordinary women of all time.

A Dominican Tertiary

Under the persuasion of her mother and her favorite sister, Bonaventura, St. Catherine indulged in a short period of "worldliness" during her early teens. She used rouge, dyed her hair, and went to the city festival in a nice dress. This brief period ended with the death of Bonaventura in August, 1362. St. Catherine wept at Bonaventura's death and over her "apostasy."

She refused the marriage her family had planned for her, and at the suggestion of Tommaso della Fonte, a young Dominican who as a boy was a foster child in the Benincasa family, she cut off her beautiful golden hair. Her punishment was to be made the servant of the house. Giacomo and Lapa did not know of St. Catherine's vow of chastity and acted out of love to try to get their strong-willed daughter to do what they thought best for her.

Eventually, after seeing a milk-white dove hovering over St. Catherine's head as she prayed, Giacomo ordered the family to leave her in peace. She was given a 15-by-9 foot street-level room in the family home, where she then lived as a hermit for the next three years, keeping silence, eating alone (and very little) and going out only to church. At this time she joined the Mantellate, or Dominican women tertiaries, the first unmarried girl to wear the famous black and white Dominican habit. It was quite a feat to obtain entry as a tertiary over her mother's original protests and the conservatism of the Mantellate. But when Catherine was very sick, Lapa, who had been finally won to her side by the threat of losing her altogether, interceded for her, and the ladies who came to assess her candidacy, seeing her almost lifeless, judged that her beauty would be no threat to the proper dignity of their membership.

The night before taking her vows, St. Catherine had a strong temptation to return to her beautiful clothes and the possibility of having a family of her own. But Our Lady appeared to her, giving her a garment that was gold-embroidered and studded with pearls. "This garment," said the Mother of God, in her soft and gentle voice, "I have drawn from the heart of my Son, and I have wrought it myself with my holy hands."

Great Temptation

Like many who receive extraordinary supernatural gifts, St. Catherine also experienced unusual torments and temptations from the evil spirits, and this throughout her entire life. God has assured us that He does not allow us to be tempted beyond our strength. But the strong He permits to be tempted mightily. St. Catherine often referred to the devil as the "Enemy," and often mentioned many devils. Her great devotion to complete truth gave her a great insight into the ways of the devil, who is a liar from the beginning.

About the age of 19, St. Catherine had a great temptation which is often recounted in biographies of her. The devil afflicted her with the thought that all she was doing offended God, rather than pleased Him. "Poor Catherine, why will you torment yourself? What is the use of all the pain you inflict upon yourself— your fasting, your iron chain around your waist and the discipline with which you make weals [a stripe or raised line] on your white shoulders? Why don't you sleep like other people? Why don't you eat and drink—in moderation, of course . . . You are simply committing slow suicide, which is a mortal sin—and an irreparable one . . . Live like other women; get a good and nice-looking husband, have children, become a happy wife and mother . . . Think of Sara and Rebecca and Rachel and so many other holy women in both the Old and New Covenant."

Then it seemed to Catherine that the room filled with sensual images. They blotted out the crucifix, dancing before her eyes, tempting her to sins of the flesh. A voice prompted her to do as they did and predicted that the temptation would last until her death. "Even if my Creator would condemn me in the end, I will not for one instant cease from serving Him . . . Of myself I can do nothing, but I trust in Our Lord Jesus Christ." At the name of Jesus, which she repeated over and over, the oppressive air of the room lifted, and all seemed again fresh and clean. A light broke out, showing Our Lord on the Cross bleeding from all His wounds.

"Where were You, O good and sweet Jesus, when my soul was being so sorely tormented?" Catherine asked. "I was in your heart, for I will not leave anyone who does not first leave Me."

"In the midst of unclean visions," she replied, "why could I not see Thee?" "Tell Me, Catherine, did these visions cause thee happiness or sorrow?"

"Oh, I hated them. I was in despair over them and over myself."

"And why do you think you felt thus but because I was present in your soul and kept all its gates closed so that those evil visions could not enter? . . . When at last you offered of your own free will to bear all the temptations and the torments and even eternal loss, rather than cease from serving Me, it was all taken from you . . . Therefore I will from henceforth show you greater confidence and be with you more."

"I Will Send Unlearned Men . . . and Women"

After three years of eremitical [solitary] life in her own home, Catherine received from Our Lord the revelation that He wanted her to lead a more active life. "Dost thou not remember that thou wouldst clothe thyself in a man's garments and become a friar preacher in strange lands?" "I am but a woman and I am ignorant. What can I do?" Catherine questioned. He replied:

> In My sight there is not man nor woman, not learned nor unlearned. But know that in these last times the pride of the so-called learned and wise has risen to such heights that I have resolved to humble them. I will therefore send unlearned men full of divine wisdom, and women who will put to shame the learning that men think they have.

During her time as a hermit at home, St. Catherine had gone out only to church, and then she had kept habitual silence. The little food she had allowed herself she had eaten alone in her cell. A lamp had burned there before the crucifix and the image of Our Lady and various Saints but her door and window had been closed to light.

After her hermit period was over, she began to join the family at mealtime, though she kept her rigorous fasts. Having trained herself to need a minimum of sleep, she still had long hours for prayer after her work. She had not done household tasks during her hermit years. But after them she often stayed up all night washing clothes or cleaning about the house. She was very efficient and quick in all she did.

She also began to visit various hospitals. Often she watched through the night at the bedside of the sick. Her ability to stay awake 20 hours or more a day made her a willing volunteer on the night shift.

One of the places she went to was La Scala, the famous hospital of Siena and house of charity for many other needs. It operated completely by donated help, which came chiefly from a confraternity of men and women who worked there and who also gave the material means of supporting it. At Mercy Hospital, St. Catherine met Matteo Cenni, its director, and won him as a friend and disciple.

St. Catherine Begins to "Raise Her Family"

As St. Catherine became more known around Siena, she made both friends and enemies. Some maligned her and said she was either mad or a show-off. The members of her own Mantellate (Third Order) complained about her ecstasies in church. The priests at St. Dominic's had a divided opinion about her. For a time she was passed by at the Communion rail. Sometimes the brothers led her out of the church in ecstasy and left her lying outside in front to be kicked at by unfriendly people. But gradually, a little band of devoted friends gathered around her, united eventually by such close bonds of friendship and spiritual union with her, and with one another, that they referred to themselves as "the family." They called St. Catherine *"Madre,"* or even more tenderly, *"Mamma"* or *"Mammina."* As time went on, and in the playful, intimate manner of perfect understanding, they often called her "our sweetest mamma." The words in English may not convey the sentiment correctly, for there was nothing weak or sentimental in these expressions, but much that for this "family" circle was refreshingly human and immediate.

Young and old, clergy, religious and lay people became St. Catherine's disciples. Her own Dominican confessors, Tommaso della Fonte, Bartolomeo Domenico, and Bl. Raymond of Capua were also her pupils. Another notable friend from the Dominicans was Tommaso Caffarini. Among the aged was Fra Santi, a lovable hermit. Another hermit was John of the Cells. Young noblemen also came to be *Caterinati* (Catherine's children), such as Neri di Landoccio, a poet; Stefano Maconi, a light-hearted and innocent young man who was later to become General of the Carthusians; Barduccio Carrigiani and Francesco de Malevolti among others. St. Catherine led Francesco from a life of sin into her little fold. Then there was the painter, Andrea Vanni. His portrait of St. Catherine, our only authentic representation, still hangs in Siena's Church of St. Dominic. St. Catherine was in her twenties when he painted her. William Flete, the famed English hermit, became one of her disciples after being introduced to her by Matteo Cenni.

Among her women disciples were her own mother, Lapa (which came about after a long uphill battle), and her sister-in-law, Lisa. Alessia Saraceni, a young widow, gave away all her wealth to the poor in order to follow St. Catherine. Close to St. Catherine, too, were Giovanna di Capo and Francesca Gori Gori, nicknamed "Cecca."

There is a new group of *Caterinati* in Siena today, devoted people so familiar with Catherine and her spiritual family that we might imagine her still living and moving among them, as with her disciples of old. They thoroughly prepare for her feast day over a nine-day period, and bread is given to the poor from her house on the vigil of the feast. The celebration continues even after the feast. There are street decorations and processions. Days after the events, school children may be heard singing

St. Catherine's hymn:

> Virgo decora et fulgida,
> Ornata Regis purpura:
> Electa puro in corpore,
> Christi referre imaginem.
> Nobis novurn cor impetra,
> Transfige dulce, et concrema
> Tecumque ad Agni nuptias,
> Sorde expiatos advoca.

> Your shining beauty, virgin, we sing,
> Adorned in purple of the King.
> Pure in body, you were elected
> To bear of Christ an image perfected.
> Beg for us a new heart
> And pierce with sweet love-dart.
> From stain of sin call us apart,
> To go with heart burned through
> To the nuptials of the Lamb with you.

The Peacemaker

As a peacemaker, St. Catherine began by helping to settle various family quarrels. Then cities invoked her aid, and eventually her work in settling arguments broadened to include Italy and Europe. In fact, one of St. Catherine's major peace-making efforts went beyond Europe. She promoted mightily the preparations for a Crusade, which was never actually launched. The Crusade was to be against the Moslems, who not only held the Holy Land, but were encroaching upon Europe itself. St. Catherine saw the Crusade as a means of stopping warfare among Christians and uniting them in a common cause and for a worthy goal.

Like others who have sought solitude, St. Catherine's love for her neighbor nevertheless gradually drew her out into public life. She had the insight to see that if one can influence policy at the place where it is initiated, he can help the greatest number of people. Therefore, she began writing to the shapers of policy. And she was listened to. She was invited to meet various leaders, and she was sent on embassies. Because of these peacemaking endeavors, her life was at times in great danger.

St. Catherine's absolute truth in God's providence and her fearlessness resulting from this trust are highlighted in an episode during her second mission to Florence. She had come to that city to promote peace, but those who wished to maintain their tyranny incited the people against her. "Let us take that wicked woman and burn her; let us cut her in pieces!" they cried. And an armed crowd rushed into the garden where she was praying. "Where is Catherine?" the leader demanded. She rose to meet him and face his drawn sword, answering: "I am Catherine; in God's name, do to me whatever He may permit, but I charge you, do not touch any of my companions." The man who threatened her now felt confused and threatened by her and called to her to flee quickly. "I am very well where I am," Catherine said . . . "I am ready and willing to suffer for God and the Church, and I desire nothing better." Confounded by her person and her plain speech, the leader and the crowd he headed withdrew in confusion. But St. Catherine wept, for she had hoped to win a martyr's crown.

From Avignon to Rome

Pope Paul VI in his address of October 4, 1970, in which he declared St. Catherine of Siena a Doctor of the Church, called her success in inducing Pope Gregory XI (1362-1370) to go back to Rome the "masterpiece of her work." As far as her external work is concerned, "it will be remembered as her greatest glory and will constitute a quite special claim to everlasting thankfulness on the part of the Church."

The obstacles to be overcome in this, her greatest achievement, were tremendous. The French Cardinals and the papal court were entrenched at Avignon, France, having been in residence there since 1309. The Pope himself was French. Italy was divided into warring sections; therefore, Rome, it could be argued, was not a safe place for the Pope and the government of the Church. Moreover, there were threats against the Pope's life and prophecies of his assassination if he returned to Rome. Gregory XI's own father (the Pope was only in his mid-forties) wept at the prospect of his son's leaving and promised to lie across the threshold to prevent him from going. And Gregory himself, who was inclined to vacillate, found it hard to make decisions.

But a thin, frail-looking young woman came to Avignon and, by her insistence, overcame all these obstacles. She induced Gregory XI to leave Avignon. And in leaving he did actually have to step over his father's body lain across the doorstep. The storms which the Papal retinue encountered at sea and the wars that were occurring on land were pointed to by critics of the move as judgments by God against the Pope's return. But Gregory XI persisted and finally effected the return to Rome in January, 1377. One of the major steps in St. Catherine's winning his confidence had been her whispering in his ear a secret known only to himself and to God. Long ago he had made a promise to God that he would return to Rome.

But Gregory XI died in March, 1378, soon after his return to the Eternal City, and the new Pope, Urban VI, pushed reform in the Church too harshly. The French Cardinals who had been influential in electing him had second thoughts about the validity of the papal election, and therefore they proceeded to elect Robert of Geneva, who became an anti-pope, taking the name of Clement VII. Christendom was divided, and the Great Western Schism, that was to last for the next 40 years, had begun. Many good men were genuinely perplexed as to who was the true Pope.

St. Catherine never doubted who the real Pope was. She pointed to Urban VI as the successor of St. Peter, calling him "sweet Christ on earth." She wrote to him, urging him to be strong but gentle. But to the Cardinals she wrote in strong, direct words. She offered herself as a sacrifice for the Church. Through Bl. Raymond of Capua, the Pope asked St. Catherine to come to Rome. She came at once, and was never to leave.

Her Sacrifice Accepted

St. Catherine saw that many devils were inciting the people of Rome to kill the true Pope. She begged the people for mercy upon themselves and upon the Pope. "You know that if this happens, not only this people, but the whole of Christendom and your Church will suffer greatly," she implored. When she understood by an inner locution that God's justice must demand this punishment, she offered herself instead. "Let the punishment of this people fall on my body!"

This prayer was answered, and Catherine entered into her final four months of life, months of intense suffering. Some of this God permitted to be caused directly by the evil spirits. She found the strength during the first part of this time to go to Mass at St. Peter's, where she would also remain praying through the day. But as usual during much of her life, she would return to her bed and lay upon it like a corpse. She had amazing swings from utter exhaustion and pain to bursts of energy, no doubt the result of spirit transcending over matter, in part due to natural causes and in part to supernatural ones. Barduccio Carrigiani described her prayer at this time: "Her prayers were of such intensity that one hour of prayer consumed that poor little body more than two days upon the rack would have done for another."

Fr. Bartolomeo offered Mass in her room on Easter Sunday, and from then on till her death, she could not go out unless carried. Easter that year was on March 25, her 33rd birthday.

St. Catherine received Extreme Unction on April 29, the Sunday before the Ascension. After this, for some time she seemed to be undergoing a final interior struggle. She called out more than 60 times, "I have sinned, O Lord, have mercy on me!" striking her arm each time on the bed. Then she repeated many times: "O God, have mercy on me! Take not away from me the memory of Thee." Apparently answering an accusation, she said: "My own honor, never! But the true glory of God and His honor." (We take these details from the account of Bl. Raymond of Capua.)

Some of St. Catherine's dear friends and disciples were present at her death; others were far away. Lapa (her mother), Alessia and Stephen Maconi were at her side. Her confessor, Bl. Raymond of Capua, was away on a papal mission to France. St. Catherine remembered them all and prayed:

> Woe is me! O sweetest Lord, Thou hast set me to govern souls, and hast given me all these beloved sons and daughters, that I should love them with a passing great love, and guide them carefully in the way of truth; and I have been to them nothing but a mirror of misery.

She confessed her faults before all present, and asked for sacramental absolution again and the plenary indulgence. One of the priests imparted these. St. Catherine, in taking leave of her "family," used many of the words Our Lord Himself had used in His final hours: "Father, they are Thine," she prayed. "Do Thou keep and guard them; and I pray that none of them may be snatched out of Thy hands." She blessed those present and those absent. "She spoke with such tenderness, we thought our hearts would cleave asunder," wrote Barduccio. True to her life-long loyalty, she again prayed for the Church and the Pope and proclaimed Urban VI as the true Vicar of Jesus Christ. A number of times she repeated the word "blood." For her it always had a mystical meaning. She may have been referring to her own life-blood, or perhaps to that which in her day she had seen so often and so recklessly spilled in conflict. But most likely she was referring to the Blood of Christ, which had redeemed us. Her final words were, "Father, into Thy hands I commend my spirit." It was the forenoon of April 29, 1380. "Then sweetly, with her face like an angel's, bowing down her head she gave up the ghost."

Pope Urban VI asked all the clergy of Rome to be present for the funeral. St. Catherine's body, lying in the Church of the Minerva in her black and white Dominican habit, was venerated by thousands. Before the Requiem on Tuesday evening, some people claimed to have experienced miracles and special favors through St. Catherine's intercession.

St. Catherine's body remains in Rome, but three years after her death, the head was detached and taken back to Siena, where it is still venerated. She was canonized in 1461 by Pope Pius II, who himself, on June 29, 1461, Feast of the Apostles Peter and Paul, wrote the office for her feast.

Mystic of the Incarnate Word

Pope Paul VI, in his speech in St. Peter's Basilica on October 4, 1970 during ceremonies proclaiming St. Catherine of Siena a Doctor of the Church, said:

> It seems to us that Catherine is the mystic of the Incarnate Word, above all, of Jesus Crucified . . . The Saint saw that Blood of the Saviour flowing continually in the Sacrifice of the Mass and in the Sacraments . . . We may say therefore that Catherine was the mystic of the Mystical Body of Christ, that is, of the Church . . . "The Church," she used to say, "is nothing else but Christ Himself." What deep respect and love, then, did the Saint not have for the Roman Pontiff! . . . In him she saw "sweet Christ on earth." To him is due filial affection and obedience, because "Whoever is disobedient to Christ on earth, who represents Christ in Heaven, does not share in the fruit of the Blood of the Son of God."

In a talk commemorating her feast day on April 30, 1964, Pope Paul VI had spoken of St. Catherine as "the humble, learned, undaunted Dominican virgin who loved the Pope and the Church with a loftiness and strength of spirit that no other is known to have equalled." During his general audience on this feast day he said, "Catherine is the Saint whose dominant characteristic lies in her love for the Church, and for the papacy in particular."

In the same discourse, he brought out the fact that St. Catherine loved the Church as it is. She did not try to separate its spiritual and mystical aspect from its institutional, historical, concrete, human aspect. She kept everything together. At the same time, as Pope Paul VI pointed out, she spoke in "free and frank language" against the ecclesiastical abuse of her time and called for reform.

St. Catherine's familiarity with Jesus, the Incarnate Word, is unique, even among saints favored with unusual gifts and visions. He even walked with her at times and joined her in the saying of the Divine Office. She would bow toward Him at the "Glory Be," saying "Glory be to the Father and to *Thee* and to the Holy Ghost." He would come to visit her, bringing St. Mary Magdalen or the Apostle Paul, St. John, St. James, or St. Dominic, talking with her in the garden or in her room. He and one of the Saints would sit on her bed holding conversation. On occasion, St. Catherine also heard the harmony of the Saints singing in Heaven. She said that the most beautiful voices were those of Saints who loved Christ most. St. Mary Magdalen's voice was beautiful and strong, rising from the heavenly choir above the others. St. Catherine loved St. Mary Magdalen especially, because she, Catherine, considered herself also a penitent.

Her Mystical Experiences

The journey of any soul toward God has its "mystical" experiences, things that can hardly be explained to anybody else. There is something elusive and mysterious in the way the Creator and His creatures come closer to each other. For the creature, it has to be both very painful and very joyful. It must be painful because the imperfect creature cannot absorb the closer presence of the Creator. Also, it must be joyful, because God is the Last End, the Real Fulfillment of His creature. The embrace of the Perfect and the imperfect, the Infinite and the finite is crushing to the creature, as well as healing.

Every soul travels on an uncharted path, and no spiritual director can judge absolutely the ways of the Holy Spirit with each particular soul. The urgings of conscience, the new surges of love, the finding of God in a new way through some life experience, the sudden new insight or the growing conviction, the impression of a voice calling, the vivid image in the mind at the time of crisis—all this has its elements of the mystical. When a person has experiences beyond the ordinary, however, we call him a mystic. St. Catherine's experiences were truly extraordinary. To dismiss them all with a shrug, or to seek completely natural explanations would be to oversimplify. It may be better just to use the word "mystical" and confess that we do not know everything about the ways of God toward a soul.

St. Catherine's growth in union with God was ceremonialized or dramatized by many unusual visions and experiences. The year 1370 stands out as her special year, a time of reaching a new plateau. "Do you not think I have become quite another?" she asked her confessor. The chief events of that year were the "exchange of hearts" with Christ, in which Christ took away her heart and gave her His own in return, and her "mystical death." In preparation for all this, there had been the "mystical betrothal" four years before, and as a development of it, there would be the invisible stigmata five years later.

In the mystical betrothal, Our Lady had taken St. Catherine's hand and presented it to Jesus. He had placed a ring on her finger (of the right hand), which she could see ever after, though it was invisible to others. This espousal was a pledge to her of remaining in the Faith.

> Behold, I espouse thee to Me, thy Maker and Saviour, in faith, which shall continue in thee from this time forward, evermore unchanged, until the time shall come of a blissful consummation in the joys of Heaven. Now then, act courageously: thou art armed with faith and shalt triumph over all thine enemies.

Present with Our Lady at the espousal were St. John, St. Paul, St. Dominic and King David.

On Sunday, April 1, 1375, in the Church of St. Christina at Pisa, St. Catherine received the stigmata, the wounds of Christ, on her hands, her feet and her side. This occurred after she had received Holy Communion. At her earnest request, these marks remained visible until after her death. About 15 months before she died, she had received also the crown of thorns from Our Lord; she pressed it onto her head with her own hands. This too had caused pain, but it remained invisible.

St. Catherine's mystical death was an experience which directly involved many of her friends. She apparently died. Her heart stopped beating and she stopped breathing. Her friends were gathered around her bed weeping, and others had also come, as reports of her death spread. In the excitement, a consumptive young friar, Giovanni, had a hemorrhage. When St. Catherine's hand was laid upon his breast, the hemorrhage stopped and St. Catherine came back to life. She wept for two days. For some four hours she had apparently been dead, and friends had already been consoling her mother and talking about plans for her burial.

Afterwards, St. Catherine explained to Bl. Raymond of Capua that her love for the Saviour had broken her heart, and that her soul had left her body and she had seen Hell, Purgatory and Heaven.

> I saw the pains of Hell and of Purgatory, [which are] so great that no tongue of man is able to declare them. I saw also the bliss of Heaven and the glory of my Divine Spouse, which only to think of fills my soul with a loathing for all things that are in the world.

She had wanted to remain with her Spouse, but He told her: "Daughter, there is a great number of souls in the world which I will have to be saved through thy means; and that is the cause why I send thee thither again." It was at this time that St. Catherine was told to leave her cell and go out to help people in an active way.

In answer to questions put to her by Bl. Raymond of Capua, St. Catherine assured him that for four hours her soul had actually been loosed from her body:

> If poor mankind only suspected what Purgatory and Hell mean, they would rather suffer death 10 times, if it were possible, than endure the pain for even one day. But above all, I saw the severe punishment of all those who have sinned in Holy Matrimony by not keeping the laws of marriage . . .

"Father, I am hungry; for the love of God, give my soul its food." St. Catherine often begged for Holy Communion with such words. Her experiences in receiving Holy Communion also involved others. After receiving, she often went into ecstasy, and not even a sharp instrument driven into her foot could disturb her. A number of priests testified that they felt the Host tremble in their hands as they were about to place It on her tongue. Bl. Raymond of Capua, her principal biographer, tells of an instance when the Particle he dropped into the chalice disappeared, much to his distress. But St. Catherine later told him not to worry or to look further for the Sacred Particle, since she had received It. "Jesus appeared to me and in His mercy offered me the Fragment that He made you lose, and I received It from His most holy hands."

If some of St. Catherine's experiences seem strange to us, we may be consoled by the words of her confessor and biographer, Bl. Raymond: "I do not think that those who have no experience of such wonders can understand them—I know I cannot. We know them only as the blind know colors, and the deaf, melodies."

After 1370, St. Catherine lived for longer and longer periods with no nourishment except Holy Communion. In her final years she ate nothing except the Host at Holy Communion, and in fact her stomach rejected food; rather than it being a penance to fast, it became a penance for her to try to eat.

In a day when this was rare, St. Catherine's great desire to receive Communion frequently helped in the gradual return of frequent Communion as a general practice in the Church.

Catherine Loved Each One Dearly

If you want to understand St. Catherine's regard for souls, you should think of the person over whom you have been most deeply concerned, whose problems stabbed at your heart, met you at your morning's waking, and left you only at the last hazy moment of consciousness before sleep. You worried and planned and prayed; and eventually, feeling helpless, you prayed the more, even to exhaustion for the person's salvation, health or security. St. Catherine's heart embraced everyone in this manner, especially in her concern for their salvation.

Nobody was unimportant. She could not be indifferent or half-concerned about anybody. Everyone was her concern. That is why criminals were favorite objects of her visits and her prayers. That is why she could write to the cruel Joanna of Naples: "Dearest Mother, I value your soul as my own." That is why she could drive herself, never reluctantly but joyfully, to care for anyone in need, be it spiritual or bodily. She was a living, breathing, walking, talking lesson on the spiritual and corporal works of mercy.

Many times when St. Catherine seemed half-dead, she could rise nonetheless, and find full energy until her task was over; then she would sink back onto her plank bed. Once, when near exhaustion, she thought of a woman in great need, gathered food and clothing for her weighing perhaps a hundred pounds, and carried it to her door in the early morning darkness. This time, however, her strength failed her before she could return, and she had to limp and crawl along until she reached home, familiarly chiding Our Lord on playing a trick on her and making her be an object of ridicule.

St. Catherine knew and loved each one of her "family" as if he or she were an only child. One of her gifts was to know a soul with its sin and ugliness, or with its beauty. Many times she went into rapture over the beauty of a soul in the state of grace. She would exclaim over it as we might over the startling beauty of sudden scenic grandeur or the fresh beauty of a child.

She could tell her spiritual family exactly what each one had been doing, especially if anyone had lost or won a notable spiritual battle. Once, when her brother was in a distant place committing a serious sin, she became aware of a strong stench. She met him on his return and urged him to quick repentance. At the papal court of Avignon, the stench of sin almost overpowered her. When a lady of this court came to visit St. Catherine, she could scarcely stand her presence. Later it was discovered that this lady, who was well-respected, was living a secret life of sin as the mistress of a priest. St. Catherine had a special reaction in particular to those who lived habitually in sin. "To sin is human, but to keep on sinning is devilish," she quoted.

Her "family" responded to her love. They reverenced her holiness and respected her wisdom because they recognized that her teacher was Christ. The number grew who called her "my little mother." Thus, even aged Fra Santi, and others, priests, scholars, political figures, monks, nuns and laymen called her "Madre," "Mamma" or "Mammina" ("my little Mother").

Her Care of the Poor and the Sick

No one could surpass St. Catherine in her care of the poor and the sick. She gave all she had in time and energy and goods. She gave more than her generous family did and even more than her indulgent father cared to give. After they became aware of her practices, they learned to lock things up. Once St. Catherine was reminded, after giving away her cloak, that the only women who went about without one in Siena were those of unsavory character, her reply was "I would rather go without my cloak than without my charity."

Her love for the poor was similar to that of St. Francis of Assisi, as was her burning love for Christ, the Holy Eucharist, the priesthood, the Church and the Holy Father. it is fitting that the Seraphic Virgin, St. Catherine, should be paired with the Seraphic Saint, St. Francis of Assisi, as co-patron of Italy. This honor was given to St. Catherine in 1939 by Pope Pius XII.

There is one instance, at least, of how St. Catherine's extreme generosity brought an immediate material favor to her own family. She had given freely to the needy from a hogshead of wine. Later, her own family began to draw from this cask, and St. Catherine continued to use it for the poor. Double and more the time passed for it to be empty. But it kept flowing freely each time anyone came to drink from it. Finally, it was said that the cask was needed for the new batch of wine in the making, and the plug was pulled. The inside was found to be as dry as though it had been empty for a long time.

In some cases St. Catherine was able to do for the sick what no doctor could do. Her prayers, the touch of her hand, brought miraculous recovery. Among those cured were some who were very close to her: Matteo, head of Mercy Hospital, and Fra Santi, both of whom were near death; Bl. Raymond and Bartolomeo, both victims of the plague; Stefano, who had a fever. St. Catherine apparently brought her own mother back from actual death. All present had seen Lapa expire. But while some thought of preparing for the funeral, St. Catherine remained praying earnestly. Her mother had not wanted to die. She had not yet confessed. St. Catherine poured out her heart to Jesus:

> Lord, my God, are these the promises You made to me, that none of my house should go to Hell? Are these the things that in Your mercy you agreed with me, that my mother should not be taken out of the world against her will? Now I find that she has died without the Sacraments of the Church. By Your infinite mercy, I beg You not to let me be defrauded like this. As long as there is life in my body, I shall not move from here until You have restored my mother to me alive. (Bl. Raymond of Capua, *Life of St. Catherine of Siena*, trans. Lamb, Kenedy & Sons, NY, 1960, p. 220).

Lapa's body began to move again, she rose up alive, and she lived to the age of 89. In her late years she wanted to die, and complained that God must have put her soul in her body crosswise, so it could not get out.

In most cases St. Catherine worked as any other devoted nurse would. Two names are often recounted among her patients: Tecca and Andrea. Tecca was afflicted with leprosy, and to such an extent that nobody wished to go near her. When St. Catherine heard she was being neglected, she hurried to the leper hospital San Lazaro, embraced the woman and offered her help. She used to come twice a day, morning and evening. But after a while, Tecca became demanding. If St. Catherine were late, she taunted her: "So at last there comes my lady, queen of Fontebranda! Were you with the friars all morning, my lady? It seems as though you can never have enough of those friars." Lapa's fears for her daughter's health were realized when St. Catherine's hands showed signs of leprosy. But nonetheless, she continued her ministrations until Tecca died, assisted by Catherine's prayers. She then washed the body and prepared it for burial. After the funeral, all trace of the leprosy disappeared from St. Catherine's hands.

Andrea was a Sister of Penance of St. Dominic, to which group (also called the Mantellate) St. Catherine also belonged. She had cancer of the breast, and her sore gave out a frightful stench. "You had to hold your nose when you went near," said Bl. Raymond. St. Catherine served the old widow, and on one occasion, when almost overcome by the odor, she overcame her own repugnance by putting her face right on the terrible sore and remaining that way until she conquered the nausea.

But as time went on, Andrea began to hate Catherine, and finally she accused her of unchaste living. The Sisters of Penance openly insulted St. Catherine and called her to account. But she insisted patiently and modestly: "I assure you, ladies and sisters in the Faith, that by the grace of God I am a virgin." Lapa insisted that Catherine should not go and help "that stinking old woman." In fact, Lapa said that if she kept going to Andrea, she would never again call Catherine her daughter. But Catherine obtained her mother's blessing by comparing her work for Andrea to the Saviour's work for sinners:

> Dearest Mother, do you expect God to stop showing His daily mercies to sinners because of human ingratitude? Did the

Saviour refuse to accomplish the salvation of the world when
He was on the Cross because of the insults that were hurled
at Him? . . . She [Andrea] has been practiced on by the devil;
now perhaps she will be enlightened by the Lord and will see
the error of her ways.

St. Catherine continued her care. And soon after this Andrea
changed when she saw a light envelop Catherine and her face
take on a look of "angelic majesty." Andrea went to Confession
and also publicly proclaimed that she had been taken in by the
wiles of the devil and had made a great mistake. But temptation again came to St. Catherine in the form of a strong abhor-
rence and nausea. "She collected into a bowl the fetid stuff that
had been used to wash the sore, along with all the pus, and
going away a little, gulped it all down." Her repugnance passed,
and she later said that never had she tasted "any food or drink
sweeter or more exquisite." After this, Christ appeared to St.
Catherine and invited her to drink of the wound in His side.
After doing so, she felt such an abundance of grace that her
body too was affected. "So, from that time forward she never
wanted food or was able to take it . . ." (Bl. Raymond of Capua,
p. 149). Also from this time onward, i.e., about the end of 1373,
says Caffarini, people called Catherine "the Saint."

St. Catherine's love for the poor and the sick was by no means
unaccompanied by affection or devoid of feeling. Her words and
her radiant face brought a message of tenderness to each person. In her letters, St. Catherine often uses the expression, "Jesus
sweet, my Lord." Her tenderness to Him is at once the echo and
the model of her sweetness to others. Each tenderness nourished the other. And her expressions of endearment for those
she cared for were also frequent. She missed her friends when
they were absent. In the last years of her life, when Bl. Raymond,
her confessor, had to leave Rome, she found it a great trial.

Her love was not abstract or ethereal. She had such tender
feeling for her nieces and nephews and other children that she
confessed, "If it were seemly, I should do nothing but kiss them."
(*Legend*, I, 6, 6). One of her favorite occupations was to gather
flowers and make them into bouquets, often in the form of a
cross, and send them out as a greeting "from a sister in Christ."

Her Love for Souls

But Catherine's chief concern was for souls. It was the soul, after all, which finally counted. To her the "invisible world" was more real than the visible world is to us. It was the soul that most linked each person with Christ, whom she loved the most. He had given His Blood for the salvation of each soul. Therefore, Catherine could say without exaggeration that she would gladly die for the salvation of any one person. In fact, she often longed to do so. After she had seen the beauty of a soul shown to her in a vision, she told her confessor:

> Father, if you could see the beauty of a rational soul, you would not doubt for a minute that you would be prepared to give your life a hundred times over for the salvation of that soul, for there is nothing in this world that can compare with such beauty. (Bl. Raymond of Capua, p. 138).

The vision had been allowed her because her earnest prayer, in which she asked to be punished for the sins of a lady named Palmerina, had saved the lady's soul. Palmerina hated St. Catherine profoundly, though during her sickness she was the recipient of much love and care from Catherine.

"Would that I could gather all the suffering in the world in a sheaf and take it upon myself!" This wish expressed St. Catherine's love for union with Christ Crucified and her love for each soul which He had redeemed. It also expressed her unselfish affection for others and the depth of her self-effacement.

When Catherine's father lay dying in August, 1368, she prayed that he would not have to go to Purgatory. "And Lord, if it cannot be otherwise, then give me the pains my father should have suffered. I will bear them for him." At the moment when Giacomo died, St. Catherine felt a sharp pain, stinging yet sweet, in her side. It stayed with her until her death.

Putting a Lid on Hell

St. Catherine bargained with Our Lord. She wanted *everyone* to be saved. He had died for everyone. Therefore, why should anyone be lost? The existence of Hell seemed like a failure for God's cause. She wanted to "lay herself down like a lid upon the entrance down to it." She even offered God to be forever lost, if all others could thereby be saved!

St. Catherine's spirit wrestled with God. She bargained with Him as had Jacob and Abraham. For weeks she grappled with the question of why anyone had to be lost. She knew it had to be because they followed their own perverse wills, but she could not understand why her prayer, her offering of taking all upon herself could not be heard. "But it is Thyself, Lord, Who hast given me these requests and desires . . . It is the goad of Thy grace that drives me on and compels me to cry to Thee!" Instead of an answer, there was only silence from her Bridegroom. She feared that she had gone too far. "Tell me, Lord, who am I, what am I? Lord, tell me also, who and what art Thou?" The answer that came back burned into her memory forever the distance between the Creator and the creature. "Daughter, thou art she who is not. I am He who is."

However, God gave St. Catherine many souls. She could not save all, as she wished, but God let her know that some who would otherwise have been lost were saved through her. To several priests who traveled with her, Pope Gregory XI gave special faculties to hear Confessions and grant absolution. Bl. Raymond, in fact, complained that at times he was much fatigued and that he and the other priests could not eat until Vespers (i.e., evening) because of the number of penitents that came to Confession due to hearing Catherine's exhortations to repentance and her vivid description of God's love and compassion. In fact, just a short contact with her, and often just seeing her, moved people to want to make a good Confession. St. Catherine was happy for the presence of these confessors, for she was acutely aware of how quickly "the Enemy," Satan, tries to snatch away from a sinner the seed of repentance before it has had a chance to grow.

A painting in St. Dominic's at Siena shows St. Catherine holding the head of a young man. The picture commemorates a moment of victory rather than of defeat. For just before his execution, St. Catherine had visited this man, Nicholas di Toldo, a young Perugian nobleman, and had won him over from raging anger at God and those who had condemned him, to repentance for his sins and a quiet acceptance of death as the door to new life and happiness. He had been sentenced to death for a few revolutionary words of advice to the Sienese, telling them to throw off their yoke. Nicholas died with the names "Jesus and Catherine" on his lips. A moment before this, St. Catherine had placed her own neck on the block, offering her life for his. When this was refused, she knelt to receive his head in her hands as the executioner severed it from the body.

One morning a cart rattled past St. Catherine's window, heading for the place of execution. Two criminals on it were blaspheming God and the Saints, instead of asking for the prayers of the people. Alessia called Catherine's attention to the scene, and after taking one look St. Catherine hurried away to prayer, to remind Our Lord of the thief He had forgiven from the Cross, of St. Peter and St. Mary Magdalen, and of others to whom He had shown mercy. "I beg You, therefore, in the name of all Your mercy, to care for these two souls and succor them." Before the cart had reached the place of execution, the criminals had received the great favor of Our Lord appearing to them and promising them forgiveness. Their blasphemies changed to hymns of praise for God. They said their tortures and death would be proofs of His mercy, for through them they would arrive at glory. After asking repeatedly for the priest, they went to Confession before they were executed. "I thank You, Lord, for saving them from a second prison," St. Catherine prayed later. She explained that she had also asked for and obtained their release from Purgatory.

Another man, who was engaged in many feuds and who was very tricky and of ill will in really working for peace, was induced by Friar William of England (William Flete) to come to see St. Catherine. He kept turning a deaf ear to her words, which were first biting, and then sweet. But as he was getting ready to go, he told her that he would make peace with one party. But when about to leave, he said: "My God, how contented I feel in my soul from having said I shall make peace." Before long, however, he burst into tears and promised to make peace with *all* of his enemies. "I realize that the devil has held me enchained. Now I want to do anything you suggest." He confessed. He was later arrested and lost much property; he was also subject to sickness. But rather than grow melancholy, he grew in spiritual strength and continued steadfast in his new way of life.

But St. Catherine also lost some battles for souls. She could not convert Joanna of Naples, nor sway the Cardinals who elected the antipope, Clement VII. There is also a strange case of one of her disciples who despaired of God's mercy—after perhaps falling in love with St. Catherine in the wrong way—and committed suicide. St. Catherine wrote in a letter to Neri di Landoccio, who was inclined to melancholy—perhaps she referred to the unhappy suicide—"Do not fear that God will permit that to happen to you which happened to that other." (Johannes Jorgensen, *St. Catherine of Siena*, Longmans, Green & Co., 1938, p. 275). With these cases as examples, we come face to face with the mystery of the human being's free will, which can reject God and His grace, even to the end.

St. Catherine's Writings

Some of the Doctors of the Church had very bad handwriting. St. Catherine is unique among them in that the question has been raised whether or not she ever actually learned how to write. She learned to read when about age 20. After making little progress in trying to teach herself to read, she prayed for help, and soon learned, though she did so in her usual whole and intuitive way, and often could not identify individual words. Though some authors still deny it, it seems that she did learn to write in the later years of her life. Fr. Tommaso Caffarini, one of her disciples, explains this as a miraculous gift.

Caffarini writes: "It chanced by sore accident that there fell into her hands one day a certain vessel filled with cinnabar, or minium, which a writer had made use of to write in red, or rather to illuminate the initial letters of a book according to the custom of the time. The Saint, moved by Divine inspiration, sat down, and taking the artist's pen in hand, though she had never learned to form a letter or to compose words in regular meter, she wrote in clear and distinct characters the following verses . . ." She then composed a prayer to the Holy Ghost in meter.

Her first letter in her own handwriting was to Stefano Maconi. It ends, "Know then, my dear son, that this is the first letter I have written with my own hand." About this time too, in late 1377, she wrote two letters to Bl. Raymond of Capua in her own hand.

The second letter to Bl. Raymond ends: "This letter and another I have sent you I have written with my own hand in the Island of Rocca, in the midst of sighs and so many tears that I could not see out of my eyes." She explains too how the gift came to her. It was after a vision of Christ, who came with St. John and St. Thomas Aquinas. St. Catherine was desolate and in need of opening up her heart. The one to whom she could do so most fully was far away, her confessor, Bl. Raymond of Capua. God in His goodness gave her the comfort of being able to write to him. Catherine too terms this gift miraculous.

St. Catherine wrote in the second letter:

> As my ignorance deprived me of the comfort of trusting any-
> one, He gave me the faculty of being able to write, so that on
> returning from my ecstasy I might relieve my heart a little
> and so prevent its bursting. He would not take me out of this
> life, and He has miraculously given me this power, as a mas-
> ter teaches the child for whom he sets a copy . . .

Ordinarily, St. Catherine dictated to one or several secretaries. She could dictate three letters to three different people at one time and never lose the thread of thought in any of the letters. Her secretaries were many, among them Stephen Maconi, Neri Landoccio, Barduccio Canigiani, Fra Santi, Crisofano and the faithful Alessia.

Her language was the Tuscan Italian idiom. Pouring out her soul in words, she had a rapid-fire flow that was volcanic. The impression she makes is powerful and moving. She had learned enough Latin to read the Divine Office, but she could not converse in it. Thus, all her original writing is in the idiomatic Tuscan Italian. It was later put into Latin.

St. Catherine's writings can be classified under three headings: Prayers, Letters and *The Dialogue*. The Prayers were taken down chiefly by friends while she spoke them in ecstasy. The letters were written to a great variety of people: to the Pope, to cardinals, to bishops, to abbots, to priests, to temporal rulers, to her disciples, to friends and to relatives. Pope Paul VI said: "Her Letters are like so many sparks from a mysterious fire, lit in her ardent heart by Infinite Love, that is, the Holy Spirit."

The one formal book written by St. Catherine was named by Bl. Raymond of Capua, who called it *The Dialogue*. It was dictated by St. Catherine while in ecstasy. She herself never gave it a name, referring to it only as "the Book." Some have called it the *Book on Divine Providence*, this being the one general topic of the first of its four parts. The other three are on Discretion, Prayer and Obedience. Literary critics say it is one of the classics of the age of Petrarch and Boccaccio.

The Letters

St. Catherine's letters, like herself, are direct, unequivocal, forceful and tender. At times there are striking passages of much beauty, with memorable figures of speech.

To Queen Joanna she writes:

> You have abandoned the counsels of the Holy Spirit to lis-
> ten to the Evil One; you were a branch of the true Vine, and
> you have cut yourself off with the knife of self-love. You were
> the beloved daughter of your Father, the Vicar of Jesus Christ,
> and now you have abandoned him.

To the Italian Cardinals:

> Before the Holy Father reproved you, you acknowledged him
> and did homage to him as the Vicar of Christ, but your tree
> was planted in pride and nourished by self-love, and it is this
> that has deprived you of the light of reason.

To the Count of Fondi, from whom Pope Urban VI had taken
his office:

> We know that Urban VI is the true Pope; so that were he
> the most cruel father possible, and had he chased us from one
> end of the world to the other, we ought not to forget or to per-
> secute the truth. But your self-love has conceived indignation
> and brought forth wrath.

To Pope Urban VI she wrote: "I hear that those incarnate
demons have elected an antichrist, whom they have exalted
against you, the Christ on earth, for I confess and deny not that
you are the Vicar of Christ." In another strain she advises him
against too much severity.

> Act with benevolence and a tranquil heart, and for the love
> of Jesus, restrain a little those too quick movements with which
> nature inspires you. God has given you by nature a great heart;
> I beg of you, act so that it may become great supernaturally,
> and that full of zeal for virtue and the reform of the holy Church,
> you may also acquire a manly heart, founded in true humility;
> then you will have both the natural and the supernatural; for
> without that, mere nature will accomplish but little; it will rather
> be apt to find expression in movements of pride and anger, and
> then, perhaps when there is question of correcting those near
> to us, it will relax and become cowardly . . . (Letter 21).

To the King of France she wrote:

I wonder exceedingly that you, a good Catholic, who would fear God and be a man, permit yourself to be led like a child, and that you do not see how you bring destruction upon yourself and others in obscuring the light of holy faith by the counsel of those who are clearly limbs of the devil and rotten trees.

Although St. Catherine went about her own spiritual life in a way that we would call immoderate, she led others in the way of moderation. She knew that souls advance by degrees and cannot be pushed too quickly from one stage to the next. Thus she led Francesco di Malevolti back from his relapses into sin. He was not completely converted until after St. Catherine's death. She calls him most dear because she had suffered so much for him.

Dearest, more than dearest son in Christ, sweet Jesus, it seems to me that the devil has carried you so far away that you will not let yourself be found and led back to the fold. I, your poor mother, go about seeking you and asking for you, and I would take you on the shoulders of my grief and compassion and carry you home . . . Do not let me implore you any longer; let not the devil deceive you; do not keep away from me, either from fear or from shame. Tear up this sling. Come, come, dearest son. Well may I call you dear, for you have cost me many tears and much care and bitterness. Come, therefore, now and return to the fold. (Letter 38, Jorgensen).

To Ristoro Canigiani, a married man with a family, St. Catherine wrote:

Think that the eye of God is ever on you and that you must die, and you know not when. Labor for the peace and happiness of your soul; that is your first duty. Relieve your conscience of everything that can burden it, forgiving injuries and repairing wrongs. Sell some of your superfluities, your sumptuous clothing, for instance, which is of no use, but rather dangerous, for it puffs up the soul with foolish pride. (Augusta Theodosia Drane, *The History of St. Catherine of Siena and Her Companions*, Burns & Oates, London, 1880, p. 447).

All those close to her St. Catherine advised to go to Confession every Saturday and Communion every Sunday. She advised Ristoro to attend Mass daily and to fast in honor of the Blessed Virgin Mary on Saturdays.

Say every day the Office of Our Lady, if you do not do so already, that she may be your refuge and advocate before God; and fast in her honor on Saturdays, as well as on the other days prescribed by the Church. (Drane, p. 447).

To Bl. Raymond, her confessor, who was somewhat too much inclined to search for the "whys" of God's providence, St. Catherine wrote:

If we would see the stars of His mysteries, we must first descend into the deep well of humility; for the humble soul casts herself upon the earth in acknowledgment of her own baseness, and then God raises her up.

To him she could also write in fully opposite strains, just as she could to the Holy Father himself. She was extremely direct in pointing out the truth, even when it might be painful. But at the same time, she was most submissive and humble, for she knew how to be both mother and daughter.

When Bl. Raymond turned away from almost sure martyrdom, she wrote: "Ah, let us lose our milk teeth, and try to get the good strong teeth of hatred and of love." (Letter 100, Drane, p. 489). Her last letter to him asked humble pardon.

And I beseech you also to forgive every disobedience, irreverence and ingratitude of which I have been guilty, and every pain and distress I may have ever caused you; humbly asking your blessing. Pray earnestly for me, and get prayers [said] for me for the love of Jesus. Pardon me if I have ever written anything to pain you. (Letter 102).

St. Catherine could also be playful with those with whom she was most intimate. When Stefano Maconi was probably acting as secretary, she referred to him in a letter being dictated as "that negligent Stefano." In a letter to him she calls him a worthless and ungrateful son. "Respond to God's grace; it is a shame to see God always standing at the door of your soul, and you not opening it to Him."

The Dialogue

Algar Thorold, who made an English translation of *The Dialogue* in 1906 (reprinted by TAN, Rockford, 1974), says of it that it is a "mystic exposition of the creeds taught to every child in the Catholic poor schools." He continues: "Every well-known form of Christian life, healthy or parasitic, is treated of, detailed, analyzed incisively, remorselessly, and then subsumed under the general conception of God's infinite loving-kindness and mercy." *The Dialogue* could well be called "The Book of God's Mercy," or "The Book of God's Kindness."

Thorold also says, "In *The Dialogue* we have a great saint, one of the most extraordinary women who ever lived, treating in a manner so simple and familiar as at times to become almost colloquial, of the elements of a practical Christianity."

Augusta Theodosia Drane, who in 1880 brought out an English Life of St. Catherine of Siena on the 500th anniversary of her death, says of *The Dialogue*: "Those who desire to know something of St. Catherine's doctrine must study it in her own pages; nor would it be easy to name any writings which combine in equal proportions the practical with the sublime."

The Dialogue outlines the spiritual life as a path to God by union with Jesus Christ, who is the Bridge. Self-knowledge and the surrender of self-will are required to begin this union. Discretion is always needed. Then proper obedience and perseverance in prayer will combine to allow Divine Providence, the ever-loving kindness of God, to bring our souls to perfection. If we can make the proper surrender of self-love, then we can avoid the common pitfall of allowing what men do to turn us away from God or to upset us and disturb our prayer and our peace. St. Catherine used to say: "Whatever happens to you, never think that it comes from men; think that it comes from God and is for your good. And then see how you may profit by it." (Jorgensen, p. 52).

In *The Dialogue* St. Catherine gives guidance, advice and inspiration for living as a true follower of Christ and coming to the closest possible union with Him. *The Dialogue* has value for the average Christian, as well as for one well advanced along the mystical way. It has value for one who follows Christ, though at a distance, and for one who has embraced Him fully and walks beside Him. Perhaps we could call her work "The Creed Come Alive," for she clothes all its articles in the rich texture and brilliant color of her own profound understanding, personal experience and deep feeling. *The Dialogue* is the *Creed* as she has lived it and felt it, and she knows how its sacred truths work on others.

St. Catherine's imagery in *The Dialogue* is rich, varied and striking. She often returns to the idea that Christ is the Bridge by which the soul goes to God. He is the Door. He is the Truth. The devil draws souls to the lower way, to the river where they are drowned in bitter waters. For he is the lie.

Foremost in St. Catherine's mind was the conviction that correct thinking, or using the light of reason, is necessary in order to stay on the Bridge. Even more necessary is the light of faith, if the soul wishes to avoid the darkness and the murky, black river of Satan. Therefore, the soul must beware of the wiles of the devil, who always presents evil in a pleasant, attractive form—under the aspect of good (*sub specie bonae*).

All through St. Catherine's writing, there are allusions to the devil and warnings about him. She knew and often felt his efforts to destroy her. She fought him regularly for the souls of others, by prayer and penance and by presenting the truth to them clearly. And there were numerous instances in her life when she drove out evil spirits from possessed persons. At the same time, St. Catherine never feared the devil, for she knew he could harm no one whose will remained united to God.

As God told her and as she recorded in *The Dialogue*,

> No one should fear any battle or temptation of the Devil that may come to him, because I have made My creatures strong, and have given them strength of will, fortified in the Blood of My Son, which will neither Devil nor creature can move, because it is yours, given by Me . . . It [your will] is an arm, which, if you place it in the hands of the Devil, straightway becomes a knife with which he strikes you and slays you. But if man does not give this knife of his will into the hands of the Devil, that is, if he does not consent to his temptations and molestations, he will never be injured by the guilt of sin in any temptation, but will even be fortified by it, when the eye of his intellect is opened to see My love which allowed him to be tempted, so as to arrive at virtue, by being proved. For one does not arrive at virtue except through knowledge of self, and knowledge of Me, which knowledge is more perfectly acquired in the time of temptation, because then man knows himself to be nothing . . . And I let him [the Devil] tempt, through love, and not through hatred, that you may conquer, and not that you may be conquered, and that you may come to a perfect knowledge of yourself, and of Me, and that virtue may be proved, for it is not proved except by its contrary. . . . (*Dialogue*, pp. 118-119).

Those who follow the devil choose Hell finally even while still alive, just as the good finally choose God and Heaven. The evil

> await no other judgment than that of their own conscience, and desperately, despairingly, come to eternal damnation. Wherefore Hell, through their hate, surges up to them in the extremity of death, and before they get there, they take hold of it, by means of their lord, the Devil. As the righteous . . . when the extremity of death comes, see the good which I have prepared for them and embrace it with the arms of love, holding fast with pressure of love to Me, the Supreme and Eternal Good. And so they taste eternal life before they have left the mortal body, that is, before the soul be separated from the body.

These are the ones who have arrived at a good degree of perfection. The imperfect embrace God's mercy, and arrive at Purgatory.

> . . . Because they were imperfect, they constrained My mercy, counting My mercy, counting My mercy greater than their sins. The wicked sinners do the contrary, for seeing with desperation their destination, they embrace it with hatred, as I told thee. So that neither the one nor the other waits for judgment, but in departing from this life, they receive every one their place, as I have told thee, and they taste it and possess it before they depart from the body, at the extremity of death—the damned with hatred and with despair, and the perfect ones with love and the light of faith and with the hope of the Blood. And the imperfect arrive at the place of Purgatory with mercy and the same faith. (*Dialogue*, p. 121).

The *Dialogue* paints a vivid picture, showing that to follow Christ is to follow the truth, and to follow the devil is to follow a lie.

> And they arrive at the Gate of the Lie, because they follow the doctrine of the Devil, who is the Father of Lies; and this Devil is their door, through which they go to eternal damnation, as has been said, as the elect and My sons, keeping by the way above, that is, by the Bridge, follow the Way of Truth, and this Truth is the Door, and therefore said My Truth, "*No one can go to the Father but by Me.*" He is the Door and the Way through which they pass to enter the Sea Pacific. It is the contrary for those who have kept the Way of the Lie, which leads them to the water of death. And it is to this that the

Devil calls them, and they are as blind and mad and do not perceive it, because they have lost the light of faith. The Devil says, as it were, to them: "Whosoever thirsts for the water of death, let him come and I will give it to him." (*Dialogue*, pp. 117-118).

The longest part of *The Dialogue* is the treatise on prayer. Part of this is a treatise on tears. From the reasons for one's tears, a person can tell what stage the soul is in. Tears come from the heart, and thus reveal the state of the soul, depending on why the person weeps. Some are merely tears of damnation. Worldly men weep when deprived of what they loved in the wrong way. But there are also four other kinds of tears, and these lead to God. There are tears which come from fear of God's punishments. Then there are tears of sweetness, which come from the hearts of men who have abandoned sin and taste how sweet the Lord is. Next there are tears that come from those who have a perfect love of neighbor and who love God with no regard for themselves. The state of soul which produces these tears implies a great detachment from creatures. The fourth stage of tears leading to salvation combines the preceding two stages, but now creatures are loved again, though with perfect detachment.

In the treatise on prayer is also included an explanation of the Holy Eucharist. One of the figures used to explain the presence of Jesus in the Holy Eucharist is "light." He is the Light which remains with the Father and yet can give Itself to everyone in the Church. God spoke to St. Catherine: "If thou hast a light and the whole world should come to thee in order to take light from it—the light itself does not diminish—and yet each person has it all."

So too each one receives according to his own capacity. Those who come with a larger candle receive more light than those with a smaller one, yet each receives the same light.

> Each one carries his own candle, that is, the holy desire with which he receives this Sacrament, which of itself [the holy desire] is without light, and lights it by receiving this Sacrament. I say without light, because of yourselves you can do nothing, though I have given you the material with which you can receive this light and feed it. The material is love, for through love I created you, and without love you cannot live. (*Dialogue*, p. 231).

In a further development of this metaphor of light, the wick of the candle, which catches the Divine Flame, is faith. Everything must start with love. The divine love is the source of all the good that comes to man through the Sacraments or in any other way. (*Dialogue,* p. 232).

The Dialogue also contains advice regarding priests who administer the Holy Eucharist.

> You should love them therefore by reason of the virtue and dignity of the Sacrament, and by reason of that very virtue and dignity you should hate the defects of those who live miserably in sin, but not on that account appoint yourselves their judges, which I forbid because they are my Christ's, and you ought to love and reverence the authority which I have given them. (*Dialogue*, p. 256).

In *The Dialogue*, God tells St. Catherine of the dignity of priests. "The angel himself has no such dignity, for I have given it to those men whom I have chosen for My ministers and whom I have appointed as earthly angels in this life." But much is demanded of priests.

> In all souls I demand purity and charity, that they should love Me and their neighbor, helping him by the ministration of prayer, as I said to thee in another place. But far more do I demand purity in My ministers and love towards Me and towards their fellow creatures, administering to them the Body and Blood of My only-begotten Son, with the fire of charity, and a hunger for the salvation of souls, for the glory and honor of My name . . . for if by sin they are cruel to themselves, they are cruel to the souls of their neighbors, in that they do not give them an example of life, nor care to draw them out of the hands of the devil, nor to administer to them the Body and the Blood of My only-begotten Son, and Me the True Light, as I told thee, and the other Sacraments of the holy Church. So that, in being cruel to themselves, they are cruel to others. (*Dialogue*, pp. 240-241).

Further, God speaks to St. Catherine of the justice which is demanded for true peace in the world—an understanding which a world reverting to paganism desperately needs to grasp.

> And this justice was and is that pearl which shines in them, and which gave peace and light in the minds of the people and

caused holy fear to be with them, and unity of hearts. And I
would that thou know that more darkness and division have
come into the world amongst seculars and religious and the
clergy and pastors of the holy Church, through the lack of the
light of justice, and the advent of the darkness of injustice,
than from any other causes. Neither the civil law nor the divine
law can be kept in any degree without holy justice, because he
who is not corrected and does not correct others, becomes like
a limb which putrefies and corrupts the whole body, because
the bad physician, when it had already begun to corrupt, placed
ointment immediately upon it, without having first burnt the
wound. (*Dialogue*, pp. 246-247).

The Cell of Self-Knowledge

"The keynote of Catherine's teaching is that man, whether in
the cloister or in the world, must ever abide in the cell of self-
knowledge, which is the stable in which the traveler through
time and eternity must be born again." (*Life of St. Catherine*,
by Edmund Gardner, 1907).

St. Catherine repeats over and over in her letters this leading idea: "We must remain in the cell of self-knowledge and
understand that we are not, but that all being is of God." St.
Catherine often quoted St. Bernard: "Destroy self-love and there
will be no more Hell." The *Dialogue* puts it plainly: "There is no
condition of the soul in which it ceases to be necessary for a
man to put his own self-love to death." (Quoted in Drane, p. 40).

One very close to St. Catherine, the Englishman William Flete,
a Hermit of St. Augustine, wrote a summary of her spiritual
doctrine. It was written in Latin in January, 1376, while Catherine
was still alive. He says,

> The holy Mother, speaking of herself as of a third person,
> said that in the beginning of her illumination she placed as
> the foundation of her whole life, in opposition to self-love, the
> stone of self-knowledge, which she separated into the three fol-
> lowing little stones: The first was the consideration of her cre-
> ation; that is to say, how she had no existence whatever of
> herself, but one solely dependent on the Creator, as well in its
> production as in its preservation, and that all this the Creator
> had done, and was still doing, through His grace and mercy.
>
> The second was the consideration of her redemption; that is,
> how the Redeemer had restored with His own Blood the life of
> grace which was before destroyed, and this through His pure

and fervent love, unmerited by man.

The third was the consideration of her own sins, committed after Baptism, and the graces therein received, through which she, having deserved eternal damnation, was astonished that out of the eternal goodness of God, He had not commanded the earth to swallow her up.

From these three considerations, there arose within her so great a hatred against herself that she desired nothing whatever conformable to her own will, but only to the will of God, who, as she already knew, willed nothing but her good. From this it followed that every tribulation or trial was to her a matter of pleasure and delight, not only because it came through the will of God, but also because she saw herself to be thereby punished and chastised. She began likewise to have the greatest dislike to [of] those things in which she used formerly to take pleasure, and great delight in what formerly displeased her; thus, the caresses of her mother, in which she had once found so much pleasure, she now shunned as she would sword or poison, whilst at the same time she joyfully embraced all the abuse and insults that were bestowed upon her.

And she also welcomed what at the same time she abhorred— the temptations of Satan; she welcomed them for the suffering they brought, and abhorred them inasmuch as they offered her sensual enjoyments. After these things, there was kindled within her an immense desire for purity, and after having made continual prayer during many months to obtain it, and that it might be bestowed on her in its highest perfection, Our Lord at last appearing to her, said: "Beloved Daughter, if thou wouldst obtain the purity thou desirest, thou must needs first become perfectly united to Me, who am purity itself, which thou shalt obtain if thou observe three things. In the first place, thou must turn thyself wholly toward Me with thine intention, and have Me alone for thine end in all thine actions, and make it thy sole study to keep Me ever before thine eyes. Secondly, denying thine own will, and paying no regard to that of any creature soever, thou must have respect and consideration for Mine, which wills thy sanctification, since I neither wish nor permit anything except for thy good. If thou attentively observe this, nothing shall sadden or disturb thee, even for an hour, but rather thou wilt esteem thyself obliged to any who insult thee. Moreover, thou shalt not judge anything to be sinful unless thou knowest it manifestly to be so, and then thou shalt be indignant against the sin, but shalt compassionate the sinner. The third thing is that thou judge the actions of My servants, not according to thine own inclination and taste, but according to My judgment; because thou knowest full well that I have

said, 'In My Father's house [there] are many mansions.'"
(Quoted in Drane, p. 646).

The "holy hatred" of which St. Catherine speaks as directed
against oneself is the result of real self-knowledge. Self-knowledge is based on our fundamental position as being created and
redeemed, and able of ourselves alone only to offend God and
deserve Hell. To her this thinking was not just abstract philosophizing, but a truth intensely personal and experienced.

We must be on guard, however, against understanding this
"holy hatred" in a one-sided way. As St. Catherine's doctrine on
tears illustrates, and as the affection in which she held her
friends shows, she came through the time of detachment to a
time of new and tender holy attachment to herself and to others. The hatred must always be holy; otherwise, it would be
wrong. And even in the lives of St. Catherine and other saints,
we can see a gradual development. When the battle against
self-love is being won, and the forces leaning to disorderly self-
love are under control, then the person in a freer, holier and
even more truly human way comes to a new love of self and
neighbor.

Perhaps, because we take the strong words of a Saint in a
one-sided way, we may want to reject the "holy hatred" idea. Or
perhaps some Saints (who said similar things) never did reach
the final stage of close union with God that allows ease and
flexibility in allowing affections to run freely and yet be under
perfect control. We may recall here, to help our understanding,
the words of Jesus Himself: "He that loveth his life shall lose
it; and he that hateth his life in this world, keepeth it unto life
eternal." (*John* 12:25).

"Hatred" of Self versus Love of Neighbor

The proper "hatred" of self flowing from true self-knowledge
and the elimination of self-will leads to a love of neighbor. In
the way that things develop according to God's plan, others, that
is, our neighbors, are the means of helping us grow in virtue
and of eliminating our defects. (*Dialogue*, pp. 39-49). God told
St. Catherine: "I wish also that thou shouldst know that every
virtue is obtained by means of thy neighbor, and likewise, every
defect; he, therefore, who stands in hatred of Me, does an injury
to his neighbor, and to himself, who is his own chief neighbor,

and this injury is both general and particular." The *general* refers to all men, even those we are not usually immediately in contact with. The *particular* refers to those who are a part of our life.

> I have told thee how all sins are accomplished by means of thy neighbor, through the principles which I exposed to thee, that is, because men are deprived of the affection of love, which gives light to every virtue. In the same way self-love, which destroys charity and affection towards the neighbor, is the principle and foundation of every evil. All scandals, hatred, cruelty, and every sort of trouble proceed from this perverse root of self-love, which has poisoned the entire world, and weakened the mystical body of the Holy Church, and the universal body of the believers in the Christian religion; and therefore I said to thee, that it was in the neighbor, that is to say in the love of him, that all virtues were founded; and truly indeed did I say to thee that charity gives life to all the virtues, because no virtue can be obtained without charity, which is the pure love of Me. (*Dialogue*, pp. 43-44).

The final development, then, of a holy "hatred" of self is the acquiring of a much greater love of God and neighbor and a proper love of self.

> When she has discovered the advantage of this unitive love in Me, by means of which she truly loves herself, extending her desire for the salvation of the whole world, thus coming to the aid of its neediness, she strives, inasmuch as she has done good to herself by the conception of virtue, from which she has drawn the life of grace, to fix her eye on the needs of her neighbor in particular. (*Dialogue*, p. 45).

God supplies for Catherine the answer to a question that many have asked: Why doesn't God give a person all he needs spiritually and materially, and eliminate so much trouble?

> I could easily have created men possessed of all that they should need both for body and soul, but I wish that one should have need of the other, and that they should be My ministers to administer the graces and the gifts that they have received from Me. Whether man will or no, he cannot help making, an act of love. It is true, however, that that act, unless made through love of Me, profits him nothing so far as grace is con-

cerned. See, then, that I have made men My ministers, and placed them in diverse stations and various ranks, in order that they may make use of the virtue of love. (*Dialogue*, p. 47).

In her final days, St. Catherine gave instructions to her disciples, especially on the dangers of self-love, the root of all evil. She echoed the thought expressed in one of her letters: "That which causes pain in us is self-will, whether it be spiritual or worldly." (*Letter* 317, Jorgensen). The *Dialogue* gives a succinct summary on self-love at the end of the "Treatise on Discretion."

It is because his love for Me is still imperfect that his neighborly love is so weak, and because the root of self-love has not been properly dug out. Wherefore I often permit such a love to exist, so that the soul may in this way come to the knowledge of her own imperfection, and for the same reason do I withdraw Myself from the soul by sentiment, that she may be thus led to enclose herself in the house of self-knowledge, where is acquired every perfection. After which I return into her with more light and with more knowledge of My Truth, in proportion to the degree in which she refers to grace the power of slaying her own will. And she never ceases to cultivate the vine of her soul, and to root out the thorns of evil thoughts, replacing them with the stones of virtues, cemented together in the Blood of Christ Crucified, which she has found in her journey across the Bridge of Christ, My only-begotten Son. For I told thee, if thou remember, that upon the Bridge, that is, upon the doctrine of My Truth, were built up the stones, based upon the virtue of His Blood, for it is in virtue of this Blood that the virtues give life. (*Dialogue*, pp. 156-157).

A Complete Love

St. Catherine's nature was to do everything completely, to grasp a truth with utter, intuitive clarity and to follow it with a logic that made extreme demands on her. There were no half-measures with her. Paradoxically, she was, to external appearances, merciless with her own poor body, and merciful beyond mercy to others.

If St. Catherine is hard to understand, it is because we are accustomed to the incomplete in vision and love. To grasp her personality, to fathom her soul requires a real sympathy for completeness in a person's thinking. Without this sympathy, St. Catherine remains one of the most fascinating and colorful women of history, but still largely incomprehensible.

"She did not stop doing anything, or leave anything half-done for the sake of something else," says Bl. Raymond of Capua. But above all, St. Catherine showed the all-out approach in love for her neighbor. "The source and basis of all she did was love; and so charity towards her neighbor surpassed all her other actions." A number of times St. Catherine's prayer for a sinner went so far as to offer to bear not only the rigors of justice for his soul, but even Hell itself. This happened in the case of Andrea Bellanti, a blasphemous, loose-living young man of Siena, who was dying impenitent.

> Lord, I desire and will that the rigors of Thy justice shall be satisfied in me, to the end that this poor man may be saved, and I am even willing to be condemned in his stead, if salvation cannot be obtained for him in any other way. I will not rise from my knees until Thou grant me my desire.

The young man did send for a priest, confessed and died soon afterwards. (*Letter* 106, Jorgensen).

God instructed St. Catherine to have a special love for priests.

> You should love them, therefore, by reason of the virtue and dignity of the Sacrament, and by reason of their very virtue and dignity you should hate the defects of those who live miserably in sin, but not on that account appoint yourselves their judges, which I forbid, because they are My Christ's, and you ought to live and reverence the authority which I have given them. You know well that if a filthy and badly dressed person brought you a great treasure from which you obtained life, you would not hate the bearer, however ragged and filthy he might be, through love of the treasure and of the lord who sent it to you. (*Dialogue*, p. 256).

Thus St. Catherine loved priests in her complete way. Encompassed in her love was the deepest respect yet the most forceful and direct pointing out of abuses. Only a complete love could have the strength and courage to correct the first priest of Christendom as a mother would, and yet to bow deeply and graciously as would a dutiful daughter.

St. Catherine was completely logical in following a complete love. Love does strange things to a person. It energizes, it overcomes obstacles, it drives one on to accomplish what seems impossible. With her whole heart and mind and soul, St. Catherine loved Christ and all others in Him.

Creatureliness

> If men knew their own nothingness, they could not be proud. The being we have, we received from God. We did not ask Him to create us. He was moved to do it out of the love which He had for His creature, whom regarding in Himself, He became enamoured of its beauty. The soul that looks within sees there God's goodness.

St. Catherine wrote this to Cardinal James Orsini. (Drane, p. 448).

The constant thought of her creatureliness made her a totality of self-giving, and her adherence to God's Will was thus forceful and vehement. She threw herself into doing all for souls and giving all to God. Her bodily chastisements were part of this giving and doing. But Bl. Raymond of Capua warns that only those who have the "fullness of spirit" can imitate St. Catherine in her stern treatment of body. (It seems that he followed this warning pretty well himself.)

Knowledge of her own status as creature helped her to see the need for complete detachment from creatures and to appreciate the joy that comes from union with the Creator. This is brought out by the one letter addressed to Countess Bianchina that has been preserved.

> We go on always forming new attachments; if God cuts off one branch, we make another. We fear to lose perishing creatures more than to lose God. And so, keeping them and possessing them against the will of God, we taste even in this life the foretaste of Hell: For God so permits that a soul which loves itself with irregular love should become insupportable to itself. It suffers from everything that it possesses because it fears to lose it; and to preserve what it possesses, there is anxiety and fatigue day and night. And it suffers from what it does not possess, because it desires what it cannot get. And so the soul is never at rest in the midst of the things of this world, for they are all less than us. They were made for us, we were not made for them. We were made for God alone, to enjoy His eternal and sovereign happiness. God alone then, can satisfy the soul; and all that it can desire it will find in Him . . . (Drane, p. 381).

Flowing from her idea of creatureliness is St. Catherine's absolute trust in Divine Providence. In taking care of the leprous woman, during the plague in Siena, amidst the rebellion in Florence, in dangerous times at sea, she left all serenely to God. In fact, she wanted to give her life for love of God, as shown in the service of a fellow creature. She wept inconsolably on a number of occasions because her desire to give her life was not fulfilled. She chided her confessor, Bl. Raymond, for turning back from what would have been the sure loss of his life while acting as envoy for the Pope.

"Whatever happens to you, never think that it comes from men, think that it comes from God and is for your good. And then see how you may profit from it." (*Legend*, II, 5,12). But she realized how men must struggle, too, and how they fear suffering. She wrote to her brother Benincasa: "For the suffering which is past we have not any longer, and that which is to come has not yet appeared. We have only the present instant." (Jorgensen, p. 91).

All suffering, because we experience only one moment at a time, is "like the prick of a needle." In fact, when we *accept* suffering, its intensity diminishes, as far as our experience of it goes. It is the rebellion against it that causes much of our pain.

> In Jesus crucified all things are possible to us, and God never lays a burden on us beyond our strength. We ought to rejoice when we receive a heavy burden, for it is then that God bestows on us the gift of fortitude. It is by the love of suffering that we get to lose the feeling of suffering. (Letter to Bl. Raymond; Drane, p. 533).

St. Catherine did not fear to give herself completely, because she trusted in God's goodness and in the love of Christ. Again, her very idea of her own abysmal nothingness as a creature made her stretch out to embrace that goodness and love. "All the way to Heaven is heaven, because He said, 'I am the Way.'" She followed the Way, because though to follow Christ crucified meant pain, the greater pain for a creature was to follow its own selfish whims. To follow Christ means sweetness and union with Him and ultimate fulfillment as God's creature raised to the level of special adoptive childhood.

St. Catherine realized that in this life we have to make a choice. She made hers early in life. Her nature and her cooperation with grace made her choice relentlessly logical and complete.

The soul cannot live without loving, for we must love either God or the world. And the soul always unites itself with what it loves and is transformed by it. But if the soul love the world, it only gains suffering, for there it finds only tribulation and bitter thorns . . . And the soul is always sorrowful and cannot endure itself . . . But God is the highest and eternal sweetness, and the soul which receives God by grace is satisfied and content, for the hunger of the soul cannot be appeased by anything but God, because He is greater than it, but the soul is greater than all [other] created things. Therefore, all that this world contains cannot satisfy man, for it is all poorer than man. (*Letters* 13, 31, 34; Jorgensen, p. 34).

Here we can see the logic of St. Catherine's rejecting all that is lesser and choosing instead to love the Creator. This is the only philosophical position that really makes sense, if we line up Creation in its proper order of dignity, with man at the top, and then direct all back to its Source, God the Father.

"That's Human Nature"

St. Catherine's story is that of a soul responding with heroic and complete generosity to God's very special graces. It is the story of a soul's inner growth, of her becoming truly and completely human in the sense of achieving perhaps the most complete possible love for God and man, and the best-ordered love of herself. All that was dross in her life was cut away. All that was good was given a chance to develop. In her hand, under the direction of God's grace, the pruning knife was sharp, and the growth was magnificent and beautiful.

The Saints were always the most human of all people because they conformed themselves most perfectly and in the most ordered fashion to reality as God made it. They were the most human because in that reality were included the truest, most perfect and highest ideals. They were most human because they won a victory over human weaknesses, which work to prevent a full flowering of ordered love. The expression, "That's human nature," has its real, its true, its fullest meaning in the person of a saint, for a saint has achieved perfection according to the divinely created order which Almighty God built into human nature when He created it. Most often, the phrase, "That's human nature," is used to explain and excuse weakness and lack of fidelity in people. However, what would be more accurate would be to say, "That's *fallen* human nature, not cooperating with the graces of Redemption obtained for man by Jesus Christ."

The true fullness of human nature within a person demands a victory of the higher faculties and aspirations over the lower. Perfect humanity will be, within its limits, a perfect reflection of the Creator. Man being made in the image and likeness of God, those who are truly the most human are those who portray that image and likeness most perfectly—following the injunction of our divine Saviour, "Be you therefore perfect, as also your heavenly Father is perfect." (*Matt.* 5:48).

Similarity to Our Lord

The most perfect and therefore complete human being who ever lived was Jesus Christ. He reflected most perfectly, even in His human nature, the image of the eternal Father. As God the Son, of course He always reflected that image with infinite perfection. In His human nature, He "advanced in wisdom, and age, and grace with God and men" (*Luke* 2:52), so that He had the most perfected human nature that ever was. Because of this, He is the model for all men. We most truly achieve the perfection of our own human nature by following Christ, and Him crucified.

St. Catherine of Siena, perhaps better than any other person we knew about, exemplified this perfecting of one's true human nature by being the Bride of the Crucified, the mystic of the Incarnate Word. And though the achievement of full perfection of human nature in Christ is an inner process, one that can have a thousand varieties of external circumstances, we are able, if we wish, to find remarkable external resemblances between the life of Christ and the life of St. Catherine of Siena.

St. Catherine died at age 33, the same age Our Lord was when He died. Like Him, she offered herself for men's souls. Her offering was as complete as she could possibly make it according to her own ardent nature, perfected by grace. Jesus Christ offered up His life on earth to found the Church. She offered up hers to preserve it in a time of crisis. He was wounded for our transgressions, wounded for our iniquities. She often asked for and received some special pain to save particular souls. At the Last Supper, Our Lord thanked God the Father that He had not lost any of those souls committed to Him. At the end of her life, St. Catherine thanked God that she had been promised the grace of salvation for each of her intimate circle of disciples. Christ had said, "Amen I say to you, as long as you did it to one of these my least brethren, you did it to me." (*Matt.* 25:40). St. Catherine identified all people, especially the least, with Christ, and she cared for them. Jesus said in reference to His salvific sufferings: "How am I straitened until it be accomplished?" (*Luke* 12:50). St. Catherine had often looked forward to martyrdom.

Christ, though God, often spoke of His creatureliness as man. He recalled over and over that He did not do His own will, but the will of Him who sent Him. He fasted and prayed, as a human being should. He used the ordinary means of speaking, giving homely examples to His Apostles and disciples in order to enlighten them. Though He fulfilled His own task completely, He left the world with much yet to be done, as any human being does, and He promised that the Holy Spirit would bring further enlightenment. He preached, and men admired, but even at the words of the Saviour they were not always convinced.

He gathered around Him His little band of disciples. St. Catherine had around her *her* little band of faithful followers. He spoke as no man had ever spoken before. St. Catherine poured forth the fullness of a heart united to God, so that without weariness, others could listen to her and be absorbed for hours. He said that He came "to cast fire on the earth." (*Luke* 12:49). St. Catherine said that her nature was fire.

Jesus had bitter enemies. St. Catherine had maligners and persecutors and those who wanted to take her life. He said of the Church: "He who hears you, hears me." (*Luke* 10:16). St. Catherine repeated over and over this identification. The Pope to her was "sweet Christ on earth." Jesus predicted unfaithfulness among those closest to Him and said that scandals would come. St. Catherine recognized unfaithfulness in those high in the Church, and she spoke so plainly of scandals that she frightened some.

"Thou art the book in which the rule of our life has been written down," St. Catherine addressed the Blessed Virgin Mary, Mother of the Incarnate Word. So it is in studying those closest to Christ that we come to understand Him and to follow Him better. We do not thereby detract from Him, but we learn how completely He can fill a human life and fulfill the yearnings and strivings of our human nature. St. Catherine has the same message today that she has had for the past six centuries. This Bride of the Crucified leads us to Him who was crucified for love of us. The more we understand her, the more we can understand Him. Every science pertaining to man has case histories. From these cases and according to the aspect of that science, we learn more and more about what the ideal man should be. Saints are case histories in the science of salvation, which is the ultimate science pertaining to man and the one that includes the purposes of all the others. St. Catherine shows us the way to Christ crucified. He gave her His Heart. Having His Heart, she shows us His life.

In a particular way, she shows us the Heart of Christ in the world today, for like our own era, her age was one of trial and change in the Church. It was a time when many people, as we say, were mixed-up, when the Pope was under attack. Loving Christ, she loved the Church. Loving Him, she saw in the Pope, as he truly is, the living voice of Christ on earth. If St. Catherine were on earth today, she would repeat what she said so often to her disciples, to her friends and to the enemies of the Church: "Follow Christ Crucified by following the Holy Father, for he is sweet Christ on earth."

St. Catherine's feast day is April 29 (April 30 in the 1962 calendar).

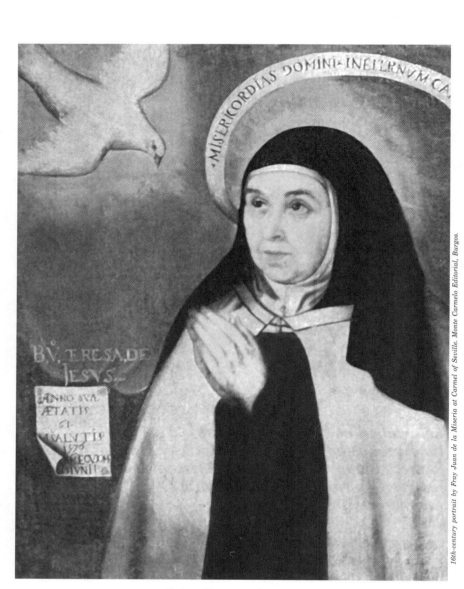

Saint Teresa of Avila

16th-century portrait by Fray Juan de la Miseria at Carmel of Seville. Monte Carmelo Editorial, Burgos.

— 26 —

SAINT TERESA OF AVILA

Doctor of Prayer

1515-1582

"WHEN I was young, I was told that I was pretty, and I believed it; later on people found me intelligent, and I believed that too; they tell me today that I am a saint. But now I have no illusions." With these words St. Teresa of Avila wittily summed up her own life. On September 27, 1970, Pope Paul VI officially declared this remarkable sixteenth-century Carmelite nun to be the first woman Doctor of the Church, thereby establishing that at least the second and third statements of her summary were not illusory. For, by definition, a Doctor of the Church must illumine the Church by both holy doctrine and a holy life. St. Teresa had been canonized in 1622.

The Pope on his own initiative decided to add two women to the select list of the then 30 Doctors, all of whom were men. The Carmelites had not asked for St. Teresa to be declared a Doctor of the Church, nor had the Dominicans asked for this for St. Catherine of Siena—who received the same title a week later, on Sunday, October 4, 1970. Both orders, in fact, were caught by surprise when the Holy Father first made the announcement of his intention on October 15, 1967. He also decided that there should be two ceremonies, a week apart, rather than one ceremony for both new Doctors. Within eight days a nineteen-centuries-old tradition was twice shattered.

Four centuries earlier, however, a contemporary of St. Teresa, Sister Mary of St. Joseph, had written: "God has given us a woman Doctor, graduated from the school of the Holy Spirit, in which this great Teresa became so wise that I hope she will be famous and great in the Church of God, not only on account of her life, but also for the doctrine she left in writing." (*Spiritual Life*, Discalced Carmelites, Washington, D.C., Winter 1970, Vol. 16, no. 4, p. 216).

In conferring the title of Doctor of the Church upon St. Teresa of Avila, Pope Paul VI confirmed a belief of many, which had in

435

fact been demonstrated for centuries. During all that time the saintly and learned, the theologians and the common people, had read and been enriched by her works. Pope Paul VI, in his September 27 homily, began by saying: "We have conferred— rather, we have acknowledged St. Teresa of Jesus' title of Doctor of the Church."

Why Women Doctors?

When Pope Paul VI (1963-1978) made his original announcement in 1967, there was much speculation about why he planned to declare two women to be Doctors of the Church and just what effect this would have on the possible future role of women as part of the teaching Church.

The Pope clearly said, in conferring the rare title of Doctor of the Church, that St. Paul's "Let women keep silence in the churches" (*1 Cor.* 14:34) still signified that women should not have hierarchical functions in the Church. Through Baptism women partake of the common priesthood of the faithful. Some, like St. Teresa, reach high summits of wisdom and, in their own distinctive, charismatic, feminine way, give guidance and enlightenment to the whole Church.

Women have their own special capacity for mystical prayer, the Pope said, and "that light becomes life in a sublime manner for the good and service of mankind." St. Teresa's light had illumined the paths of many. The highest official recognition of this fact would encourage others to follow it.

"We have taken care to see that, having been adorned with this magisterial title, she may have a more authoritative mission to perform in her religious family, in the praying Church and in the world, through her perennial, ever-present message— the message of prayer."

In a strong and masterful statement, the Holy Father showed how much St. Teresa's message of prayer is needed in today's world.

> Teresa's message of prayer comes to us children of the Church at a time marked by a great effort at reform and renewal of liturgical prayer. It comes to us who are tempted by the great noise and business of the outside world to yield to the frenzy of modern life and to lose the real treasures of our souls in the effort to win earth's seductive treasures. It comes to us, chil-

dren of our time, just when we are losing, not only the habit of conversation with God, but also the sense of the need and duty to worship and call on Him . . .

Psychoanalytical exploration is breaking down the frail and complicated instrument that we are, in such a way that all that can be heard is, not the sound of mankind in its suffering and its redemption, but rather the troubled mutterings of man's animal subconscious, the cries of his disordered passions and his desperate anguish.

Doctor of Prayer

St. Teresa's message about prayer has something in it for everybody, the beginner as well as the most advanced in the art of praying. Writing about mental prayer, she says in her autobiography:

> Anyone who has not begun to pray, I beg, for the love of the Lord, not to miss so great a blessing. There is no place here for fear, but only desire. For even if a person fails to make progress, or to strive after perfection, so that he may merit the consolations and favors given to the perfect by God, yet he will gradually gain a knowledge of the road to Heaven. And if he perseveres, I hope in the mercy of God, whom no one has ever taken for a Friend without being rewarded; and mental prayer, in my view, is nothing but a friendly way of dealing, in which we often find ourselves talking in private with Him whom we know loves us. (Vol. I of *Life of the Holy Mother Teresa of Jesus,* trans. E. Allison Peers, Sheed & Ward, London, 1950, ch. 8, p. 50).

St. Teresa warns against discouragement and giving up because a person finds he is still sinning. She had the same temptation, and says that the devil tried to lead her by the road of false humility.

> I can say what I know by experience—namely, that no one who has begun this practice, however many sins he may commit, should ever forsake it. For it is the means by which we may amend our lives again, and without it, amendment will be very much harder . . . If we repent truly and determine not to offend Him, He will resume His former friendship with us and grant us the favors which He granted aforetime, and sometimes many more, if our repentance merits it. (*Life,* ch. 8).

It is comforting to know that this "Mistress of Prayer," as her contemporary, the Dominican Fr. Garcia of Toledo, called her, experienced over many years how distractions come into prayer. She compared the darting ideas to wild horses pulling the mind here and there. St. Teresa knew that the very structure and balance of body and spirit lead to distractions. In fact, distractions are inevitable. Therefore, we must not fret over them. For more than 18 years in the convent St. Teresa experienced aridity in her praying, and she was often restless. "I could not enter into myself, could not lock up myself within myself." (*Life*, ch. 7).

She also recognized that the devil enters into the picture to persuade people not to pray—even to fear it. She knew too that some of her fear and distraction came from lack of mortification and from lack of silence, as well as from too much interest in the world and in vain things. ". . . More than 18 of the 28 years which have gone by since I began my prayer have been spent in this battle and conflict, which arose from my having relations both with God and with the world."

Praying, for her, was hard work:

> I was more occupied in wishing my hour of prayer were over and in listening whenever the clock struck, than in thinking of things that were good. Again and again, I would rather have done any severe penance that might have been given me than practice recollection as a preliminary to prayer. It is a fact that, either though the intolerable power of the devil's assaults or because of my own bad habits, I did not at once betake myself to prayer; and whenever I entered the oratory, I used to feel so depressed that I had to summon up all my courage to make myself pray at all . . . (*Life*, ch. 8).

St. Teresa warns against the wiles of the devil, who can also play the other side of his record. A person may think he is making progress in prayer, and yet be deceived by the devil. Dryness and desolation of spirit may often be better signs of progress than sweetness. "The pleasures and joys which the devil bestows," says St. Teresa, "are, in my opinion, of immense diversity. By means of these pleasures he might well deceive anyone who is not experiencing, or has not experienced other pleasures given by God." (Peers, p. 160).

When God takes over the faculties in the higher stages of prayer, it is like suddenly finding that one knows something without having studied it. "He has no idea how or whence it has come, since he has never done any work, even so much, as was necessary for the learning of the alphabet." (*Life*, ch. 27). God favors the soul by this "dark knowledge," which is a shaft of great light. There may be at times visions and locutions. The soul advances in the "Prayer of Quiet" to the prayer of Mystical Union. The soul is passive and God takes over, doing the work.

But we must not imagine that once this happens, all effort and distractions are gone forever. We must not imagine that the person remains in a constant ecstasy. He has to return to ordinary "self-propelled" prayer. St. Teresa says that "there is no state of prayer so lofty that it will not be necessary to return many times to the beginning."

Some of Her Prayer Hints

In order to pray well or to keep the peace, which is necessary for leading an interior life, St. Teresa gives three recommendations. They are: 1) real but regulated love for one another, 2) detachment from all created things and 3) true humility. She goes on to say, "Although I put it last, humility is the most important of the three, and embraces all the rest." (*Way of Perfection*, ch. 4).

Embracing the Cross from the beginning is necessary in order to make progress.

> There must be many who have begun some time back and never manage to finish their course, and I believe it is largely because they do not embrace the cross from the beginning that they are distressed and think that they are making no progress. When the understanding ceases to work, they cannot bear it, though perhaps even then the will is increasing in power and putting on new strength without their knowing it. (*Life*, ch. 11).

According to St. Teresa, therefore, determination is necessary for mental prayer and advancement in the spiritual life, and one must push ahead even when things are difficult. The devil likes to turn people away from mental prayer on the grounds that they are too weak and sick. St. Teresa found out that the less she bothered about her health, the more it improved.

> As I am so sickly, I was always tied up and good for nothing until I resolved to take no account of my body and my

health . . . But as it pleased God I should see through this
trick of the demon, I would say, when he put before me the
loss of my health, "It little matters if I die . . ."

Still, St. Teresa advises us that at times a person should turn
from prayer to seek relief in legitimate recreation.

> At such times the soul must render the body a service for
> the love of God, so that on many other occasions the body may
> render services to the soul . . . Sweet is His yoke, and it is
> essential that we should not drag the soul along with us, so to
> say, but lead it gently, so that it may make the greater progress.
> (*Life*, ch. 11).

From childhood St. Teresa had been fond of the story of Jesus
and the woman by the well. "Give me this water, that I may not
thirst," the Samaritan woman had asked of Jesus. Many times
little Teresa had echoed in her heart the words, "Lord, give me
this water." Later, in her writings, she dwells on the example of
water to explain prayer. She had a special love for water, which
is so simple and clear and takes such a variety of forms and is
good for so many needs.

> The beginner [in prayer] must think of himself as of one set-
> ting out to make a garden in which the Lord is to take His
> delight, yet in soil most unfruitful and full of weeds. His Majesty
> will uproot the weeds and put in good plants. . . . We must con-
> sider how to water the garden. . . . There are four ways to have
> this accomplished.

St. Teresa explains that we draw water laboriously from a
well, or we have a waterwheel and buckets, which is less trouble. Our garden may be near a stream or brook, or finally the
Lord may send a heavy rain. (*Life*, ch. 11). St. Teresa follows
out this figure of the water, showing that as the soul advances,
prayer becomes less of a labor, God does more work, and the
fruits become greater. True contemplative prayer may itself result
in fruitful apostolic work, or it may powerfully sustain the work
of others.

She mentions a friends of hers, Fr. Pedro Ibañez, who made
more progress in prayer in four months than she did in 17 years.
He did so, she thought, because he prepared better, evidently
by laying better the foundation for what she called her three

special requisites: love for neighbor, detachment from creatures, and humility.

Her Confessors

The fabric of St. Teresa's life of prayer, her development in the art of prayer, is bound up with her confessors. She had about 25 different confessors and directors over the years. She tells us that most were Jesuits. Others came from the Carmelites, Dominicans or diocesan clergy. A famous Franciscan whom she consulted was St. Peter of Alcantara. Of the Carmelites, St. John of the Cross and later Fr. Gracian were for some years her regular confessors. The Dominican, Fr. Vincent Barron, helped her very much in the period after her father's death, getting her back into mental prayer, which she had left off. He had also been her father's confessor.

William Thomas Walsh, in his biography of St. Teresa, sums up her thinking about confessors: "She prized intelligence and learning above all other qualities in her confessors, and she had a peculiar distrust of holy men who were stupid." (*St. Teresa of Avila*, Bruce, 1943; TAN, 1987, p. 75). At least one quite learned priest, however, caused her unusual suffering by misunderstanding her. He was Don Pedro Gaspar Daza of Avila, who concluded falsely that St. Teresa's mystical experiences were not genuine. When her good friend Don Francisco de Salcedo, who had encouraged her in mental prayer, brought this news to her and said he also agreed with Don Pedro's opinion, St. Teresa burst into tears. "I was so frightened and pained that I did not know what to do. All I could do was weep." (Peers).

Throughout her works, St. Teresa speaks often of confessors. Her idea, of course, of a confessor was not one who just absolves, but one who gives real spiritual direction. She paints a moving picture of the trials and the anguish of mind some confessors had caused her. They did not understand her visions, locutions and ecstasies. She gives detailed advice about confessors to her sisters, for she knew that confessors could either hinder or greatly help a nun's spiritual development.

Some confessors, she said, were too afraid of the devil. St. Teresa, who spoke often of the wiles of the devil and who for a time feared him too much herself, said:

> I am quite sure that I am more afraid of people who are themselves terrified of the devil than I am of the devil himself. For he cannot harm me in the least; whereas they, especially if they are confessors, can upset people a great deal, and for several years they were such a great trial to me that I marvel now that I was able to bear it. (*Life*, ch. 25).

Others, she thought, were too imperceptive to recognize when God wanted to lead a soul into the passive states of prayer.

> I have met souls who were penned in and afflicted because he who taught them lacked experience, and they made me sad; and another who didn't know what to do with herself, for when the spirit is not understood, both soul and body afflict one and prevent improvement. One told me that her *maestro* kept her in leash for eight years, and that he would not let her give up self-knowledge, and yet the Lord held her in the Prayer of Quiet; and so she endured much woe. (*Life*, quoted by Walsh, p. 90).

In her own time of greatest trouble, after the announcement by her friend Salcedo and the learned Fr. Daza that they thought she was led by a devil, someone suggested that she consult a Jesuit. The Jesuits had recently come to Avila and were held in much esteem. Fr. Juan de Padranos came to hear St. Teresa's story and correctly sized up the matter. This sickly but wise young Jesuit gave her the direction she needed. She then found more peace of soul in meditating on the Passion and grew more in love with the Sacred Humanity of Our Lord.

Some of Fr. Padranos' advice might sound strange to us. For instance, he told St. Teresa that despite her morning and evening vomitings and heart trouble, which she had had for 20 years, she should do some mortifications. Perhaps God sent her sickness because she did no penance, he suggested. Under this treatment, the morning vomitings stopped and St. Teresa's health improved.

St. Francis Borgia, another Jesuit, visited Avila about this time—in 1554. He also heard St. Teresa's Confession and agreed with her that her mystical experiences were genuine gifts of God.

But her troubles were not over. There was a short period of peace for her soul, but whispering that was going about Avila had it that she was another Magdalena of the Cross. This lady had been a Poor Clare nun of Cordoba who in childhood had made a pact with the devil and who had feigned even the stigmata. Thousands had asked for her prayers, including Isabella, wife of Charles V. But the Inquisition finally exposed her as a fraud, and the shock was felt throughout Spain. It affected even St. Teresa, and at times she had painful self-doubts about the genuineness of her own experiences.

The doubts of her good friend Fr. Francisco de Salcedo returned and grew into a conviction that she was deceived. St. Teresa tells of her suffering from being talked about concerning this:

> I have been caused great distress by the indiscretion of certain persons with whom I have discussed my experiences in prayer. By talking about them to each other they have done me great harm, divulging things which should have been kept very secret, for they are not meant for everyone to know, and it looked as though I were publishing them myself. The fault, I believe, was not theirs: the Lord permitted it that I might suffer. I do not mean that they divulged what I had told them in Confession, but nonetheless, as they were people whom I had consulted about my fears, so that I might obtain light from them, I thought they ought to have kept silence. (*Life*, ch. 23).

St. Teresa's young new Jesuit confessor, Fr. Baltasar Alvarez, understood her and helped her. But St. Teresa experienced several years of extreme pain and suffering nonetheless. Even Fr. Alvarez, who believed in her, caused her much pain, because in the face of so much talk to the contrary of his own judgment, he did everything possible to test her, and he treated her with much severity. Many times St. Teresa wanted to leave him.

The devils, too, took a hand in tormenting her, trying to sow doubts in her mind. But not succeeding in that, they took on external appearances and at times severely beat her.

St. Teresa was at once a very independent thinker and also a very submissive and humble penitent. It has been said that she often directed her directors. She did require them to study in order to understand her, and she did put forth her own reasonings. She tells us that several were spiritually improved as a result of their work with her. They learned from her and she learned from them—and she also suffered much from them, as she reports. At times they advised differently from what she had learned directly from God. But God, in time, changed their minds.

A priest who had dealings with the "*Madre*," as St. Teresa

was often called, said dourly that she never did anything except what her superiors commanded, but they never commanded anything except what she wanted. Fr. Gracian, her Carmelite superior and confessor, for some time observed:

> It often happened to me to talk over some matter with her and to be of contrary opinion, and afterward at night to change my purpose; and [upon my] going back to tell her it should be done as she had thought, she would smile; and [upon my] asking her why she did, she would say that, having had a revelation from Our Lord that it should be done as she said, though the Prelate told her the opposite, she would go to Our Lord, saying, "If You want it done, move the heart of my Prelate that he may so command me, for I cannot disobey him." (Quoted in Walsh, p. 446).

Her final advice is: "We must describe the whole of our spiritual experiences and the favors granted to us by the Lord to a confessor who is a man of learning, and obey him." (*Life,* ch. 26). She said this even though some men of learning had misunderstood her greatly, and even some very spiritual and holy confessors had greatly tried her spirit. She knew that despite this, God would sustain her soul in its suffering. Her obedience, however, was not one that traveled blindly and never questioned advice given. That is why she suffered. She tried to make those who misunderstood her, understand so that she could have the security of obedience. Thus she advanced and her soul grew strong and was purified.

Born in Avila

St. Teresa was born in Avila on Wednesday morning, March 28, 1515, the third child of Don Alonso Xanchez de Cepeda and Dona Beatriz Davila y Ahumada. She was to be one of nine children, and she also had a half-brother and sister from the earlier marriage of her father. St. Teresa's favorite brother, Rodrigo, had the same birth date as hers, but four years earlier.

It was with him that she ran off one day when she was seven, so that they both could be martyred by the Moors. Why not? For the joys of Heaven would last forever, she had reasoned. *"Para siempre!"* "Forever and forever and forever," she made Rodrigo repeat with her. Why not get there the quick way by martyrdom? The journey to this happy, early victory, however, was interrupted by an uncle. This matter-of-fact gentleman found the children traveling on the road from Avila and brought them back to their parents, who hugged and kissed them.

As a child St. Teresa already had a strong devotion to St. Joseph. She took her many requests to him with complete trust, and he never let her down. She also had great devotion to Our Lady, and used to find a quiet place in the house where she could pray the Rosary.

> She was a shapely, graceful child. Like so many of the Castilians, she had the fair rosy skin of the North, and her well-marked brows, straight rather than arched, retained a somewhat reddish tinge even when darkened by time. Her curly brunette hair, on the other hand, suggested a southern strain, while her eyes, which seemed to laugh and dance when she smiled, were almost black, and the small symmetrical nose, with its sensitive nostrils, ended in something like a little hook. Her face was plump and roundish and marked with three tiny moles that were considered highly ornamental in that day: one below the middle of the nose, the second over the mouth on the left, the third beneath it on the same side. Her hands were small and singularly beautiful. (Walsh, p. 7).

St. Teresa was only 13 when she lost her mother. But to console herself at this loss, she sought comfort in thinking nightly of the agony of Jesus in the Garden. Her love for Our Lord grew as it fed on her own loneliness. She also went to Our Lady.

> When I began to realize what I had lost, I went in my distress to an image of Our Lady and with many tears besought her to be a mother to me. Though I did this in my simplicity, I believe it was of some avail to me; for whenever I have commended myself to this sovereign Virgin, I have been conscious of her aid; and eventually she has brought me back to herself.

But before long, sentimental reading and vanity, abetted by idle companionship, also came to fill the vacuum created by her mother's death. Throughout the rest of her life she bewailed the sins of this teenage period. St. Teresa's sins during this time seem not to have been grave in the usual sense, but they are something which she later considered to have threatened her entire spiritual development. Her sorrow over her life during this period, as well as over her later failures to give herself fully to God for years while in the convent, remained throughout the rest of her life. Commentators on this aspect of her life at times dismiss her sorrow as so much pious exaggeration. But once in a vision she was shown the place in Hell that might have been hers had Christ not rescued her from the logical downward path of these infidelities.

At age 16 she became a boarder in the Augustinian Convent at Avila, which she liked, but at this time she had a feeling of positive hostility against becoming a nun herself. But under the influence of the saintly Sister Maria Briceno, her love for prayer and her sense of the need for unselfishness grew. After a year and a half, because of illness, she had to leave this convent and return home. But later, a visit to an uncle's home, plus conversation with him and the reading of some spiritual books he had, led her to the decision to become a nun. Her choice came only after a conflict within herself that had gone on for three months. Reading the letters of St. Jerome gave her the courage to tell her father of her decision. He had opposed the idea of losing the company of his favorite daughter. But she went secretly and entered the Carmelite Convent of the Incarnation at Avila in November of 1536.

Life for the more than 100 sisters there was not too strict. They could continue to own property, go out to visit, and have frequent callers in the *locutorio* or "speaking room." St. Teresa, a lively, brilliant conversationalist, enjoyed the speaking room, but later said that her excessive use of it had hurt her spiritual growth. Some fashionable lady boarders at the convent who liked the opportunity to meet people there, plus the convent's general atmosphere, did little to improve the monastic spirit. Yet St. Teresa spent the next 20 years chiefly at this convent.

Her story during these years is one of struggle toward spiritual maturity. Pain and infirmity of body, anguish of mind, restlessness that sought both solitude and companionship (she keenly needed both), the co-existence of remarkable mystical experiences with faults and a certain lack of mortification: all entered into her growth. But eventually she reached a peaceful synthesis, and she was ready for her great work of reform of the Carmelite Order. While carrying out this reform, her soul would continue to grow to spiritual maturity, she would compose her writings, and she would attain a more complete and uninterrupted union with God.

A Daughter of the Church

St. Teresa founded the last of the convents of the Carmelite reform at Burgos, Spain in April, 1582. Leaving there near the end of July, she never completed the trip back to Avila. She died in the Carmelite convent at Alba de Tormes at 9:00 in the evening on October 4, 1582. "I am a daughter of the Church," she repeated over and over again, giving thanks to God that this was so. Thankfulness for the gift of faith was a dominating trait in St. Teresa's life. Her era was one in which many had fallen away from the ancient Church. Over them she had wept, had done penance and had prayed. The thought of those who had lost the Faith and of all in the New World who had never received it, spurred her on, and she passed this enthusiasm and solicitude along to her sisters.

St. Teresa's face looked young and beautiful in death, and a sweet odor pervaded the room where her body lay—an odor so strong that windows had to be opened. Nine months later, when her body was exhumed, moist earth was found to have fallen on it through the broken casket. But the body bore the self-same appearance as when it had been buried, firm in flesh and giving off a sweet odor. Today the major portion of her remains are at Alba. As mentioned above, St. Teresa was canonized in 1622—along with St. Ignatius Loyola, St. Francis Xavier and St. Isidore. Her feast day is October 15.

Hard to Sum Up

Pope Paul VI said that St. Teresa "escapes from the descriptive outlines in which we might wish to contain her." She is hard to sum up. Her biographer, Ribera, says that at the corner of her lips, "which were very beautiful," there was always a slight ironic smile, yet an indulgent one. (*St. Teresa in Her Writings*, Rodolphe Hoornaert, Benziger, NY, 1931, p. 121). She recognized life on earth as terribly serious, because it was man's only chance to win a happy eternity. But she saw life's emptiness; it seemed a "poor farce," "a comedy." But with her customary gaiety, "she hastened to laugh at it lest she should be forced to weep." One day St. Teresa read the thought of a sister who, at her request, was copying some of her verses. The sister was wondering how the Madre could occupy herself with such trifles. St. Teresa answered the unspoken question:

"All *that* is necessary to make life endurable."

"God deliver me from gloomy saints," St. Teresa used to say. (Walsh, p. 310). She was cheerful and witty at recreation. She loved the neat turn of words in popular sayings, and on her many journeys she regaled the muleteers with stories and witticisms, winning their loyalty and affection. At times she would be so filled with joy that she would take a tabor and dance and sing. Her voice, ordinarily "harsh and untuneful, became wonderfully sweet and melodious." (Hoornaert, p. 252). The sisters would clap their hands or shake castanets to the rhythm.

But the dance and St. Teresa's accompanying joy could easily change to a mournful adagio. "How I miss you and how lonely I am here!" she wrote to Luisa de la Cerda in 1572, when she was 57 and in the maturity of her mystical gifts. A year before her death she wrote about how she could find no consolation in those who were with her at Avila. "I am very lonely here at Avila, without anyone to give my soul a little consolation; the older I grow, the less reason I have for expecting any in this life." (Hoornaert, p. 133).

St. Teresa tended to be stricter with those she had the most affection for. "I am uncompromising with those I love. I wish them to be faultless." (Hoornaert, p. 142). Completely detached from people in any way that could interfere with her union with God, she grew more in affection toward others as a result. But she found it hard to deal with those who did not love God or who did not practice mental prayer. "I have not derived comfort from any others or cherished any private affection for them." (*Life*, ch. 24).

A Saint of Common Sense

St. Teresa has been called "common sense canonized." One of her biographers said that she had "the most perfect good sense that ever lay concealed within a human brain."

St. Teresa, moreover, had an extraordinary sense of proportion. She saw all things in relation to one another. This was the gift of an intelligence illumined by mystic favors. "A sense of proportion is the characteristic note of her intelligence, as compassion is the dominant trait of her emotional life." (Hoornaert, p. 170).

St. Teresa knew that we are not angels and that we should not try to play the part of angels. Sometimes people accused her of fastidiousness in food—even of immoderation. But she fasted rigorously. The Reformed Carmelites, for instance, ate no meat. But when eating or celebrating, St. Teresa believed in enjoying God's gift of food, and on occasion she would express a wish for exactly some particular dish.

Her ability to see things in proportion helps explain her sense of humor and her keen, penetrating judgment of people. She knew the heights and depths of the human soul. She warned Fr. Gracian of woman's whims and wiles:

> Don't trust too much to nuns: I can tell you that if they want anything, they will make you see it in a thousand different aspects. [She laughed at those who] think they are dispensed from choir one day because they have a pain in their head, and the next day because they have had one, and the third day in case they may get one. (Quoted in Hoornaert, p. 166).

Her affection, charity and obedience could not prevent her from seeing that some confessors hurt their convent penitents. They were "miserable, sanctimonious men, destroyers of the spouses of Christ." (Hoornaert, p. 169). St. Teresa had bitter personal experiences, but never herself became bitter. Her sense of proportion and her compassion prevented that. But she did write, without rancor and for the benefit of her sisters:

> If you should chance to have a revelation, you will scarcely be believed by any confessor. And there are very, very few of them who will not put you into a fright. And really, they seem to be less afraid at hearing you say that the devil has suggested blasphemous temptations to you, or is urging you on to extravagant and unbecoming actions. These things scandalize them less than if they hear you say that an angel appeared to you and spoke to you, or that Christ has shown Himself to you on the Cross. (Hoornaert, p. 169).

Concerning the secrecy of her first foundation she said, "I thought it of great importance to do nothing against obedience, but I knew that if I told my superiors about it, everything would be ruined." (Teresa did, however, have the permission of the Bishop.)

St. Teresa knew that we are supposed to become perfect, but she knew too that we do not get that way all at once. In any human endeavor, in any part, you do not treat beginners like those more advanced, and this is true especially in the art of growing in union with God. She said of one priest she consulted:

> He began with the holy determination to treat me as though
> I were strong . . . But when I saw how determinedly he was
> attacking these little habits of mine . . . and that I had not
> courage enough to live more perfectly, I became distressed, and
> realizing that in spiritual matters he was treating me as though
> I were going to become perfect immediately, I saw that I should
> have to be much more careful . . . I, though advanced in divine
> favors, was, as regards virtues and mortification, still quite a
> beginner. Really, I think if I had had nobody else to consult,
> that my soul would never have shown any improvement, for
> the distress which it caused me to find that I was not doing
> what he told me, and felt unable to do so, was sufficient to
> make me lose hope and give up the whole thing. (*Life*, ch. 23).

St. Teresa's balance and sense of proportion rested on a conviction of God's goodness. She suffered much, but counted it little. For it *was* little in comparison to the joy of closer union
with God which the suffering brought.

> All things fail, but Thou, O Lord of them all, failest never.
> Little is the suffering that Thou allowest to those who love
> Thee . . . Thou seemest, O Lord, to give extreme tests to those
> who love Thee, but only that, in the extremity of their trials,
> they may learn the greater extremity of Thy love. (*Life*, ch. 25).

St. Teresa's faith in the teachings of the Church was absolute
and rock-firm. Therefore, in seeking the Sacraments of Confession
and Communion she was esteeming things that were absolutely
real to her.

> The Lord had given this person [herself] such a lively faith
> that when she heard people say they wished they had lived
> when Christ walked on this earth, she would smile to herself,
> for she knew that we have Him as truly with us in the Most
> Holy Sacrament as people had Him then, and she would won-
> der what more they could possibly want. (Peers, Vol. II, p. 147).

The force of this faith drove her to find the complete inner unity
she needed for her unusual common sense. The Sacraments were
the visible instruments, not only in their supernatural efficacy,
but in the very efforts they occasioned and the conquering of
self they demanded, as she sought for understanding from her
spiritual directors in the confessional.

St. Teresa had a complete trust in God's providence. "To those who give up everything for Him, God gives Himself," she wrote. (*Life*, ch. 27). "Nothing is insignificant in our lives. Every event represents a divine opportunity, a divine call, a definite contribution to the intricate design of God's providence." (*SL*, Vol. 16, no. 4, p. 254). She says that God is watching and will care for you; therefore, she advises: "Cease to be anxious for yourselves, for He bears your anxiety and will bear it always." (Peers, Vol. II, p. 146).

To Suffer or to Die

St. Teresa had a longing for affection and understanding that could find fulfillment only occasionally, but most often she was left with an emptiness. Even while enjoying affection, she would recall its passing nature. When her father was dying, he asked the children to look at him and see how quickly he had reached his last day, reminding them that they should therefore serve God alone. He impressed upon them that nothing else matters. All things pass. We must soon part from our dearest ones on earth. These words of his left a lasting impression on St. Teresa.

Her conviction of the passing nature of life on earth, her sensitiveness, her tasting of emptiness, all helped to create a vacuum in her soul that could be filled only by God. This vacuum was increased immeasurably by her mystical experiences. As the hall is emptier and stiller after the play is over, and as the house is emptier and lonelier when a loved one goes away, so the soul of one who has mystical experiences suffers when her contact with the Infinite has passed. At the same time, the lingering "fragrance" of that experience gives joy and security. St. Teresa experienced the full range of mystical experiences: visions, locutions, raptures, levitations, spiritual marriage and the transverberation of her heart. (Her heart was pierced by the arrow of God's love. She actually saw it enter her breast and felt the pain as it entered her heart. When she had died and her heart was removed, it was found to have a hole in it.) These experiences began when she was about 40, and in her writings she has minutely and movingly described these favors from Almighty God. She has set forth in vivid words the anguish and the joy, the darkness and the light of a soul that willingly throws itself into the arms of the Infinite.

St. Teresa's soul had a natural disposition for the Infinite, trying always to do the utmost. Her mystical experiences magnified this disposition and also accentuated the feeling of loss, loneliness and emptiness that she felt when she was afterwards left to her ordinary human resources. She crystallized her feelings in this regard by the famous sayings: "I die because I do not die," and "To suffer or to die!" Whatever exact interpretation may be given to such sayings, they express a longing to do the utmost, to give her all, to return an immeasurable love for an immeasurable love received.

St. Teresa the Reformer

Archbishop Luigi Raimondi, in ceremonies at the Shrine of the Immaculate Conception in Washington, D.C. on September 27, 1970, remarked that "Teresa envisioned her great work of reform as beginning with herself, and even made a vow always to follow the more perfect course." (*S.L.*, Vol. 16, no. 4). Her whole life prior to the founding of the first convent of the Discalced Carmelites, St. Joseph's at Avila, may be looked upon as a preparation for the crowning activity of her life, which was the reforming of the Carmelite Order, both among the male and female religious.

Her work of reform began relatively late in her life; she made 21 foundations in her last 20 years—from the time she was 47 till her death at age 67. Among these were 17 convents for nuns and four monasteries for the Reformed or Discalced Friars, as they were called. St. John of the Cross, working with St. Teresa, is considered the Father of the men's reform.

St. Teresa made her foundations against extreme difficulties. There was a tangle of misapprehension, slander and open opposition to this work. Moreover, she had no funds. No doubt the devil used to the best advantage against her all the human weaknesses of those who surrounded her. St. Teresa purposely chose August 24 for opening San Jose in Avila because it was the feast of St. Bartholomew, who is invoked against the snares of Satan.

The first convent of the Reform, founded in Avila in 1562, was dedicated to St. Joseph. It was "home base" for Teresa for most of the rest of her life. The majority of the later convents were also dedicated to "the glorious St. Joseph," to whom was attributed St. Teresa's cure from paralysis. She said,

I wish I could persuade everyone to be devoted to this glorious saint, for I know from long experience the benefits he obtains from God. I have never known anyone who was truly devoted to him and performed particular services in his honor, who did not advance greatly in virtue . . . I only ask, for the love of God, that anyone who doubts what I say make a test of it himself, and he will see, from actual experience, the great benefit it is to commend oneself to this glorious Patriarch, and to have devotion to him. (*Life*, VI, 11-12).

St. Teresa had suffered from heart trouble and upset stomach for more than two decades. In her twenties she had been paralyzed for three years. She was very happy afterwards when she was able just to crawl again. Now in her fifties, she crisscrossed Spain by foot and on muleback or by mulecart. Her remarkable series of journeys began with that connected with the foundation at Medina at 2:00 a.m. on the Feast of the Assumption in 1567. Mass was offered at dawn, and thus the Lord came to San Jose de Medina. St. Teresa was determined to start this foundation at daybreak on this feast day.

Teresian Carmelites came to the U.S. in 1790, settling at Port Tobacco, Maryland, and later moving the site of the convent to Baltimore. They are now once again at Port Tobacco.

As of 1991, there were approximately 11,400 Discalced Carmelite nuns in the world. Of the 764 convents, some 67 were in the United States. Plus, there were approximately 3,700 Carmelite Friars in 426 monasteries worldwide as of 1991.

I Have Confided My Soul to You

"I write as I speak, and have no other care than to use words that clearly express what I wish to say, and I say this as simply as possible; affectation befits no language." (Hoornaert, p. 257). St. Teresa simply poured forth her soul in her writings. "Remember, it is my soul I have confided to you," she wrote when asking Louisa de la Cerda for a return of the manuscript of her *Life* (autobiography).

St. Teresa had no ambitions as a writer. She wrote not for publication, but for some immediate and private need. She had a great volume of correspondence in later years. "These letters are killing me." She wrote them to obey the directives of her superiors or confessors, but she wrote the *Life* and *The Way of Perfection* to provide practical guidance for the nuns of her communities.

This future Doctor of the Church asked Fr. Gracian (Jerome of the Mother of God),

> Why do they wish me to write? Let the theologians do it. They have studied, and I am only a simpleton. What do you want me to say? I shall put one word instead of another and so do harm. There are plenty of books on prayer already. For the love of God, let me go on with my spinning, go to choir, and follow the Rule like the other Sisters; I am not made to write; I have neither the health nor the intelligence for it. (Hoornaert, p. 229).

St. Teresa said she should rather spin than write, but with words she has spun out a delicate, beautiful portrait of her own soul, and in so doing she has traced out a pattern for other souls to follow who are striving toward fulfillment in God. For four centuries people have admired and tried to copy that portrait of hers in their own souls, and to follow her pattern in their own lives.

As one writer states, "there is probably no other spiritual writer who continues to address the great reading public just as naturally as when she first wrote. At the level of simple reading, needing neither study nor specialization, the level of that dialogue which fuses the thought of writer and reader, neither St. Thomas nor the Fathers of the Church have had the success of this enclosed nun." (*Mt. Carmel*, p. 23; Vol. 17, Summer 1969).

St. Teresa of Avila was declared the Patron of the Catholic writers of Spain on September 18, 1965.

She is also admired outside the Catholic Church. Patriarch Athenagoras of the Greek Orthodox Church said his most frequent spiritual reading was from St. Teresa and St. John of the Cross. Dr. Michael Ramsey, Primate of the Church of England, listed St. Teresa as one on whom Anglicans build their spirituality. Trueman Dicken, another Anglican scholar, in *The Crucible of Love* (1963), synthesized the doctrine of St. John of the Cross and St. Teresa on prayer. Even beyond Christian circles St. Teresa has won acceptance, for example, among Shintoist and Buddhist Japanese. The Communist R. Garaudy said: "For us Marxists, the two Spanish mystics, St. Teresa of Avila and St. John of the Cross represent the highest example of human love." (*The Pope Speaks*, Our Sunday Visitor, Huntington, IN, 1970, p. 223).

Saint Teresa's Writings

During the four centuries since her death, "There have been over 2,015 editions of her books in more than 22 languages." (*S.L.*, Vol. 16, no. 4, p. 215).

St. Teresa's major works are *The Life of Teresa of Jesus* (also called her *Autobiography*), the *Relations, The Way of Perfection, The Interior Castle* or *The Mansions,* and *The Foundations.* The smaller works include the *Constitutions, Exclamations of a Soul to God, Thoughts on the Canticle of Canticles, Manner of Visiting Convents of Discalced Carmelite Nuns,* and *Verses.* English translations include those by David Lewis, by the Benedictines of Stanbrook, by the Anglican scholar E. Allison Peers, and by the Institute of Carmelite Studies, Washington, D.C.

St. Teresa wrote her *Life* as a series of "Relations" or "things related" for her confessors, directors or Church authorities. She referred to it as the "big book" or the "book of the Mercies of God." The major manuscript of some 200 yellowed leaves, in a firm, masculine hand, is in the Escorial near Madrid. It was first written, then added to several times and finally recast during the years 1561-1565. The chapters on prayer are the heart of the work and make up a beautiful separate treatise.

The Way of Perfection St. Teresa called the "Little Book of the *Pater Noster.*" *The Way of Perfection* is really two small books. The first is an extended ferverino to the Sisters at St. Joseph's in Avila to follow the evangelical counsels (poverty, chastity and obedience) and make reparation for the sins of Catholics and the falling-away of heretics. The second is on the *Our Father* and gives a good idea of prayer in its various forms and degrees. Three chapters on the Holy Eucharist are very beautiful, "among the most beautiful and lyrical of all her writings." (Hoornaert, p. 228).

The Interior Castle or *The Mansions* was the best planned of St. Teresa's writings. She wrote it from June to November of 1577 at the insistence of Fr. Gracian, her friend and the regional Carmelite superior. The manuscript is at Seville in the Carmelite monastery there. St. Teresa pictures the seven degrees of prayer, by which a soul advances in perfection, as seven concentric mansions of a castle. The King of Glory dwells in the center, illumining all of them. Outside there are darkness and filth, vipers and ugly creatures. None of these can enter the Castle while the soul is in the state of grace. But if there is mortal sin in the soul, they have the power to penetrate the walls of the castle. In the first mansions, the soul commits many venial sins and sometimes falls back into mortal sin; in the second mansions, it is beset by and suffers more from the devil as it tries to be more purified; in the third, the soul progresses toward detachment even from venial sin. In the fourth and up through the sixth mansions, God intervenes in the soul with particular help, and it undergoes purifying "nights." The "mystical marriage" is celebrated in the sixth mansions, and "transforming union" takes place in the seventh mansions. This is the highest favor God can give a soul on earth, and a human being has then reached the apex of spiritual progress in this world.

"It is estimated that Teresa wrote about 15,000 letters, of which fewer than 500 have been preserved." (*S.L.*, 16, p. 214). Her letters always have "IHS" at the top, and she signs them "Teresa of Jesus," her name in religion. Only one preserved letter has the signature she used in her earlier days, Dona Teresa de Ahumada. The letters "deal with all subjects, her gravest concerns, such as the defense of the Reform, and her daily preoccupations, such as ordering fowl for the community dinner. She writes, burdened as she always is with business affairs, in haste, encroaching on her night's sleep, never, save most rarely, rereading what she has written, and with that charming conversational ease in which she excelled." (Hoornaert, p. 253). She wrote long letters to her brother. "Now I begin to write to you. I never know where to stop. God forgive you, for you are making me waste my time." About half her extant letters (240 out of 450) were written within a five-year period of comparative rest, with by far the greatest number being written in the 13 months (1576-1577) that she spent at Toledo.

New Insights from St. Teresa

One of today's over-worked words is "insight." Perhaps this overuse indicates an unconscious effort on the part of a bored society to express the thrill of childhood discovery. When new insight is obtained into a person or a thing or a situation, there is the thrill of discovery. It is the jump into the unknown and the finding of a safe and almost unexpected landing. Sometimes, when speaking of discoveries about people, there is the chill of discovery when something bad is uncovered. The human heart has strange depths of selfishness, and even the tears of old age often witness to new insights here.

St. Teresa shows how an expert in prayer gradually develops through new insights into his own interior. He discovers that he is selfish, tied by a thousand strings to inconsequential things, victim of a thousand dependencies on the opinions of others. Gradually, he purifies himself, becomes less and less attached to sin—which is another name for selfishness, or *is* selfishness in a variety of guises.

She shows that after a while, when enough insight (or self-knowledge) and detachment have been gained, God begins to take over. He gives new insights, and at greater depth. But these deep stirrings in the soul are knowledge in darkness. For a time, the person seems lost, and even his ordinary faculties seem to be confused or suspended. But an unknown peace and certitude pervade him. Then the intelligence begins to grasp this new knowledge and relate it to other conscious knowledge. Now there is conscious new insight. There is both the thrill and the chill of discovery.

There is the thrill of knowing more about God's love and goodness, of having a truer sense of values about all creation. But there is also the chill of knowing how far away the soul is from properly returning God's love. Step by step, God gives ever new and fresh knowledge in darkness, until finally the purified, self-knowing soul is able to enter into a state of constant union with God. Those who advance like this in mystical knowledge have a rare wisdom and often know much about various subjects, especially those arts and sciences that refer to understanding man.

The "prayer expert" is powerful in apostolic action, full of love for God, loving others far beyond the ordinary, selfish way typical of most people. He is truly a man of insight and wisdom. His knowledge of self, of others and of God makes him a human being developed to the fullest possible extent. His insight into God's creation is greater than that of the expert in any other field, and his value system puts each part of creation into the proper perspective.

The great artist or scientist does not always attain wisdom, for often he sees his own art or science in an over-emphasized way. He is in fact a person who may lead us the furthest astray from real truth. The prayer expert, however, sees things in better relationship to one another because his close union with the Creator gives him a better overall view of creation and the division of knowledge into the various fields of study. He knows man and other creatures better because he has a union with the Creator that gives him a sweeping vantage point from which to view things.

> Teresa's large heart, full of charity for all, originated many a shrewd psychological observation, while her sense of humor often brightened a simple, daily event into its true supernatural significance. The many disordered elements in human living were integrated by her rich personality . . . (*Mt. Carmel*, Vol. 17, pp. 85-94).

The Mystic Sees Total Reality

If one does not see reality in its totality, one does not really see reality. He sees a part, and his judgment about that part may be way off because he does not look on it as a whole. This happens when one operates on the principle that only the visible, material world is real, and when the invisible world is ignored or shrugged off, denied or decried.

Now Heaven, Hell and Purgatory, Angels, Saints and devils are either real or they are not. If they are not, then they *should* be denied and decried. If they are real, then they must be taken into consideration if we want to understand ourselves and know how we fit into God's creation, if we want to know how to direct ourselves and our thinking, if we want to know how to shape our values. The question of accepting or rejecting these things is really not one of religion only, but of psychology and mental health as well, of moral goals and the directives that shape human conduct. (It is often a question too of bodily health.) In short, looking at reality in its totality belongs to the full development of a human being.

It is in this respect that St. Teresa of Avila, who recalls to us the proper approach through prayer to the great and very real spiritual and invisible world, has a great role to play in the world today. Because she described so well and in such a realistic, detailed way the complete reality of life as she experienced it, she has a valuable gift to bestow upon us. She shows us the struggle that must take place within the soul before an harmonious interaction can occur between the visible and the invisible worlds. She shows us that there is an interplay and an exchange among body, emotions, mind, will, supernatural grace and mystical experience. And she shows how a person may succeed in his struggle to harmonize all these elements into a beautiful unity.

The Prayer Expert Knows Man

Our age is interested in man; it is proud of its going forward into new frontiers of knowledge in general and of knowledge of man himself in particular. Medical doctors, for example, know more now than ever before about the inner workings of man's body and how it functions. Man's mind and emotions have been given new and intense scrutiny by psychologists and psychiatrists. All that relates to man's environment, comfort and social welfare is under constant investigation. But in all this advancement of knowledge and in all this intense new looking into man, error has crept in. Many fundamental facts about man in relation to his final destiny have been forgotten. And this leads to a constant distortion about what man really is and how he should act, which in turn leads to errors that reach over into the observable part of God's creation. In other words, everyone today can see that there is something terribly wrong with man, but the vast majority do not see what it is.

St. Teresa of Avila has a message for our age, that to have a whole view of man, we have to look at him in relation to his final destiny. All things here on earth are passing. Therefore, man's spirit reaches out for that which will last. Many are looking for their pills when they would find a far better, and indeed lasting cure, by looking for their prayerbooks.

We Are Born to Be Mystics

St. Teresa of Avila calls out to our times to take a new, and to most of us, untried step toward knowledge of God. For we are all called upon by God to prepare ourselves for the gift of mystical experience. There are undoubtedly many mystics who are going about their daily work, but who could not even spell or define the word. Yet they too dip into that closeness with God in prayer where God takes over in a mysterious way. And they thereby grow in wisdom and understanding and charity, or divine love.

True mystical knowledge is a challenging frontier for our age. It is not, as some might think, something separated from all other kinds of knowledge. Rather, it integrates all other knowledge. It is not something for just a few. Rather, many, if they cooperate with God's grace, can dispose themselves for it. True mystical knowledge is not a psychological quirk, but is something that will integrate and pull together the elements of the personality and will turn one, in a newly found simplicity, to a strong and true love of God and of neighbor.

There is another way to say all this. St. Teresa's message for the modern era is, "Learn to pray." Prayer is the highest art. It requires perseverance, insight into self, insight into others, mortification and that humble spirit whereby the creature constantly looks up imploringly to the Creator. For by prayer does God fill His creature's emptiness with a new fullness, his darkness with a new light—that at first is a seeming darkness. And this new light illumines all creation. Then man, knowing that he is little and weak, becomes great and strong by leaning on the power of his Creator. Prayer, carried to the highest degree, will unite us with God and will also make us the most fully developed human beings. And St. Teresa of Avila, unlikely Doctor of the Church, is our sure guide on this path.

St. Teresa of Avila's feast day is October 15.

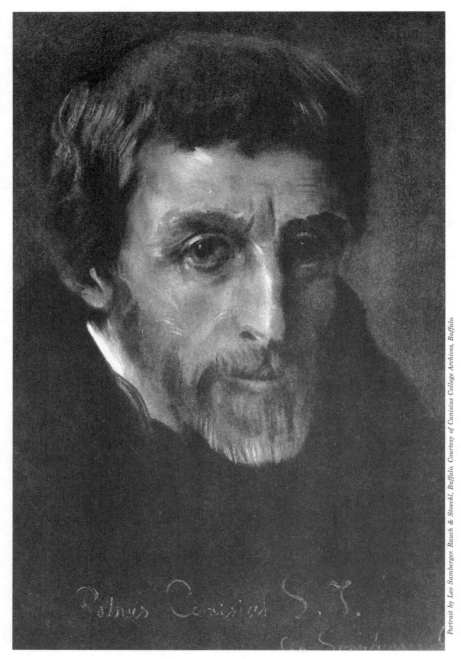

Portrait by Leo Samberger. Rauch & Stoeckl, Buffalo. Courtesy of Canisius College Archives, Buffalo.

Saint Peter Canisius

27

SAINT PETER CANISIUS
Doctor of the Catechism
1521-1597

ON a spring day in 1558, the Father Provincial of the Jesuits in southern Germany and a companion stood outside the door of the Jesuit house in Loreto, Italy. The porter would not let them in because they had no letter from their major superior. The explanation that one of them was himself the Provincial Superior left the porter unconvinced. He closed the door, and the weary Fr. Provincial sat on a bench to rest. About an hour later, one of the resident Fathers returned and was amazed to see Fr. Peter Canisius and his companion. Amid the apologies that followed, Fr. Canisius, Provincial of Southern Germany, excused the porter and commended him: "I have nothing to pardon; he has only done his duty."

The incident very likely made St. Peter Canisius the first Jesuit Provincial ever to be locked out of a Jesuit house. He also has a claim to other "firsts." He was the first German Jesuit; he became the first Jesuit to publish a book—when he put out a new edition of St. Cyril of Alexandria in 1546; he was the first prefect of studies when the Jesuits opened the first school of the Society at Messina in 1547; he founded the Jesuit house of studies in Cologne, the first Jesuit educational institution in Germany; he founded the first Jesuit university, at Dillingen, rescuing the almost defunct university of Cardinal Truchsess of Augsburg.

Born at the Beginning of the Reformation

St. Peter Kanis, or Canisius, was born May 8, 1521 at Nijmegen, an independent city then, and now a part of Holland. On this same day, Martin Luther was put under ban of Empire by the Edict of Worms, which marked the formal start of the Protestant Reformation. St. Peter's biographers point to the coincidence, for he was to become the leading figure in the Catholic Counter-Reformation in Germany.

St. Peter's mother, Aegidia, died when he was a child, leaving her husband Jakop (James) with three small children—Peter and his two sisters, Wendelina and Philippa. Jakop married again, and from this second marriage there were at least eight more children. St. Peter wrote of his stepmother, Wendelina, that nobody "could have been less of a stepmother to him than she." One of his half-brothers, Theodoric, followed him into the Society of Jesus.

In an account known as his *Confessions* (*c.* 1570) and his *Testament* (*c.* 1596), St. Peter Canisius accuses himself as a boy of contentiousness, fits of anger, jealousies, secret hatreds, arrogance, inconsiderate expressing of opinions on weighty matters, "like a blind man discoursing of colors," and carelessness in resisting temptations against purity arising from thought, desire and the conversation of the boys he associated with. His intense humility can be expected to underscore his faults, but his words tells us that he did have a nature that needed to be tamed and controlled. In early youth he also had the inclination occasionally to be deeply stirred spiritually and to give signs of his future vocation by playing priest, acting out the Mass, preaching, singing, and praying, all this sometimes before a group of playmates. He also liked to serve Mass. (*Confessions*, p. 12 of Braunsberger, Vol. 1).

A great factor in St. Peter's vocation was the friendship of a holy young priest, Fr. Nicholas van Esche, who gave him spiritual direction when he went to Cologne to study. St. Peter Canisius was then in his fifteenth year. In his *Confessions* he gives thanks to God, who had provided him with "such a master and daily counsellor of piety." Not only did he confess to Fr. van Esche, but he used to go to him often before retiring and tell him about all his falls, his foolish behavior and the things that might have stained his soul during that day. This openness and willingness to be directed would certainly lead him to great spiritual progress. (*Confessions*, Braunsberger, Vol. 1, p. 18).

On his birthday in 1543, while making a retreat under Fr. Peter Faber, one of the original nine Jesuits, St. Peter Canisius made a vow to enter the newly founded Society of Jesus. He did so and began his novitiate soon after. In that same year he had to hasten to the deathbed of his father. On June 12, 1546, he was ordained a priest at Cologne. The next two years he taught at Messina.

In 1549 St. Peter began a 30-year period which was spent

chiefly in Germany, where he accomplished the major work of his life. In his encyclical of August 1, 1897, Pope Leo XIII calls St. Peter Canisius "the second apostle of Germany after Boniface." He says that he cannot describe, but only mentions in passing,

> the details of this man of outstanding holiness; with what effort he labored to recall the Fatherland, torn by dispute and strife, to its ancient harmony and concord; with what zeal he entered the fray against the teachers of error; with what sermons he aroused souls; what troubles he endured, how many regions he traveled to, how grave were the positions of legate he took in the cause of the Faith. (*Acta Sanctae Sedis*, 1897, p. 4 of encyclical).

An important part of St. Peter Canisius' career can be summed up under the heading of education. He was "the most influential agent in establishing the Jesuit system of education in central Europe." (Hugh Graham, Ph.D., in *Jesuit Religious Instruction*, Vol. 16). He founded or helped in founding Jesuit colleges at Cologne, Vienna, Prague, Ingolstadt, Strasburg, Freiburg in Breisgau, Zabern, Dillingen, Munich, Wuerzburg, Hall in Tyrol, Speyer, Innsbruck, Landshut, Landsberg and Molsheim in Alsace. (*America*, Vol. 89, p. 107-108). In the last part of his life, he overcame unusual difficulties in starting the famous college at Fribourg in Switzerland. His English biographer, James Brodrick, S.J., remarks:

> By the close of the century, when he had been dead only three years, his brethren had forty flourishing colleges or missions in northern lands, scarcely one of which but owed its existence, directly or indirectly, to his influence with secular princes or dignitaries of the Church. (*St. Peter Canisius*, James Brodrick, S.J., London, 1935; Carroll Press, Baltimore, 1950, p. 337).

St. Peter Canisius had considerable influence in turning Pope Gregory XIII into "the Pope of the Seminaries." Gregory had given his name to the famous Gregorian University in Rome and had pushed the seminary movement, "the soul of the counter-Reformation" (Brodrick, p. 726), throughout the Catholic world. St. Peter's influence behind the scenes touches many other events of importance and can hardly be overestimated. At the later sessions of the Council of Trent, for instance, he kept the Emperor, Ferdinand, from pursuing a course that could have broken up that Council.

In 1580, at the age of 59 and considered an old man in those days, St. Peter Canisius went as a substitute to Fribourg, Switzerland to found a college. At Fribourg, he engineered the founding of the university, and there he spent the last 17 years of his life. His coming to Switzerland made a great difference to the faith of that country. "If the Swiss," said Pope Benedict XV in 1921, "have kept the Catholic Faith, after God, it must be attributed especially to the watchfulness and wisdom of this holy man." Above his portrait in the Church of St. Nicholas at Fribourg are the words: Patriarch of Catholic Switzerland.

Thirty years before, St. Peter Canisius and two fellow Jesuits had come to Germany. When he left it in 1580, never to return, he left behind him more than 1,100 members of the Society of Jesus. St. Peter Canisius was interested in the term "Jesuit" and wrote to Ribadeneyra (who had earlier sent him his biography of St. Ignatius for criticism) asking for a statement that the Society members had never arrogated the title for themselves. The origin of this name is still shrouded in mystery; whether it was first used in contempt or in compliment has never been settled. (p. 722). (In German, *Jesuwider* means something like "anti-Christ."

St. Peter Canisius was of medium height and somewhat stockily built. His face was ascetic, giving the impression of both severity and mildness. His nose was a bit aquiline, and his eyes very direct and open. Portraits show him with thick hair and a short beard, almost grizzled in the cheeks.

A Tireless Worker

Throughout his career St. Peter Canisius displayed amazing industry and versatility. It is hard to classify him during his different assignments. He was one thing officially, and he was many others unofficially. Whether he was a teacher, a legate or an administrator, he was still a confessor, a preacher, a visitor of the poor and sick. And he was always a writer.

Besides composing formal books, he engaged in a huge correspondence, and his letters were not little notes about private affairs. In his *Litterae Decretales* of May 21, 1925, Pope Pius XI says: "The same copiousness of his learning and doctrine, his same tireless striving for the divine glory, the same zeal for souls are breathed forth in the almost innumerable letters of this blessed man (you might better term them theological or ascetical tracts), which were lately edited in eight volumes." This document at once made St. Peter a Saint and a Doctor of the Church. (*A.A.S.*, Vol. 17, pp. 349-365).

The eight-volume work referred to was edited by Fr. Otto Braunsberger, S.J. It contains 2,420 letters either by or to St. Peter Canisius, as well as his *Testament and Confessions* and other biographical material classified as "Acts." The collection, which is entitled *Beati Petri Canisii Societatis Jesu Epistulae et Acta* (*The Acts and Letters of Blessed Peter Canisius of the Society of Jesus*), *1896-1923*, has 7,550 pages. "Certainly no saint in the calendar of the Catholic Church has had his correspondence edited with more devotion and scrupulous accuracy than Peter Canisius." (Brodrick, p. xv). Relatively little of this monumental work is available in English; however, many representative and important letters are quoted in the life by Fr. James Brodrick.

The vast correspondence of St. Peter Canisius attests to his industry and far-flung influence. It also provides a window that gives a personal and behind-the-scenes view of the turbulent civil and religious events of the sixteenth century.

Among St. Peter's correspondents were St. Ignatius, St. Francis Borgia, St. Francis de Sales, St. Charles Borromeo and Blessed Peter Faber. There were also three popes, two emperors, 12 cardinals, many bishops and other men of prominence. (Braunsberger, Vol. 1, p. xxvi).

In the last 10 years of his life St. Peter Canisius wrote many lives of saints, especially those honored among the Swiss. Included are St. Fridolin, St. Beatus, St. Meinrad and St. Nicholas of Flüe. His lives are not scientific and are historically uncritical, but they are aimed at promoting devotion. Yet even in this (for him) relatively easy kind of writing, he asked for prayers, "while I sweat with my pen." (He was working at the time on the life of St. Ursus and made his request to the people of Soleure, where the relics of the Saint were supposed to be.)

When St. Peter Canisius was working on his book about the Blessed Virgin, his half-brother, Theodoric, wrote:

> It is incredible how much the good Father fatigues and torments himself and many others with this business. We and all who know his studies consider it almost a miracle that he has not been overwhelmed and killed some time ago by the immensity of his labors . . . (Brodrick, p. 743).

The Provincial, Fr. Paul Hoffaeus, often a thorn in the side of St. Peter Canisius, became especially exasperated while Canisius was working on the *Opus Marianum*, entitled "Five Books on the Incomparable Virgin Mary and Most Holy Mother of God." He wrote to the General, Fr. Mercurian: "Father, that *Opus Marianum* of Fr. Canisius was a most grievous burden on this province for eight or nine years on end . . ." Fr. Paul said that St. Peter's various assistants

> groaned under his yoke and at last deserted him. Then he had recourse to extern assistants, but neither could they help him in the way he wanted, and the result was that he nearly killed himself with overwork . . . He submits all his writings to our professors of rhetoric, who find the imposition a nuisance. Finally, he is never able to get done with the matter under his hands, and in consequence distresses the printers, who have to look on while their work is altered throughout. If your Paternity can discover even one rector in this province who is ready to put up with such annoyances from Father Canisius at his college, I shall not oppose in any way, but rather help to promote the arrangement . . .

St. Peter's reaction was very mild: "I think that Fr. Provincial does not regard my writing activities with a very favorable eye . . ." (Letter to Fr. Mercurian, p. 733 of Brodrick). It might be surmised that Fr. Provincial was not exactly a patron of writers. He made short shrift of Fr. Peter Canisius' suggestion for a college of writers. "The whole world is full of books already. What we need are examples . . . Many of our men evade more necessary labors through a pretext of and itch for writing . . . In my opinion non-Jesuit writers are more diligent, accurate and careful in their work than our people . . ." (Brodrick, p. 732). Fr. Paul Hoffaeus, the Provincial, was not, however, unfeeling. In 1571 he wrote to Fr. Nadal concerning St. Peter Canisius: "His health now needs attention more than ever. He should not be allowed to kill himself as he does with his writings."

Preacher of the Word

Preaching was an almost constant task of St. Peter Canisius. Extant notes of his sermons cover 12,000 large sheets of paper. And his sermons were not mere 10-minute homilies, but long discourses, which use Scripture to such an extent that it may not be wrong to surmise that he knew the Bible largely by heart. Often the sermons were given to the most learned audiences in Christendom. At age 32, St. Peter was court preacher at Vienna. Often his sermons were given to men leaning away from the Church, to those who had already left or to those confused by the new religious teachings of the Protestants.

He usually wrote out the sermon in order to get things clear in his own mind; often he made a revision or several revisions. He had alternate beginnings and conclusions. Many times he worked much of the night preparing his sermons. At Augsburg, where he was the official city preacher from 1559-1566, he gave 90 sermons during the nine months of 1560 that he actually spent in the city. Even in his declining years, when he could no longer speak in public, he still gave exhortations to the Jesuit community on special occasions.

So great was the reverence people had for St. Peter Canisius at Augsburg that they knelt during his sermons. A visitor from Cologne found this especially remarkable, since in his own city a man who went down on one knee for the elevation was considered a devout Catholic.

St. Peter's sermons were direct and colloquial, aimed at leading people to piety and penance. Often tears flowed freely in the eyes of his audience; yet St. Peter Canisius was not an orator, nor was his language flowery; he was simple and plain, clear and sincere. But his sermons were effective, leading people to the Sacraments. The Christmas after he arrived in Fribourg, six people received Communion. Three years later there were 600 who received on this feast day. Even today his spirit lives on in this Catholic university city; he is truly Fribourg's Saint.

His sermons were very effective, too, in bringing about conversions and a return to the Faith among those who had quit their religious practice from carelessness or who had gone over to the Protestant Reformers. St. Peter's sermons were a bulwark among the people in holding the line against further losses to the Faith, and were a strong tonic in strengthening the faith of those who were weak.

His sermons and all his work was of course effective because of the good example of his life, and also because he stormed Heaven by prayer and penance in order to win graces for those he was trying to help. He relied a great deal on fasting as an aid to his ministry. As Pope Pius XI observed:

> . . . He rarely gave himself to unusual austerities, but relied
> often on vigils and fasting as arms for quickly and effectively
> overcoming the difficulties that would hinder his sacred min-
> istry. (*Decretal*, p. 18).

St. Peter often chided and spoke sternly, but compassion was
his keynote.

> We show our devotion to him [St. Nicholas of Fribourg] by
> stuffing ourselves and getting drunk—to him indeed who was
> such a pattern of Christian abstinence and moderation. We
> have forsaken our ancient patron and adopted Bacchus . . .
> (Brodrick, p. 781).

Concerning bad priests, he advised that when they gave Holy
Communion "it is the same Bread and the same Sacrament,
whether dispensed by Judas or Peter."

> If the minister of the Sacraments leads an evil life, think of
> him as an old basket in which good bread is carried. Permit
> that the bread be given you and leave the basket alone. Good
> pears and apples taste good even if taken from a dirty wooden
> dish. And is not he a fool who despises a gold piece or a gem
> because he found it in the mud. (Brodrick, p. 687).

A Man of Compassion

St. Peter Canisius was a man of tender feeling. This showed
in his care of the sick and the poor. He was much concerned
over the health of his fellow Jesuits for whom he was responsible. He was a great believer in "native air" as an aid to health,
and at various times he sent some ailing priest or brother back
to his home town, to reap the benefits of the climate.

To a priest who had caused him grave trouble, he wrote when
both were old and sick:

> I beg and shall gladly continue to beg that He may increase
> in you holy patience, which is the medicine you now most
> urgently need . . . I shall look forward with desire to seeing
> you in our heavenly fatherland, where we shall embrace one
> another affectionately.

St. Peter Canisius speaks often in his sermons about those
in want, and they are always referred to as "the dear poor." He

asked magistrates to investigate the condition of the poor and do something for them. He suggested that the money spent on large wedding banquets and other festivities might be better given to the poor. The merry-making before Lent he thought should include providing recreation and refreshment for those who were poor, infirm and troubled.

"Is it not inexcusable that there should be so many people in rags while our clothes chests are stuffed with abundance of garments?" he asked in a sermon. "And what defense can there be for women who are never done acquiring jewels and aids to beauty, who are always thinking of something new in hopes of outshining rivals . . .?"

In another place he says:

> Remember the words of the angel Raphael: Prayer is good with fasting, and alms more than to lay up treasures of gold; for alms delivereth from death, and the same is that which purgeth away sins and maketh to find mercy and life everlasting. On this St. Cyprian comments that without alms our prayers and fastings have little power with God. Many works of piety have been commended in the faithful, but no persons have been singled out by Christ so conspicuously or will be praised by Him at the Last Day so openly as those who have shown themselves kind and helpful to the poor. (Brodrick, p. 798).

St. Peter Canisius favored the southern demonstration of affection over the more stolid northern customs.

> I would like all members of the Society to receive an embrace before setting out on a journey . . . On the arrival or departure of our brothers. Italian charity rather than German simplicity should be our practice." (Brodrick, p. 415).

His attachment to friends was very real. "Without friends there is no living, and to take friendship away is nothing else than to take the sun out of the sky." (Brodrick, p. 833). To a Jesuit nephew he wrote about a year before his death: "See that you do not forget old Canisius, who is now a sick man, incapable of helping other people." (Brodrick, p. 832).

A Man of Simple Piety

St. Peter Canisius composed many devotional books, such as his *Manual for Catholics*. He did not in fact consider himself a learned writer, but rather he aimed at inspiring devotion. "There is nothing more excellent, more pleasing to God or more serviceable and necessary to men for the leading of a good and holy life than diligent and constant meditation on the life and sufferings of our Lord Jesus Christ." (Brodrick, p. 237).

He was forever asking for prayers for himself. At the beginning of a sermon, he would ask the people to join him in an *Our Father* and a *Hail Mary*, "that I may deal with the Word of God rightly, and that you may hear it fruitfully." (Brodrick, pp. 779-780).

He himself ordinarily prayed about seven hours a day: four hours in the morning, beginning at 4:00 A.M., and three hours in the evening. This custom he continued through his last illness, when he was hardly more than skin and bones and it was torture for him to remain long in any one position. And yet he fretted: "I am become for all to see a useless, fruitless sluggard, undeserving of the bread which I eat and the kindness which my brethren show me." (Brodrick, p. 815). He prayed the Rosary several times a day and murmured a prayer whenever he heard the hour strike. He had a routine at retiring: after getting into bed, he would draw five deep breaths, saying a special prayer at each breath, which expressed the sighing of a full heart after the glory of God and the good of mankind. "Strengthened by these five sighs, you will sleep happily, and He who can deny nothing to the longings of a loving soul, will in His divine power, fulfill these desires." (Braunsberger, Vol. I, p. 59).

When he offered Mass, St. Peter Canisius said the words "with an actor's precision." His Mass lasted about an hour.

In 1549, before leaving for Germany, St. Peter Canisius prayed in St. Peter's at Rome. He received a special grace then, which he describes in his *Testament*:

> Thou, my Saviour, didst open to me Thy Heart in such fashion that I seemed to see within it, and Thou didst invite me and bid me to drink the waters of salvation from that fountain. Great at that moment was my desire that streams of faith, hope and charity might flow from it into my soul. I thirsted after poverty, chastity and obedience . . . (*Testament*, p. 125).

Several times in his life he received some very special grace. These graces spurred him on to his extraordinary and persevering efforts. With St. Peter Canisius, as with all great servants of God, it should be remembered that these occasions *were* extraordinary. They were like the sudden insight of the poet, catching a vision of rare understanding and beauty. But the poet must labor to confine his bursting vision in the narrow limits of words and to express what can hardly be said. So too the receivers of some extraordinary grace must bend their natural powers and use the ordinary graces in an heroic manner, trying to shape events and other human wills according to the divine pattern of their momentary vision. It must not be imagined that because some holy person is raised to the heights that for him all becomes easy and that he stays on those heights. Cast back onto the plains, he keeps working and trying harder, just because he remembers the heights he has at times seen.

Devotion to Mary

In the explanation of the *Hail Mary* given in St. Peter Canisius' large *Catechism* (The edition of Antwerp 1587 is in St. Louis University Library), St. Peter Canisius expresses much confidence in the intercession of the Blessed Virgin Mary.

> To be sure, walking in the footsteps of the Holy Fathers, we not only salute the praiseworthy and admirable Virgin, who is as a lily among thorns, but we also believe and profess her to be endowed with such great power that she can listen to, assist and favor poor mortals as long as they especially commend themselves and their desires to her and suppliantly expect daily grace through her motherly intercession.

At the end of his *Opus Marianum,* he wrote expressing the love that kept him to this laborious task:

> Most August Queen, and most true and faithful Mother Mary, whom none implores in vain, I beg of thee reverently from my heart that thou, to whom all mankind are bound in everlasting gratitude, wouldst deign to accept and approve this poor testimony of my love of thee, graciously measuring its littleness by the good will that went to its making . . .

To a sodality at Cologne which offered public thanksgiving on the appearance of St. Peter's work on Mary, he wrote:

> By the same never-to-be-sufficiently-honored Virgin Mother, I most earnestly beg and entreat all who have embraced this sacred Sodality to be resolute and generous in their undertaking, assuring themselves that God's wonderful graces and protection will be with Mary's clients, not only at the beginning of their course, but much more abundantly as they go on in her service . . . (Brodrick, p. 755).

He told them that devotion to Mary was the surest ground for hope for the restoration of Catholicism.

St. Peter Canisius was active in founding and promoting sodalities of the Blessed Virgin Mary. At least one, which he founded in 1581 at Fribourg, Switzerland, has continued uninterrupted through the years. In his old age St. Peter Canisius used to climb to the shrine of the Blessed Virgin Mary at Bourguillon near Fribourg. This little shrine, located on a 2,000-foot eminence, is still in existence.

Pope Pius XI focuses attention on the title of St. Peter's Marian work and says: "For 800 pages, beside the exquisite learning, the tender piety by which Blessed Peter was enkindled toward 'the incomparable Virgin Mary and most holy Mother of God' (to use his own words) is poured forth with disarming candor." (*Decretal*, A.A.S., Vol. 17). The Pope also mentions that St. Peter Canisius died, "as it is piously believed, [with] the Mother of the Lord herself standing by." On the text of *Genesis* 3:15, St. Peter Canisius wrote in his *Opus Marianum*:

> To Christ alone has she [the Church] attributed the honor that He by a certain absolute and excellent power should tread the serpent underfoot and, at the same time, endow others, and above all his Mother Mary, with similar power. Nor do we thus make the Mother the equal of the Son, but rather proclaim His greater glory, in that not only personally, but through His Mother and many others, He acts against the old serpent so powerfully that they, though by nature weak, triumph over so great a foe and reduce all his strength and cunning to nothingness. (Bk. 5, ch. 9, cited in Brodrick, p. 646).

A Man of Moderation

One of St. Peter Canisius' finest traits was moderation. The bishops of Switzerland in a letter of May 1, 1921 said: "It is remarkable that in his large catechism, namely in the work which he wrote to defend the Faith of tradition against [then] current objections, he never mentions an opponent." (*St. Peter Canisius: A Champion of the Church*, by William Reany, D.D., Benziger, NY, 1931, p. 169).

He wrote to Lindanus, an aspiring young writer:

> Men of learning agree with me that much in your writings might be expressed with greater restraint, especially where you make unfair play with the names of Calvin, Melanchthon and similar people. It is the mob-orator's privilege to riot in such blossoms, not the part of the theologian. With such medicine we do not heal the sick, but render them the more incurable. The truth must be defended wisely, seasonably and soberly . . . (Brodrick, p. 339).

Again he wrote to the same fiery young man:

> I beg you to tone down any harsh passages there may be in the book, that we may admonish the erring in a spirit of meekness, rather than provoke them . . . (Brodrick, p. 341).

In Rome he cautioned a commission of cardinals who proposed severity in Germany to act rather with "*lenita et piacevolezza.*" (Brodrick, p. 690). He considered St. Charles Borromeo too strict in some ways and wrote to Aquaviva, the Jesuit General, "I prefer to be out of Cardinal Borromeo's company rather than in it, because I consider him too rigorous a physician for the spiritually weak and delicate Swiss." (Brodrick, p. 808).

As an administrator and superior, St. Peter Canisius was much easier on his subjects than he was on himself. When relieved of the office he wrote to the Fr. General: ". . . I have no doubt but that this change of provincials will be, not only a comfort to me personally but a pleasure and advantage to others in Christ Our Lord . . ." St. Francis Borgia was touched, and he commented on the way St. Peter Canisius laid down the burden "borne for 14 years so patiently in the continual stress of government, and with so much good zeal, integrity and prudence."

The Catechism

Even in our times, in some parts of Germany, parents were still asking their children: "Have you learned your Canisius?" The Saint's name became synonymous with the Catholic Catechism, and more than anything else he is remembered for his catechisms.

Pope Leo XIII wrote in his encyclical *Militantis Ecclesiae* (1897):

> And so it happened that for 300 years Canisius has been held the common teacher of the Catholics of Germany, so that in popular speech these two have the same meaning, to know Canisius and to remember your Christian doctrine. (Cf. *The Papal Encyclicals: 1740-1981*, 5 vol., ed. Claudia Carlen, IHM, McGrath, Raleigh, NC, 1981).

Pope Pius XI wrote of St. Peter Canisius' large catechism, *Summa of Christian Doctrine:*

> Clearly and concisely made up, always expressing genuine Catholic teaching, one can hardly express how much this book, almost up to our own times, has helped in the formation of the clergy and in refuting errors.

Even in St. Peter Canisius' own lifetime his catechism reached more than 200 editions and had been translated into 15 languages. A modified English version had appeared already in 1567. By 1582, the large Latin catechism was "common to be seen and solde" and "every man might have and reade" it in England.

Besides his largest catechism, the *Summa of Christian Doctrine*, he composed a little catechism for the very young and a smaller catechism for the groups that in age or education would be in between the other two. The large catechism in its original edition had 213 questions, the one for beginners had 59 questions, and the intermediate one had 124.

The catechisms were all written originally in Latin, even the smallest one, where religious truths were joined to the learning of grammar. In doing this St. Peter Canisius imitated Melanchthon, "the Teacher of Germany," who had attached Protestant doctrine to school books. Latin at that time was still the language of books throughout Europe, and in those days high school boys were required to speak only Latin during school hours. (We have fallen a long way on the language road, for today it is considered too great a task for a man with eight years of schooling after high school to acquire even a reading knowledge of Latin.)

The first catechism of St. Peter Canisius was published in the spring of 1555. The shortest one came out in 1556; it included prayers for meals, for morning and night, for when the clock strikes the hours, and others as well. At Christmastime of 1558 the *Smaller Catechism* was published. German editions soon followed. The edition of the *Smaller German Catechism*, combined with prayers and instructions, published in 1564 became the most famous of the Canisius catechisms.

Luther's *Shorter Catechism*, "a work of genius in its lucidity and conciseness," was first published in 1528. It had a great effect in promoting the Reformation. An authority on the writings of Luther has said that "the catechisms of Canisius had certainly as much significance for the Counter-Reformation as the catechisms of Luther for the Reformation." (Quoted in footnote, Brodrick, p. 251). Another writer said, in reference to Canisius' *Summa of Christian Doctrine*, "No other summary of the Christian Doctrine has had such a successful history." (Hugh Graham, Ph.D., *Jesuit Religious Instruction*, Vol. 16).

It is interesting to note that St. Peter Canisius' original catechism, the *Summa of Christian Doctrine*, was a substitute for a larger work, a *Summa Theologica*, which he had worked on unsuccessfully and gladly relinquished. It was to have been a manual for students of theology. The Jesuits had been ordered by King Ferdinand to compose a theological compendium, and St. Peter Canisius' unsuccessful effort was an answer to the King's desire.

St. Peter Canisius' success as a catechetical writer was not accidental. He succeeded in producing a work of marvelous simplicity because, for one thing, he labored much. Over 3,000 references to Scripture, the Fathers or Church Councils and other writers back up his text. His genius was to be simple in stating religious truths. He saw these truths in their most essential and simplest form. He was not what we would consider today a speculative or original thinker. But he was able to get to the heart of the matter and present it clearly.

The Protestant scholar, Dr. Drews, has stated:

> The catechism of Canisius has taken his name through the
> world and down the centuries. Hardly any other book has had

such a huge circulation as this, for 130 years after the date of its first appearance, it had gone into nearly 400 editions . . . The whole plan and lay-out of it is skillful in the highest degree, and the execution a model of lucidity and exact statement, unequalled among Catholic books. All the moral doctrines and commandments of the medieval Church [sic] here come to life again, and the strong emphasis laid on them makes one feel that the age of the Counter-Reformation has dawned.

He Answers the Magdeburg Centuriators

Flacius Illyricus, a disciple of Melanchthon, gave to the world about 300 writings; he was surpassed in productivity among Lutherans only by Martin Luther himself, who wrote about 400 works. Flacius was introduced to Luther's writings by a cousin who was a Franciscan Provincial. Under Flacius' direction a history of Christianity was planned and begun at Magdeburg. It was divided according to centuries, and so became known as *The Centuries of Magdeburg*; its authors are known as the Magdeburg Centuriators. The purpose of *The Centuries* was to discredit the Catholic Church, and especially the Papacy. Flacius pirated much of his material from the monasteries he visited, tearing and cutting out pages of manuscripts. Hence the term, "the Flacian knife."

St. Peter Canisius was much disturbed by *The Centuries* and expressed his wish many times for a thorough and competent answer to "that most pestilent work of the Magdeburgers." He considerd it a "great shame and crime that ecclesiastical history should be distorted in so many ways by the sectaries."

Eventually, and much against his wishes, he was himself commissioned by Pope St. Pius V to answer the Centuriators. He considered himself entirely unequal to the task and urged various reasons against it.

> My own unfitness, too, is to be considered, for being sorely distracted by the external cares of the Province, I feel a distinct repugnance to these graver studies. In addition, I am by nature an extremely slow and plodding person when it comes to serious writing . . .

It is true that one of the most distinctive traits of St. Peter Canisius was the meticulous and unremitting care he gave to his writing. He was forever revising, to the distress of printers.

His handwriting, too, is precise, giving evidence of an unusually careful person, laboring over every detail.

He planned to bring out three volumes, building an historical refutation around three persons: St. John the Baptist, the Blessed Virgin Mary, and St. Peter. St. Francis Borgia, the Jesuit General, relieved St. Peter Canisius of the office of Provincial so he could devote more time to this writing. For eight years he labored and worried his way through the first two volumes— never satisfied, always revising, held by obedience, wanting to do a good job and yet feeling inadequate. It was a real purgatory for him.

As usual he continued his schedule of preaching, visiting the sick and hearing confessions. Often some special task took him away from the writing for longer periods. Working at Dillingen on this book commissioned by a pope, he answered a call for help in hearing confessions at Augsburg. He also gave all the time he could to the instruction of children and illiterate persons. Many nights he spent keeping company with some poor sufferer. He thought nothing of traveling several days to help an individual family settle a quarrel.

The first volume, the one on St. John the Baptist, came out in 1571, and the *Opus Marianum* in July, 1577. The planned volume on St. Peter was never finished, as the author was mercifully relieved of the task. The volume on the Blessed Virgin had 780 pages and was divided into five books. Evidence of the immense work that went into it is attested by the more than 10,000 references to the Fathers and scholastic writers and the 4,000 Scriptural texts (in the revised edition of 1583).

A modern critic calls the work on the Blessed Virgin "a classical vindication of the whole body of Catholic doctrine on the Blessed Virgin" (Scheeben in *Manual of Dogma*, Freiburg, 1882, Vol. III, p. 478), and another ranks it "among the most important books which devotion to the Blessed Virgin has ever inspired." (Jansens, quoted in Brodrick, p. 748). (Bishop Jansens was a long-time rector of the Benedictine College of St. Anselm in Rome.)

That St. Peter Canisius was aiming his work especially at the people of his own time can be judged from the fact that he mentions Luther 140 times, Calvin more than 100, and Melanchthon 70 times. His efforts at this work and his zeal in the Catholic cause earned him from the Centuriators various unhistorical charges of misdemeanors and crimes and a choice list of epithets.

He was "the Pope's own donkey," "an impudent and miserable devil," "a gross blockhead," "a fearful blasphemer of God." Because in Latin his name is similar to the word for dog, he was often the subject of puns, being called such things as "a dog of a monk."

Colloquy at Worms

The Emperor Ferdinand wanted a conference at Worms, and he wanted St. Peter Canisius there. Canisius was against it, because he knew that no good results would come of it. The colloquy was to take place between leading exponents of the Catholic and Lutheran religions.

Nevertheless, St. Peter Canisius went as one of the six chief Catholic theologians. Philip Melanchthon was one of the six chief Lutheran representatives. The Colloquy of Worms opened September 11, 1557. When it ended, the last attempt of any great moment at bringing together Catholics and Protestants also ended. The historian Ranke gives the reason: "It is humiliating to be forced to record that the Conference was not broken up by disputes between the two great parties; it never got so far—the divisions among the Protestants themselves put an end to it altogether." (Brodrick, p. 418).

In the fifth session of the Colloquy, St. Peter Canisius asked for a clear statement in regard to Melanchthon's *Augsburg Confession*.

> In view of the fact that doctrines held by those who adhere to the Confession vary a great deal, and that at times they are in conflict with some of the Confession's most important articles, we ask those who stand by it to condemn openly and plainly, in common with ourselves, all teaching contrary to such Catholic truths as we defend and they do not repudiate.

In the sixth session St. Peter Canisius spoke again and pointed out the need for a fixed criterion of judgment if arguments were to be settled. "Where the sense of Scripture is clear and unambiguous, we do not appeal to the Church, but in doubtful places we prefer the common agreement of the Church to the private exegesis of changeable man."

St. Peter Canisius pointed out that important passages in Scripture, such as the words of Christ, "This is my body," were under dispute.

The Scriptures provide different men with different views, which they puzzle out in all sorts of ways and quarrel about among themselves. If all the mysteries of the Bible and all its evidences are so manifest, why do men find contradictory meanings in it?

Whenever the Bible is clear and distinct in itself, we gladly submit to its testimony and ask for no other authority or evidence. But as soon as conflict arises about the meaning of an obscure passage and it is difficult to decide rival claims to the true meaning, then we appeal with perfect justice to the constant agreement of the Catholic Church and go back to the unanimous interpretation of the Fathers. (Brodrick, p. 405).

After the sixth session, Melanchthon tried to eliminate the Flacians from the Conference. When he could not oust this powerful Lutheran group in the seventh session, Melanchthon and the ones who favored him walked out. Melanchthon is the man best known after Luther as the establisher of Lutheranism. Brodrick says: "Melanchthon is a great puzzle. Despite his unimpressive appearance, his stammering tongue and diffident manner, he had a fine brain and a character not only noble but in many ways full of charm." (Brodrick, p. 392). Melanchthon grew more bitter as he grew older. Brodrick comments: "Somewhere in his soul there seemed to be chained a protesting Catholic whose voice so troubled his conscience that he cried his heresy the louder in hopes of drowning it." (Brodrick, p. 393).

A Frequent Traveler

In those days, when "travel was travail," St. Peter Canisius made five trips from Germany to Rome. And his trips north of the Alps are so numerous that a map marking them can be clear only if it traces none but the longer and more important ones.

Very seldom did St. Peter Canisius say anything about the adventures or the troubles of his journeys. Once, sick with a fever, he complained about being forced to stay in bed for a day. Then he added: "May the Lord do what seems good in His eyes and make use of us, either sick or well, for His greater glory."

When Pope Pius V made St. Peter legate for promulgating the decrees of the Council of Trent in specified parts of Germany, he kept moving so much that he wore himself to exhaustion. During 1565 he walked or rode on horseback more than 5,000 miles. His comment about all this travel was laconic. "Troubles on the road and from the wintry weather were not wanting to us . . ." When writing to the Fr. General, he thanked God for the strength to complete these journeys, and confessed: "For the last few days I have been feeling exhausted and without my usual vigor." The grueling trip through Germany had begun at Innsbruck, with St. Peter spending eight days in bed with a high fever. His delicate tact had much to do with the acceptance of the decrees of the Council of Trent in the territory he had visited. (Brodrick, p. 640).

Quite often St. Peter and his companions had just enough funds to take them to the next Jesuit house. Then they would beg or borrow more. But St. Peter was very conscientious about repaying debts as soon as possible, even to the extent of borrowing (at least once) from one Jesuit house in order to repay another.

Although utterly poor, he never stopped for a moment in launching some project that would cost great sums, such as the founding of a college. (Brodrick, p. 345). He might at times have hardly enough money to buy a book, but he thought nothing of writing to the Pope to suggest his subsidizing of printers. Books he had ordered were forever missing him at one place after another, following him around. Then, to his huge joy, they would turn up unexpectedly somewhere else.

St. Peter's travels did not interfere with his writing as much as one might imagine. He could turn from the distractions of the road to concentrate on his work. One day he was dictating to a lay-brother companion when the brother had to leave on some errand. Later St. Peter Canisius heard someone enter the room and, without looking up, began to dictate again, saying: "You were certainly quick about your business, Brother." Still later, when his lay-brother companion did re-enter, St. Peter was much surprised to see Duke William of Bavaria taking his dictation. St. Peter asked the Duke's pardon. "I have nothing to pardon," said the Duke. "I willingly consent to be your secretary, deeming myself happy to be able to contribute to such a work." At this particular time, St. Peter Canisius was writing his much labored-over treatise on the Blessed Virgin. (Reany, p. 92).

A Patron for Many Causes

St. Peter Canisius received Holy Communion early Sunday morning, December 21, 1597. During the night he had had a fit of trembling, but he sent away the brother who had become alarmed at this. After receiving Communion, St. Peter Canisius, whose eyes were still good, read some prayers for about an hour; he was anointed about 3:00 in the afternoon. About an hour later he breathed his last so quietly that even those in the room could not tell the exact moment of his death. Two Capuchins were present at the death of St. Peter Canisius: Fr. Anthony de Canobbio, Guardian of the Monastery at Lucerne, and Bro. Leander Renaud, a novice.

St. Peter's relics are in the chapel of St. Peter Canisius in the Church of St. Michael at Fribourg, Switzerland. They were last identified in 1924, some months before his canonization.

On August 1, 1897 Pope Leo XIII issued an encyclical entitled *Militantes Ecclesiae* setting forth his ideas on the necessity of a full Catholic education at all levels for Catholic students. It was issued on the occasion of the third centenary of the death of Peter Canisius, at that time revered in the Catholic Church as "Blessed." Pope Leo extolled the role that Peter Canisius had played in many different ways in saving the Faith in Germany— in particular by his promoting Christian education, by his writing and by his founding of so many schools. In itself the issuing of an encyclical commemorating the anniversary of one not yet canonized was remarkable, and perhaps unique. Pope Leo XIII expressed a strong desire "that his grand example may be taken to heart, and may incite [in us] his love of wisdom, which never stopped seeking the salvation of men and protecting the dignity of the Church." (*Encyclical*, par. 9).

In his sermon for the canonization of St. Peter Canisius on May 21, 1925, Pope Pius XI seemed to register a mild complaint against his eminent predecessor, Pope Leo XIII. Pope Leo, he said, had spoken of St. Peter Canisius "with praise which seemed hardly to be suitable for one to whom the title of Doctor had not yet been assigned." (Reany, p. 199). Pope Pius XI, however, quickly came to the rescue of Leo XIII. For on Ascension Day of 1925 he both canonized St. Peter Canisius and declared him to be a Doctor of the Church, thus endorsing the words of Pope Leo XIII.

In 1897 Pope Leo XIII had commended "the valiant leader, Peter Canisius, as a model to all who fight for Christ in the army of the Church, so that they be convinced that the weapons of science must be joined to the justice of the cause . . ." He did so because he saw a resemblance between the times of St. Peter

Canisius and his own day, when "the desire for innovation and freedom in religious thought were followed by a decrease in Faith and very great laxity in morals." (Reany, p. 10-11).

Pope Pius XI saw St. Peter Canisius as "one of the creators of the Catholic press and especially of the Catholic periodical." (Reany, p. 158). In the last part of his document (*Litterae Decretales—Misericordiarum Deus, A.A.S.*, vol. 17) he expressed confidence in St. Peter Canisius' intercession as a patron of unity.

> And finally, what is closest to our heart, and which, relying on the very powerful prayers of St. Peter Canisius, we do not judge it rash to hope for—and this all are obliged to join us in fervently beseeching: that all the sheep of the Lord who have strayed from the True Fold of Christ . . . may hear the voice of His vicar, no matter how unworthy, and hasten to return to the saving pasture of truth, happily fulfilling in themselves that divine, infallible promise: "There shall be one fold and one shepherd." (*Encyclical*, par. 24).

These are some suggestions from the Popes that attest to the many-sided activity of St. Peter Canisius. He would indeed be a good patron for many causes: for those who fight for the Church with the weapons of science, for writers, for publishers, for librarians. And he would be a most proper patron for unity.

St. Peter Canisius would be at home in this day, when the printed word is so powerful, when there is admiration for the man of science, the man of moderation. He left no scientific or diplomatic stone unturned in his efforts for religion—not that he himself was expert in many fields, but he did recognize the need for expert scholars to bring out the truth. He was a great buyer of Protestant books, so they might be read by the proper persons and discussed by experts in the field. In the name-slinging age in which he lived, he was so noted for moderation that, despite his intense Catholicity, many people believed various reports that he had turned Protestant.

St. Peter used human means to the full, but he relied most on prayer, and he remained a man of utmost simple piety. If one will think of people living today who have that mixture of sternness and lovableness united to deep, tender piety, which was characteristic of the "old-time" German, he will see St. Peter Canisius. His spirit, especially as shown in his *Catechism* and his books of devotion, has left an indelible impression on the character of Catholic Germany.

Though our age can admire St. Peter Canisius in many different ways, perhaps it can best imitate him by a return to the sort of living, pulsating faith that animated his soul and drove him, for the sake of the salvation of others, to exert himself to such incredible limits. In our age, when faith has grown cold in the hearts of mankind, the life of St. Peter Canisius is a burning example for all to emulate, that we may bring true Christian meaning and perspective back into our lives.

St. Peter Canisius' feast day is December 21 (April 27 in the 1962 calendar).

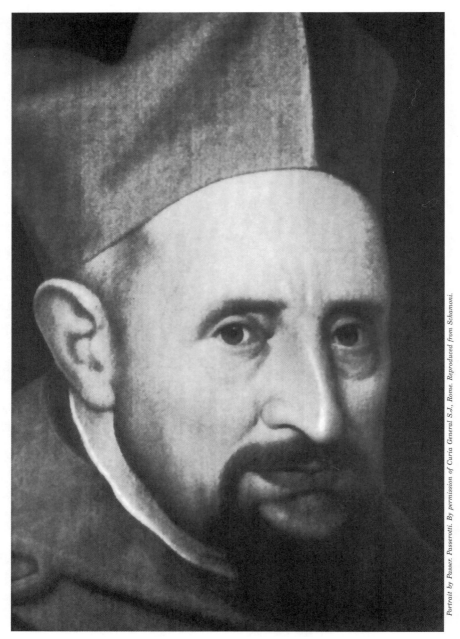

Saint Robert Bellarmine

28

SAINT ROBERT BELLARMINE
Prince of Apologists
Gentle Doctor of *The Controversies*
1542-1621

HIS first ambition was to be a doctor of medicine. His final triumph was to be declared a Doctor of the Church. He lived in an age of religious controversy, and he had the unflagging zeal, the capacity for work, and the intellectual equipment to make him a great champion. From what friends and enemies alike have written about him, the historical picture of St. Robert Bellarmine is that of a strong man, a fearless and brilliant defender of the Papacy, a great fighter for the Church. The name Bellarmine itself has a strong sound.

St. Robert Bellarmine deserves his reputation, but paradoxically he was a man whose great ability as a controversialist was equalled only by his strong distaste for controversy. Basically he was meek, compassionate, humorous, even whimsical, and very tender of heart. He felt the troubles of others so personally that he could burst into tears upon hearing of the death from starvation of a poor, unknown girl in Rome. Whereas his knockout intellectual punches were the talk of Europe, those who lived closest to him knew him most as a man of great heart.

Born into a Large Family—
He Enters the Jesuits

At the instance of two Jesuit friends, St. Robert Bellarmine wrote a small autobiography of 7,000 words. He tells us that he was born in 1542 of pious parents. He was the third son in a family of five sons and seven daughters. The family was noble, but of very modest means. The house in which the family lived still stands at Montepulciano in the hills of central Italy. Robert's father was Vincent Bellarmine, and his mother's name was Cynthia. St. Robert Bellarmine says of her: "She was devoted to almsgiving, to prayer and contemplation, to fasting and corporal austerities. As a result of these she contracted dropsy and died holily in the year 1575, 49 years old." With her accent on piety and her hope of giving the children an untarnished Christian character, she counselled her sons to play together rather than mingle with other boys. When Robert was about 14, his father wrote: "Times are so bad and expenses so great that I think I must have despaired had not God in His mercy come to my aid." Within the family Robert was especially close to his sister Camilla, in whom he confided as a child and whom he later often found it necessary to help when she married a husband who seemed not quite able to make a living.

Through acquaintance with Fr. Paschase Broet, a Jesuit priest who had come to the region for his health, Robert's mother conceived a strong liking for the Society of Jesus. She hoped that all her sons would become Jesuits. St. Robert first started to prepare for the study of medicine, but later, when the Jesuits opened a school at Montepulciano, he transferred to this school and at the age of 16 decided to enter the Society. For a time his father strongly opposed this because he had ambitions for Robert to become a cardinal if he chose a clerical and religious life, and the Jesuits forbade their members to accept such dignities. But Vincent finally gave in, and Robert entered the Jesuits at Rome in 1560 at the age of 18.

During his three years at the Roman College Robert was sick, suffering extreme fatigue, violent headaches, and being judged tubercular. Still, he made excellent progress in philosophy. Because of poor health he was given time off from study, but instead of convalescing taught humanities at Florence and Mondovi during the years 1563-1567. It was at Mondovi that he was assigned to teach Greek classics, although he knew no Greek. He simply told the students that he would first review grammar with them. In doing this, he learned while they reviewed, and when their review was finished he was ahead enough to teach Demosthenes. The secret of his success was not just in his talent, but also in his long hours of intense study during the night while others slept.

For three years his theological studies were made at Padua, but they were completed at Louvain, where he taught theology for seven years. Even in the years before his ordination, St. Robert Bellarmine preached. He was a powerful speaker, much sought after in his early years and indeed throughout his life. Even in the closing years of his life he gave exhortations to the

Jesuit novices and community. Because of his short stature, he stood on a stool in the pulpit. People who met him were often surprised because they had thought of him as a commanding figure as they listened to him in church.

St. Robert Bellarmine gives his ideas on preaching in a short essay, and among other items mentions that

> Three things are necessary for the attainment of the preacher's ends, three qualities of the soul without which his efforts will be unavailing. They are a great, vehement zeal for the honor of God, wisdom and eloquence. The fiery tongues which appeared above the Apostles when God made them the first preachers of His Evangel are the symbols of these things: the burning fire, betokening zeal; the light, wisdom; and the form of a tongue, eloquence. Eloquence without charity and wisdom is only empty chattering. Wisdom and eloquence without charity are dead and profitless. And charity without wisdom and eloquence is like a brave man unarmed. (Quoted in Brodrick, *The Life and Work of Robert Francis Cardinal Bellarmine, S.J., 1542-1561*, 2 Vols., by James Brodrick, S.J., London: Burns, Oates & Washbourne, 1928, p. 33. Also *Robert Bellarmine: Saint and Scholar*, by James Brodrick, S.J., London, Burns & Oates, 1961).

In 1576 St. Robert Bellarmine, again in poor health and thought by the doctors to have little time left to live, was recalled to Rome. Precise instructions given to him said he was to avoid Milan, where St. Charles Borromeo was most anxious to have him. St. Robert Bellarmine as a result spent most of the rest of his life in Rome, as teacher at the Roman College (1576-1588), as rector of the Roman College (1592-1594), and as a cardinal and theologian to the Pope (1597-1621). His longest stays away from Rome were as Provincial Superior of the Jesuits at Naples (1594-1597), and as Archbishop of Capua (1602-1605).

His father's dream and his own dread were realized on March 3, 1599 when he was made a cardinal. His brother Thomas, however, rejoiced in the place of their father, for he had been urging this honor for years. St. Robert Bellarmine was created a cardinal before he was made bishop. Pope Clement VIII left him no choice, for he announced the dignity and conferred the red hat both on the same day.

"We elect this man," said Clement, "because he has not his equal for learning in the Church of God." In a letter to the Society three days later, the Jesuit General, Aquaviva, wrote to the heads of the 32 provinces: "When he [Bellarmine] attempted to urge them once again, just before receiving the biretta, the Pope commanded him in severe tones to accept the dignity and to make no further protest." (Brodrick, p. 157). St. Robert Bellarmine himself wept during the ceremony.

Almost Elected Pope

St. Robert took part in three papal conclaves, the last one shortly before his death. In the first two, and especially in the second one, he was himself a prominent candidate for the Papacy. In his autobiography he says that in the second conclave, which eventually elected Pope Paul V in 1605, his prayer was: "From the Papacy, deliver me, O Lord." Others at the conclave noticed that he stayed to himself and was quite gruff, in contrast with his usual gaiety and affability, and that he walked around saying the Rosary. These were hardly maneuvers apt to win him any votes. "If picking up a straw from the ground would make me Pope," Bellarmine said, "the straw would remain where it was."

During the historic siege of Paris by Henry of Navarre in 1590, St. Robert Bellarmine happened to be in the city as theologian to Cardinal Cajetan, the Pope's envoy there. On this occasion, he predicted Pope Sixtus V's death to the worried Cajetan, who feared the Pontiff's wrath upon their return. "Your Lordship, he will be dead before the end of this year," St. Robert said. And events turned out as he had prophesied. He displayed on various occasions this same ability to prophesy correctly. In his autobiography he says of one such instance that it just came into his mind to predict something at the moment he actually said so.

Later in his life, when St. Robert Bellamine was a cardinal, a member of his household asked him in curiosity: "Your Lordship predicted the death of Pope Sixtus while you were in France, that of Pope Clement while in Capua, and now that of Pope Paul. How do you do it?" This was in 1619, when he was in much pain and not expected to live. St. Robert Bellarmine laughed: "Oh well, I'll tell you. All the popes either think themselves, or other people think for them, that they will reign such and such a number of years. Now what I do is to take away a third of that number, and thus I hit the mark." (Brodrick, p. 239). This, obviously, was a facetious way of drawing attention away from his gift of prophecy.

Referring to the time he was kept in Paris during the siege, St. Robert Bellarmine mentions dog-broth and a horse's leg as part of the menu. In the starving city, people ate dogs and cats; they dug up corpses and ground their bones into a flour which they baked; grease from cartwheels also served as food.

Bellarmine was connected with many men whose names are famous in history; he had much to do with events of long-range interest and importance. Under Pope Gregory XIV (1590-1591), he exercised a strong influence in revising the Latin Vulgate version of Scripture, as corrected by Pope Sixtus V, and wrote the preface for this revision. He was a close friend of Cardinal Baronius, the great Church historian, and he was the spiritual director of St. Aloysius Gonzaga. He worked closely with the Popes of the period, especially with Sixtus V (1585-1590), Gregory XIV (1590-1591), Clement VIII (1592-1605) and Paul V (1605-1621). He was a friend of Galileo and made known to him the decision of the Holy Office which said that the Copernican system could be taught as an hypothesis only. (St. Robert Bellarmine held to the Ptolemaic system taught by Aristotle, which was the current expert opinion.) Galileo was not unhappy about the decision of the Holy Office; it was later developments, after St. Robert Bellarmine's death, that caused the trouble. Till the end of his life Galileo always kept a certificate which St. Robert Bellarmine had issued to him, defending him against calumnies that had arisen. The statement is dated May 26, 1616.

> We, Robert Card. Bellarmine . . . declare that the said Signor Galileo has not abjured in our hand, nor in the hand of anyone else here in Rome, nor, so far as we are aware, in any place whatever, any opinion or doctrine held by him; neither has any penance, salutary or otherwise, been imposed on him. (Brodrick, p. 376).

Work in Spite of Sickness

One of the amazing anomalies about St. Robert Bellarmine is his immense output of work despite being sick a great deal of the time. He was near death a number of times in his younger years. On the way back from the siege of Paris, he almost died of a fever. He was amazed when he reached his middle seventies. He had thought that surely he would have died in his sixties. Certainly St. Robert Bellarmine did not continue to live because he coddled himself. One person who worked for him for 17 years testified that during that time St. Robert Bellarmine had never taken a siesta, although practically nobody in Rome could do without an afternoon nap in the hot months. He fasted three times a week and often dined on chicory and garlic, the food of the poor.

In 1584 he wrote to Salmeron:

> Last Whitsuntide, a disease of the nerves attacked me in the head and right arm and caused me the most dreadful pain I have ever experienced. For some days I was unable to make the slightest movement in bed and could not obtain a wink of sleep, even with the aid of opiates . . .

He was like St. Francis of Assisi in the scant attention he gave to his bodily needs, often enduring the cold, from which he suffered much, with no effort to warm himself. "The little loves of the flesh, of food and drink and pleasant converse with one's fellows," he said, "became like a bitter cross to St. Francis because his heart was filled with that love whose horizons are not closed by the Ganges or Caucasus." He used to say that he found it very difficult to attend to his most ordinary bodily needs, for "the more the love of God fills a man's heart, the less room is there in it for any natural desire."

When his brother Thomas kept bringing up the hope that he would be made a cardinal, St. Robert gave a number of good reasons why he could not accept this honor. He was not quite 57 at this time, and cited physical handicaps. "I have had to wear spectacles for the past two years, and the hearing of my left ear is almost completely gone. With the right one I can hear well enough if people speak up." (Brodrick, p. 140).

St. Robert's day, while a cardinal, began long before dawn. After several hours of prayer and Mass, he received visitors or attended meetings and functions. He served on most of the Roman Congregations. His Divine Office was said at such regular hours that his household attendants could always predict the order of his day, as other events followed on the completion of the various Hours. If he was with a visitor when the time for a canonical Hour came, he would courteously ask to be excused, and pray; this he did even when the visitor was another cardinal. If St. Robert Bellarmine was not seeing a visitor, attending a function or praying, he was reading or writing. When he retired he fell asleep instantly.

A summary of his writings drawn up in 1930 at the Pontifical Gregorian University cites 37 published works and an autobiography. Some are small; some run into many volumes. Among these works his catechisms should be mentioned. They proceeded from the instructions which he gave to lay brothers of the Jesuit community. They have been translated into 62 languages and have been used "from China to Peru." The small one is for children, and the larger one is a handbook for teachers.

In the last years of his life, wondering why he did not yet die, he brought out each year a treatise on the spiritual life. These books became popular with both Catholics and Protestants. The title of the first of these was *The Ascent of the Mind to God by the Ladder of Created Things*. It reveals much about St. Robert's cast of mind, which saw in all Creation a sacrament drawing man to his Creator. He wrote *The Eternal Happiness of the Saints,* and *The Mourning of the Dove or The Value of Tears*. All these books were written in his own hand except one brought out nine months before he died: *The Art of Dying Well*. From them we can see that his thoughts were primarily on eternity and his heart was sad at the troubles of the Church.

As might be expected from a man who suffered so much from sickness, St. Robert's mind throughout his life was often occupied with thoughts of sorrow and suffering. In his younger years he had written a treatise called *My Lady Tribulation*. Therein he told why a Christian should gladly suffer in this life.

> As in time nothing is present but a brief indivisible now, so the burden we bear can never in a true sense be more than momentary. We sip our chalice slowly and gradually, God putting the tiny drops of sufferings to our lips one by one . . . (Brodrick, p. 35).

The Imitation of Christ with its sadly serious outlook on this life was his favorite book.

St. Robert Bellarmine's unpublished letters run into the thousands. He was a busy man who wrote at high speed, and his handwriting is very hard to decipher. He also has a large, unpublished commentary on the *Summa Theologiae* of St. Thomas Aquinas which runs to more than 3,000 pages.

A Lovable Character

At times St. Robert was accused of being too meek. Once a poor stonemason was brought before him; the man had stolen a piece of porphyry from the cathedral. St. Robert admonished him, but then instead of a penalty, he gave him some money and made him promise never to steal again. To aid the poor fellow in his resolution, he sent him some money every month. On another occasion, when the poor priests of Capua could not pay a city tax, he went to the authorities and paid it himself. They took the hint and dropped the unjust tax.

St. Robert gave each person the impression that he or she was the only one who counted, and that his time belonged entirely to them. His expression and manner were consistently very friendly. St. Robert Bellarmine played the violin skillfully, as well as several other instruments; he also did some musical composition. As rector of the Roman College, he cleverly changed words of love songs to make hymns of them, and he had the students sing them for recreation.

St. Robert Bellarmine was often taken for 10 or more years younger than his actual age. When he was 52, he was visited by Fynes Moryson, an English Protestant, who left the following description:

> I came into Bellarmine's chamber, that I might see this man so famous for his learning, and so great a champion of the Popes: who seemed to me not above 40 years old, being leane of body and something lowe of stature, with a long visage and a little sharpe beard upon the chin of a browne colour, and a countenance not very grave and for his middle age wanting the authority of grey hairs.

His memory was photographic. He once told the English Jesuit, Thomas Fitzherbert, that he could memorize a Latin sermon of more than an hour's length by reading it over once. His powerful memory gave him great confidence as a speaker.

He was not too interested in speculative thinking. When he began his task of lecturing on controversial theology in Rome on November 26, 1576, he said in the inaugural address:

> Our concern will not be with little things that make no difference however they stand, nor with the subtleties of metaphysics, which a man may ignore without being any the worse

for it, but with God, with Christ, with the Church, with the Sacraments, and with a multitude of other matters which pertain to the very foundations of our faith. (Brodrick, p. 53).

St. Robert ends his *Autobiography* (which was not intended for publication, but was published anyway 132 years after his death) with a statement indicating his matter-of-fact humility.

These things *N.* wrote, being asked by a friend and confrere in 1613, the month of June. He has said nothing of his virtues because he does not know if he really has any; he has been silent about his vices because they are not proper to write about, and oh, that they may be found erased from the book of God on the day of judgment!

A person who watched St. Robert Bellarmine at prayer in his room said that during prayer he was as immobile and still as a statue. No doubt a man with his powers of concentration would readily lose himself in conversation with God. Yet he has very practical advice for those who cannot do so:

Since we find it difficult to pray because our souls are hard and dry and devotionless, then let us do as the parched earth does which yawns open and in a manner cries out for the rain. A humble recognition of our need is often more eloquent to the ears of God than many prayers. (Brodrick, p. 126).

Another witness wrote that Bellarmine celebrated Mass "with as much fervor, reverence, care and holy intentness of mind as if he saw God Our Lord standing there before him." The vividness of St. Robert Bellarmine's language about the Real Presence of Christ in the Holy Eucharist shows the simplicity and clarity of his faith in this great mystery.

When a testator says, "I leave my house to my son John," does anybody or will anybody ever understand his words to mean, "I leave to my son John, not my home itself standing foursquare, but a nice painted picture of it." In the next place, suppose a prince promised one of you 100 gold pieces and, in fulfillment of his word, sent a beautiful sketch of the coins; I wonder what you would think of his liberality. (Brodrick, p. 38).

Perhaps St. Robert Bellamine gives us a glimpse into the secret of his constant placidity when he explains the importance of bearing with one another's faults.

> When two pieces of wood are placed together in the shape
> of an inverted V, if each supports the other, both will stand;
> but if they do not, both fall to the ground. As this matter is
> one of such great consequence, try to look upon the defects of
> your companions as a kind of special medicine and [a] cross
> prepared for you by God. There are many people who willingly
> practice penances which they have chosen for themselves, but
> who refuse to put up with their neighbors' faults, though that
> is the penance which God wants them to bear . . . (Brodrick,
> p. 127).

The Father of the Poor

St. Robert Bellarmine was born on October 4, 1542, the Feast
of St. Francis of Assisi, and he died on September 17, 1621,
which is the commemoration of the stigmata of St. Francis. His
middle name was Francis. Like St. Francis, St. Robert Bellarmine
loved all creatures. He would rather walk than risk overtiring
a horse. He was like St. Francis in his life of constant prayer
and in his complete loyalty to the Holy Father. But above all
St. Robert Bellarmine was a man who treasured the riches of
poverty, who had a tender and compassionate heart for the poor.

He had this love as an endowment of nature; he had deepened it from the example of his generous mother; and he brought
it to perfection by striving to imitate his patron, St. Francis of
Assisi. As he remarks:

> St. Francis was not ashamed to go out and beg meat and
> other things for the sick, and he used to procure little delica-
> cies for them which he would never have accepted for himself
> . . . Indeed he could not look upon anyone in affliction with-
> out his heart melting within him . . . That is the test of real
> charity, to love the poor, the wretched and the loveless. It is
> easy enough to feel drawn to good, healthy people, who have
> pleasant manners, but that is only natural love and not char-
> ity. (Brodrick, p. 126).

As a cardinal, St. Robert Bellarmine had an almoner (dis-
tributor of alms) named Peter Guidotti, to whom he gave charge
of all his financial matters. When Guidotti complained about
having to pay a good sum to rescue a deserter from the army

who had appealed to St. Robert, he was told, as he himself relates: "I ought not to be so terribly cautious and strict about the merits of a case; that if we gave freely and generously, God would see that we did not become bankrupt; that if I did not have money at the moment, I could pawn something and get it that way." Guidotti said that he could easily write a book about his "experiences . . . [concerning] his Lordship's instructions and doings" in the matter of almsgiving.

The Cardinal's own ring was often in pawn to help out some poor person. So were some silver candlesticks and other silver pieces given him as presents when he received the red hat. Two times he gave away the mattress from his own bed, the second time with careful instructions to avoid meeting Guidotti on the way out. Even for his parents' graves St. Robert wanted just a simple memorial. "Let it be a simple memorial, for poor living men have greater need of my money than dead men have of rich tombs."

St. Robert Bellarmine had always suffered much from the cold. However, he did not go near the fire, nor did he wear gloves, until in the last years of his life his hands bled a good deal from the cold and he was forced to wear gloves. Once he was into his old age, his legs were so swollen that his gaiters would no longer fit. Asking the price of a new pair, he was told that they cost about 5 or 6 guilii, a trifle. He replied that this amount would not be a trifle in some poor man's pocket, and continued to use the old gaiters with longer strings.

When he gave away some drapes, his almoner—"Peter of little faith," as the Saint called him—complained very forcibly. "The walls won't catch cold," was St. Robert's laconic reply. When he would return home from some function, as many as 300 people might be awaiting him, seeking alms. He would answer Peter Guidotti's beseeching look heavenward with the reassurance: "These are the people who will get us to Heaven."

St. Robert Bellarmine received such people the same as he did friends or important personages. When a beggar came into his presence, he would stand up and remove his cap. He was generous too with those who worked for him, giving them free medical care and always paying their wages in advance. He himself never used the word "servant." When any member of his household conferred with him, he always accompanied him to the door, as he would any guest. Cardinal Bellarmine was easy on servants who broke household items, but he was very stern to anyone who broke the Commandments by cursing or impure or slanderous talk.

Not only did he give freely to those who asked, but he remembered those who were too embarrassed to ask, too reserved to beg. He sent out men to find such cases and helped them. He was often "taken in" by beggars who were not deserving. Some came back in disguise to receive a second alms. He knew this, but his principle was that it is better to be deceived a hundred times than miss one genuinely in need. No wonder the people of Rome called him "the new Poverello," referring of course to St. Francis of Assisi, his patron.

The Controversies

If an author is honored by the stir his books cause, then St. Robert Bellarmine was indeed much honored in his time when he published his most famous work, *The Controversies*. Under Elizabeth I in England, possession of this work was punishable by death, although a London bookseller claimed he had made more money "by that Jesuit than from all his other books."

The impact of *The Controversies* was so great that within a century almost 200 full-length books of reply had been written to refute it. In Bellarmine's time practically every Anglican theological writer in England wrote a reply from the Anglican viewpoint. A worried French Calvinist wrote: "Methinks it is not one Bellarmine who speaks in these pages; it is the whole Jesuit phalanx, the entire legion of them mustered for our destruction." (Brodrick, p. 76).

A backhanded tribute to St. Robert Bellarmine's greatness as displayed in *The Controversies* also came in the many names he was called: He was likened to the giant Goliath, who frightened the army of Israel. He was a "braggart dunghill of a soldier, a furious and devilish Jebusite." The dictionary still carries the word "bellarmine" for a pot-bellied jug made to deride him. No wonder that when Bellarmine visited England, the people came in crowds to view him. They were surprised to see a mild, scholarly-looking man, certainly no fierce gargoyle as the popular picture of him had it. He stood in the minds of many Protestants as the greatest champion of the Catholic Church, and some unintentionally paid him a compliment, as people in the fourth century had done to St. Athanasius. As in that earlier era some would pin the name "Athanasians" on Catholics, so in the late sixteenth century some referred to Catholics as "Papists" or "Bellarminists."

Bellarmine's writing of *The Controversies* developed from his lectures as professor of controversial theology in the Roman College. The fame of the lectures brought about a demand for printing them. St. Robert Bellarmine wrote out in his own hand the two million words of the three volumes. They were published in 1586-1593 at Ingolstadt. The lectures had been given during the years 1576-1587, when he was between the ages of 34 and 45.

Though the title indicates a negative approach, the material is chiefly a positive explanation of Catholic doctrine. Pope Pius XI said, in declaring St. Robert Bellarmine a Doctor of the Church, that *The Controversies* "embrace almost the whole theological field in their massive bulk." (*A.A.S.*, Sept. 17, 1931, p. 435). Another Doctor of the Church, St. Francis de Sales, when reduced to minimum baggage while traveling and preaching in the hostile and mountainous Chablais region of France, just south of Switzerland, tells us that he carried "no other books except the Bible and those of the great Bellarmine," meaning *The Controversies*.

The whole work of *The Controversies* can be summed up as a defense of the articles of the Apostles' Creed: "I believe in . . . the Holy Catholic Church, the Communion of Saints, the forgiveness of sins . . ." Volume I treated of the Church; Volume II dealt with the Communion of Saints through the Sacraments; and Volume III, on the remission of sins, concerned itself with grace.

In Volume I is found Bellarmine's defense of the Papacy. Pope Pius XI says: "He stood as such a defender of the authority of the Roman Pontiff, even to our own times, that the Fathers of the Vatican Council [Vatican Council I, 1869-1870] used his writings and ideas most fully." The decree declaring St. Robert Bellarmine a Doctor of the Church called him "the prince of apologists and strong defender of the Catholic Faith, not only for his own time but for all future ages." Fr. James Brodrick, S.J., the English biographer of St. Robert Bellarmine, says: "At Trent the Bible and St. Thomas ruled the debates; at the Vatican, the Bible, St. Thomas and Bellarmine."

In his own time St. Robert had the happiness of knowing that his clear-cut arguments had helped to bring a great number of people back into the Catholic Church. The Anglican Archbishop Laud spent much time in seeking flaws in St. Robert Bellarmine's arguments. He concluded that "If I could swallow Bellarmine's opinion that the Pope's judgment is infallible, I would then submit without any more ado. But that will never go down with me, unless I live till I dote, which I hope to God I shall not."

In doing his work, St. Robert Bellarmine had read practically all the Protestant works of his own century. An Anglican bishop called him a "man of stupendous reading." And contemporary spokesmen for Protestants said that Bellarmine's description of their opinions was "strikingly complete and faithful."

A fellow Jesuit criticized *The Controversies*, saying: "The Lutherans and Calvinists will have no further need of Luther's and Calvin's books. They can find all they want here." This shows the extent of the fair-mindedness of St. Robert Bellarmine in stating the Protestant case. Far from trying to distort the position of Protestantism, he quoted it very thoroughly. Then he proceeded to explain the teaching of the Catholic Church to refute it.

Dispute with King James

One of the points brought out in the process of the beatification of St. Robert was his reluctance to have his works published. *The Controversies*, for instance, were brought out in published form after much urging from friends. The lectures required a great amount of re-writing and editing before they were ready for the press.

Bellarmine's writings always flowed from the need at hand: his teaching, his preaching, giving spiritual direction, answering questions proposed by friends, or finding a solution to the difficulties brought up by books attacking Church doctrine. Many times he was designated by the Popes to write solutions for difficult problems.

Archbishop Goodier has commented on the way St. Robert Bellarmine's writings evolved from the need of the hour.

> Newman said of himself that, except for two books, he wrote nothing that was not forced on him by the circumstances of the moment. The same with even more significance must be said of Bellarmine. He wrote a Hebrew grammar because he was teaching Hebrew; he wrote his great book on the controversies because he had been appointed to the chair in the German College; he wrote his treatise *De Scriptoribus Ecclesiasticis* because he needed something accurate to fall back

on in his lectures; he wrote his ascetical works entirely as the outcome of the spiritual retreats and instructions which he had to give as spiritual Father in his old age. (*Catholic Mind*, 29, 429-38).

A famous example of how St. Robert worked can be seen in his two books against the proposition of James I of England. The King first wrote anonymously, and then under his own name in defense of the divine right of kings. He held, in accord with this theory, that kings are accountable to God alone, and that written law is merely whatever the king willed, a concession or a clarification of his will. The practical point at issue was the Oath of Supremacy which all English subjects were required to take, and which the Pope had condemned. Most English Catholics thought it against conscience to take the oath, and many died rather than take it.

King James wrote anonymously in his book, known as *The Apology*, that "the great and famous writer of *The Controversies*, the late un-Jesuited Cardinal Bellarmine, must adde his talent to this good worke, by blowing the bellowes of sedition and sharpening the spur to rebellion." He concludes, "Christ is no more contrary to Belial, light to darkness, and heaven to hell, than Bellarmine's estimation of Kings is to God's." (Brodrick, p. 278).

St. Robert Bellarmine answered the book under a pseudonym. Later the King wrote under his own name, and Bellarmine answered under his own name. In each instance St. Robert Bellarmine wrote under strict orders from the Pope and contrary to his own wish in the matter.

It is interesting to note that St. Robert Bellarmine held that the Pope's authority over temporal affairs was only indirect. The Pope could correct an erring king when his wrongdoing was opposed to the spiritual good of souls. St. Robert Bellarmine had had trouble by stoutly opposing the idea of the Pope's direct power in temporal affairs. Pope Sixtus V had in fact put the first volume of *The Controversies* on the *Index of Forbidden Books* because of this opinion, though the book was dedicated to him. (Another source states that the Pope threatened to put Volume One on the Index but died before doing so.)

Writing on the relative positions of pope, king and people, St. Robert Bellarmine dealt with the authority of the people. He held that the people have authority (from God) as a group, and that they single out one person to exercise it.

> Men are born naturally free in an earthly republic, and hence the people themselves possess political power immediately, unless they have transferred it to some king. (*De Clericis*, 1, 7). This power is in the whole multitude immediately, as in a subject, because this power is by divine right. And the divine justice has not given this power to a particular man; therefore, it has been given to the multitude. *De Laicis*, 6 (Quoted by von Kuehnelt-Leddihn in *The Tablet*, 195, 446, 1950).

A number of discussions have been carried on as to what effect St. Robert Bellarmine may have had on the thinking of the framers of the American Constitution. No direct connection has been shown, though the ideas are similar.

Devotion to the Blessed Virgin Mary

It may be more than a happy coincidence that on December 25, 1931 Pope Pius XI instituted the Feast of the Maternity of the Blessed Virgin Mary, and in the same year declared two great servants of Mary to be Doctors of the Church. The Divine Maternity is certainly the greatest privilege of Mary, and the two Doctors, St. Albert the Great and St. Robert Bellarmine, were certainly two of her greatest servants.

St. Robert Bellarmine's petition of August 31, 1617 for a definition of the Immaculate Conception makes him most likely the first bishop to ask formally for this declaration. When Pope Pius IX defined the doctrine of the Immaculate Conception in 1854, he did it as St. Robert Bellarmine had suggested in his 3,000-word petition—by means of a Papal Bull, rather than a General Council.

St. Robert, who was ordinarily the mildest of men, could be very incisive on occasion. He took Luther to task for comparing himself with the Blessed Virgin (Sermon 42, on The Nativity of the Blessed Virgin Mary). Then he proceeded to state strongly the position of Mary in the Mystical Body.

> The Head of the Catholic Church is Christ, and Mary is the neck which joins the Head to its Body . . . God has promised that all the gifts, all the graces, and all the heavenly blessings which proceed from Christ as the Head, should pass through Mary to the Body of the Church. Even the physical body has several members in its other parts—hands, arms, shoulders and feet—but one head, and one neck. So also the Church has

many apostles, martyrs, confessors and virgins, but only one Head, the Son of God, and one bond between the Head and members, the Mother of God.

St. Robert Bellarmine was strong in his statements on the place of Mary in distributing grace. She began her role as mediatrix, he says, with the free acceptance of the Angel's message. She then cooperated in every detail of the Saviour's infancy, the years at Nazareth and the Public Life; and finally and especially, she cooperated in His offering of Himself on the Cross. Christ wanted His Mother to share in that final agony.
"The Blessed Virgin," St. Robert says,

> suffered extremely when she beheld her Son hanging on the gibbet of the Cross; but she loved the honor and glory of God more than the human flesh of her Son . . . Thus did she blend her own affections with those of Christ, who also preferred His Father's glory and our salvation to the temporal safety and security of His human body.

On another occasion he wrote incisively to the nuns of San Giovanni in Capua.

> If the Blessed Virgin were on earth and wanted to become a nun, she would never be able to get into your convent, being a carpenter's wife . . . This will show you in what favor you will be with the Queen of Heaven and her divine Son, if you persist in such a spirit of worldly vanity. (Brodrick, p. 227).

St. Robert used to recall fondly that having been ordained on Holy Saturday of 1570, March 25, the Feast of the Annunciation, he celebrated his first Mass to honor the Annunciation. As a cardinal he made it a rule that his household should go to the Sacraments six times a year. Three of these were for feasts of Mary: the Annunciation, the Immaculate Conception, and the Assumption. His titular church in Rome was fittingly named Our Lady of the Way. His sermons on the various feasts of the Blessed Virgin thoroughly cover the field of Mariology.

It is in his own life, however, that the greatest evidence of his love for Mary can be found. Every day after finishing the Divine Office, he recited the Office of the Blessed Virgin. Every day he used to recite a Rosary after dinner, and again in the evening after Compline. He usually said the Rosary while walking back and forth. This in fact was his daily exercise and recreation. Every Saturday he fasted in honor of the Blessed Virgin.

St. Robert's confidence in Mary was a personal expression of his strong belief in her role as Mediatrix of all Graces. Logically, his confidence was unbounded:

> As Queen of Heaven and earth, she has only to ask the King for anything she wants, and it is already given to her. If therefore in spite of our Mother's power and willingness to help us, we sink beneath the waves of sinful desperation, we have only ourselves to blame for not having called upon Mary.

In *The Mourning of the Dove*, he tells about a person appearing to St. Lutgarde all clothed in flame and in much pain. When the Saint asked him who he was, he answered her,

> I am Innocent III, who should have been condemned to eternal Hell-fire for several grievous sins, had not the Mother of God interceded for me in my agony and obtained for me the grace of repentance. Now I am destined to suffer in Purgatory till the End of the World, unless you help me. Once again the Mother of Mercy has allowed me to come to ask for your prayers.

Then St. Robert drew this conclusion from the story:

> From this we may gather that there is not one of us who is so exalted in dignity or advanced in virtue that he does not need the maternal care of his Blessed Mother. Christ in His agony on the Cross had said to her: "Behold thy son." For centuries now she has been faithful to this commission, never allowing anyone finally to perish—provided he also has been mindful of those other words spoken to him by the Saviour, "Behold thy Mother."

The Famous Argument about the Operation of Grace

The end of the sixteenth century and the beginning of the seventeenth found a very bitter dispute raging about a fundamental theological issue. The dispute was known as the *De Auxiliis* controversy. It began in 1588 with the publishing of a book on free will by the Spanish Jesuit, Luis Molina. It ended in 1607 after two decades of stormy dispute. Two great religious orders were on opposite sides, the Jesuits and the Dominicans.

The book by Molina, *The Harmony of Free Will with the Gifts of Grace (Concordia liberi arbitrii cum gratiae donis)* was attacked by the Dominican, Domingo Bañez, the spiritual director of St. Teresa of Avila. Bañez first tried unsuccessfully to have the publication of the book prohibited. Before the dispute was over, the original principal contenders were dead. Molina had died in 1600 and Bañez in 1604.

Both positions affirmed both grace and free will. However the Dominican position favored efficacious grace whereas, the Jesuit position favored free will. Bañez and the Dominicans said that God by a *"praemotio physica,"* a "prevenient motion of grace," moves the will, independently of circumstances or person. Molina and the Jesuits said that by a *"scientia media,"* an "intermediate knowledge," God knows the decisions a person will make in a particular circumstance. He gives grace to those He knows will use it. He is like a prince who gives a horse to the man he knows will ride it to the right destination.

Pope Clement VIII asked St. Robert Bellarmine to write out an opinion, and Bellarmine did this, giving several suggestions: 1) the Pope should counsel brotherly love, and 2) each party should be forbidden to term the teaching of the other as heretical or even rash. He also stated that the question was as yet not capable of solution. The Pope rejected this advice and instead appointed a commission to solve the matter. Later he tried to delve into the matter himself. St. Robert Bellarmine reminded him that Sixtus V, in trying to correct the Vulgate, had caused much trouble; and that John XXII had held the opinion that the Blessed in Heaven do not yet have the Beatific Vision (until the Last Judgment and Resurrection of the body), "and slammed the door of truth in his own face." (Brodrick, p. 209). When Cardinal Del Monte told St. Robert Bellarmine that the Pope had made up his mind to define the matter, St. Robert replied that yes, the Pope had the power, but would not exercise it. "Why?" asked Del Monte. "Because he will die before he gets the opportunity."

In the end the final decision reached was very much the same one that St. Robert Bellarmine had suggested many years before. It is quite possible that in the influence he did exercise, he helped stem a movement against the Society of Jesus which could have ruined the Order. This theological dispute has still never been settled.

"The Art of Dying Well"

During his last illness, many cardinals and the Pope himself came to visit St. Robert. He never complained about the treatment of the doctors, which included bloodletting and making blisters on his legs; nor did he complain about the food, which most often he could not retain. His only complaint was that he could not offer Mass nor say the Breviary. He was even denied his rosary, but he won that back, although he was told to pause between decades and rest a bit. St. Robert Bellarmine complained: "Methinks I am become a mere secular man, and am no more religious, for I neyther say Office nor Masse, I make no prayers, I doe no good at all." (Coffin, quoted by Brodrick, p. 406). He was conscious to his last breath and kept praying, saying softly the name of Jesus. When he died on September 17, 1621, he was just a few weeks short of 79 years old.

The simple funeral he wanted did not turn out that way. People flocked to the church day and night. Thousands of rosaries were touched to his body. Two prelates stole his red cardinal's hat—though only temporarily. The brother infirmarian, appropriately named Finali, expressed surprise that so many distinguished men, ordinarily exact in conscience, did not scruple to strip the house of its linen, to catch relics of the blood at the embalming. "There were pious thieves so cunning that some of them cut away pieces of his miter that he wore, others the tassels and knots of his cardinal's hat, others the skirts of his vestments, others, other things, and what each would get, with great devotion he kissed the same, lapping it up in cleane linen, silke, etc." (From *A True Relation of the Last Sickness and Death of Cardinal Bellarmine*, by Fr. Edward Coffin, an eyewitness of these events).

St. Robert Bellarmine was originally buried in the Jesuit Church of the Gesù in Rome. In 1923 his body was transferred to the Church of St. Ignatius in Rome and placed near the body of St. Aloysius, whom he had loved and directed in the spiritual life.

The process of St. Robert Bellarmine's beatification dragged on for three centuries, despite the instantaneous proclamation of the people that this man was a "Santo." St. Robert Bellarmine had many opponents who fought his being declared a Blessed, urging all kinds of objections. Some objections, for instance, were based on his autobiography, in which with the utmost simplicity he tells of his intellectual achievements. This was pointed to as pride. But eventually Pope Pius XI declared Robert Bellarmine Blessed in 1923, and a Saint in 1930, finally declaring him a Doctor of the Church in 1931. His feast day is May 13, the date of the first appearance of Our Lady at Fatima, a fitting day for one who had such a childlike and complete devotion to the Blessed Virgin Mary.

It is also very fitting that a man with such a clear grasp of the eternal realities should be declared a Doctor of the Church. With regard to the virtue of charity, St. Robert Bellarmine had written this while at the University of Louvain in Belgium:

> Who is there in this illustrious home of learning who does not think daily as he goes to the schools of law, medicine, philosophy or theology, how best he may progress in his particular subject and win at last his doctor's degree? The school of Christ is the school of charity. On the last day, when the great general examination takes place, there will be no question at all on the text of Aristotle, the aphorisms of Hippocrates, or the paragraphs of Justinian. Charity will be the whole syllabus.

The following quote regarding preaching gives an insight into his thoughts on that subject:

> In order to stir in men's hearts the love of holiness, it is not enough to get angry with sinners and shout at them. Empty clamoring of that kind may, indeed, terrify simple folk, but its only effect on the educated is to make them laugh. In neither class will it produce any solid fruit. Therefore we must first of all appeal to the minds of those who listen to us, and endeavor by sound reasons deduced from Holy Writ, by arguments of common sense, by examples and by similes, so to convince them that they will be forced to acknowledge the ideal of living which we propose as the only one becoming a reasonable man. (Brodrick, p. 33).

On the transitoriness of life and the fleeting passage of time St. Robert Bellarmine had written:

> Once upon a time a poor fellow stumbled over the edge of a dizzy cliff. By a lucky chance, he managed in his fall to grasp hold of a little bush which grew from the side of the rock, but hope died in his heart when he peered into the crevice to examine the roots of his frail support. For what was it he saw? Two

mice, a black one and a white, gnawing ceaselessly at the roots, and already halfway through them. And such is human life, pitched perilously between two eternities. Day and night eat into it with never a pause. Soon they will be through, and what will happen then?

St. Robert Bellarmine is a great and yet a lovable patron. Those who bear his name will think of him less as the redoubtable Bellarmine, and more as St. Robert, "Father of the Poor," a man of kindly humor and ready wit, and of utmost consideration for others. The sick may forget about his being a strong fighter for the doctrine of the Church and think of him rather as one whose life was one long struggle with disease and pain. But anyone can take personal petitions with confidence to this Saint who in life never refused admittance to anyone who came asking for a favor and who would doff his Cardinal's hat and rise to meet a beggar.

St. Robert Bellarmine's feast day is September 17 (May 13 in the 1962 calendar).

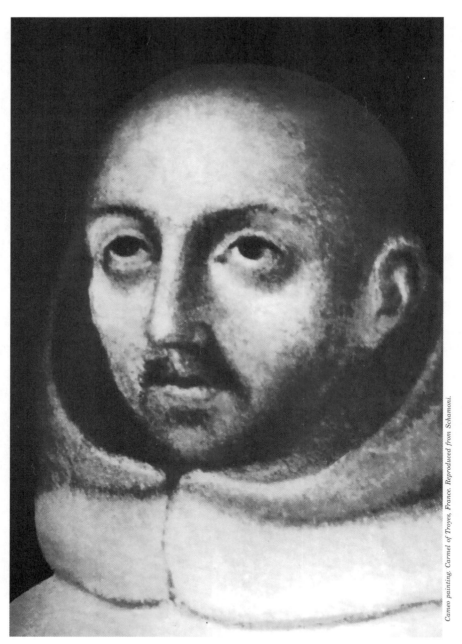

Saint John of the Cross

29

SAINT JOHN OF THE CROSS
Doctor of Mystical Theology
1542-1591

WHEN a young woman came very fearfully to his confessional at Avila, he encouraged her: "*I* am not so, but the holier the confessor, the gentler he is, and the less he is scandalized at other people's faults, because he understands man's weak condition better." Sometimes as superior in the monastery he coughed or rattled the rosary hanging from his belt, to warn an offending friar of his approach. This was St. John of the Cross, often and even commonly thought of as the utmost in severity.

St. John was essentially a very gentle person, yet very intense. If he drove a generous and well-disposed penitent and spiritual child hard, it was only to lead him to greater union with God. He was not anxious to catch anybody breaking silence or infringing on some other monastic rule. He was willing to look the other way; yet he never closed his eyes to what really needed correcting. His strong sense of justice and the desire to see others advance led him to impose punishments that were on occasion severe.

When his vice-rector at the College of Baeza, without consulting him, accepted an invitation to preach, he sent another priest instead to give the sermon. He could never compromise, but his sense of balance between justice and love was delicate. He hoped to lessen the punishments he imposed, when the charity of a third party would come forth to intercede. At times he even complained when none of the brethren would ask for mercy for one of their fellow religious. St. John of the Cross dipped deeply into the wells of contemplation, and his union with God reflected some of the justice and mercy of God, which to most mortals often seem apparently contradictory—unless a person can look far below the surface of things.

St. John of the Cross was a many-sided man—in both his character and in his teaching. He was a great lover of nature, perhaps more so than any noted Saint, except perhaps St. Francis of Assisi. Still, he taught that all natural goods and all natural beauty must be forsaken if we wish to find God. He was affectionate and attached to friends, yet he said we should love and be forgetful of all in an equal way. Even by his biographers St. John has been interpreted from opposite viewpoints: "It is a striking reflection," says E. Allison Peers, (Anglican) scholar of the University of Liverpool and translator of and commentator on St. John of the Cross, "that critics and panegyrists have in turn associated St. John of the Cross, more or less exclusively, with every one of the principal elements of his teaching." (*Tablet,* July 4, 1942).

From a Poor Family

St. John of the Cross was the third and last child of a nobleman father who had been disinherited when he married a common working girl. The father, Gonzalo de Ypes, died when St. John was an infant; and the mother, Catalina, had a hard time trying to support her three sons, Francisco, Luis and Juan, by her work at the loom. The boys had all been born at Fontiveros, then a town of 5,000 people, about 24 miles northwest of Avila. Luis died in childhood, and when Francisco was about 20 and Juan six, the widow and two boys moved to Arevalo. Three years later, poverty again forced a move, this time to Medina del Campo.

It was in this business center of 30,000 that "Juan de Ypes" went to school. He was placed as a boarder in the Catechism School, a kind of orphanage, whose program afforded him a chance to learn something about tailoring, woodcarving, carpentry and painting. A sketch he painted of a crucifix is still preserved at the Convent of the Incarnation of Avila. St. John was not really skillful in any of these trades, but throughout life he liked to work with his hands. From the orphanage he went to live at the hospital of Nostra Señora de la Concepcion, where he worked as a male nurse and also where he collected alms for the upkeep of the institution. While living and working here, he was also permitted to attend the Jesuit College in the city. After a very busy four years, he graduated in 1563.

It was poverty that forced these boarding arrangements. St. John was very close to his mother and brother. Later, when Francisco, also noted for his holiness, was helping as a laborer, building the monastery of Los Martires at Granada, St. John always introduced him as "my brother, who is the treasure I value most in the world." Not long before his death, St. John sent for Francisco to come and spend some time with him. When Francisco wanted to leave, St. John made him stay a few days longer, knowing this would be their last time together on earth. "Don't be off in such a hurry, for you do not know when we shall see each other again." Their mother had died during an influenza epidemic at Medina del Campo in 1580. At the time, St. John of the Cross had been far away in Andalusia.

He Joins the Carmelites

In his boyhood St. John had twice been saved from drowning, once when he fell into a pond at Fontiveros and later when he was pushed into a well at Medina del Campo. He himself has told us that the Blessed Virgin saved him both times. It is not surprising, therefore, that he was attracted to the Order of Our Lady of Mount Carmel. He entered this order at St. Anne's in Medina del Campo in 1563 at the age of 21 and received the name, John of St. Mathias.

After his novitiate, he spent four years studying at the Carmelite College of St. Andrew and at the University of Salamanca. His training in literature, philosophy and theology was very thorough, and he was a diligent and brilliant student. He was ordained in the spring of 1567 during his theological studies; the exact date is not known. At the time he offered his first Mass at Medina, in September, the great favor of being confirmed in grace was granted to him. His first assignment was as tutor to the young Carmelites of St. Anne Monastery in Medina del Campo.

He was still a newly ordained priest of 25 when he met St. Teresa of Avila, who was visiting Medina. At the age of 52, she was then just over twice his age. St. John was thinking of joining the Carthusians so he could lead a more retired and prayerful life. But the reforming Madre Teresa saw in St. John of the Cross the man she had been looking for. She told him he could find what he wanted in religious life by helping her launch a reform of the Carmelite friars.

After their first meeting, St. Teresa hurried to tell her Sisters: "Help me, daughters, to give thanks to our Lord God, for we already have a friar and a half to begin the reform of the Friars." (This could have been a way of emphasizing St. John's worth, if it refers to him alone. As usually interpreted, it refers to his small stature; he would be the "half," while Antonio de Heredia, to whom St. Teresa had already spoken about the reform, would be the "whole" friar.) St. Teresa used to refer to St. John affectionately as "my little Seneca." She also wrote in a letter: "He is not tall, but I think he is of great stature in God's eyes."

The Reform of the Carmelite Friars

The Father General of the Carmelites had already given permission to found two reformed monasteries in Castile. On November 28, 1568, the first house of male Discalced ("shoeless") Carmelites opened at Duruelo. Antonio de Heredia, the former prior at Medina, came there to be the first superior, under the name Fray Antonio de Jesus. From this time onward, St. John signed his name, "John of the Cross." St. John, his brother Francisco and a lay brother had done the work of altering the little farmhouse given to St. Teresa at Duruelo. The chapel was so small that one could stand only in the center of the room, but toward the rear he would have to sit or kneel.

St. John of the Cross was the first to wear the rough habit of the Reformed Carmelite Friars. It was actually he who shaped their spirit, and he must be considered as the first of the Discalced Carmelite Friars and the Father of the Reform. The elderly Padre Antonio just happened to be the first local superior, and a little later, the first prior.

Duruelo was found to be just too far out of the way and was therefore abandoned in less than two years, the Friars going to Mancera, three miles distant. Another monastery was founded at Pastrana, and this became to a large extent the nursery of the Reform. When things were going badly at Pastrana, St. John of the Cross went there for awhile to organize matters and give a more steadying direction to the new novitiate.

St. John of the Cross, the Prisoner

It was at Toledo that St. John went through the greatest and most dramatic crisis of his life. He underwent a severe test of his courage, endurance and faith. He was caught in the vortex of a dispute between the Carmelites of the Mitigated Observance and the Carmelites of the Reform. There were good men on both sides of the disputed question, and the correct answer was not so clear in the heat of the argument. The key to the trouble was a conflict of authority between the Prior General of the Carmelite Order and the Papal Nuncio in Spain. In 1575 at Piacenza in Italy, the General Chapter of the Order suppressed those monasteries of the Reform which had been founded without authorization of the General. Nothing was done to put this decree into effect, however, as long as Ormaneto, the Papal Nuncio, who was friendly to the Reform, was in office. After his death, however, and with the coming of Sega, a nuncio hostile to the Reform, the Calced Carmelites (Carmelites of the Mitigated Observance), calling on the civil arm of the law, had a number of the Reformed Carmelite Fathers arrested.

St. John of the Cross was taken prisoner in December, 1577, from his chaplain's house at the Convent of the Incarnation in Avila and brought to Toledo. He judged rightly that the decrees of Piacenza, which were read to him, referred only to houses founded without the Prior General's permission. But he would not renounce the Reform, as he was called on to do. Therefore, he was termed rebellious and contumacious.

He was imprisoned in the monastery in Toledo in a room ten feet by six, with a very small slit high in the wall being his only source of light. The room was really nothing but a large closet. Here St. John was locked in for nine months, suffering from the cold in the winter and the stifling heat in the summer. When he was brought out, it was to take his meal of bread and water and sometimes sardines, kneeling in the refectory, and to hear the upbraidings of the Prior. After the meal on Fridays, he had to bare his shoulders and undergo the circular discipline for the space of a *Miserere*. Each person present struck him in turn with a lash. St. John bore the scars of these beatings throughout his life.

There were other cruelties, for the conversation outside the dark cell dwelt on the complete crushing of the Reform. All the letters of St. Teresa of Avila to the King of Spain, Philip II, and others were to no avail. No one even knew where John was kept. "I do not know how it comes about that there is never anyone who remembers this holy man," she complained in one letter.

In the darkness of this cell, St. John of the Cross composed and committed to memory some of his greatest poems, including most of his book, *The Spiritual Canticle*, which is 40 stanzas in length. On August 14, when the Prior, the stern Fray Maldonaldo, came to St. John's cell and asked what he was thinking about that he did not rise, St. John replied: "That tomorrow is Our Lady's feast and how much I should love to say Mass." "Not while I am here," the Prior replied.

The Escape

Later, after his incarceration was over, St. John of the Cross never said a word against those who had treated him so badly. "They did it because they did not understand," he said in excuse. He bore no ill-feeling toward his "jailers," for his soul in its most inward part was unruffled and at peace and dwelt with God.

A change in jailers after six months brought a more lenient friar to be his keeper. But he was torn by doubt as to what was God's Will: Should he try to escape, or was it the will of God for him to die here? His searching prayer was answered by the conviction that he should escape. So he began to plan. While the others were at table, the more lenient young Father, Juan de Santa Maria, allowed St. John to help clean the cell. This included the liberty of walking down the corridor outside the room onto which his prison closet opened in order to empty the night pail. The jailer had also given St. John a needle and thread to mend his clothing. He tied a small stone to the thread and measured the distance to the ground from a window in the corridor. Back in his cell, he sewed his blankets together and found that they would, if used as a rope, reach to within 11 feet of the ground— close enough to permit a jump. Little by little he had also loosened the screws in the padlock outside the cell. On the night he planned to escape, two visiting friars happened to be sleeping in the room outside. They awoke when the padlock fell when St. John shook it, but they went back to sleep again, their sleepy eyes perhaps being closed by a wide-awake angel.

St. John stepped between the friars and silently let himself out through the window and down on his improvised rope. Had he landed two feet farther out from the building, he would have fallen to the rocky banks of the Tagus River below. He next found himself in a court surrounded by walls; he was almost ready to give up, but he finally succeeded in climbing one of the walls and was able to drop into an alleyway of the city. After daybreak, he found the convent of the Discalced Carmelite nuns, who sheltered him and later found a temporary refuge for him in the Hospital of Santa Cruz, very close to the monastery from which he had escaped. The friars from the monastery had come to the convent looking for him while he was there, and now little knew that the emaciated, nearly dead object of their search was being nursed back to life not a stone's throw away.

The Holder of Many Offices

St. John of the Cross escaped from his prison in August; in October he rejoined the brethren of the Reform in their meeting at Almodovar. When the results of this chapter were made known to the new Papal Nuncio, Philip Sega, he excommunicated all who had taken part in it. St. John, then enroute to his new appointment as Prior of El Calvario near Beas in the south of Spain, also fell under this penalty. However, the Reformed Carmelites finally obtained autonomy as a province in 1580 and as a religious order in 1593.

Meanwhile St. Teresa of Avila, that "vagabondish" woman, had been confined to the first convent founded at Avila; she had been greatly concerned over the outcome of the whole Reform of the Friars, which seemed to be tottering and ready to collapse. But in the height of the trouble, St. John of the Cross predicted a favorable outcome for the mission of the two friars who had been sent to Rome to present a petition for autonomy for the Reformed Order.

One of the striking aspects about the life of St. John of the Cross is the great variety of offices and places to which he was assigned. Before his imprisonment he was novice master at the early foundations, rector of the first College of the Reformed Carmelites at Alcala, and chaplain of the Sisters of Avila. After his imprisonment, he founded the Carmelite College at Baeza, was Prior successively at El Calvario near Beas in Andalusia, Los Martires near Granada, and Our Lady of Carmel at Segovia. St. John was Prior three times altogether at Los Martires and built the monastery near the Alcazar outside Segovia. He was also a definitor and counselor of the Reformed province. From 1585 to 1587 he was Vicar Provincial of Andalusia and as such traveled extensively, visiting the monasteries of the Discalced, both men and women.

It was during the five-and-a-half years he spent at Avila that St. John of the Cross was the spiritual director of St. Teresa of Avila. He had always spent a fair part of his time in the spiritual direction of nuns. He used to go to the convent at Beas, for instance, every Saturday and return on Monday. He spent his time there giving spiritual direction and conferences and hearing Confessions. In between he would work in the garden. Wherever he happened to be, he was consulted by many lay people in their spiritual problems, including both the most humble and the most distinguished. Whatever the official office he held, he was always actively and primarily a spiritual director.

A New Storm

In 1591 St. John came to the chapter of the Discalced in Madrid as First Counselor. Opposing the views of the Vicar General, Doria, he upheld at this Chapter the desire of the nuns to be free of subjecting their affairs to the council of the friars; he also wanted an inquiry about Father Gracian to be conducted more privately. As a result, the Vicar General decided to exclude him from any post of influence. St. John's offer to go to Mexico was accepted, and he was appointed to take 12 religious to the country. In the meantime, until the arrangements could be made for this trip, Father Doria thought of appointing him Prior of Segovia. But St. John wanted to be free from office. He was then sent to Andalusia, but assigned to no particular place, so he went to the monastery at La Penuela.

When in this isolated spot he developed a fever and ulcers on his leg, he was given a choice of two places to go: Baeza, where he was known and loved, or Ubeda, where he was little known and where the local superior, Padre Francisco Crisostomo, who had been corrected at one time by St. John, was hostile toward him. John chose Ubeda.

As a result of this, a storm broke over his head. Padre Diego Evangelista, along with Father Crisostomo, had suffered correction from St. John many years before. St. John had insisted that both of these men, who were outstanding preachers, spend more time in the monastery. Father Diego Evangelista, now in the position of definitor, worked to have St. John of the Cross cast out of the Reform. He set forth a process of defamation. News of this had already reached St. John at La Penuela. St. John wrote in a letter: "They cannot deprive me of the habit except for being incorrigible or disobedient, and I am more than prepared to make amends for anything in which I may have erred and to accept whatever penance they may give me."

Matins in Heaven

At Ubeda St. John's illness grew worse. The inflammation spread to his back. Father Crisostomo assigned him to an unsuitable room and grumbled about the growing interest in him of the people of the town and about the expense of keeping him. The medical and surgical treatment of the ulcerated leg was painful. Padre Antonio, now past 80 and the Provincial in Andalusia (who had started the Reform with St. John), came to visit him. Twenty-four years had elapsed since they had opened the first tiny house at Duruelo.

St. John asked pardon of Father Francisco Crisostomo for all the trouble and expense he had caused; Father Crisostomo, finally moved, left the room in tears, to become a more humble man and eventually to die with a reputation for holiness.

"What time is it?" St. John asked repeatedly on Friday night, December 13, 1591. "Tonight I have to go to say Matins in Heaven." At 11:30 p.m. he called for the friars to come and pray with him. He pulled himself up on the rope hanging from the ceiling above his head and prayed with them. As the bell of the church clock struck midnight, he kissed his crucifix and said, "Into Thy hands I commend my spirit," and quietly breathed his last.

St. John of the Cross had written that when the soul burns gently, having reached the ninth step of the mystical ladder to God, it departs from the body. (*Dark Night of the Soul*, Bk. 2, Ch. 20). Men attribute the person's death to some disease, but the person really dies because of mystical love and knowledge of God. When St. John died at midnight on that Saturday morning, he merely stepped to the tenth and final rung of the mystic ladder. Only St. Augustine can challenge him for the title of "The Greatest Mystic of the Church." And no one has written more clearly than St. John of the Cross on the mystical and "dark" ascent of the soul to God. Jacques Maritain, in his book *The Degrees of Knowledge*, says concerning mystical knowledge: "I hold St. John of the Cross the great Doctor of this supreme incommunicable knowledge."

The Doctor of Mystical Theology

A mystic is a person who is given knowledge about God, about Creation and about himself in a way that is beyond the ordinary manner of knowing. The ordinary process of knowledge is for the intellect to operate by way of abstraction from the "material" impressions presented by the senses. Memory and reason are employed in this normal operation of the mind. Mystical or contemplative knowledge, on the other hand, is communicated by God directly to the soul. The ordinary faculties of the soul are not operative; mysterious forces work within the soul which it cannot grasp or understand with its usual powers of memory, understanding and reason. St. John of the Cross therefore calls this contemplation "dark knowledge."

Contemplation, or mystical knowledge coming from God, is like a ray of light; it is loving wisdom. But when it enters the soul, it becomes "dark" contemplation. St. John asks the question: Why is it called "dark" if it is a divine light? "In answer to this," he says,

> There are two reasons why this divine wisdom is not only night and darkness for the soul, but also affliction and torment. First, because of the height of the divine wisdom, which exceeds the capacity of the soul. Second, because of the soul's baseness and impurity; and on this account, it is painful, afflictive, and also dark for the soul. (*Dark Night of the Soul*, Bk. 2, ch. 5).

If a person tries to experience what is actually going on, he cannot.

> This contemplation is active while the soul is in idleness and unconcern. It is like air that escapes when one tries to grasp it in one's hand. (*Dark Night*, Bk. 1, ch. 9). If a model for the painting or retouching of a portrait should move because of a desire to do something, the artist would be unable to finish, and his work would be disturbed. (*Dark Night*, Bk. 1, ch. 10).

Thus, the soul that tries to assist the process of contemplation can only interfere.

The Two Dark Nights

There are *two* dark nights of the soul caused by contemplation. The first is the "night of the senses." The second is the "night of the soul." The *night of the senses* is the loss of satisfaction and fervor in prayer and in serving God; it is what we ordinarily call dryness. This "sensory night" happens to many souls, and is relatively common among those who are striving for spiritual perfection.

> The spiritual night is the lot of very few. This night, which as we say is contemplation, causes two kinds of darkness or purgation in spiritual persons, according to the two parts of the soul, the sensory and the spiritual. Hence, the one night, or purgation, will be sensory, by which the senses are purged and accommodated to the spirit; and the other night, or purgation, will be spiritual, by which the spirit is purged and denuded as well as accommodated and prepared for union with God through love. (*Dark Night*, Bk. 1, ch. 8).
>
> The first purgation or night is bitter and terrible to the senses. But nothing can be compared to the second, for it is horrible and frightful to the spirit. (*Dark Night*, Bk. 1, ch. 8).

The first night brings the benefits of self-knowledge. With this will go a new awareness of the soul's own misery and weakness and a greater respect for and dependence upon God, plus a greater love of and esteem for one's neighbor. And the soul is ready to proceed. It has gone through the first purgatory, which aligns the senses with the spirit. The second will align the spirit with God. The first night is only the gate to the second. (*Dark Night*, Bk. 2, ch. 2). About this time, the person can be called a "proficient" instead of a beginner. About this time, too, raptures and dislocation of bones can occur; these are a sign of imperfection, because they represent a sensory reaction to a morsel of the deeper, "dark" contemplation. (*Dark Night*, Bk. 2, ch. 1).

As God continues to communicate loving knowledge of Himself to the soul, the soul goes through the darkness of the second night. It feels that it is hanging in mid-air, unloved by friends and forsaken by God; it feels empty, oppressed, tormented. "Only at intervals is one aware of these feelings in their intensity." (*Dark Night*, Bk. 2, ch. 6). Otherwise, death would result. The dark night will last for some years. In conformity with the degree of union God wants to grant to the soul, "the purgation is of greater or lesser force and endures for a longer or shorter time." (*Dark Night*, Bk. 2, ch. 7).

Psychologists may find one particular sentence of St. John of the Cross to be especially interesting. It describes how, shaken to the depths by divine communication, the person may show traumatic effects that are usually diagnosed as coming from an unhealthy disturbance.

Furthermore, he frequently experiences such absorption and profound forgetfulness in the memory that long periods pass without his knowing what he did or thought about, and he knows not what he is doing or about to do, nor can he concentrate on the task at hand, even though he desires to. (*Dark Night,* Bk. 2, ch. 8).

Union with God

St. John returns many times to the example of fire and a burning log. (*Dark Night,* Bk. 2, ch. 10). Mystical knowledge or contemplation is the fire; the soul is the wood. As the pure flame touches the wood, it dries up; impurities, like tar, run from it. The wood suffers, we might say, until it is purified and becomes like the flame itself, glowing and hot. The purgation of a soul on earth is similar to that of the soul in Purgatory. "The soul that endures it here on earth either does not enter Purgatory or is detained there for only a short while." (*Dark Night*, Bk. 2, ch. 6).

This process of communication by God of Himself to the soul goes on in ever deeper stages. Despite the suffering the person undergoes, he enjoys an abiding serenity and peace. At times there is a high degree of happiness. This happiness would represent a time when the soul was temporarily resting and not being favored by God with contemplative communication. When God again teaches the soul mystically, the person feels a misery greater than before. (*Dark Night*, Bk. 2, ch. 7). In the later stages of union with God, communication will be made "in the delight of love." (*Living Flame of Love*, Stanza 3, no. 34).

St. John says that the same process goes on in Purgatory and that the souls there for that reason have great doubts about whether they will ever leave; for each time God raises them by a new communication of loving knowledge of Himself, they feel that they have lost all that went before, just as the mystic soul on earth feels lost at each deeper communication of God. (*Dark Night,* Bk. 2, ch. 7).

Thus, the ordinary procedure in the contemplative life of the soul is one of communication, which produces pain, along with a mysterious loving knowledge, and of rest, which allows at times a high state of happiness. "This is the ordinary procedure in the state of contemplation until one arrives at quietude; the soul never remains in one state, but everything is ascent and descent." (*Dark Night*, Bk. 2, ch. 18).

As the soul grows closer and closer to divine union, its certainty and its strength and happiness in God remain more constant. The soul on earth can advance nine rungs on the mystical ladder. Only at the seventh step will the soul be daring enough to bargain with God for great favors. To do so before, and even here without real assurance that God wants this, may make the soul tumble back down the rungs it has advanced upon. (*Dark Night*, Bk. 2, ch. 20). At the ninth step, the soul will separate from the body; the mystic who comes to this stage always dies of love for God. The tenth stage of knowledge of God remains for Heaven.

Not many go on to the higher degrees of union with God, St. John says.

> It should be known that the reason is not because God wishes that there be only a few of these spirits so elevated; He would rather want all to be perfect, but He finds few vessels that will endure so lofty and sublime a work . . . As a result He proceeds no further in purifying them. (*Living Flame of Love,* Stanza 2, no. 27).

After outlining this process, it should be noted that the progress of contemplation in an individual person will be varied. There is no exclusiveness in the various stages; the activities of several stages may be transpiring at the same time. But at any one time the person is nonetheless primarily at one stage, that is, on one particular rung of the mystical ladder to union with God.

The Doctor of Nothingness

St. John refers often to a "nakedness of spirit." This means the most complete awareness of the soul's misery and the most ready submission to God's plans for it. It means the freedom from any attachment that may hinder it. Even a single attachment can stop its progress. "It is the same thing if a bird be held by a slender cord or a stout one; for both equally prevent it from flying away." Even a single attachment is enough also to "hinder the experience or reception of the delicate and intimate delight of the spirit of love which contains eminently in itself all delights." (*Dark Night*, Bk. 2, ch. 9).

St. John keeps insisting on complete detachment from things to assist in this activity within the soul, so much so that he has

been called "The Doctor of Nothingness." Everything less than
God must be rejected. To a nun who asked for direction, he wrote
"nada," "nothing," several times in succession across the paper.
In the drawing he made showing the ascent to Mount Carmel,
he used the word *"nada"* to substitute for every good of earth
and Heaven. The perfect soul goes to Mount Carmel, where it
meets God, by the path of nothingness. Nothing must be sought,
enjoyed or used for its own sake.

The poem that accompanies the drawing explains why and
shows that St. John of the Cross could just as easily be called
"The Doctor of the All," or "The Doctor of Everything."

> To reach satisfaction in all,
>   desire its possession in nothing.
> To come to the knowledge of all,
>   desire the knowledge of nothing.
> To come to possess all,
>   desire the possession of nothing.
> To arrive at being all,
>   desire to be nothing.
> To come to the pleasure you have not,
>   you must go by a way in which you enjoy not.
> To come to the knowledge you have not,
>   you must go by a way in which you know not.
> To come to the possession you have not,
>   you must go by a way in which you possess not.
> To come to be what you are not,
>   you must go by a way in which you are not.
> When you turn toward something,
>   you cease to cast yourself upon the all.
> For to go from the all to the all,
>   you must leave yourself in all.
> And when you come to the possession of all,
>   you must possess it without wanting anything.
> In this nakedness, the spirit finds its rest,
>   for when it covets nothing, nothing raises it up,
>   and nothing weighs it down,
>   because it is in the center of its humility.

St. John of the Cross says essentially the same thing as St.
Thomas Aquinas on this need for complete detachment from
creatures. Thomas Merton writes: "It will come as a surprise to
many to learn that the fiercely uncompromising principles on
which St. John of the Cross builds his doctrine of complete

detachment from creatures in order to arrive at union with God are sometimes quoted word for word from St. Thomas in these questions on beatitude. Practically the whole of *The Ascent of Mount Carmel* can be reduced to these pages of the Angelic Doctor." The reference is to the six opening questions of the *Prima Secundae* of the *Summa*. (*Ascent to Truth*, by Thomas Merton, Harcourt, Brace & Co., 1951, p. 132).

St. John speaks as a poet and as one who has personally experienced the things of which he writes. His writings are autobiographical. Bishop Alban Goodier comments on this theme:

> To interpret his works aright, one needs to keep in mind all the time the author himself and his experiences; then it will be seen that what he writes is not so much an exhortation to spiritual surrender as a continual cry telling what God has taught him by means of a suffering that is not easily paralleled. (*The Month*, London, Vol. 154, pp. 1-9).

A Safe Spiritual Guide

St. John is a practical, thorough and safe spiritual guide. The bull declaring his canonization says that he is a "guide of the faithful soul seeking to attain to the most perfect life." His treatment is clear and orderly and is based on Scripture and scholastic philosophy. "No other Christian mystical theologian builds on such clear dogmatic foundations, or with so powerful a framework of thought." (Thomas Merton in *Ascent to Truth*, p. 121).

Though St. John of the Cross wrote from experience, he relied on Scripture and Catholic doctrine and tested his experience in this way.

> . . . My intention will not be to deviate from the true meaning of sacred Scripture or from the doctrine of our holy Mother the Church. If this should happen, I submit entirely to the Church, or even to anyone who judges more competently than I about the matter. (Introduction to *Ascent of Mount Carmel*).

He puts the scholastic position on acquiring knowledge as plainly as anyone could do it.

> . . . As the scholastic philosophers say, the soul is like a *tabula rasa* ("a clean slate") when God infuses it into the body, so that it would be ignorant without the knowledge it receives

through its senses, because no knowledge is communicated to it from any other source. Accordingly, the presence of the soul in the body resembles the presence of a prisoner in a dark dungeon, who knows no more than what he manages to behold through the windows of his prison and has nowhere else to turn if he sees nothing through them. For the soul, naturally speaking, possesses no means other than the senses (the windows of its prison) of perceiving what is communicated to it. (*Ascent of Mount Carmel*, Bk. 1, ch. 3).

In declaring St. John of the Cross a Doctor of the Church on August 24, 1926, Pope Pius XI said:

Although they deal with difficult and learned questions, *The Ascent of Mt. Carmel*, *The Dark Night of the Soul*, *The Living Flame* and other works and letters of his abound in such great spiritual doctrine and are so adapted to the insight of readers that with merit they can be seen as a codex and a school for the faithful soul which strives to attain to a more perfect life.

In the same decree Pope Pius XI remarks that writers and holy men have found in him "a master of holiness and piety, and in treating of spiritual matters, have drawn from his doctrine and writings as from a limpid font of the Christian sense and the spirit of the Church."

Pope John Paul II issued an Apostolic Letter entitled *Maestro en la Fe* ("Master in the Faith") on December 14, 1990 for the fourth centenary of the death of St. John of the Cross. In it he recalls that he himself did his doctoral thesis in theology on the subject of Faith according to St. John of the Cross. In the thesis he gave special attention to what he calls the central affirmation of St. John: "Faith is the only proximate and proportionate means for communion with God." In the Apostolic Letter the Pope also portrays the Mystical Doctor as a saint for our times. "His writings are a treasure to be shared with all those who seek the face of God today. His doctrine speaks to our times, most especially in Spain, his native land, whose literature and name he honors with his magisterium of universal reach." (*The Pope Speaks*, Vol. 36, no. 4, pp. 217-228).

Misleading Warnings

There have been too many warnings in times past against the works of St. John of the Cross, as though they were dangerous or misleading. St. John merely spells out in remarkable and clear detail the path of the soul that takes seriously the words of Christ: "Amen, amen I say to you, unless the grain of wheat falling into the ground die, itself remaineth alone. But if it die, it bringeth forth much fruit. He that loveth his life shall lose it; and he that hateth his life in this world, keepeth it unto life eternal." (*John* 12:24-25).

St. John in his own lifetime was an unparalleled guide to holiness, and he brought many nuns especially to a high spiritual development. When Madre Ana de Jesus, the prioress at Beas, complained that so young a priest would call St. Teresa of Avila his daughter, St. Teresa answered:

> You have a great treasure in this holy man, and all those in the convent should see him and open their souls to him, when they will see what great good they get and will find themselves to have made great progress in spirituality and perfection, for Our Lord has given him a special grace for this. (*Life of St. John of the Cross*, by Crisogono de Jesus, O.C.D., translated by Kathleen Pond, p. 132).

In some places St. John speaks to beginners and in others to proficients; but he distinguishes carefully as to which he is addressing. Only those who would unwisely pick out a sentence here and there and use it indiscriminately to attempt to direct themselves or others, will get into trouble using the works of St. John of the Cross. Those just starting out on the way of spiritual progress must not vainly imagine that they can immediately ascend the final steep slope of Mt. Carmel. St. John's entire career shows that he considered spiritual direction very much an individual matter for each person.

There is something for everybody in St. John's writings. (Introduction to *The Ascent of Mount Carmel*). But he had a particular group of people in mind.

> My main intention is not to address everyone, but only some of the persons of our holy Order of the Primitive Observance of Mount Carmel, both friars and nuns, whom God favors by putting them on the path leading up this mountain, since they are the ones who asked me to write this work. Because they are already detached to a great extent from the temporal things of this world, they will more easily grasp this doctrine on the nakedness of the spirit. (Introduction to *The Ascent of Mount Carmel*).

St. John's eyes are always on the mountaintop, and he guides others that way. Those who want to follow him with care will find in him a good guide; those who do not wish to be guided by him can at least come to understand better the road they are walking on.

In sixteenth-century Spain, men spoke of "God's Indies," meaning the supernatural world of the mystic. This world awaits exploration by those willing to adjust their lives to high standards. The writings of St. John of the Cross are a map for those who are striving for the heights. "Only such as were bound upon a heroic adventure were bidden to strive after a heroic detachment, and none who believe a mountain in the heavenly realms to be indescribably the better worth climbing than a mountain in the Himalayas will begrudge those who set out to climb it, either their due preparation or the perils and hardships of the way." (*Tablet*, 159, 661. The article tells of Peers' Rede Lecture at Cambridge, May 12, 1932).

St. John of the Cross is no lover of mortification for its own sake. Rather, he is a lover of the fuller life to which mortification is a necessary path. Fr. Goodier says: "Juan taught them as one who knew, not as a hardened ascetic, but as a lover of life who had discovered a new world. This was the meaning of his Obscure Night and of his encouragement to men to brave it." (*The Month*, 154, 1-9).

One very important point of St. John's teaching should also be recalled. He wanted complete detachment from creatures, not absolutely, but only until they could be loved and used in such a way as to further the love of God. Even love for a friend or relative, if inordinate, is like excess baggage, definitely keeping a man from making progress up the heavenly mountain.

> Until a man is so habituated to the purgation of sensible joy that at the first movement of this joy he procures the benefit spoken of [that these goods turn him immediately to God], he must necessarily deny his joy and satisfaction in sensible goods in order to draw his soul away from the sensible life. (*Ascent of Mount Carmel*, Bk. 3, Ch. 26).

The conclusion one would draw is that when creatures can be loved completely in and for God, then they may be accepted along with the joy they bring. One writer says: "*Nadas* are not in the Saint's mind an end but a means, to be used in the beginning of the spiritual life to avoid the danger of inordinate affection in a heart which is still imperfect. Once purification has been effected, however, the need for this attitude ceases to exist, for the heart now purified and under control will draw good from it all. Then it not only can but must love all things, and the predilections imposed by the difference of persons and the nature of the heart—which in the saints is more genuinely human and sensitive than in others—will come to the fore, just as through this purification the disfigurements of passion will have disappeared, while the energies for good of the passions become confirmed and strengthened." (*Crisogono*, p. 311).

About Spiritual Directors

St. John warns very strongly against confessors and directors of souls who are ignorant and cannot distinguish between what is caused by sickness, the devil or the hand of God. He lists ignorant spiritual directors, along with the devil, as destroyers of spiritual progress. St. Teresa of Avila complained bitterly of directors who had harmed her. Of St. John of the Cross she said after he had left for Andalusia: "After he went there, in the whole of Castile I didn't find anyone like him."

St. John has a chapter in *The Ascent of Mount Carmel* (Bk. 2, ch. 18) on the harm caused by spiritual directors who misunderstand visions. He quotes the words of the Saviour (*Matt.* 15:14), "And if the blind lead the blind, both fall into the pit." Using the words of Scripture, he then discusses through three additional chapters the bad results that can flow even from visions and locutions from God, and how God is angered at our quest for revelations.

He includes strong words against spiritual directors who hinder souls:

> They are like the builders of the tower of Babel. When these builders were supposed to provide the proper materials for the project, they brought entirely different supplies, because they failed to understand the language . . . It will happen that, while an individual is being conducted by God along a sublime path of dark contemplation and aridity in which he feels lost, he will encounter in the midst of the fullness of his darknesses, trials, conflicts and temptations, someone who in the style of Job's comforters (*Job* 4:8-11) will proclaim that all of this is due to melancholia or depression or temperament, or to some hidden wickedness . . . (Prologue of *Ascent*, No. 4).

Discernment of Spirits

Once when in Lisbon, St. John of the Cross was urged to see Sister Maria de la Visitacion, a Dominican nun who had the marks of Christ's wounds in her hands, feet and side, and who was reported at times to be surrounded by light and suspended in the air. She was held in respect by many learned men. St. John's companion, Padre Bartholomew, came back with pieces of cloth dipped in her blood, as well as other relics. St. John refused to go to see her. Later, when the Inquisition revealed that the nun was a fraud, St. John explained that he did not go to see her because he knew that she was moved by no good spirit.

When he was confessor to the nuns at Avila, St. John of the Cross was called in by request of the Augustinian Father General to consider the case of a young Augustinian nun who, though uneducated, could explain the Scriptures in a wonderful way. Noted professors from the University of Salamanca had listened to her and had been favorably impressed. After St. John heard her Confession, he announced that she was possessed by the devil. The exorcisms which St. John was authorized to perform lasted several months and were attended by dramatic incidents of the nun's foaming at the mouth, going into convulsions, throwing herself on the ground and flinging insults at St. John. On one occasion, the devil even assumed the look of St. John and his companion and went to hear the nun's Confession. The deception was discovered when the nun told the Mother Superior that the confessor had thrown her into confusion, telling her things opposite to the usual advice. St. John of the Cross was sent for to set her right. Eventually, a script, written in her blood when she was six years old and made as a pact with the devil, was recovered.

In another case, St. John of the Cross exorcised a possessed nun on the feast of the Holy Trinity. He interrupted the exorcism to go to Vespers with the community. During the chanting, the possessed nun suddenly gave a leap and remained suspended in the air upside down. While all those who were praying stopped in amazement, St. John of the Cross commanded in a loud voice, "By the power of the Most Holy Trinity, Father, Son, and Holy Spirit, whose feast we are celebrating, I command you to return this nun to her place." The nun turned over and took her normal position in the choir.

St. John paid for all the good he had done in these exorcisms by temptations and physical assaults from the devil. Many times his bedclothes were ripped off in the cold of the night. But the devil paid tribute to St. John through the mouths of the possessed: "Nobody has tormented me since the time of Basil as this little man." "Now little Seneca is coming to do me harm," he said through the mouth of the possessed Sister Assuncion at Granada.

On one occasion St. John was sent to carry out an exorcism at Medina. After hearing the Sister's Confession he said: "This Sister is not possessed by the devil, but is weak mentally."

When as a young woman in Granada, Isabel de la Encarnacion wanted to join the convent, she had a long struggle with her relatives. Finally she won the day and was about to enter the convent. Then violent doubts and scruples took hold of her. St. John of the Cross, who was to give her the habit, heard her Confession, gave her Communion, prayed for her, and then led her by the hand to the convent door, telling her that her scruples would disappear. This happened as soon as she entered.

Proof that even the greatest of spiritual directors cannot foresee or pre-arrange all things, however, can be seen in the case of Sister Catalina Evangelista. St. John had chosen her along with others from several convents when he founded the convent at Malaga in 1585. Just a few months later, she lost her reason and threw herself through a window.

Some Practical Guidance

St. John always tried to inspire in the brethren complete confidence in Divine Providence. This was one of his own strongest characteristics. Juan Evangelista, second novice at Los Martires and St. John's companion on many trips and a cherished friend, once came as procurator to say that there was no food in the monastery. Could he go to seek an alms? St. John asked whether or not they could not do without food for a day or even more "if God wishes to prove our virtue." Soon Juan Evangelista was back again to say that there were sick in the house. Even then, St. John chided him for his lack of confidence in God. When Juan Evangelista came back a third time to say, "Fr. Prior, this is tempting our Lord," St. John told him to go, take a companion, and see how God would confound his little faith. Just beyond the monastery door, Juan Evangelista met a man who was already bringing them a large alms. "How much more glory would have been yours," St. John told him kindly, "had you stayed in your cell; there God would have sent you what was necessary, without your being so solicitous. Learn, my son, to trust in God."

It should not be imagined, however, that St. John of the Cross was impractical or presumptuous. As a youth he had begged for the hospital where he lived; and he had often gone out to seek some special food for the sick and made arrangements with benefactors for building monasteries and for other needs. It is up to the man of fine discernment to know when to go out and beg and when to stay at home and pray—or just wait for Providence to supply what is needed.

When St. John was Vicar Provincial in Andalusia, he sent seven novices with two brothers from Cordoba to Seville while a larger monastery was being constructed. When Brother Martin complained of having no provisions, St. John of the Cross had six loaves of bread and a few pomegranates put in a saddlebag. Gifts and alms met the group at every stop on the journey, and Brother Martin returned with 300 reals to hand over proudly to St. John. For this he received no congratulations, but rather a scolding: He should have returned home "more holy and with less money."

An example given by St. John brings out very well the value of learning how to get along without sensible devotion. He says that God

> is like a nursing mother who warms her child with the heat of her bosom, nurses it with good milk and tender food, and carries and caresses it in her arms. But as the child grows older, the mother withholds her caresses and hides her tender love; she rubs bitter aloes on her sweet breast and sets the child down from her arms, letting it walk on its own feet, so that it may put aside the habits of childhood, and grow accustomed to greater and more important things. (*Dark Night*, Bk. 1, ch. 2).

In line with this thinking, St. John was always quick to point out the value of suffering and mortification. The words "Do not seek Christ without the cross" crystallize his teaching. He wrote this in a letter to Juan de Santa Ana:

> If . . . someone, whether he be a superior or not, should try to persuade you of any lax doctrine, do not believe in it nor

embrace it; even though he might confirm it with miracles. But believe in and embrace more penance and detachment from all things, and do not seek Christ without the cross.

To Mother Ana de Jesus he wrote:

Things that do not please us seem to be evil and harmful, however good and fitting they may be . . . Now, until God gives us this good in Heaven, pass the time in the virtues of mortification and patience, desiring to resemble somewhat in suffering this great God of ours, humbled and crucified. This life is not good if it is not an imitation of His life. May His Majesty preserve you and augment His love in you, as in His holy beloved. Amen.

He consoled Maria de la Encarnacion, who grieved at his great, final afflictions and persecution: "Think nothing else but that God ordains all, and where there is no love, put love, and you will draw out love . . ." Practically all the marriage problems of the world would be solved if people would put this advice into daily practice. So too would the disturbing grievances in religious communities be eliminated.

Some of St. John's maxims point out the same thinking: "Whoever knows how to die in all will have life in all." "Suffering for God is better than working miracles." "Love consists not in feeling great things, but in having great detachment and in suffering for the Beloved." "Anyone who complains or grumbles is not perfect, nor is he even a good Christian."

St. John of the Cross often taught others how to mortify even good desires. Once on Ash Wednesday, when the Sisters were waiting to receive, he did not give them Holy Communion. "Today is a day for ashes," he explained. When St. Teresa of Avila expressed a preference for a large host, he gave her half a host. When a prior of a needy monastery asked St. John as Vicar Provincial to allow the novices from the two wealthiest families to stay there, he assigned to him two from the poorest families. We can readily believe that at times others would share the sentiment of St. Teresa: "Although . . . I have been vexed with him at times, we have never seen an imperfection in him." The little man so intent on teaching detachment could not help meeting a few less-than-willing pupils.

One can be sure, however, that St. John's words and actions were not chosen indiscriminately. "God leads each one along different paths so that hardly one spirit will be found like another in even half its method of procedure." (*Living Flame of Love,* Stanza 3, No. 59). Souls, he said, must not be tyrannized.

For some, meditation and active work will be better; for others, more contemplation will be proper. "Seek in reading, and you will find in meditation; knock in prayer, and it will be opened to you in contemplation."

A soul that has reached a certain degree of union with God may be harmed by external works.

> After all, we were created for this goal of love. Let those who are very active and who think to encircle the world with their preachings and external works learn then that they would give much more profit to the Church and please God much more, quite apart from the good example they would give, if they spent even half this time in remaining with God in prayer, even though they had not arrived at such a high point as this. It is certain that they would then do more and with less labor with one work than they do now with a thousand, for their prayer would merit this, and they would have gathered spiritual strength in it; for to act in any other way is to hammer vigorously and accomplish little more than nothing, and at times nothing at all, and it may even sometimes do harm. (*Spiritual Canticle*).

His Writings

St. John's major prose works are *The Ascent of Mount Carmel, The Dark Night of the Soul, The Spiritual Canticle* and *The Living Flame of Love*. All were written in response to requests for more detailed explanations of his poems and his conferences. St. John's poems, composed for the most part in prison, and his sentences, written on slips of paper and given to individual nuns, marked the beginning of his writing career. Since nothing of his writings was published until 27 years after his death, St. John of the Cross never saw any of his own books in print.

St. John's four major prose works offer a complete ascetical and mystical theology. They could be considered as one work.

The Spiritual Canticle and *The Living Flame of Love* (especially the latter) deal with the higher states of union with God on earth through contemplation.

The Ascent of Mount Carmel and *The Dark Night of the Soul* in a certain sense really form one work. Both titles comment on the same poem. *The Ascent of Mount Carmel* treats the poem from the viewpoint of active purgation and spiritual development in knowledge and love of God. *The Dark Night of the Soul* comments on it from the viewpoint of passive purgation and growth in the loving knowledge of God. The poem is just eight stanzas long and contains the essence of all St. John's thought. Because of its importance, it is quoted here in its entirety:

1. One dark night,
     Fired with love's urgent longings
     —Ah, the sheer grace!—
     I went out unseen,
     My house being now all stilled;

2. In darkness, and secure,
     By the secret ladder, disguised,
     —Ah, the sheer grace!—
     In darkness and concealment,
     My house being now all stilled;

3. On that glad night,
     In secret, for no one saw me,
     Nor did I look at anything,
     With no other light or guide
     Than the one that burned in my heart;

4. This guided me
     More surely than the light of noon
     To where He waited for me
     —Him I knew so well—
     In a place where no one else appeared.

5. O guiding night!
     O night more lovely than the dawn!
     O night that has united
     The Lover with His beloved,
     Transforming the beloved in her Lover.

6. Upon my flowering breast
     Which I kept wholly for Him alone,
     There He lay sleeping,
     And I caressing Him
     There in a breeze from the fanning cedars.

7. When the breeze flew from the turret
     Parting His hair,
     He wounded my neck
     With His gentle hand,
     Suspending all my senses.

8. I abandoned and forgot myself,
     Laying my face on my Beloved;

All things ceased; I went out from myself,
Leaving my cares
Forgotten among the lilies.

The poem, of course, requires explanation, for it is so packed with meaning that St. John could write more than 300 pages about it. His prose is very lucid and easy to follow, considering the sublimity of what he writes about.

The fact that he purposely wrote directly for individuals whom he knew gives his words a clarity, directness and simplicity that is free from all affectation and rhetoric-for-its-own-sake. This fact also gives his words a much greater value for directing individuals today.

St. John of the Cross had studied mystical writers with much interest. Even in his student days he made a study of the mystical works of St. Denis and St. Gregory. In composing his own writings, however, he referred very little to other books. His works were largely the expression of the experiences of his own daily life. And he wrote very prayerfully, requesting the assistance of Almighty God. At least some of *The Spiritual Canticle*, for example, he composed while on his knees.

Very little of his writing is preserved in its original, and much has been lost altogether. We have only the *Sayings of Light and Love* and a few letters in St. John's own handwriting. There are no letters extant of the correspondence between St. Teresa of Avila and St. John of the Cross. Only 33 letters, or fragments of letters, of St. John are known, compared to 450 for St. Teresa. A good bit of what St. John wrote was destroyed by Madre Agustina, a nun of Granada, during the last days of his life because she feared that Padre Diego Evangelista might use it against him. The resulting loss is immense and irreparable.

As a poet St. John of the Cross ranks with the greatest. Many literary critics consider him Spain's greatest lyric poet. "He was a supremely great artist, endowed with a very full measure of natural skill." (E. Allison Peers, *The Tablet*, July 4, 1942, p. 6).

As in his own lifetime St. John of the Cross was known and yet unknown, revered and yet forgotten, loved and yet persecuted, so in many respects have his writings fared since his death. Between 1703 and 1912 hardly any of his works were reprinted. A pall hung over his name. But in our own era, there has been a great revival of interest in and understanding of them. All of his works, e.g., now are offered in English in one volume, translated and commented on by Kieran Kavanaugh and Otilio Rodriguez, O.C.D. (published by Institute of Carmelite Studies, Washington, DC.)

St. John's books were written to further his own work of spiritual guidance and in most cases in response to a request by one of his spiritual children for more explanation. *The Living Flame of Love*, for instance, was written for the noble lady, Ana de Penalosa, whom he had directed and brought to vigorous spiritual life.

His Personality

St. John of the Cross was short, only about five feet tall, and quite thin. His features were ascetical; he had large, deep eyes, a broad forehead and a somewhat aquiline nose. The oldest description of him comes from Fray Eliseo, who had made his profession of vows under St. John, who was then Prior at Los Martires. Eliseo's testimony, dated March 26, 1618, was taken in Mexico:

> I knew our Father, Fray John of the Cross, and had to do with him on many and diverse occasions. He was a man of medium height, with a serious and venerable expression, somewhat swarthy and with good features; his demeanor and conversation were tranquil, very spiritual, and of great profit to those who heard him and had to do with him. And in this respect he was so singular and so effective that those who knew him, whether men or women, left his presence with greater spirituality, devotion, and affection for virtue. He had a deep knowledge and a keen perception of prayer and communion with God, and all questions that were put to him concerning these matters he answered with the highest wisdom, leaving those who consulted him about them completely satisfied and greatly advantaged. He was fond of recollection and given to speaking little; he seldom laughed and when he did so it was with great restraint. When he reproved others as their superior (which happened frequently), he did so with a gracious severity, exhorting them with brotherly love, and acting throughout with a wondrous serenity and gravity. (*St. John of the Cross*, by Leon Cristiani, Doubleday, 1962, p. 290).

St. John of the Cross was above all else a contemplative soul, and as with others much given to prayer, he required little sleep. It seems that a well-ordered soul, closely united to God, keeps the body better ordered and less in need of sleep. He had a strong devotion to St. Joseph, and a very tender devotion to the Blessed Virgin Mary. Hairbreadth escapes from danger were rather numerous in his life, and he usually attributed his safe-keeping in the face of danger to the help of the Blessed Virgin. Workmen at Cordoba toppled a building in the wrong direction, and it crushed a small house where St. John was staying. When they dug through the debris, expecting to extricate his dead body, they found him huddled in a corner and laughing. He said that he had great support because the Blessed Virgin of the White Mantle had protected him. (Crisogono, p. 240).

He had a good sense of humor, and often he entertained and cheered his fellow friars with his stories. On one occasion when helping the aging Padre Antonio to mount a donkey, St. John pinned his habit in place—by accident also sticking him in the leg. When the good Padre protested, St. John of the Cross countered facetiously, "Don't say anything, Father, for thus it is more securely fastened." When a Sister praised St. John before others and referred to him as the Prior of the monastery, he rejoined in a humorous reference to an avocation: "There I was actually cook."

He liked to work with his hands and often put in long hours helping to build and care for the monasteries. As Prior he took delight in preparing and serving some special dish for a sick friar.

He was affectionate by nature. Besides cooking for the sick, he spared no expense for medicine or other care for them. When he noticed a friar sad, he would take him out to the garden or into the countryside for a walk. His affections caused him some trouble with bouts of loneliness and with a longing to see old friends. His closest human bond was with his brother, Francisco. The friars, for their part, held St. John of the Cross in affection and missed him when he was absent, even though he was quite strict in his management of the friary.

He wrote to Juana de Pedrazza, a young lady who had been his penitent in Granada and who felt cut off when he was transferred: "How could I, do you think, forget one who is in my soul, as you are? . . . If there is something worrying you, write to me about it, and write to me soon and more often . . ."

Even with those who justly deserved hard treatment, he was not unfeeling. When he was living in the chaplain's quarters at Avila, a young noblewoman came at night to tempt him, climbing over the wall of the garden while he was eating supper. St. John created no scene, but met her with a calm but forceful reprimand. She went home repentant. Another time, when he was at an inn, a woman of loose morals came to solicit him. When he refused, she threatened to denounce him. He simply said, "That does not matter to me," and more or less ignored her, rather than going through the expected procedure of chasing her off. She soon left, having no one even to argue with her. St. John's methods always showed tact, even in the most unusual circumstances. On another occasion, a woman accused him in the streets of being the father of a baby, which she held out to him. "How old is the baby?" St. John asked. When he was told that the baby was about a year old and the mother had lived in that area all her life, he laughingly pointed out that he himself had come there for the first time less than a year before. The bystanders joined in the amusement.

There are many instances of miracles quietly worked. Once when a certain Brother fell and broke his leg, St. John and Brother Martin helped him mount their mule. When they finished their trip, St. John said, "Let us help you down." The Brother protested that there was no need, since he had no pain; the leg was completely healed. When a Sister died and all the nuns in the convent were saddened because she had not had a chance to receive the Sacraments, St. John called her back long enough to hear her Confession and give her Holy Communion.

Toward the end of his life there were a few dramatic evidences of his power with God. At La Penuela he once traced four crosses in the air at the four points of the compass, and a gathering storm disappeared. Also, while he was living there, a field fire threatened the chapel and monastery. He sent some to pray in the chapel, and others he sent to fight the fire on one side. He himself went to where the flames were advancing toward the buildings and knelt in prayer. The flames came to him, and then changed their direction. "Are you very tired?" he asked the friars who had been praying in the chapel, "with a laughing face that stole your heart away," reported one of the friars.

As mentioned earlier, it has been said that, among the Saints, St. John of the Cross showed a love for nature second only to that of St. Francis of Assisi. (Gilles Mauger, quoted in Cristiani, p. 206). He loved to sit at the side of a brook and watch the running water. Many nights he would spend at the window of his cell looking into the starry sky as he prayed. When he was a prior, he often took the friars outside for their hour of meditation, saying it was not too good for them to be too confined. They would pray together, and then walk apart, each one in solitary prayer. The surroundings of nature had a profound effect on St. John, for he was sensitive to beauty and scenic grandeur.

He Points to the Cross

The renown of St. John of the Cross has emerged in recent years more than ever before. His life and his works are becoming better and better known. The Church has acknowledged him by the high honor of Doctor of the Church. And in God's wisdom there is reason for this. In one way the reason may be found in his name; again, it may be summed up in one of his maxims: "Do not seek Christ without the cross."

Our age is exploring the mind of man as never before, trying to look deeply into the hidden forces that make the mind healthy or unhealthy. There is much talk of disturbing inhibitions, of the need for complete freedom, for the finding of a full life. St. John of the Cross explored the human mind at even greater depth and discovered that there must be conflict if man is to advance, that there is a need for restraint if the soul of man is to find the freedom to love God, that there is a dying that must precede the "full life" of the spirit.

Our age is making an approach never made before to the world at large. There is an effort to give full value to the natural goods God has created and to develop human nature to the full capacity of its talents. This is good if the natural is not cherished to the detriment of the supernatural, if natural knowledge and wisdom, garnered from study, are not ranked above that given directly and supernaturally by God to good, humble, simple and prayerful souls.

There is need to assist those suffering from poverty, ignorance and injustice. But the human spirit craves much more than material comforts, literacy, political freedom and whatever these bring in themselves. Many of those who have all these benefits are occupied in nothing but a ceaseless round of activities. There must be leisure in a person's life for the seeming inactivity of contemplation, more respect for the "mountain climbers of God" and more respect for the goods of the soul which these people bring from the heights.

According to St. John of the Cross, all who make an honest

attempt to love and serve God are contemplative in a limited sense. God communicates Himself directly to such souls in a "morsel of contemplation," that dark knowledge that so raises and so agitates man's presently imperfect soul. The direct communication of God to man is something that is interwoven with the fabric of daily life. No matter what other goals are sought, no matter how much one's natural talents are used and developed, this slow, joyful and agonizing process should proceed in each individual. The generous and truly courageous souls will reach the heights.

St. John of the Cross is the matchless leader in guiding us along those mystical paths where man has a touch of Purgatory and of Heaven while yet in this life. He shows those who would find heaven on earth that it can never be truly found here unless a person is willing to accept his purgatory along with it.

St. John of the Cross's feast day is December 14 (November 24 in the 1962 calendar).

BIBLIOGRAPHICAL NOTE

The Collected Works of St. John of the Cross. Translated by Kieran Kavanaugh, O.C.D. and Otilio Rodriguez, O.C.D. Copyright © 1979, 1991 by Washington Province of Discalced Carmelites, ICS Publications, 2131 Lincoln Rd. N.E., Washington, DC 20002-1199, U.S.A.

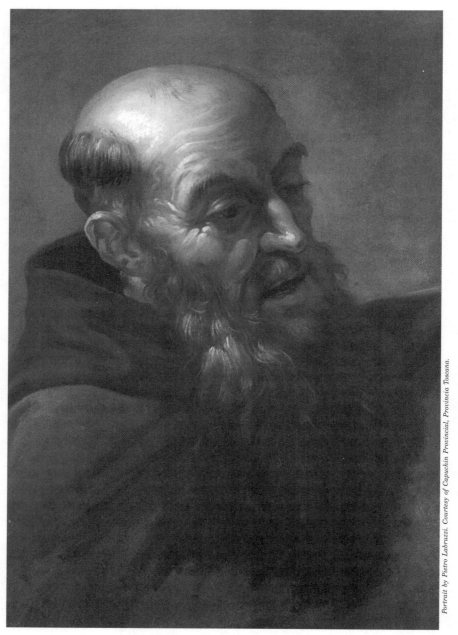

Saint Lawrence of Brindisi

30

SAINT LAWRENCE OF BRINDISI
The Apostolic Doctor
1559-1619

"**H**EAVEN has sent us a son, and what a son! His countenance is so wondrously beautiful that one cannot help recognizing in him a child of benediction. Nor must you imagine that such language is prompted by parental fondness. All who have seen your little nephew are agreed that he is more like an angel than a human being."

So wrote William Russo to his brother Peter, a priest at Venice, concerning his first-born and only child. Neighbors agreed with the parents in calling him "the little angel," especially when from his toddling years he showed signs of a serious, thoughtful nature.

William Russo (or Rossi) and his wife, Elizabeth Masella, named their boy Julius Caesar, probably after two Christian martyrs of Nero's persecution. The father's interest in the military could have had some bearing on giving him a name also borne by the great military strategist who had described the Gallic wars. Little Giulio Cesare was born July 22, 1559 at Brindisi, a seaport on the Adriatic in the heel of Italy, terminus of the famous Appian Way, and death place of the Latin poet Virgil. The parents were both descendants of noble families who had moved there from Venice 60 years before.

The father died when little Giulio was age 6 or 7, leaving him to a widowed mother who showed a quite natural tendency to cling to her child when he displayed early indications in favor of a religious vocation. He attended the day school of the Conventual Fathers at Brindisi, and later wore the habit of an oblate and stayed at the monastery. After about five years as an oblate, and not long after the death of his mother, he went in his early teens to Venice, to attend the private school of his priest-uncle.

The Young Capuchin

At Venice he used to serve Mass at the Jesuit church in the morning on Sundays and holy days and go to the Capuchin church in the evening for the sermon. From his contacts at these two churches his choice of a vocation developed. On February 18, 1575 Giulio Cesare became Brother Lawrence of Brindisi in the Franciscan Capuchin novitiate house at Verona. The priest who was Vicar Provincial there had given the boy his own name.

Brother Lawrence entered into the life of his order so fervently that near the end of his novitiate year his health was impaired and only his dogged determination kept him going. Because of his poor health, he passed the voting for admission into the Order by just one vote, and his profession in the Order was delayed for a few weeks. He recovered his health and was professed on March 24, 1576.

His studies in philosophy were made at the University of Padua, where he learned to distrust Aristotelianism and where he adopted a Platonic way of thought. (His distrust may have stemmed from evidence of atheistic leanings in some professors who derived their own philosophy from Aristotelian principles.) He studied theology at Venice. Here his health again grew poor and he was sent to rest for a while at Oderzo. After recovering his health, he finished his studies and was ordained a deacon while still under 23 years of age.

The confidence his superiors felt in Brother Lawrence was shown when, though not yet a priest, he was given the assignment to preach the Lenten course at San Giovanni Nuovo in Venice. Before Lent had progressed very far, the whole city was talking about the marvelous young speaker who could move his listeners to repentance and who held their rapt attention. Like St. Francis of Assisi, St. Lawrence of Brindisi felt unworthy to be ordained a priest, but when commanded by his superiors, he was ordained on December 18, 1582.

St. Lawrence's first assignment was to be lector of theology and Scripture in the Capuchin school at Venice. He taught there and also directed the spiritual life of the young Capuchin students from 1583 to 1586. In 1586 he was appointed Guardian at Bassano del Grappa, the novitiate house. As was the custom at the time, he also acted as master of novices during his three-year term.

Many Careers

St. Lawrence's life and activities were unusually varied and are not easy to enumerate. He was always a preacher, continuing this activity no matter what his other duties were. He was often employed as a diplomat, being sent on official missions for the Pope. He was a powerful behind-the-scenes confidant of many people. He was for a time a military chaplain. The Capuchin Order gave him a remarkable variety of positions of authority, including the highest, that of Vicar General. And he was Definitor General five times; he was elected Vicar Provincial four times, in four different provinces, and he served actively three of these times. He was Commissary General of the German Missions. He was guardian, spiritual director of clerics, and novice master. Throughout his life he was idolized by the lay people, who not only were enchanted by his preaching, but who followed him as a hero, often besieging the monastery where he was staying.

But St. Lawrence's life was not all adulation and success. He did not always attain the result he aimed at in his diplomatic efforts. He had powerful enemies who tried to thwart his work. Despite his popularity within the Capuchin Order, he had opposition there too from certain groups. He suffered insults and bodily beatings on the streets of Prague and elsewhere from heretical factions. His life was at times threatened and sought by political and religious enemies.

To follow his fast-moving steps in chronological order requires painting a very complex picture. For the sake of clarity, it is better, then, to drop a strictly chronological sequence, and to look at some of the high points in the life of this man of many careers.

Major Superior

In 1589 at the age of 30, St. Lawrence of Brindisi was elected Vicar Provincial of Tuscany. He must have had a trying time in this first office as a major superior; some dissatisfied friars complained to the Cardinal Protector, Giulio Antonio Santori, who disliked Lawrence, and called a special chapter in January 1590, hoping to oust St. Lawrence and elect a new provincial. But Fr. Girolamo of Polizzi, the Vicar General, arrived in time to stop the proceedings.

From 1594-1597, St. Lawrence was Vicar Provincial of Venice. During this time he was also elected a Definitor General for the first time. Since at that time Definitors General did not reside in Rome, he continued in his office as Provincial. In 1598 St. Lawrence was elected Vicar Provincial of Switzerland, but he did not go there, the province being ruled by a pro-Vicar Provincial.

Still another term as provincial superior was to come in his final years, 1613-1616, in Genoa. When he wanted to refuse this office and appealed to the Fr. General, the matter was referred to the Cardinal Protector and finally to the Pope. Pope Paul V replied to St. Lawrence's objection that he could not make the visitation on foot as prescribed: "A good head is better than two legs." In this last provincial term as in his first, in Tuscany, St. Lawrence was beset by painful troubles both inside and outside the Order. A group within wanted to divide the province; St. Lawrence opposed this, but after his term the division was made anyway. Charles Emmanuel, Duke of the Piedmontese part of the province, interfered with the government of the friars and told St. Lawrence that no "foreign" superior could make official visitation of houses in his territory.

From 1602 to 1605 St. Lawrence served as Vicar General of the Franciscan Order. During this time the Capuchin Order was legally subject to the Conventual Franciscans; autonomy and the full title of General came in 1619 under Pope Paul V. (Provincial superiors were also properly called Vicars Provincial.) In the three years of his generalate, St. Lawrence literally walked all over Europe, following the prescription of the Rule of St. Francis which forbade riding. He often walked 25 or 30 miles a day, allowing himself nothing beyond the ordinary fare of the monastic table and still arising at midnight for the Divine Office. Within the first year of his term, he had visited the provinces of France, Switzerland, Belgium and Spain.

St. Lawrence, who considered the chief of the four official marks of the Catholic Church to be Holiness, was considerate but quite strict in demanding an exact and holy life among the Friars. He was especially strict in enforcing poverty and very forthrightly corrected abuses in this and any other matter, even when his words directly concerned Vicars Provincial.

On one occasion, he was much concerned over the sumptuousness of a certain monastery. Finding that the person responsible was dead, he prayed for his soul. Then he addressed the monastery as the religious listened in terror: "Ill-starred monastery, unfitted by your sumptuousness to be the dwelling of these religious, professors of the most rigid poverty, I, in the name of Jesus Christ, of His most poor servant Francis, whose unworthy vicar I am—I curse you." (*Life of St. Lawrence of Brindisi: Apostle and Diplomat*, by Anthony Brennan, O.F.M. Cap., Benziger Bros., 1911, p. 101). He told the stunned friars to have no fear for themselves. A few days later, while all the friars were absent at a procession, the building collapsed from top to bottom. In another instance, he took a pick and ordered some of the friars to help him destroy a part of the building he thought too fancy.

Severe attacks of lumbago and other infirmities curtailed St. Lawrence's work for a time, and one attack was so severe that he almost died. Before the end of his three-year term, however, he had paid official visits to all the provinces of the Order, most of which were in Italy.

His Work in Germany

St. Lawrence spent the years 1599 to 1613 chiefly in Germany, except for the three years when he was Vicar General (1602-1605). Here he acted as Commissary General of the Capuchins. From 1606 on he was also in Germany at the request of the Emperor, and as Commissary General at the request of the Pope, to preach throughout the Empire. He resided chiefly at Prague and Munich.

Clement VIII had commanded the Capuchins to go to Prague after having received repeated requests from within the Empire for their services as missionaries. For many people there had fallen away from the Ancient Faith. St. Lawrence and a band of 11 companions set out in July, 1599 as 12 apostles eager for martyrdom.

Exhaustion, sickness and plague delayed them. But even strong opposition from heretical factions, which included insults, blows and, at Vienna, the firing of shots, did not stop them from founding friaries in Vienna, Prague and Graz. At Prague, the mentally unstable Emperor, Rudolph II, was persuaded that the Capuchins wanted to kill him, and he tried to have them expelled. But St. Lawrence was a fighter and fought back with prayer, mortification and diplomacy. Finally Rudolph changed his attitude. St. Lawrence was soon acting for him as a diplomat and an envoy in an effort to rally the various princes of the Empire to the cause of fighting the Turks.

St. Lawrence's mission to Prague began a new chapter in Capuchin history; from this beginning the Order spread throughout southern Germany, soon forming six provinces. The preaching, the charity to the poor and the sick, the edifying life of prayer and penance of these missionaries, and at times their diplomacy, played an important role in saving the Catholic Faith in that region. Ludwig von Pastor, historian of the Papacy (Vol. XI, p. 281), says that the Capuchins were among the strongest bulwarks of the Faith against the Lutheran and Hussite heresies.

Thomas Neill, an expert on the history of this period, gives us an insight into the mentality of the age and the role played by St. Lawrence of Brindisi. The men of that time, he says, looked on the Protestant Reformation and the Catholic Counter-Reformation as warfare.

"Both [sides] believed they were God's legions, and their enemies were God's enemies. . . . They struggled primarily for men's souls and minds, but also for their bodies, their churches, their lands, and even their cemeteries. This idea of struggle or warfare is a key idea to understanding the age. It gives us a better understanding of the otherwise somewhat scandalous relationship between argument from the pulpit and the employment of diplomatic action and military force. Most important here, it enables us to see St. Lawrence's work in Germany as a whole rather than [as] a series of spectacular but uncoordinated adventures. For establishing monasteries, reforming sinners, refuting heretics, arranging alliances, and defeating the Turks were all parts of the same struggle." (*St. Lawrence of Brindisi: Doctor of the Universal Church—Commemorative Ceremonies,* Capuchin Press, Pittsburgh, PA, 1961, pp. 51-52).

A Man of Vast Influence

To describe St. Lawrence's work only in terms of his official positions would be to over-simplify it. Officially, he was an administrator and a missionary. At times he was also officially a diplomat, and at other times he was a military chaplain. But he was also a confidant and friend of influential men; he was a zealous man of prayer, a fiery orator, a miracle-worker and a powerful personality with a wide following.

St. Lawrence's friendship with Maximilian, Duke of Bavaria and "the most forceful princely leader in the Catholic Counter-Reformation in Germany" (Neill, *Comm. Cer.*, p. 53), gives us a concrete idea of how his influence was exerted.

Maximilian, who knew Lawrence by reputation and had probably met him earlier, asked him to perform an exorcism on his wife, Elizabeth of Lorraine. She seemed to be possessed; at least, she showed signs of mental turmoil. After much prayer and penance by St. Lawrence and others, Elizabeth was cured. St. Lawrence then became the close friend and the spiritual director and adviser of Maximilian. When St. Lawrence resided in Munich, Maximilian and his wife often came to his daily Mass. The Duke would drop in to see St. Lawrence at practically any time, to consult with him about his various affairs, whether personal or public, religious or political. The net result of this close friendship, which helped to shape the man who largely shaped the Catholic League, must have been very great. (The Catholic League was the Southern German Catholic political alliance that opposed Protestantism in the early 17th century and formed the Catholic side in the Thirty Years War—1618-1648.) Maximilian himself declared: "All Germany and all Christendom owes an eternal debt of gratitude to Fr. Brindisi, because through him was established the Catholic League from which, as is evident, so much good has ensued." (Brief of Pope Paul V, Oct. 28, 1610 and quoted in Brennan, p. 155).

St. Lawrence's influence was often multiplied dozens of times by a similar combination of circumstances. What the man was himself—with his many talents and his capacity for friendship—must be considered. He had a strong effect in shaping the religious and political outlook of the men who in turn shaped the religious and political events of his time. A great deal of this influence has obviously never been recorded.

Donauwoerth

One specific instance of St. Lawrence's influence can be seen in the Donauwoerth incident. Contrary to the terms of the Peace of Augsburg (1555), freedom of worship for Catholics in Protestant areas was not allowed in practice. St. Lawrence himself was vilified as he went through the city streets. On St. Mark's Day, during a religious procession, Benedictine monks had been struck, their banner and cross broken. Their appeal to authority was not acted on. St. Lawrence proceeded to Prague, where he brought the matter to the authorities. He then began hinting in his preaching about this weak policy, and eventually, getting no results, he publicly denounced it. The result was that the Emperor was goaded into action, and Maximilian was entrusted to secure by military force the rights of the Catholic minority in Donauwoerth.

History points to this Donauwoerth incident as the fuse which started a reaction by Protestants, whose forces gathered in the Evangelical Union or the Protestant Union centered in the northern part of Germany. Later, the Catholic League arose to combat the Union, and eventually the opposing forces began the drawn-out struggle known as the Thirty Years War. A great many other opposing interests and motives would go into that struggle, and it would end as chiefly a political battle. Yet St. Lawrence of Brindisi's strong stand in the Donauwoerth incident and his consistently strong stand for Catholic rights helped to line up the forces in the preliminary stages.

The Diplomat

At the same time, one of St. Lawrence's great tasks as a diplomat had the effect of delaying the Thirty Years War. Theodore Roemer, O.F.M. Cap., Ph.D. says that St. Lawrence helped defer the Thirty Years War and might have prevented it if "the heart of the Empire had been more thoroughly Catholic." (*Historical Bulletin*, Vol. 24, pp. 27-28).

In 1609 St. Lawrence was sent as the envoy of the Catholic League to Philip III of Spain to seek financial and military help. At the time he was chaplain to the Bavarian army, Nuncio of the Pope to the Catholic League, and Ambassador of Spain to Duke Maximilian. He won his plea and obtained a promise of help from Philip, despite powerful maneuverings on the part of others to prevent this. Returning to Rome, he found that Philip had gone back on his word and was demanding fulfillment of conditions St. Lawrence had already argued against. Working strenuously and bearing the brunt of much criticism, St. Lawrence was able to secure a working agreement, which brought Spain's help to the Catholic League and made that alliance a power to be reckoned with.

His influence with Philip III depended, again, not only on his persuasive ability as a diplomat, but on the respect and confidence which came to him as a man of God. During his stay in Spain, the Queen, for instance, often sought his help in private conferences. The boy prince, later to become Philip IV, took a liking to St. Lawrence and, when sick, wanted him to visit every day. St. Lawrence would oblige, also bringing along a little gift.

Stuhlweissemburg

In October, 1601 there occurred to St. Lawrence of Brindisi the most remarkable event of a truly remarkable career. He was chief chaplain in the imperial army under Archduke Mathias, the brother of the Emperor, Rudolph II. The Christian army was greatly outnumbered by the Turks, having perhaps 18,000 to oppose more than 60,000 of the Turks. The contending armies were drawn up near Stuhlweissemburg (now Szekesfehervar), about 35 miles southwest of Budapest.

At the request of the Archduke, St. Lawrence spoke to the men. He said he would march at their head with the cross, to fight the enemies of the Cross. This stirring address he made after two days of skirmishing on October 9 and 10. On the 11th there was a full-scale battle, a lull on the 12th and again a heavy battle on the 13th. St. Lawrence rode into the thick of the battle, holding the cross aloft. Cannonballs, bullets, arrows whizzed all around him. Scimitars flashed at him, yet he went through it all unscathed. On the last day of the battle, this man who always humbly traveled on foot, following the rule of St. Francis, either wore out or had five horses shot from under him.

The field commander, the Duc de Mercoeur, conceded that "the victory, which was truly miraculous, was, after God and the Blessed Virgin, due to the Capuchin Commissary." (Brennan, p. 91). (The Duc de Mercoeur's funeral oration, the next year, was preached by another Doctor of the Church, St. Francis de Sales.) The events of the battle, which was a decisive and important one, were witnessed by Catholic, Protestant and Turk. Some of the Protestant witnesses became Catholics because of St. Lawrence's part in the battle; the Turks thought he was a magician.

Dr. Thomas Neill describes St. Lawrence's exploits.

> He rode back and forth in front of the troops, holding aloft his crucifix as the sign of victory. He encouraged the soldiers to attack relentlessly, and he himself rode headlong into the Turkish lines, once being completely surrounded by Turks. Whether by good fortune, poor Turkish marksmanship, or a series of miracles—or a combination of all three—he rode through a literal shower of bullets—much of the time without ever being hit . . . (*Comm. Cer.*, p. 55).

More Adventure

St. Lawrence of Brindisi returned to Spain in 1619 on a diplomatic mission. He went, as he had often gone on diplomatic missions before, under obedience and contrary to his own wishes. But he went strongly believing in the cause that he represented.

The nobles of Naples had asked him to go to Philip III as their envoy and tell the Hapsburg king of the oppressive rule of his appointee, the Duke of Osuna, who was viceroy at Naples. St. Lawrence had to leave the city disguised as a Walloon soldier and riding a horse, in order to escape the clutches of Osuna, who had given orders to stop him, dead or alive. Later, while Osuna's boats patrolled the sea, St. Lawrence set forth on a dark, stormy night to continue his trip. Intrigue delayed him from October, 1618 until April, 1619. Eventually, however, he reached Philip III on May 25 near Almeda.

As usual St. Lawrence stated his case forcefully, and the King was inclined to act on his recommendation that Osuna be dismissed. But Osuna and his supporters were resourceful and powerful and soon swayed the King the other way. At the time, the King was also distracted with the festivities connected with the crowning of Philip IV as King of Portugal.

St. Lawrence prophesied to King Philip III that for his lack of enforcing justice he would die within two years. He also said that he was as certain of the King's death as he was of his own imminent death. Later, in a letter, St. Lawrence repeated that God would take the King's life for failing to administer justice, and also the Pope's for failure to intervene in the just cause of the Neapolitans. History shows that Philip III and Paul V both died within two years.

His Death at Lisbon

Even the doctors did not believe St. Lawrence when he predicted his own death. On July 14 the young Philip IV had been crowned King of Portugal at Lisbon. St. Lawrence lay sick in the city residence of his friend, Don Pedro de Toledo. He went to Confession almost daily, and received Holy Communion. Often he prayed: "Praise be to God and Mary!" After asking pardon for all the trouble he had caused them, and after asking them to beg pardon of all the friars through the Father General for his faults, he gave them his cross. "Tell the Father General that this most holy cross which I wear was given me by the Duke of Bavaria, and His Highness wishes that after my death it should be placed with the other relics belonging to His Highness in the church at Brindisi. Take the cross, therefore, to the Father General and, when he so wills, go with it to Brindisi . . ." This was on July 21st. The famous cross is today in the possession of the Capuchin Generals at Rome. They have carried it with them when making visitation. St. Lawrence of Brindisi used to wear it about his neck.

On July 22 St. Lawrence announced that this was his last day. He received Viaticum in the morning, and asked for Extreme Unction about noon. A witness, his friend Count Melzi, describes the scene:

> When I entered the sick room, I saw that the Father had commenced his agony. His face and eyes were raised toward Heaven. I remained in the room all the time, and I never noticed in him the slightest sign of uneasiness or restlessness. Throughout he preserved his habitual gravity, recollection, and attention. A little before he expired, I went to the left of the bed, and I beheld in his countenance, not without emotion, a peace and a calm that presaged the flight of his blessed soul to the bosom of God. In expiring, he raised the left knee two or three times as if trying to rise, and this was the only movement he made.

St. Lawrence of Brindisi died about sunset on July 22, 1619; it was his birthday, and he was just 60 years of age.

The people of Lisbon came in great crowds to view his remains, and they succeeded so well in cutting away pieces of his habit as relics that soon a new habit had to be found. Because of the suspicion that poison was the cause of his death, an autopsy was conducted; this revealed no traces of poison. While the monasteries of Conventual and Observant Franciscans in Lisbon discussed who should have the body, Don Pedro quietly arranged to have it taken to Villafranca. The Poor Clares there, including the daughter of Don Pedro, welcomed it as the body of a saint.

The two friars who had been companions of St. Lawrence, Frs. Jerome and John Mary, asked for the heart, which, after the autopsy, had been buried in the parish church at Lisbon. The Archbishop of Lisbon approved, and they carried the heart, divided into halves, back to Italy. One half is at Brindisi in the convent of the Capuchin nuns. Part of the other half was given to Maximilian of Bavaria and is preserved at Munich, at the Capuchin church there. The other portion is presumably in Rome.

After his death, miracles through his intercession continued to occur, and appearances by St. Lawrence were recorded. One of these appearances has a special interest because it helped an artist produce a good portrait of St. Lawrence. The artist, Melchior Dona of Venice, had been commissioned by the Fr. Guardain of Mantua to make a portrait of him, but everyone was disappointed at the results. The artist was going by descriptions, having never himself seen St. Lawrence. The artist prayed and was joined in prayer by the friars there. The next morning after awakening, he saw before him the face of a Capuchin priest, the head circled with light. He recognized it as that of Fr. Lawrence, and with this image in mind, he made a portrait that pleased all who had actually known St. Lawrence of Brindisi during his life.

"Lawrence was tall and well proportioned. He had a grand musical voice, an impressive appearance, a dignified bearing. His beard was long and full, even when a young man. In his late fifties, it was white as snow." (*Irish Ecclesiastical Record*, Vol. 92, pp. 49-59).

> Lawrence was tall and well proportioned; his expression grave but tempered with kindness; the forehead large and high; the look keen and penetrating. A pleasant smile played about the lips, indicating perfect peace of soul. The beard was long and full, and in his latter years white as snow. The face was oval and strikingly spare. Altogether he was a most imposing personality, stamped by nature as a leader of men. (Brennan, pp. 229-230, from details supplied by contemporaries).

"Ah, Simplicita!"

It has been said that St. Lawrence of Brindisi, like many great men, has suffered from his biographers. His exploits in battle, his work as a public figure and his miracles have been told. But not enough has been said of his *personal* traits, of his undoubted personal struggles. We know him well as a kind of superman, but not well enough as a mere human. Though he wrote many letters, only a few have been brought to light, or perhaps even preserved. Eighty-five are published in Appendix II of his *Opera Omnia* (Padua, 1964—all in Italian), and these are chiefly about business matters.

His favorite expression was *"Ah, simplicita!"*—"Ah, simplicity!" which is not quite what would be expected from a renowned diplomat. In Prague he and two other friars were beaten, kicked, and had their beards pulled by ruffians. When rescued by several young men who rushed in with drawn swords asking if he were hurt, St. Lawrence replied: *"Ah, simplicita,* what harm have they done me?" In the battle at Stuhlweissemburg he took a bullet from his hair, where it had come to rest, and patting the bullet, said: *"Simplicita,* so you meant to kill me." Brother Michael, who was nearby, picked up the bullet and kept it as a souvenir. The expression shows a profound depth of understanding and kindness and a constant viewing of all things in their ultimate relationship to the divine plan.

St. Lawrence needed an unusual amount of simplicity and trust in Providence to continue his work despite frequent sickness. Throughout much of his life he suffered from gout, lumbago, arthritis and "stone." A number of times he was at the point of death. Sometimes he had to delay a trip because he was too sick to go on. But as soon as he regained strength, or the pains abated, he continued. He had little use for medicine, however, and took it only with persuasion and in extreme need. *"Ah, simplicita!"* was his reaction when offered medicine—as if to say, how little need God has of such aids in restoring health.

Though he suffered much from the cold in Germany, he asked for no relaxations. He did express a wish in 1610 that he might be relieved from his assignment there, as he feared that he might become a useless cripple in that northern climate. When word came back that he could either return to Italy or stay, he chose to stay.

An Intense Man

Everything St. Lawrence did was done with energy and wholeheartedly, whether in his work, or in his own spiritual life. A clue to the depth of his spiritual life at an early age can be seen in what he replied to the Father Provincial, Lawrence of Bergamo, who was trying to impress him and another applicant with the strictness of the Capuchin life. "Father, there will be nothing difficult here, provided we have a crucifix." (Brennan, p. 20).

His intensity is shown in the way he observed the Capuchin Rule, especially in his regard for poverty. He himself wore only one garment, his habit, and that next to the skin, in both heat and cold. He walked everywhere he went, and made no exceptions for himself. Even as Fr. General of the Capuchins he thought nothing of doing menial tasks, such as washing dishes. When worn out and urged to rest, he would say: "One should not accept an appointment unless one is prepared to discharge at all costs its obligations." (Brennan, p. 43).

Tears came easily to St. Lawrence, as it seems they did to many of the Church Doctors. These would appear to have resulted not from emotions too strong for control by thought, but rather from thoughts too strong not to involve an emotional outlet. When St. Lawrence read the Scriptures, he knelt. When he prepared his sermons, he knelt before a picture of the Blessed Virgin, reading the Bible, and from time to time making notes. Often copious tears accompanied his thoughts. In the pulpit, tears often streamed down his face. At Mass he used a half dozen or more handkerchiefs. When preaching, he had a brother sit behind the pulpit to watch the time and warn him with a pin when he was going too long. Sometimes the Brother had to draw blood to catch his attention.

St. Lawrence's simplicity and intensity were evident in his willingness to obey. When he was first made a Guardian, he appointed a lay brother to check on him, hoping to keep the practice of obedience alive for himself. The good Brother fulfilled the task quite willingly. As a superior, St. Lawrence was kind, being easier on others than on himself. Coming to a monastery after a hard day's travel, he nibbled at any special dish that had been prepared, hoping to encourage his traveling companions to partake of it. But when in authority, St. Lawrence never hesitated to command.

His Popularity

It seems that St. Lawrence was sensitive to criticism, because he reacted vigorously when he was maligned. As a diplomat often opposed by unscrupulous men who used any means to present a false picture, he must have had much to endure. As a superior, too, though a widely revered one, he could not have escaped dislike and criticism from various individuals or groups. His biographers, painting a picture all with glorious colors, have not said much of this, but there is some evidence.

But St. Lawrence had much more to endure on the opposite

side. He was an immensely popular man. Very often his journeys from one place to another were more like triumphal processions. People literally overran the monasteries where he stayed.
At times he had to be bodily protected or spirited away. Instances
where he had to be accompanied by a military escort were not
uncommon. At Venice, people put up ladders against the
monastery wall and climbed to the window of his room. "For
God's sake, give over tormenting me. Go away!" he urged. Other
people climbed trees. (Brennan, p. 195). At Venice, too, the fence
around the church and the doors of the monastery were broken
down. People who got close enough to St. Lawrence thought
themselves lucky if they were able to snip off a piece of his habit
or a few hairs from his beard. At Eversa, even the Poor Clares
were not above taking his mantle and skull cap, and would not
return them though he later asked for them.

At Milan it was not unusual that 300 carriages would be
stretched out in a long line leading to his monastery. Leaving
Mantua in a weakened condition one time, he accepted the offer
of a carriage, hoping that he might leave unnoticed. But a great
crowd soon surrounded the carriage and stopped it. He alighted
to give his blessing. At Padua, St. Lawrence hoped to escape
recognition by trying to pass as a Brother Questor. He pulled
his capuche over his head and put a sack on his shoulders. But
soon some people recognized him and followed him, shouting:
"Behold the Saint! The Saint!"

His Miracles

St. Lawrence's popularity can be explained in part by his mag-
netic personality. Beyond this he was by common estimation also
a holy man, "a saint," as the people frankly proclaimed. There
were, too, accounts going around of the miracles he had worked
and the diabolical possessions from which he had freed people.
A striking point about these accounts is that in many instances
there was a considerable number of witnesses. Besides St.
Lawrence's military exploits at Stuhlweissemburg, two similar
instances of smaller-scale battles are recounted in connection
with him. Once while in Germany he charged with his group of
25 soldier escorts into a regiment of 700 that had wanted to
ambush them. In 1616, not long after he had received Viaticum
and preparations had been made for his funeral, he recovered
quickly and went to the front lines in a battle between Spaniards

and Savoyards. Don Pedro de Toledo, commander of the Spaniards, attributed the victory to Fr. Lawrence.

Before he entered religion, St. Lawrence was returning one evening from Vespers at the Capuchin church in Venice. A severe storm threatened the small boat he and the others were in. He made the Sign of the Cross over the water with the *Agnus Dei* he wore, and the tempest in the canal subsided. There were many witnesses of this miracle. While the Franciscan Provincial of Tuscany, he cured a blind man—again in the presence of many people. At the court of Philip III, he cured a woman of paralysis; later, before the King and Queen and many members of the court, he placed a few grains of soil from Calvary on a corporal to give to the Queen. As he did so, fresh drops of blood appeared on the corporal. Stopping at an inn in Germany, St. Lawrence and his companions were made the butt of jokes and insulting remarks by one of the diners there. Later, the man began to blaspheme and curse St. Lawrence's cross. St. Lawrence held up the cross and said: "To vindicate the honor of this cross which you have blasphemed, may God punish you!" Immediately after these words, the man fell dead right before the crowd in the inn. (Brennan, p. 92). At Milan, among others cured, there was a boy six years of age, Christopher Caimi, who was deformed and covered with running sores; his head rested on his left shoulder and his right arm was fast against his chest. Many neighbors watched his limbs and his head straighten out and the sores dry up when the boy came home after receiving the blessing of St. Lawrence of Brindisi.

His Love of the Mass

St. Lawrence's love for the Holy Sacrifice of the Mass was extraordinary. Especially in his later years, after 1606, he spent an unusually long time at the altar. When he returned to Germany at this time, he was armed with all the dispensations he needed to offer Mass in the manner he liked. The length of his Masses was most evident on the feasts of Our Lord and the Blessed Virgin Mary. The longest Mass he ever offered was in 1618 on the last Christmas of his life. This Mass took 16 hours! His Masses often lasted six, eight and 10 hours during these years. Even when he was quite sick, his Mass would last for several hours. In the latter part of his life, as his pains increased, sometimes he was confined to bed and could not stand or move. But carried to the altar, he was nonetheless able to offer Mass. In Venice a doctor who came to see him predicted that St. Lawrence could not last another day, but later that day he found his patient offering Mass.

Nothing could keep St. Lawrence from saying Mass. One morning he walked 20 miles while fasting in order to reach a place where he could offer Mass—after having walked 20 miles the preceding day for the same reason. During his Mass he would shed many tears and his face would mirror a variety of emotions, ranging from great sorrow to intense joy.

Francis Visconti, a colonel who commanded a military escort of 25 horsemen sent to protect Lawrence during a missionary tour, went to Confession to him. His penance, he tells us, was to serve Fr. Lawrence's Mass on his bare knees. The Mass began as customary, not long after midnight. At the Offertory, the officer already felt uncomfortable and showed an inclination to leave. A warning finger from St. Lawrence, as Visconti brought the wine and water for the Offertory, showed him that his thoughts were being read. So he continued to serve the Mass. Near exhaustion after several hours, he forgot his pain as he noticed the celebrant raised about three feet above the floor, a position which he maintained for about an hour and a half. Visconti, having no air cushion nor anything but the hard floor to kneel on, nevertheless persevered to the end. The Mass lasted over 10 hours.

The Preacher

If there is one thing to remember about St. Lawrence of Brindisi, it is that he was one of the greatest preachers in the history of Christianity. Those who heard him considered him to be the greatest preacher of his time. He had the natural endowments of a great orator: a good voice, an imposing appearance and a photographic memory. He tells us that when he stood in the pulpit, his sermon was there before him, completely clear in his mind. But St. Lawrence also possessed the personal magnetism that would attract people to him. Besides these endowments, his long-range and immediate sermon preparations were strenuous and painstaking.

He knew the original languages of the Bible. And he usually wrote out his sermons in Latin. Then, at least before his formal sermons, he would spend three to five hours in prayer just before preaching. He was then a man eminently ready and on fire to give a message. A contemporary witness gives his impressions of St. Lawrence of Brindisi in the pulpit:

> He seemed wholly melted with the love of God, and his zeal and earnestness in denouncing sin touched the inmost hearts of his hearers and drew from their eyes an abundance of tears. So bright was his countenance that one could not bear to look at it, and his eyes sent forth a flame of [both] severity and sweetness that at once terrified and attracted. Copious tears and perspiration ran down his cheeks [while he preached], and the people were so moved by his words that they implored aloud forgiveness of their sins. (Brennan, p. 39).

One characteristic of his preaching was its fearlessness. St. Lawrence of Brindisi came out in strong terms against those in authority when they neglected their duties. Even when these eminent persons might be in his audience, he did not hesitate to denounce their vices in a way that left no doubt about whom he spoke.

In 1592, Pope Clement VIII appointed St. Lawrence as preacher to the Jews in Rome. He continued in this office, the longest of several such appointments, until 1594. Jews 12 years of age and over were obliged by papal decree to come to these sermons, a fact that may seem strange to today's thinking; but this arrangement was prompted by charity, which sought to save the souls of these people by bringing them to the truth. Preachers were appointed with extreme care and urged to speak in Hebrew. St. Lawrence spoke Hebrew so well that the rabbis thought he was a converted Jew.

Wherever he went, St. Lawrence was a friend of the Jews and gave many instructions to them throughout his career, besides those during his official appointments. In Ferrara he helped the Jews by persuading the Duke to give them a ghetto, or an assigned quarter in the city, to protect them from insult and injury. St. Lawrence made many converts among the Jews; he also made some enemies. At Venice, for example, the rabbis who could not refute him are said to have plotted his assassination. He had met several rabbis in public debate, and taking the Hebrew bibles they brought, read many passages to prove to them the truth of Christianity.

Some of the Jews called St. Lawrence "the living Bible." In the twentieth century, Rabbi Umberto Cassuto wrote in a letter:

The Hebrew learning of St. Lawrence was truly extraordinary. He was familiar not only with the Old Testament Hebrew text, and its Judaeo-Aramaic versions ("Targumim"), but also with the medieval commentaries, which he cites often and interprets, even in their most difficult passages, with masterly sureness and precision. (*IER*, Vol. 92, pp. 49-59).

In St. Lawrence's collected sermons, which make up the bulk of his writings, there are 52,000 quotes from the Bible. Of his sermons, 800 are in Latin, and just nine in Italian. When he preached, however, he spoke in the vernacular of the place—usually German or Italian—in the various dialects.

Besides giving his sermons to Jews, his many Lenten courses and his Sunday sermons, St. Lawrence would go on mission tours; he would be invited everywhere by bishops and priests to address their people. (In one instance at Pavia, the Bishop was caught in the crowd and had to stand during the sermon.) Many of St. Lawrence's sermons were not written out, and others that were written out have undoubtedly been lost. Those that remain testify to St. Lawrence's unremitting zeal and ability, and they constitute a goldmine for theologians and preachers.

"He looks like St. Paul," the people said of St. Lawrence in the pulpit. Cardinal Cajetan, a contemporary of his, said of St. Lawrence that he was "an incarnation of the old apostles, who, speaking to all nations, were understood by all. He is a living Pentecost." (*Extension*, Chicago, Vol. 54, p. 13).

His Writings

It is only in the twentieth century that the works of St. Lawrence of Brindisi have been published. He himself probably intended to publish only one work, that on Lutheranism, but he did not do even that. The *Opera Omnia (Complete Works)* were published in 10 quarto volumes at Padua between 1928 and 1964. They are contained in 15 tomes, plus two appendices. The last appendix, of 83 pages, contains his letters and regulations. Volume XI contains indices.

One of the hindrances to publishing the works of St. Lawrence of Brindisi was the great difficulty involved in reading his manuscripts. Various attempts were made at different times, only to end in failure. He had his own system of shorthand and wrote in a racing fashion. The clear sweep of the pages, with hardly a correction on them, indicates a mind of great brilliance, clarity and concentration. A commission of Capuchin priest scholars of the Venetian Province was established in 1926 to publish his works, and the task was tackled once again—this time successfully.

The first volume to appear was the *Mariale*, in 1928; it was reprinted in 1964. Volume 2, the *Lutheranismi Hypotyposis (The Image of Lutheranism)* appeared in three parts, from 1930 to 1933. The *Explanatio in Genesism (Explanation of Genesis)* came out in 1935. Three volumes of Lenten sermons were issued from 1936 to 1941. Volume 7, containing Sunday sermons, was published in 1943; Volume 9 was sermons on the Saints; Volume 8 containing Advent sermons, appeared in 1942. The Vienna Codex, containing Lenten sermons in Part One and seasonal sermons and small works in Part Two, appeared as Volume 10 in 1954 and 1956. Appendix I, containing notes on the *Lutheranismi Hypotyposis*, came out in 1959.

Other works definitely attributed to St. Lawrence which have not yet been found are: 1) six familiar letters to Francesco Cerratto; 2) four letters concerning observance of the Rule which were sent to the Order while the Saint was serving as the General; 3) a tract on the method of preaching; and 4) an exposition of the book of *Ezechiel*. This last was unknown until 1786. Some scholars also think St. Lawrence of Brindisi wrote a *Direttorio di Diritto (Guide for Punishments)* from which came the *modus procedendi* (literally, "the manner of proceeding") of the Capuchins.

The *Explanation of Genesis* covers only to the first 11 chapters. It is St. Lawrence's only professedly exegetical work known to be extant, though he had a long-nursed ambition of writing commentaries on the whole Bible and managed to use some 90,000 quotes from Scripture in his various works. Pope John XXIII in his Apostolic letter of March 19, 1959, said: "Especially pleasing to us is the book *Explanation of Genesis*, in which Lawrence, employing the doctrine of the Jewish masters, the Fathers of the Church, and that of the schoolmen, examines the divine truth, and as a most severe judge, passes judgment on various opinions and controversies." R. F. Smith, S.J. thinks that St. Lawrence's "use of Jewish commentators makes the work unique in the writings of the Doctors of the Church." (*Review for Religious*, Vol. 46, pp. 46-52).

His method of first going to great pains to establish the exact text by comparing various readings, and then weighing previous commentaries before making his own, is quite modern and can serve as a model method of procedure even for present-day scholars. Fr. I. Voste, O.P. says that "for his age, he showed himself an exegete endowed with extraordinary philological knowledge."

The *Lutheranismi Hypotyposis*

St. Lawrence's one apologetical work grew out of a controversy with Polycarp Laiser (variously spelled Leyser or Layser), a Lutheran theologian and preacher. Laiser was a man of some renown, had revised Luther's bible and had won from contemporary readers commendatory titles, such as "light of theologians." On July 8 and 11, 1607 he delivered two sermons from a window in the castle of the Catholic emperor at Prague, setting forth strongly the Lutheran stand. On July 12 St. Lawrence answered him, using *Acts* 13:10 for an opening text, and finally sending copies of the Bible in Greek, Hebrew and Syro-Chaldaic to Laiser, challenging him to read them. Laiser did not take up the challenge, but left the city. Back at home in Dresden, Laiser published his two sermons in a pamphlet, which was widely circulated in Prague. The pamphlet was entitled *Hypotyposis (The Image) of Martin Luther*.

Laiser even sent an autographed copy to St. Lawrence. St. Lawrence replied to the pamphlet first in a sermon and then himself began to write a pamphlet in rebuttal. This pamphlet kept growing until it became the large apologetical work, entitled *Lutheranismi Hypotyposis (The Image of Lutheranism)*, which covers 1,500 pages of his works.

The word *hypotyposis* means "image." St. Lawrence's work has three parts. Part I, *The Hypotyposis of Martin Luther*, is an historical study of Luther and the rise of Protestantism. Part II, *The Hypotyposis of Lutheranism*, is a doctrinal study of the teachings of Lutheranism and their refutation. Part III is *The Hypotyposis of Polycarp Laiser* and is a study of the effects of Lutheranism in practice.

As he wrote in the free-swinging style of the day, St. Lawrence of Brindisi may sound rough to modern ears. Luther, says St. Lawrence, was indeed a Paul, but a Paul turned Saul. But compared to many of the Reformers, St. Lawrence was actually quite mild.

St. Lawrence has his own style of apologetics, "a certain kind of method between the oratorical and the scholastic." It allows him more freedom and gives the material an interesting personal flavor.

The most important part of the work is the doctrinal part. St. Lawrence says there are two Lutheran principles: 1) Scripture alone must be believed, and 2) faith alone is necessary for justification and salvation. He says that if "1" is true, then "2" is false; for Scripture nowhere says that man is saved by faith alone, but rather, the opposite, in *James* 2:14. St. Lawrence also says that "1" destroys itself, for nowhere does Scripture say that nothing can be believed except what is contained in it. (Cf. Volume II, pp. 346-57 of St. Lawrence's *Opera Omnia* for a statement of and refutation of Lutheran principles. Reference here is from *Round Table of Franciscan Research*, St. Anthony Friary, Marathon, WI, 1960, Vol. 25).

The ultimate judge of truth, says St. Lawrence, is the Church.

> We do not consider the Word of God written in the heart of the Church by the Spirit of the Living God to be of less authority than that written by pen on parchment. Nor does the application of the pen to parchment give authority to the Word of God, but the belief of the Church does. The Word of God written on paper has authority only from the Word of God written in her heart. (Quoted in *American Ecclesiastical Review*, Vol. 143, pp. 117-120).

Elsewhere, St. Lawrence says: "God is in the Church as the driver in the chariot, the sailor in the ship, the father in the home, the soul in the body, the sun in the world." (*Quad.* I, p. 257, quoted in *Comm. Cer.*, p. 88).

St. Lawrence wrote the work on Lutheranism from September 1607 to December 1608, and revised some parts of it in 1610. The work was not yet completed when Laiser died. St. Lawrence's ambitions to appear in print must have been about nil, for he did not publish this large work, over which there had been so much labor. In preparing for this writing, St. Lawrence had read all the Latin and German works of Martin Luther and had translated much of the German into Latin. He had read, and quoted, about 40 authors among the Reformers. (*Homiletic and Pastoral Review*, Vol. 60: pp. 129-133 gives this number; article by C. Gumbinger). The nuncio at Prague and Cardinal Dietrichstein made efforts to have the work published, but it remained in manuscript form for more than three centuries.

St. Lawrence's tripartite *The Image of Lutheranism* is the most complete criticism, based on Scripture, ever written on the subject. For St. Lawrence accepted the Lutheran thesis of relying only on Scripture as a starting point and used his knowledge of the original languages and his vast acquaintance with Scripture in launching his refutations. Perhaps he wrote the book that was so wanted in Catholic circles and which another Doctor of the Church, St. Peter Canisius, had labored so long and painstakingly to accomplish. But St. Lawrence's work lay neglected and practically forgotten, when it could have served as a very valuable manual of apologetics.

Speaking of the *Lutheranismi Hypotyposis*, Pope John XXIII said:

> Therefore, those who teach theology, and especially those who explain and defend Catholic doctrine, have a work with which they can nourish their minds and equip themselves for protecting and relishing the truth and thus prepare themselves for leading others to salvation. If they follow this man who dispelled errors, explained obscurities and solved doubts, they may be sure they follow a secure path. (*Comm. Cer.*, p. 26, from the Apostolic Letter).

A Devout Marian Scholar

If we were limited to calling St. Lawrence of Brindisi either a great Marian scholar or a great lover of the Blessed Virgin Mary, it would be hard to make a choice. In him scholarship and devotion went together. His *Mariale*, consisting of 84 sermons, is the outstanding Mariological work of his time. His personal devotion to Mary and his love for her were the outstanding features of his own life.

St. Lawrence was a profound theologian as well as a Scripture scholar, so that when he spoke of Mary, he always stood on the rock-solid ground of Catholic doctrine. His own heart-felt love and devotion came to him as gifts of his youth. They deepened and intensified as his studies gave him greater acquaintance with the plans of God for Mary and how these affect men.

St. Lawrence of Brindisi explained more clearly than any writer before him the fundamental principle of Mariology, which is the divine maternity. (C. Vollert, *Comm. Cer.*, p. 65). All of Our Lady's privileges, offices and glory are related to the unique fact that she is the Mother of God.

With St. Lawrence this fundamental fact took on a special meaning and beauty in light of the absolute primacy of Christ. Since you cannot separate mother and child, Mary was included in the divine decree of the universal primacy of Christ. If Christ was first in the plan of God as the Model and Head of all creation, then Mary must have been included in this same decree. This concept paves the way to a sweeping view of Creation and of the re-creation that came with Redemption, in which Christ and Mary always act together and are viewed together.

St. Lawrence viewed Christ and Mary as inseparable in God's plans. Therefore, Our Lady is in all ways similar to Our Lord. Christ and Mary are considered as a pair in securing the Redemption, as Adam and Eve were in man's fall.

> Through the first woman and the first man the world was condemned; through the second Man and the second woman it was saved. Thus the principle of our reparation corresponds wonderfully with the principle of our ruin. As then a demon in the bodily form of a serpent was sent by the devil to lead Eve astray, who was at that time both a virgin and espoused to a man, so an angel was sent by God in bodily guise to Mary, likewise a virgin and spouse. And as Eve, by giving ear to the serpent, became the origin of our fall, so Mary—by believing the angel—became the origin of our restoration. The former inaugurated sin and death; the latter inaugurated grace and life. Through the former we lost the earthly paradise; through the latter we gained the heavenly paradise. (*Mariale*, p. 91, quoted in *Comm. Cer.*, p. 72).

On her own plane as a creature, acting with free will, yet associated with Christ by the divine maternity, Mary joined in the sacrifice on Calvary.

> . . . In the Passion of Christ, although the Most Holy Virgin stood near the Cross of Christ, she did not give forth unthinking sighs from a helplessness of soul, as women ordinarily do, but with the strongest of souls bore the greatest sorrow, saying within herself as Christ prayed in the garden: I have already offered my Son to God. I have given Him to God; if it so pleases the divine Majesty, may His will always be done. This is the perfect fruit of love, to offer God that which we love the most— freely from the mind, truly from the heart . . . (*Mariale*, p. 536).

The Blessed Virgin Mary's association with Christ in the Redemption has often been spoken of. Less heard of and so perhaps more striking are St. Lawrence's thoughts on her association with her Son in the universal primacy. "Every gift, every grace, every good that we have and that we receive continually, we receive through Mary. If Mary did not exist, neither would we, nor would the world." (Quoted in Carmignano-Barrett, p. 129). Such words as these of St. Lawrence reveal a mind that saw the beauty of Mary everywhere, logically following from the original divine decree.

The well-known Mariologist, Msgr. Emilio Campana, declared that "few have spoken of the Madonna as well as St. Lawrence, and none better." (*IER*, Vol. 92, July 1959).

St. Lawrence attributed everything to Mary—his vocation, his restoration to health as a student, his knowledge of Hebrew, all his successes. He always went to her in all his needs. When made General of the Order, he first went to Loreto, his favorite shrine, and he went there again at the conclusion of his term. In fact, he thought nothing of making a trip to Loreto or to other shrines of the Blessed Virgin, taking a few days detour and setting aside the time from his many occupations.

He said the Rosary and the Office of the Blessed Virgin daily; from his student days onward, he fasted every Saturday in her honor, and from 1610 on he had an indult to say her votive Mass every day except on the chief feasts of the year. He often sang her hymns while he was walking along; his favorite was Petrarch's *Vergine Bella*. In his later years especially, the mere mention of Mary's name was apt to send him into a state of rapture in which he would lose track of what was happening about him. St. Lawrence used to bless the sick with the words, "May God deliver you through the names of Jesus and Mary." His favorite blessing for the friars was, "May the Virgin Mary bless us with her loving Child!"

The *Mariale*

The life of St. Lawrence of Brindisi can be called a Marian canticle of the heart. His *Mariale* can be called a canticle of the mind. It was not composed as a tract, but its 84 sermons form a complete Mariology, including material on the Immaculate Conception and the Assumption, which were defined only centuries later. Points which he treats about Mary's relation to the

Church and her universal motherhood are still being developed. Pope John XXIII said that the *Mariale* contains "the most complete doctrine regarding the Mother of God." (*Apostolic Letter*, in *Comm. Cer.*).

Of the 84 sermons, two are on Our Lady of the Snows, three on the Assumption, two on the Visitation, 11 on the Immaculate Conception, five on the words "Blessed is the womb," six on the text *Fundamenta ejus* (Her Foundations), six on the Purification, six on the *Salve Regina*, 16 on the text *Missus est* ("He was sent"—namely, the Angel), 10 on the *Hail Mary*, 10 on the Canticle of the Virgin (the *Magnificat*) and seven on other topics.

St. Lawrence's great use of Scripture in the study of the Blessed Virgin Mary's role in the divine plan is very modern and received new emphasis with Pope Paul VI's recommendations to the Mariological Congress in March, 1965. In fact, the future course of study about Mary is likely to be based much more on Scripture than on speculative theology. St. Lawrence's *Mariale* can therefore be a resource even for non-Catholic scholars, as well as a source of inspiration for preachers and of delight for lovers of Mary.

Fr. Clement, the Capuchin Fr. General, in his letter of April 16, 1959 said of St. Lawrence and his work on Mary, "His *Mariale* is truly a Marian poem, the most beautiful, I should say, and the most comprehensive ever written these 2,000 years since the beginning of the Christian era." Fr. Clement also stated that in this Marian age, "The Mother of God herself must have desired the name of her ardent, lofty minstrel, heretofore unknown to most of the faithful, to be associated with her in her glory."

Fr. Cyril Vollert, S. J. concluded his address at the Commemorative exercises honoring St. Lawrence of Brindisi in Washington, D.C. in October, 1960 by saying that his sermons had not become worn with age.

> All of us, especially preachers and theologians, could profit immensely if we would delve deeply into the treasures of doctrine, piety and eloquence of the eminent Capuchin, a glory of the Catholic pulpit so long unknown. Without exaggeration, we can safely say that St. Lawrence of Brindisi is the outstanding Mariologist of his own time, and unquestionably ranks with the great Mariologists of all time. (*Comm. Cer.*, p. 77).

We may get the truest picture of St. Lawrence as scholar and lover of Mary by remembering that, when he saw a mother and child, he often caressed the baby and was moved to tears as he remembered the Blessed Virgin Mary and her Divine Child. In his way of thinking, this mother and child were there before him only because they could represent and grow more like the supreme models, the first in God's plan, Our Lord and His Mother Mary. God planned the inimitable Mother and Child, and then, in a continuing outpouring of love, His creative hand has never ceased making copies stamped in their image. Over each one broods the paradoxical divine wish that this one may become more like the originals, which are the perfect ideal.

The Incarnational Circle

St. Lawrence has five sermons on St. Joseph which combine to present a Josephology of much importance for all future thinking about the place of St. Joseph in the divine plan. St. Lawrence places St. Joseph with Mary and Jesus in what may be called the *Incarnational Circle*. Fr. Blaine Burkey, O.F.M.Cap., says that St. Lawrence of Brindisi "is signally deserving of credit. More than three centuries ago he unfolded a Josephology which, like his Mariology, is 'surprisingly modern.'" (*The Theology of St. Joseph in the Writings of St. Lawrence of Brindisi*, Center of Research & Documentation, St. Joseph's Oratory, Montreal, 1973, p. 1).

The Incarnational Circle comes first in God's plan to create. Before there was anything, before time began, God decided to link all creation to the Incarnational Circle. There were no stars, no sun, no moon. Everything was vast and empty. Then God said: I will make *a* man. He will have a virgin-mother and a virgin-father. He will be joined as one Person with My Son, the Second Person of Our Trinity. His Mother will conceive of the Holy Spirit. All else that is made will be below this Incarnational Circle—all material things, all living things, birds, animals, fish, all the universe, yes, even all angels and men. All will be made for My own Son, conceived by a virgin-mother who is united to a virgin-husband.

What we read in St. Paul (*Col.* 1:12-20), what the celebrant says at Mass, guides us into this grand decision of the Creator. It establishes the Absolute Supremacy of Christ. Through Him, with Him, in Him, all honor and glory are given to Almighty God. Jesus is not an after-thought in creational planning, but the first thought, *the* man united to the Second Person of the

Trinity, for whom all else will be made, and through whom all return of honor and glory will come to the Creator.

The theology of St. Lawrence of Brindisi would draw both Mary and Joseph into an unbreakable, absolutely unique Incarnational Circle. It is this Incarnational Circle that sheds its light on all Creation, brings all else a glow of beauty and gives reason for all other created things and persons.

Fr. Burkey sums up St. Lawrence's teaching (pp. 75-78):

1. Joseph was predestined in the eternal plan of Creation in the first place after Jesus and Mary. (explicit)
2. His predestination, always subordinate in every way to Christ and Mary, was:
   a) to the highest dignity, grace and glory (explicit), even prior to the foreknowledge of Adam's sin;
   b) for his own excellence rather than for other creatures, and therefore, other creatures were created for his greater glory;
   c) as mediator and exemplar in predestination and grace of all other creatures. (in principle)
3.a Even if Adam had not sinned, Joseph would have existed, because Christ and Mary would have. (implicit)
3.b Joseph was to participate in a limited, yet most sublime, way in the work of our Redemption; the effects of the Redemption were also to his greater glory. (in principle)
4. Joseph was predestined as the Spouse of Mary and [virgin] Father of Christ. (explicit)

The above four points Father Burkey lists in conclusion as belonging to eternity. He follows this list with a list of 29 points about St. Joseph in time. Finally, Fr. Burkey cites St. Paul (*Rom.* 8:29-30) as he gives two final paragraphs that provide all lovers of St. Joseph with sublime material for future meditation.

> Lawrence has surely covered all the principal facets of Josephology. Moreover, his Christocentric conception of creation has given a new insight into Joseph's position in creation. It emerges as the most stupendous position imaginable for a mere man.
>
> God predestined Joseph, He called him to be Christ's true [virgin] father and Mary's true husband, He justified him and glorified him above all the elect save Mary, not only men but also the angels. Through it all, Lawrence safeguards the unique privileges and prerogatives, the more perfect predestination, grace and glory of Joseph's Immaculate Spouse. The *Apostolic*

Doctor was certainly a Giant of Josephology, and more comprehensively, the *Doctor of the Incarnation*.

The Apostolic Doctor

In his Apostolic Letter *Celsitudo ex humilitate (Sublimity from Humility)* of March 19, 1959, Pope John XXIII said that the elevation of St. Lawrence of Brindisi to the rank of Doctor of the Church was opportune.

> Now, at a time when infectious diseases are rampant and men are being trapped by false teaching and all sorts of corruption, it is again necessary that this man be placed in the spotlight. It is expedient that Christians be encouraged to do good by the splendor of his virtue and draw strength from the precepts of his salutary doctrine.

The Pope presented St. Lawrence as a man "who inflamed the hearts of his listeners with the fire of his burning heart and genius; with the force of his tears he shook their calmness."

"In this exalted and excellent man," said Pope John XXIII, "two things were outstanding: apostolic zeal and mastery of doctrine. He taught by word, he instructed with the pen, and he fought with both." From this papal pronouncement, as well as from the whole tenor of St. Lawrence's life, the title of "Apostolic Doctor" is aptly chosen to describe him.

St. Lawrence's life was varied; his career had many facets. But whether he preached or went on a diplomatic mission, whether he wrote or urged his Capuchin confreres on to a life of prayer and penance, he was always doing but one work. He was laboring with apostolic zeal for the salvation of souls. In a particular way he spent his energies for the reunion of Christendom. Whether he spoke to Jews or wrote against Protestantism, whether he corrected or instructed Catholics, he aimed at the restoration of the Church. Foremost in his mind was the image of the Church as Christ present in the world. This demanded unity among believers in Christ.

Perhaps St. Lawrence's greatest success was the stamping of his spirit on the branch of the Franciscan Order to which he belonged i.e., the Capuchins. Pope John XXIII said,

> Very many competent historians maintain that the Capuchins, with Lawrence of Brindisi as their leader, through a singular

providence of God, preserved the lower classes immune from the evil opinions of the dissidents and even restored unity to the Church by dispelling the darkness of error.

St. Lawrence of Brindisi was a man who could not brook compromise or weakness in pursuing justice. He could do nothing but take an unyielding stand on essential religious truth. So he thundered forth with apostolic zeal. His writings proclaim him as a man of love, a man much more for something than against anything. His writings are positive in their tone and content, setting forth the traditional teaching of Christianity through the centuries, illumining and bolstering doctrine with prolific use of Scripture—which he knew by heart in its entirety. He grieved over the sins of Catholics and the divergent teachings of Protestants. He poured out his energies as a true reformer, a man inspired by love for Christ and aching for the salvation of souls. He spoke freely and strongly like the father of a family, because he loved much.

> The most skeptical historian must accept as fact that St. Lawrence was a striking, magnetic personality . . . a man of outstanding holiness, a tremendous leader, loved by his followers and both respected and feared by his opponents. We know that St. Lawrence was the well-rounded ideal of his age: a biblical scholar and theologian, a man of prodigious memory and cogent logic; an eloquent, persuasive preacher, an intrepid missionary; a counselor of princes and a diplomat; and finally a warrior who gave no quarter to the enemy and who considered any form of compromise wrong. (Thomas Neill, *Comm. Cer.*, p. 49).

In 1881, Pope Leo XIII said of St. Lawrence:

> There were resplendent in him all virtues, especially those which bring us close to God—faith, hope, and charity, from which all the other virtues spring and derive their supernatural value. Hence his diligent and fervent love of prayer, during which he was frequently rapt in ecstasy; hence his remarkable devotion to the Blessed Sacrament and his constant grief over the sufferings and death of Our Lord; hence his most tender love for the Mother of God, to whom he credited all that he had received from Christ; and hence also his stalwart love of the Catholic faith, his horror for heresy and error, and his rock-firm fidelity to the See of Peter. (*Rev. Rel.*, Vol. 14, p. 46).

Not under a Bushel

The official steps in recognition of St. Lawrence by the Church were slow, considering his great fame in his own day. The difficulties in publishing his writings were one important factor in the delay. Seven years after his death, Cardinal Frederick Borromeo, nephew of St. Charles Borromeo, said: "Like the sun, he sent the piercing rays of his light far and wide. In the judgment of the most eminent men, his light should not be kept under a bushel, but set on a candlestick by legitimate authority." (*IER*, Vol. 92). In the process leading to his beatification in 1783, his works were already judged worthy of a Doctor of the Church. Canonization did not come until a century later, in 1881, under Leo XIII. As noted earlier, the crowning accolade, the title of Doctor of the Church, was given by Pope John XXIII on March 19, 1959.

More than 400 Capuchins of the United States and Canada gathered at Catholic University in Washington, D.C. on October 11, 1960, then the feast of the Maternity of Mary, to celebrate this signal honor. After a number of lectures on St. Lawrence and his teaching, Francis Cardinal Spellman offered a solemn pontifical Mass in the National Shrine of the Immaculate Conception. The Archbishop of Washington, Patrick A. O'Boyle, was in attendance, and Bishop John Wright of Pittsburgh delivered the sermon. Adding a special touch reminiscent of St. Lawrence's military service was the presence in the sanctuary of a score of uniformed military chaplains.

"Thus it has come to pass," wrote Fr. Clement, the Capuchin Fr. General, in his circular letter, "that, as we look back over the past three and a half centuries, we Friars Minor Capuchin find that his figure towers above all the members of our family, however illustrious they may have been by reason of holiness or doctrine or other endowments . . ."

It is likely that St. Lawrence of Brindisi was the greatest linguist among all the Doctors of the Church. He knew the Scriptural languages of Hebrew, Chaldean, Syriac and Greek. He was well versed in Latin, German, Bohemian, French, Spanish and Italian. "Truly God gave the gift of languages to St. Lawrence," said Pope Leo XIII, "just as He gave it to the Apostles, so that he who was destined for the salvation of many spoke in the tongues of many." (*Comm. Cer.*, p. 26).

St. Lawrence of Brindisi was the 30th man in history to be

declared a Doctor of the Church. He was the third from the Franciscan family, the others from that order being St. Bonaventure and St. Anthony. Moreover, he is the first (and so far the only) Capuchin.

Pope John XXIII, who declared St. Lawrence a Doctor of the Church, did not act lightly. John XXIII was well acquainted with Venice, whose ecclesiastical history he had written, so he knew well of St. Lawrence of Brindisi. St. Lawrence was the one Doctor that Pope John gave the Church. The Pope knew that St. Lawrence of Brindisi had spent his life for the restoration of the Church and for the conversion of Protestants and Jews to the one Fold. St. Lawrence should have a special meaning for the current era in the Church. The example of his life and of his works, which were the fruit of great learning and of even greater zeal, can help us today in working toward a true renewal of the Church and in paving the way toward true Christian unity.

St. Lawrence of Brindisi's feast day is July 21.

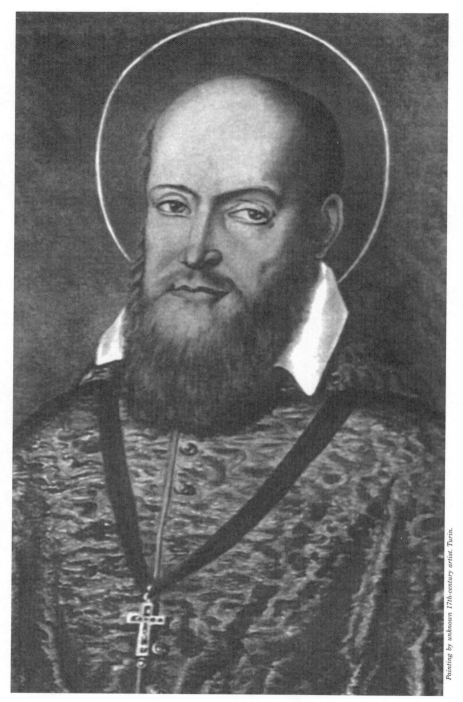

Saint Francis de Sales

31

SAINT FRANCIS DE SALES

The Gentleman Doctor
Patron of the Catholic Press
Everyman's Spiritual Director
1567-1622

"I AM a man and nothing if not a man. My heart has been broken in a way I could not have believed possible." Thus St. Francis de Sales expressed his grief at the death of his youngest sister, Jeanne, who had died at age 14. He was then 40 and a bishop. In expressing his grief, he also gives us a glimpse into his character and his life. He was a man totally dedicated to God, but he was nothing if not completely human.

Because of his qualities of affability, meekness and constant charity, St. Francis de Sales has been called "the gentleman saint." St. Vincent de Paul said of him: "And he so governed the passions of the soul and the movements of reason that not only did he ever preserve the same tenor of his way of life, but even his countenance showed no change in prosperous or adverse circumstances." (*Irish Ecclesiastical Record*, Vol. 59, pp. 209-228).

There is always a danger in summarizing a person's life or giving a short description of him. Therefore, it is hard to give a true and adequate picture of St. Francis de Sales in summary form. There is the danger of making him appear sugary and weak because of his frequent expressions of affection and because of his great charity. We may recall that he raised his hat to his own servants (*Deposition of St. Jane Frances de Chantal . . .* Burns and Oates, London, 1908, p. 132), yet at the same time we might forget that he defended himself against the anger of a Cardinal Prince of the Church at Turin: St. Francis' tears and sweat had dropped onto the Holy Shroud, which he was helping to unroll. He replied to the Cardinal's indignant correction by telling him that "Our Lord was not so touchy" and that "He had not poured out His sweat and blood but that they should be mingled with ours, that these might win us the price of eternal salvation." (*Francis de Sales*, Michael de la Bedoyere, Harper & Bros., 1960, p. 193).

Because he emphasized interior mortification more than exterior penances, St. Francis de Sales has been thought of as an easy spiritual guide. Yet to follow his basic philosophy completely, "To ask for nothing, to refuse nothing," takes true heroic virtue. One woman he directed for some time was surprised that anyone could think of him except as quite strict. He was stern in correcting abuses among both clergy and people. (*de la Bedoyere*, p. 104). He forbade sending Valentines because this was done in a way that treaded on the sanctity of marriage. "I do not understand sympathy which provides a pillow for vice and a cushion to ease sin," he said. "No, but I do understand that we must accommodate ourselves to the reach of each person, yielding something, not to the malice, but to the weakness. Souls do not wish to be bullied, but gently brought back; such is the nature of man."

A Wealth of Available Detail

We are fortunate in having a wealth of testimony about the life and character of St. Francis de Sales. His only spiritual son, the one whose life he directed most closely and who visited back and forth with him, was the neighboring Bishop of Belley, Jean Pierre Camus. Camus was a voluminous writer of some 200 volumes, including 50 novels. The work by which he is remembered today, however, is his *The Spirit of St. Francis de Sales* (1639-1641), originally a six-volume work, but now ordinarily presented in an abridged form. (In English, it is in one volume edited, translated and introduced by C. F. Kelley, published by Harper & Bros. in 1951). *The Spirit of St. Francis de Sales* is in itself a classic and rather neglected; it is the work which has fixed the character of St. Francis in our minds.

Two canonized Saints gave testimony in the official process of his beatification and canonization. Both knew St. Francis de Sales intimately. St. Vincent de Paul gave his testimony in Paris in 1628; it is fairly short. St. Jane Frances de Chantal gave her testimony at the convent in Annecy in 1627, and it makes in itself a fair-sized book. St. Francis de Sales had once written to St. Jane Frances: ". . . My heart cannot hide anything from yours. It cannot be different or other than yours—but just one with yours." The sworn testimony of a woman so closely united with another Saint in affection and the pursuit of holiness is surely unique. Her writing, therefore, should surely be well known and readily available.

The abundance of testimony by close associates, plus the more than 2,000 extant letters and other writings of St. Francis de Sales, afford a picture of his character and inner life replete with detail. Biographers do not have the problem of finding enough interesting material, but rather the task of knowing which interesting and worthwhile material to exclude.

He Starts His Career in Law

On August 21, 1567 in the castle of Sales near Annecy in Savoy (now in southeastern France), the firstborn child, St. Francis, came after seven years of marriage to rejoice the hearts of his soldier father and noble mother, Francis de Sales and his wife Frances. (They had been aged 42 and 15 at their wedding.) The boy was named after the Poverello, St. Francis of Assisi, and one of his early followers, Francis Bonaventure.

Of the two boys in the family closest to him in age, Louis was his favorite brother, and Jean-Francis later was to be his successor as Bishop of Geneva. St. Francis de Sales said of himself and these two brothers: "We three would make the dressing of a good salad: Jean-Francis would be the vinegar because of his strength; Louis would be the salt because he is so good, while Francis who is a kindly lump of a fellow would serve for oil, so fond is he of peace."(*St. Francis de Sales* by Mildred V. Woodgate, Newman Press, Westminster, MD, 1961, p. 14). To Jean-Francis, then, the "vinegar of the salad" and later to be his coadjutor when he was bishop of Geneva, Francis remarked one day, "I am thinking there is one very lucky woman in the world." Asked innocently for an explanation, St. Francis said: "The lucky woman is the one you did not marry." (*de la Bedoyere,* p. 227).

His father's ambition for Francis was that he be a lawyer and attain political renown. So Francis was sent to the University of Paris, where he studied for seven years. There he learned all the proper skills of the day, including dancing, riding and fencing. But as he tells us, "In Paris I studied many things to please my father, and theology to please myself." (*The Story of St. Francis de Sales, The Patron of Catholic Writers,* by Katherine Bregy, Bruce, Milwaukee, 1958, p. 18).

St. Francis then went to the University of Padua for a little more than three years; here he won a brilliant degree as a doctor of law. His study of theology continued at Padua; he found a good spiritual director in the Jesuit, Antonio Possevino, who approved his mortified daily rule of life. St. Francis had begun this type of life under the influence of several Capuchins, especially Ange de Joyeuse, Benet of Canfield and Père Archange of Pembroke. About this time it is likely that he was considering the Capuchin life for himself. (*de la Bedoyere,* p. 30).

Though St. Francis was popular and readily participated in social occasions, he avoided moral dangers. This and his prayerful piety drew on him the wrath of some students. A group of them waylaid him in a deserted street and threatened him with drawn swords. Francis drew his own sword and wielded it so well that the young toughs were soon ready to apologize.

Vocation to the Priesthood

It was no easy matter for St. Francis to make known to his ambitious and strong-willed father his decision to become a priest. Since the age of 12 he had carried this hope without saying anything to either of his parents. On his return from Padua, his father had begun arrangements for a marriage, and St. Francis had even gone to meet the girl chosen for him.

About this time St. Francis had confided his hope to his cousin, Louis de Sales, a canon of the Annecy cathedral. Louis quietly and quickly secured papers from Rome making St. Francis the Provost of the diocese, a position next to that of the bishop. St. Francis himself was astounded when the papers were shown to him. Armed with these and the remarkable story of the three crosses, he approached his father. Coming back from Chambery not long before, St. Francis had been unseated three times from his horse; and each time his sword and scabbard, clattering to the ground, had formed a perfect cross.

St. Francis first bore the stern reproof of his father and then received the blessing of Monsieur de Boisy, Bishop of Geneva, though residing at Annecy due to the Calvinist stranglehold on Geneva. But his father recognized the hand of God, and his faith proved stronger than his ambition.

Following his vocation, even for St. Francis, was not without temptation. "I have been suffering from a temptation against my vocation. The devil has tempted me in all parts of my spirit, even to the tips of my hair." He referred to the regret he felt at losing his curly blonde hair in the tonsure ceremony making him a cleric. He was ordained a week before Christmas, on December 18, 1593. The first Baptism he performed was that of his sister Jeanne, the thirteenth child in the family, who had been born three days before his ordination.

The Apostle of the Chablais

Much against the will of his father, St. Francis volunteered to work in the Chablais, a country region in the northern part of his diocese which lies south of Geneva, Switzerland and north of Annecy. Conditions here were dangerous. By treaty the territory was legally Catholic, but the local authorities were Calvinists and strongly resisted allowing the Catholic Church to exercise her civil rights. In Thonon, a city of over 3,000 people, there were only about 20 Catholics. St. Francis would go from door to door both here and through the hill country about the region.

In the first year there was a very hard winter, and more than once attempts were made on St. Francis' life. Not being able to get his message across to the people by gathering large groups, he started to write and publish tracts. These he distributed by slipping them under doors and posting them in public places. They were written at night, in a cold little room, after long, weary days of trudging the countryside. St. Francis called these explanatory sheets on the truth of the Catholic Faith "Meditations." Thirty-six years after his death, they were gathered together and published under the title of *Controversies*, and later as *The Catholic Controversy* (Burns and Oates, London/Cath. Publ. Society, NY, 1886; TAN reprint., 1989). These tracts mark St. Francis de Sales as the forerunner of the modern pamphleteer. In these lonely years of much work against great odds St. Francis also found time to publish a book defending the use of crosses. Its full title was *The Defense of the Standard of the True Cross of Our Saviour, Jesus Christ.*

Mass could not be offered publicly in church in the Chablais. At Christmas of 1596, however, St. Francis erected an altar and celebrated Mass publicly in Thonon. Yet in the following Lent, when he decided to restore the custom of putting ashes on the heads of the faithful, they themselves so threatened him in the church that he had to leave the church and flee for his life. Calvinist teaching had made them suspect this ancient custom as gross superstition. The incident gives a clue to the heart-break St. Francis must have often experienced in dealing with his flock, even when he could gather them together after painful effort.

In his early, rugged period of missionary activity in the Chablais, he worked alone or with just a few priests. This major effect of "The Apostle of the Chablais," as he came to be called, was accomplished when he was between the ages of 27 and 31.

Eleven years after this mission began, while he was returning from an episcopal visit, St. Francis wrote to St. Jane Frances de Chantal:

> For three years I was quite alone there, preaching the Catholic faith, and God has granted me on this journey the very fullest consolation, for whereas formerly I could only find a hundred Catholics in the whole of the Chablais, I was now not able to find a hundred Huguenots. (*Deposition of St. Jane Frances de Chantal*, p. 81).

In a report to Pope Clement VIII in 1603, St. Francis summed up his work in the Chablais:

> Twelve years ago, in 64 parishes near Geneva and almost under its walls, heresy was in occupation. It had invaded everything. Catholicism held not even an inch of territory. Today the Catholic Church in those places everywhere spreads its branches and with such vigor that heresy can find no room. Before, it was hard to find 100 Catholics within all those parishes taken together; today, it would be just as hard to find 100 heretics . . .

The problems were not all solved, however, for at this same time he was almost poisoned by enemies who were jealous over his converting prominent Calvinists. Warned in time, he took an antidote and escaped with a bad case of upset stomach.

His "Poor Wife"

St. Francis de Sales was examined before Pope Clement VIII and a board of examiners which included St. Robert Bellarmine as a preliminary to being named coadjutor to Bishop Granier of Geneva. The Pope stated that never before had a candidate for a bishopric given him more cause for satisfaction. This was in

1599. The consecration actually took place only after Granier had died, on December 8, 1602. St. Francis then became Bishop of Geneva; nevertheless, he visited this city only once as a bishop, since all Catholic worship was forbidden there, it being the capital and hotbed of the Calvinist heresy. He had been there as a priest and had had several interviews with Theodore Beza, the Calvinist leader, in an effort to convert him. At the time Beza was 80 and St. Francis 29. The diocesan seat for the Geneva diocese was actually the city of Annecy, some 65 miles south of Geneva in France; and here St. Francis spent most of his time as bishop. He resisted all efforts to give him a more prominent bishopric or the office of cardinal. He had only accepted the idea of becoming a bishop after several refusals. "The episcopate for me cannot be thought of. I am not born to command; it would be quite enough for me to have charge of a parish." (Woodgate, p. 42).

In additional to trips made during his student days, St. Francis had made two more visits to Paris, both on business for the Duke of Savoy, Charles Emmanuel. One visit lasted most of the year 1602, just preceding his consecration as bishop, and the other took place 17 years later. The first visit brought him contacts that were refreshing and valuable for widening his outlook, both on the spiritual life and on the ways of statesmen. During his first visit he became known as *"Monsieur de Geneve,"* "the gentleman from Geneva," and established himself as a much sought-after preacher, even in the royal chapel. King Henry IV liked him very much and desired to establish him in a more important see. When he broached this idea to him, St. Francis answered with the famous reply: "Sire, I have married a poor wife and I cannot desert her for a richer."

This answer pleased the King exceedingly, and Henry said of St. Francis, "A rare bird, this Monsieur de Geneve. He is devout and learned, but also at the same time a gentleman, a very rare combination."

During his second visit, St. Francis became friends with the royal family of Louis XIII and was appointed chaplain to the Princess Christine. One man in particular interested him in the royal entourage, the Bishop of Luçon. St. Francis recognized his vast spiritual possibilities. St. Francis wrote of him: "He promised me the fullest friendship and told me that henceforth he would place himself on my side, in order to think only of God and the good of souls." The world remembers the Bishop of Luçon as

Cardinal Richelieu. Louis XIII referred to St. Francis as "my good Father and saintly bishop."

The Visitation Order

One of the great works of St. Francis' life was the founding with St. Jane Frances de Chantal of the Visitation Sisters. The story of the founding of this order is a lesson in the wisdom of God, which so often confounds the prudence of men. When he first made the decision that he would found with her a new order, she was a widow with four children, the youngest being just six. After telling her his decision, he told her that there were many obstacles, and that six or seven years would pass before they could start. "Yet I can give you my word," St. Francis said, "that divine Providence will see to it by ways hidden from His creatures." To add to the difficulties, St. Jane de Chantal was living with and caring for her strong-headed father-in-law 200 miles distant from Annecy, where the foundation was to be made.

Events shaped themselves, however, in such a way that after three years the time was ripe for starting, though still not without unusual obstacles to be overcome. No scene more dramatic can be imagined than the tender-hearted mother, Jane Frances, stepping over her 15-year-old son, Celse-Benigne, who, perhaps coached by relatives, had thrown himself at her feet, saying: "Mother, I am too weak and too unhappy to be able to stop your leaving, but at least let it be said that you have trampled on your son at your feet." (*de la Bedoyere*, p. 166). (In those days a boy of 15 was often separated from his parents when he was sent away to school.) More heart-rending than dramatic was St. Jane's parting from her youngest daughter, Françoise. The separation was not, however, long nor complete, as she and the next in age, Marie-Aimée, already married, were often at the convent with their mother. The first convent, a damp, cold house called La Galerie, was opened on Trinity Sunday, June 6, 1610.

St. Francis felt so helpless in the face of the odds against starting the Visitation Order that he said that "God made it out of nothing, as He made the world." "This new Institution," wrote St. Jane, "brought down upon him much censure, contradiction, and contempt. It was openly declared to be a folly, and many persons of high standing asserted this, some even telling him to his face that this was so."

St. Francis de Sales and Women

The many letters of St. Francis, especially those to St. Jane Frances de Chantal, show him as a man who could harbor the tenderest of human affections together with the most complete and sacrificial dedication to God. "Who but God, my dear daughter, could cause two spirits to mingle so perfectly that they have become one only spirit, indivisible, inseparable, for He only is one by His very essence." (*de la Bedoyere,* p. 186). Referring to his work in the Chablais, he wrote to her: "I tell you all this, because my heart cannot hide anything from yours. It cannot be different or other than yours—but just one with yours." (*de la Bedoyere*, p. 133).

In her deposition, St. Jane Frances said that St. Francis draws his own portrait in his *Treatise On the Love of God*. (*Deposition* of St. Jane Frances, p. 90). She relates too that St. Francis said to one he loved as himself: "If God were to command me to offer you up in sacrifice as He commanded Abraham to sacrifice Isaac his son, I would do it."

St. Francis summed up the relationship between himself and St. Jane Frances when he addressed her, as he did so many other women with whom he corresponded, as "Daughter." "And by the way, in regard to that word 'daughter,' I do not want you to use in your letters any other title than that of 'Father'; it is stronger, more pleasing, more holy, more glorious for me." (*de la Bedoyere*, p. 137). The relationship between these two Saints proves beyond doubt that a full and flowering affection between a man and a woman is compatible with a life of perfect chastity and the truest love of God.

St. Francis once expressed amusement over the arrangement of a young bishop who had built a parlor next to the chapel of his residence and spoke to women through the grating between them. He said that a prelate who separated himself from half his flock was only half a shepherd. When the young bishop asked how he should act, St. Francis said:

> Do not see women alone. Arrange for someone from your household to remain in sight when you receive them—not within hearing distance, however, when your meeting concerns matters of conscience. Ask your chaplain to give you friendly hints should you slip in speech or action, and believe me, you will guard yourself far more effectively than by any iron bars. (Camus/Kelley, p. 186).

When someone criticized St. Francis to his face, saying that he was continuously surrounded by women, he replied, "It is not that I wish to make a presumptuous comparison, but it was similar with Our Lord, and the Pharisees engaged in much gossip about it." When the friend continued, saying he did not see why the women gathered around him, since he seemed to have little to say to them, St. Francis explained that they came because he was a good listener. "Don't they talk enough for us both?" he asked his friend. "And nothing is more pleasing to great talkers than a patient listener."

Death in Lyons

St. Francis de Sales was not able to realize his cherished plan of retiring from the bishopric and spending his last days in a monastery. He had always had an inclination to the monastic life, and had almost before ordination made up his mind, it seems, to join the Capuchins. As events turned out, he did not even spend his last days quietly at Annecy but was away from home at Lyons. His last days were a whirlwind of activity. Christmas Eve and Christmas were unbelievably busy, and he collapsed on the afternoon of December 27, 1622. To the Sister Superior who asked for a last word of advice from the exhausted man after he had said Mass that same day he handed a card on which he had three times written the word "humility."

In those days the medical profession thought it dangerous to let a man in his condition fall asleep. They had diagnosed his sickness as a brain hemorrhage. So they pinched, rubbed and slapped him, and eventually sat him up in a chair to keep him awake. After this, they applied a plaster of blister beetles which soon raised blisters on his bald head. While this set, the doctors applied the final remedy, pressing a red-hot iron against the back of his neck. The plaster was then torn off, and with the poor man submissively telling them to do what they thought best, they pressed a red-hot iron on the blistered and bleeding head. St. Jane de Chantal said the skull itself was injured. After the final treatment by the doctors, he was returned to his bed, where he died at 8:00 in the evening, December 28, 1622. He had been anointed earlier in the day. Asked at that time to beg God then to spare him, his reply had been, "No, I will not do it, for I know that I am absolutely useless." He died in the gardener's cottage attached to the convent of the Visitation.

Immediately, the people of Lyons came to venerate the body as that of a saint. The heart was kept at the Visitation convent in Lyons, where St. Jane said five years later that it had the same color and substance as in life, and from the heart flowed a liquid which was soaked up and given to people who asked for it. The heart was later brought to Venice. The tombs of St. Francis de Sales and St. Jane Frances de Chantal now flank the main altar of the new monastery of the Visitation at Annecy.

Patron Saint of the Catholic Press

St. Francis was beatified in 1662 and canonized three years later. Pope Pius IX declared him a Doctor of the Church on November 16, 1877, in the Brief, *Dives in Misericordia*. The Bull says:

> Acknowledging himself the debtor of the wise and the ignorant, being made all things to all, he strove to teach the simple and rude in simple language; among the wise, he spoke wisdom. He also gave forth the most prudent counsels regarding preaching and obtained that the vitiated eloquence of the times should be restored to the ancient splendor set forth in the example of the Holy Fathers; and from this school came forth most eloquent orators from whom the richest fruits have redounded for the universal Church. Therefore, he has been held by all to be the restorer and master of sacred eloquence.

On January 26, 1923, Pius XI fulfilled the wish of his predecessor, Benedict XV, by issuing an encyclical on St. Francis de Sales, entitled, *Rerum Omnium Perturbationem*. He proclaimed the rest of the year, until December 28, the tercentennial of the death of St. Francis de Sales. In his encyclical, Pope Pius XI also designated St. Francis de Sales as patron of the Catholic Press.

> But we wish that all those Catholic men who, by publishing newspapers or other writings for the public, illustrate, advance and protect Christian wisdom, may receive a special and useful fruit from these solemnities . . . Since, however, it is not evident that St. Francis de Sales has been given as a patron by a public and solemn document of the Apostolic See to these Catholic writers whom we have mentioned, we, seizing this happy occasion, after study and mature deliberation, now give,

confirm and declare by our apostolic authority, through this encyclical epistle, that St. Francis de Sales, Bishop of Geneva and Doctor of the Church, is for all of them their Heavenly Patron, all things to the contrary notwithstanding. (Cf. *The Papal Encyclicals*, Vol. 3, McGrath, Raleigh, NC, 1981).

The Catholic Bishops of the United States of America acted on this declaration in their annual fall meeting and designated the Sunday nearest St. Francis' feast day, January 29, as Catholic Press Sunday, which was first observed in 1924. Since, to be effective, a program emphasizing Catholic reading needed a longer time than one day, the whole month of February, during which the program continued, came to be called Catholic Press Month.

St. Francis gives this advice to writers: "Use simple, homely words; likewise the transition between ideas should be simple and readily grasped by all."

Introduction to the Devout Life

St. Francis de Sales was one of the great letter writers of history, penning 20 to 30 per day in his own hand, which was quite legible, according to facsimiles. Some letters ran to as much as 7,000 words. The most noticeable thing about all his writing is its direction to an individual, just as the whole pattern of his life and character showed an intense interest in each person. "One should not be surprised that every plant and flower in a garden requires its own particular care," he explained. St. Francis did not consider himself a professional writer, and though he planned to write several books after retiring, he really wrote only one in a formal manner. On a great question raging in his own day, the relationship between Church and State, he expressed his full opinion in a private letter to Madame Brûlart, one of his spiritual daughters. (*de la Bedoyere*, p. 189).

His most famous work, the *Introduction to the Devout Life*, was originally a series of letters which he then arranged and adapted in a way to make up a practical guide to Christian perfection. Many of the letters had been sent to Madame Louise de Charmoisy, whom St. Francis described (in a letter to St. Jane de Chantal) as "a lady sterling throughout and infinitely suited for the service of our Saviour."

In preparing his second edition, St. Francis asked St. Jane Frances for the letters he had sent to her. The *Introduction to the Devout Life* is addressed to "dearest Philothea," and is sometimes published under the title "Philothea," meaning "Lover of God," or "Soul who loves God," or "Woman who loves God." The first edition was published about the end of 1608. St. Francis published the *Introduction* at the suggestion of Père Fourier, a Jesuit to whom he often went for spiritual advice. The book was also an answer to an earlier request by Henry IV of France that St. Francis write a book of spiritual guidance suitable for all classes of people.

The *Introduction* contains much detailed advice for people living in the world who wish to advance in holiness. It is basic to St. Francis' way of thinking, of course, that holiness is compatible with all the demands and conditions of living in civilized society. How to pray, how to meditate, how to choose friends, what recreations to have, what virtues to strive for in particular, how to act against sadness and lack of peace and temptation—all are treated in a direct and personal way. Though addressed to women and solving their specific problems, the advice, with occasional adaptation, applies equally to men. The examples used in illustrating are often very striking, though the ones taken from botany and biology are naturally based on information those sciences proclaimed in the early 17th century. Today they may sound quaint or laughable, but the point they set forth still comes through very clearly.

This book has been an all-time devotional best-seller in many languages. Even James I of England and John Wesley, founder of the Methodists, usually carried a copy in their pockets. Pope Pius XI said of the *Introduction*:

> And would that this book, which in its own day was considered unequalled by any in the same line, be used today by all as it once was in the hands of all, and then truly, Christian piety would revive throughout the world, and the Church could rejoice in the widespread holiness of her children. (Encyclical).

Treatise on the Love of God

The Patron of Writers' one formal book was his (*Treatise*) *On the Love of God*. Giving so much of his time to the immediate need of each person who sought him out prevented St. Francis from fulfilling his plans for further writing. At the same time, his intense interest in each person is the quality that today makes his writings alive, interesting and personal to each reader.

The *Treatise* contains the fullness of his teaching. St. Vincent de Paul said of this work:

> . . . He published the immortal and most noble work, *On the Love of God*, a faithful witness of his most ardent love for God; a truly admirable book, which has as many heralds of the suavity of its author as it has readers; and which I have carefully arranged shall be read in our community as the universal remedy for the feeble, the goad of the slothful, the stimulus of love, the ladder of those who are tending to perfection. Oh, that all would study it, as it deserves! There should be none to escape its warmth. (*Deposition of St. Vincent de Paul* in *Irish Ecclesiastical Record*, Vol. 59, pp. 209-228).

St. Francis de Sales took more than four years to write the *Treatise*, publishing it in August, 1616. It was written, like all his works, in French, and was translated thereafter into many languages, the first being English, in 1630. The *Treatise On the Love of God* is a good book for lay people as well as for religious. It is a guide for all who would advance in knowledge of the love of God and in actually loving Him.

St. Jane Frances de Chantal said of the *Treatise*:

> Often when he was composing, he used to say that he should try to write as much on his own heart as on the sheets of paper before him. Humble souls, who receive from God special and abundant light, find there all that they could desire to guide them to a perfect union with God. (*Dep.* St. Jane, p. 213).

Pope Pius XI says that this book was not written in dry terms,

> but in conformity with his fertile and ready genius, adorning the *Treatise* with so much pleasure, with such unctuous sweetness and illustrating it with such a variety of comparisons, of examples and citations, taken for the most part from the Sacred Scriptures, as to make it appear that what he has written flowed not only from his mind, but from his heart and from the inmost fibers of his being.

An Inspired Writer

St. Francis de Sales left his mark on French literature. He was a stylist whose limpid and free-flowing prose expressed his own soul and the thoughts and feelings of others so well that his appeal is still fresh today. He has followed his own recommendation of hiding the art and setting forth the thought, so that his words seem deceptively simple and effortless. Yet they are correct, elegant and polished.

But beyond the power of his style, his words have a special power to raise the reader to God. They came directly from a heart full of love for God and neighbor. And with St. Francis, writing and prayer were never far apart. He himself confessed, with the simple truthfulness of the humble, that he shed tears reading his own books. He told St. Vincent de Paul that he wept because he saw that his books had been infused by God rather than by his own genius.

The particular flavor of Francis de Sales' writing springs from his positive view of the Incarnation and his own intensely affectionate nature. If the Incarnation is first in God's planning, then all the things of God's creation take on a more joyful and lovable aspect. For one thinks of them as planned from the very beginning as illustrations of and a preparation for the grand climax of creation: the humanity of Christ. St. Francis de Sales, like his namesake, St. Francis of Assisi, had the kind of heart that can respond fully to the wonder of this concept.

We might picture a young man building a house for his bride-to-be. She is always first in his intention. He has the heart to respond with affection. So he watches every bit of material that goes into making the house, and he sees in it the lovable light that she sheds on it. Her name is on every brick and every board.

This is how St. Francis de Sales thought of Christ and of all men and of other creatures. They were all for Him and because of Him. Thus, everyone and everything is very lovable. God must be praised for all these wonderful works, and they must be rejoiced in. They are beautiful and good in themselves, and much, much more beautiful and good because they illustrate and prepare the way for God's final masterpiece of creation, His own Incarnation.

In the *Treatise On the Love of God* (Bk. 2, ch. 12), and in his last sermon for Christmas, St. Francis speaks of this viewpoint of the Incarnation, which had previously been set forth by St. Cyril of Alexandria and elaborated by the great Franciscan philosopher, Duns Scotus:

The heavenly Father planned the creation of this world for the Incarnation of His Son. The end of His work was also the beginning. Divine Wisdom saw from all eternity that the Eternal Word should assume our nature and come into this world. Before Lucifer and the world were created, before our first parents had sinned, all this had been determined.

A Man of Great Devotion

With this background in mind, it is not surprising that St. Francis de Sales should have had much to do with the development of devotion to the Sacred Heart of Jesus and to the Blessed Sacrament. He did not write an express treatise on the Sacred Heart, but his writings abound with references to that devotion. They were used extensively in obtaining papal approval for the Sacred Heart devotion which flourished as a result of the visions and messages from Our Lord received by St. Margaret Mary.

In launching the Visitation Order, St. Francis wanted it "to be founded on the virtues of the Sacred Heart, meekness and humility." The sisters should be adorers, imitators and servants of the Sacred Heart. St. Francis' work with regard to devotion to the Sacred Heart was crowned in the above-mentioned appearances and revelations of Our Lord to a Sister of the Visitation community at Paray le Monial in France, St. Margaret Mary Alacoque (1647-1690), in the latter part of the 17th century, 50 years after St. Francis' death. The Mass Preface granted to the Sisters of the Visitation in 1847 renders thanks to God, "who raised up for His Church St. Francis, a shepherd according to His own Heart, who by his writings, sermons and example might strengthen piety and make smooth the rough ways . . ."

"To die or to love," the motto of St. Francis de Sales, expresses the plea of one who knew something of the loving Heart of Jesus. One day St. Francis told St. Jane, "I wish that I could tell you the feeling which I had today at Holy Communion; the sweetness of my hope—nay, rather, of my certainty—that my heart will one day be wholly swallowed up in the love of the Heart of Jesus." (*Dep.* St. Jane, p. 86). Looking back at this history, we can see the gradual working of God's plans to develop devotion to the Sacred Heart of Jesus, which was brought to fullness in the messages of Our Lord to Margaret Mary.

St. Francis de Sales introduced the Forty Hours Devotion to

Savoy as a public demonstration of faith in the Real Presence of Christ in the Eucharist, which was denied by Calvinists. The first year this devotion was practiced there, the procession went 18 miles through the countryside, from Thonon to Annemasse, near Geneva, gathering people as it advanced. The second year, the Forty Hours devotion was celebrated in Thonon, and it is reported that at this time the prayers of St. Francis de Sales restored to life a baby long enough for it to be baptized. The Protestant mother and her entire family became Catholic. This is the only miracle of St. Francis de Sales recorded during his Chablais missionary years. During the rest of his life many people attributed extraordinary favors to the prayers of St. Francis de Sales, including other restorations to life of those who had died.

"I am surrounded by people, yet my heart is solitary," wrote St. Francis. (*Dep.* St. Jane, p. 155). He lived in the divine presence and felt at ease in the royal company, he explained, because he thought of a more majestic Presence than that of kings. His mind was never far from the Holy Eucharist. During his retreat just before ordination, St. Francis made a resolution to make "every moment of the day a preparation for tomorrow's Mass: so that should anyone ask me 'What are you doing at this moment?' I could truly answer, 'Preparing to celebrate Mass.'" (*Bregy*, p. 24).

St. Jane Frances de Chantal describes St. Francis de Sales at Mass:

> When the holy bishop was at the altar, it was easy to see how deep was his reverence in the presence of God. His eyes were modestly cast down; his face full of recollection, and so calm and sweet that those who looked at him attentively were touched and thrilled with devotion. Especially at the moment of Consecration and Communion the peaceful radiance of his countenance filled every heart with emotion. Indeed this Divine Sacrament was his true life and strength, and in this action he appeared like a man wholly absorbed in God. He said his Mass in a grave, gentle, even tone of voice, without the least hurry, however busy he might be. He told me, many years ago, that from the moment that he turned to the altar he had no distraction of any kind. (*Dep.*, pp. 160-161).

His Love for Mary

As a youth of 19, St. Francis underwent a severe spiritual crisis, brought on by a temptation regarding the Calvinistic teaching on predestination. The thought plagued him: perhaps he was destined for Hell, and could do nothing about it. With valiant prayer he fought this temptation, but it continued. It caused him six weeks of great mental anguish and ruined his health. He finally prayed: "Whatever happens, Lord, may I at least love You in this life if I cannot love You in eternity, since no one may praise You in Hell. May I at least make use of every moment of my short life on earth to love You." As he made this plea in a more extended way in a chapel of the Blessed Virgin, he picked up a card nearby containing the *Memorare* prayer. When he finished praying this prayer, his doubts vanished. He felt suddenly at peace. This happened at Paris during his student years. Later, under stress of illness at Padua and still later during an illness in 1597, he experienced again a return of some of the horror that he might be predestined for Hell.

In gratitude to the Blessed Virgin Mary for deliverance from this terrible trial, he promised to say a Rosary daily. As St. Jane tells it,

> . . . Our Blessed Founder also told me that while he was still a student he made a vow to say the Rosary every day of his life, in honor of God and of the Blessed Virgin, to obtain deliverance from a grievous temptation which molested him, and from which he was delivered. He always carried it in his belt as a sign that he was the servant of Our Lady. (*Dep.*, p. 61).

When he was so busy that he feared he might forget to say his daily Rosary, he put it around his arm as a reminder. The day before he died, he asked that his rosary be twisted around his wrist. St. Vincent de Paul tells us that St. Francis was always "sweetly intent on the Rosary." He took an hour each day to pray the Rosary, taking so long because he meditated on the mysteries as he said the *Hail Marys*. St. Francis also wrote several short instructions on the manner of saying the Rosary.

His heart is revealed in a remark he made in 1621 while visiting a hermitage near Talloires: "Dear God, what a good and agreeable thing it is for us to be here! Yes, surely, my coadjutor must be left with the burden and heat of the day, while I serve God and the Church here with my pen and my rosary."

Another favorite prayer of St. Francis was the *Angelus*, which he prayed three times a day; when the bells announced it, he would kneel down wherever he happened to be at the time.

His devotion to the Blessed Virgin Mary was tender and full of confidence. After recovering from a near-fatal illness in Padua, and being reminded to thank the lady who had nursed him, he announced with a play on words that he was going to Loreto "to thank the Lady who gave me the most help during that time." To Our Lady he gave the thanks for all the success of his labors. While dying, he murmured over and over the names of Jesus and Mary.

> I have been feeling most strongly how great a blessing it is to be a child, though an unworthy one, of this glorious Mother. Let us undertake great things under her patronage, for if we are ever so little dear to her, she will never leave us destitute of what we are struggling to attain.

St. Francis confided this to St. Jane de Chantal. She tells us further:

> In all his necessities our holy bishop had recourse to the most glorious Virgin, and advised the same to his penitents. He made pilgrimages in her honor to the Chapel of Loreto, to Our Lady of Compassion at Thonon, whither he went on foot, and to many other places where our dear Mother is specially honored . . .
>
> He placed our Order, which he himself instituted, under her protection and named it after the sacred mystery of the Visitation, procuring for us the privilege of saying the Little Office of the Blessed Virgin only . . . The intention of our Blessed Founder in doing this was that there should be an Order in the Church of God specially consecrated and dedicated to sing day and night the praises of that sovereign Queen of whom he speaks so worthily and in such high terms in his books, and to whom he has even dedicated his *Treatise On the Love of God*. (*Dep.*, pp. 161-162).

Human in Suffering

St. Francis was originally of strong and robust health, but throughout most of his life he suffered from poor circulation. While still a youth, he had two near bouts with death. In fact, he gave orders at Padua in 1590,

As for my body, let it be given after my death to the medical students. Seeing that it has been useless during my lifetime, I should like it to be of some use after my death. I am happy to think that I may be able in this way to prevent one at least of the fights and killings to which the students resort when they are trying to get hold of the corpses of the executed for dissection.

Of St. Francis' first sermon, St. Jane relates: "When he heard the bell ring for the sermon, he was seized with such violent spasms and intense physical pain that he was obliged to throw himself upon a bed." The victory, however, went to mind and will over the poor instrument of the body, and he went out to deliver a sermon that made a good impression.

St. Jane summarizes the ailments of St. Francis, which sound amazing considering his more than full schedule of work.

All through the 19 years during which I had the great honor of his acquaintance, I knew, both from hearsay and from my own personal observation, that he suffered from all sorts of maladies; from attacks of fever, quinsy, and catarrh, and from internal abdominal weakness which greatly exhausted him, accompanied as it was for many years with severe hemorrhage. All these ailments increased with his advancing years, and in addition to excruciating pains in the head and body, he suffered from weakness and even open wounds in the legs [he had varicose veins], making walking so difficult and so fatiguing that it was grievous to see him wearily struggling along. Yet, in spite of all these sufferings and many more of which nothing was known, he made no change whatever in his manner of life and so controlled his countenance that he was only known to be ill by his change of color, especially as he never took to his bed except when overtaken by very serious illness. (*Dep.*, pp. 147-148).

St. Francis de Sales was not by any means a worrier about his ailments. "Since we must die," he said, "what do ten years more or less signify?"

An Affectionate Man in Daily Life

St. Jane Frances said that St. Francis did not talk like a book, that his conversation was much admired for its agreeableness. He never criticized, but rather made excuses when somebody was criticized in his presence. If he could make no excuse, he would shrug his shoulders, raise his eyes and murmur, "Human misery, human misery! This is but to remind us that we are men." Sometimes he told amusing little stories, but never at anybody's expense; he could not stand having somebody ridiculed.

At the same time, he freely expressed his opinion in the cause of God and the salvation of souls. He even mildly disapproved of the opinion of another contemporary Doctor of the Church.

> I have not found to my taste certain writings of a saintly and most excellent prelate [St. Robert Bellarmine] in which he has treated of the indirect power of the Pope over princes—not that I have thought what he wrote not to be to the point, but because in this age when we have so many enemies outside, I believe that we should not disturb anything within the body of the Church.

St. Francis de Sales' manner of speaking was accurately revealing of his character. "He spoke in a low voice, gravely, steadily, gently and wisely, and always to the point, but without any attempt at fine language or any affectation; he loved artlessness and simplicity." (*Dep.*, p. 222).

Children liked to be near him, and he very much enjoyed teaching them. His vivid imagination, his store of interesting facts about nature, and his ready affection made him a favorite as an instructor in catechism. At his last meeting with St. Jane Frances de Chantal shortly before he died, he spoke to her as usual through the grille of the convent enclosure. As the door to the outside was half open, he got up after a while to close it against the cold. Then he noticed a few children standing there and enjoying the strange sight of a man apparently talking to a wall. He returned to his chair, leaving the door open for their benefit.

In All Ways Human

The balance of St. Francis de Sales in all things is his greatest characteristic. He was most tender, yet he was iron-willed. He could wait with endless patience, yet keep driving relentlessly for his goals. His sweetness seems, at least to English sensitivities, almost feminine, but his courage in danger and his constancy in difficulty show the toughest masculine spirit. He could write to St. Jane that his heart was with hers a thousand times a day, and yet go about his duties for several years without actually seeing her. By nature slow in speech and in action, he was quick in thought and great in accomplishment. He kept his eye incessantly on Heaven, while neglecting no social, civic or human values.

St. Francis did not urge exterior mortifications, but counseled adaptation to the ordinary problems of life that would require heroic interior mortification. As a result, his advice seems deceptively easy, and those who examine his teaching superficially will misinterpret him. It is not easy to follow the advice, for instance, which he gave in a sermon:

> My friends, people are making a mistake when they attach little value to a small act of surrender to the bad humor of another, to the gentle endurance of other people's faults: of an insulting glance, of preference shown to another, of contempt or importunity; to a kind answer to an unjust or harsh reproach, to the patient acceptance of refusal, to the showing of kindness to others. All these things are small in the eyes of the world, which appreciates only dramatic virtue, but they are great in the eyes of God. (Quoted in *Catholic Digest*, March, 1946).

He managed the affairs of his diocese with much order, yet hated worldly prudence. "We must never permit our lives to be guided by worldly prudence, but rather by faith and by the Gospel." St. Francis' prudence was "in the simplicity of a perfect confidence and total dependence on the Providence of God." (*Dep.* of St. Jane, p. 109). He did not allow people to complain about the weather being too hot or too cold, for he said that this was finding fault with Divine Providence.

St. Francis was inclined to lose his temper, but learned to govern it so well that popularly meekness is often thought of as his chief virtue. As a child he was inclined to fear dark places, but he learned little by little to force himself to be alone in the dark until he actually felt better there because there he remembered more the presence of God. In later life, crossing the Lake of Geneva in a small boat, he said that he felt more secure with just a little plank between him and the sea, for then he knew that he was more in God's hands. (*Dep.* St. Jane, p. 88). His great temptation to despair he counteracted with a stronger and firmer belief in God's love, and thus restored his hope.

St. Francis was not a person so one-sided or strong in one

direction of thinking that he missed half the struggle of life. He has in fact been accused in some quarters of suffering during much of his life from depression. It is true that often in his letters an underlying sadness shows through. Yet he was essentially the optimist, looking on the good and happy side of things. However, this often meant making a great effort.

His virtue came with slow development, as he learned to balance within himself the conflicting forces of nature and to settle the apparently opposed tugs of Catholic teaching. As far as poor humans go, there must always be a tension in reconciling God's mercy and His justice, God's will for man's happiness and man's present sorrow and possible future damnation. To St. Francis, not to have any trouble with such questions is either the sign of a great grace or of superficiality. To settle them in this life is to crush some part of nature.

A Safe Spiritual Guide for All

St. Francis de Sales never crushed anything. His spiritual guidance was based on allowing each soul to develop according to its own capacity and as God Himself gave it inspiration.

His whole effort was always bent to the individual soul. He would preach to a handful of people, or even go to the end of his diocese to hear the Confession of a dying man who asked for him. He valued the liberty of the individual and believed in conversion as a free acceptance of God's truth and law by each person. The early years of his priesthood were spent in a courageous seeking out and instructing of individuals in the Chablais region of eastern France. But he soon recognized the great damage that could be done to conversions by an unfriendly civil authority, and so he asked for soldiers to preserve order, lest his converts be threatened and lest others fear to follow their conscience.

The individual soul must be free to choose the poverty of Christ. He wanted his clergy to be poor; he himself lived as a poor man. At the same time he could see in the civil establishment of his day the need for state support for Church activities. He asked Charles Emmanuel of Savoy for the support due, for this was just according to the law, and also necessary if the Catholic religion was to enjoy real freedom and respect among the people.

Whereas St. Francis directed many people, he did not think that they should find their full direction from him. They should pick up some hints from reading, from sermons, from others, and chiefly from communing with God in prayer and meditation.

He was for method and for a rule of life, but he was against being overly methodical. "True love scarcely goes by method," he said. He was for being exact, but against too much examination. He was not too much in favor of looking back over one's faults, but more in favor of "forward examination," preparing for dangers to come, planning what to practice in the future.

"Salt and sugar are both excellent things, but too much of either spoils the dish." (*Camus/Kelley,* p. 183). This statement of St. Francis reported by Bishop Camus sums up the Saint's way of thinking.

Asked one day who his spiritual director was, he took a copy of Scupoli's *The Spiritual Combat* from his pocket. Questioned about this, he explained that although he was in favor of having a living spiritual director, "he must be chosen out of 10,000." He quoted an ancient emperor who had said that his best advisers were the dead, meaning books. "In the same way," St. Francis concluded, "devotional books are our best guides." (*Camus/Kelley,* pp. 194-195). It is of interest that the Salesian Library on Lawrence Street in Washington, DC has possibly the best collection of books in the U.S. by and about St. Francis de Sales (about 600 volumes).

The Church sets St. Francis de Sales before us as a special and excellent guide to perfection for everybody, but especially for the laity. In the words of Pope Pius XI, St. Francis de Sales shows

> that holiness can be very well reconciled with all the duties and conditions of civil life, and that each one can live according to the moderate customs of his own age in a way harmonious with attaining salvation, as long as he does not himself drink in the spirit of the world.

In our modern era of change and of emphasis on human values, St Francis de Sales, the completely supernaturalized man of perfectly balanced humanity, is an unerring guide. Today the pendulum may be swinging, paradoxically, now at one time too far to the side of the intellect and now at another too far to that of emotionalism. But a knowledge of St. Francis de Sales' approach to the spiritual life will help restore the balance between the two that we all need and will lead men by means of his books to a greater love of God and to a truer service in His cause. St. Francis de Sales has a direct, personal way of speaking from heart to heart. Those who use his works will happily find in him a safe and understanding spiritual guide.

St. Francis de Sales' feast day is January 24 (January 29 in the 1962 calendar).

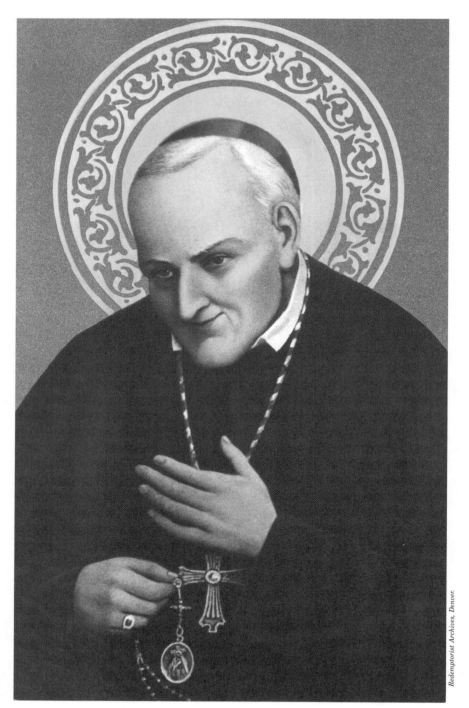

Saint Alphonsus Liguori

32

SAINT ALPHONSUS LIGUORI

Prince of Moralists

Most Zealous Doctor

Patron of Confessors and Moral Theologians

1696-1787

S T. ALPHONSUS de Liguori was born at the country house of the Liguori family at the town of Marianella, two and one-half miles north of Naples. The house still stands. The noble parents, Don Joseph Liguori, captain of a royal galley, and Anna Cavalieri, showed a hard-driving, take-no-chances Catholicity in providing the first of their eight children with patrons. Born on September 27, 1696, he was baptized two days later and named Alphonsus Mary Anthony John Francis Cosmas Damian Michaelangelo Gaspar de Liguori.

Two of his brothers would also become priests: Anthony a Benedictine, and Cajetan a diocesan priest; and two of his sisters became nuns: Mary Louise and Mary Anne. His sister Teresa married, as did Hercules, the brother Alphonsus was most associated with and attached to. Magdalen died as an infant. The children all gave testimony to the strongly religious, saintly character of their mother, who prayed with them in the morning and evening, carefully watched their companionship, and took them to Confession weekly. Little Alphonsus did what many other boys from devout families still do; he pretended to set up an altar and imitated the priest in offering Mass.

A Brilliant Lawyer

Don Joseph decided that his oldest son, Alphonsus, would be a lawyer and whatever beyond that he could attain in government. The ambitious father had much reason for honest pride and the hope of a brilliant career for his son when the boy won degrees in canon and civil law at the age of only 16. After visiting the courts for two years, he began active practice at 18, still two years under the ordinary legal age for attaining a degree. His complete honesty and hard logic made him very successful. As a Neapolitan knight, St. Alphonsus wore a sword, and as a member of the Parliament of Naples, due to family influence, he attended its meetings.

For about a year during young manhood, St. Alphonsus was somewhat careless in keeping up his custom of daily Mass and other spiritual exercises; he hurried off to many receptions, met influential people, and went often to the theater. But even at this time, his conscience was so tender that he took off his glasses at the theater and listened only to the music. "I used to go to the theater, but thanks be to God, I never thereby committed a venial sin. I would go to hear the music, which so occupied my mind that I paid no attention to anything else."

This period could, however, have been the beginning of a mediocre spiritual life. But a retreat made in March, 1722 at a house of the Vincentians recalled him to his early fervor. St. Alphonsus decided that there could be no half-measures in serving God. He began his lifelong habit of visiting the Blessed Sacrament daily. Besides the great effect these visits had in shaping his own vocation, their fruit has come down to us in the book, *Visits to the Most Blessed Sacrament and the Blessed Virgin Mary.*

Don Joseph twice chose a bride for Alphonsus. The first time, he rather cold-heartedly called off the marriage when a male heir was born into the wealthy family of the bride. The second time, the intended bride left the room rebuffed when St. Alphonsus would not look at her as she sang and he accompanied her on the harpsichord. "It appears as if the brilliant young lawyer has lost his mind," she flung back. Alphonsus had already decided to remain celibate, but had been using the excuse of his asthma for not being interested in marriage.

From the Court to the Altar

It is said that St. Alphonsus never lost a case in court until his last one. In an important lawsuit involving the equivalent of a half-million dollars in today's money, he overlooked a document on which the case hinged. In his unflinching honesty he admitted publicly that he was wrong. For three days he ate nothing, locking himself in his room. "Let him die," said Don Joseph when Anna worried that Alphonsus might starve. During the ensuing bitterness between father and son when St. Alphonsus announced he was giving up the practice of law, he one day returned for comfort to an old custom, visiting the sick. While doing this, when leaving the hospital, and later in the Church of Our Lady of Ransom, he felt himself surrounded by light and urged to renounce the world by becoming a priest. He took off his sword and laid it on the altar of Our Lady. The date was August 28, 1723.

"I pray God to take either myself or you out of the world, for I cannot bear the sight of you." This was the reaction of Alphonsus' father upon hearing the news. But when he saw that the battle was lost to his strong-willed son, Don Joseph himself presented Alphonsus to the Archbishop of Naples with the petition for acceptance as a candidate for the priesthood. Don Joseph was basically a good Catholic and parent, albeit ambitious and financially hard-headed.

Chiefly to please his father, St. Alphonsus pursued his studies for the priesthood while living at home, and he continued to reside there during the early years of his priesthood. Just shortly before he was ordained on December 21, 1726, he had been so sick that the Last Sacraments were administered. After becoming a priest, he did missionary work for five years in the Naples area as a member of the diocesan Congregation of Apostolic Missions. He belonged at the same time to the White Fathers, a group of priests who wore white mantles when visiting prisoners.

Part of St. Alphonsus' activity consisted in street preaching, and when this led to a troublesome incident for one of his associates, he went indoors, forming the "Association of the Chapels." The people in this organization met first in private houses and shops, and later in chapels, to pray and to hear instructions on the spiritual life. In time the members added care of the sick to this daily intensive program of piety.

Founding of the Redemptoristine Sisters

St. Alphonsus and some of his fellow priests took off three or four days each month and went to a secluded place outside the city to spend the time in spiritual renewal. In June, 1729, St. Alphonsus went to live at the newly organized Chinese College in Naples. Members were being gathered by Fr. Mathew Ripa, with the ultimate purpose of going to the Far East as missionaries.

About this time St. Alphonsus met Fr. Thomas Falcoia, who in time became his spiritual director and was to exercise a determining influence on his life by getting him started in the foundation of religious congregations, first for women, and then for men.

In 1730, when Fr. Falcoia was the bishop-elect of Castellamare, he asked St. Alphonsus to take his place in visiting a community of Sisters at Scala, 20 miles south of Naples. Bishop Guerriero of Scala then designated St. Alphonsus to conduct an inquiry among the nuns about revelations being given to the Sisters; the revelations were chiefly to Sr. Maria Celeste, a former Carmelite whose convent had been dissolved. St. Alphonsus decided that the revelations and the rule based on them were coming from God, and he won the disbelieving members of the community to his view. A bitter controversy of five years was thus happily settled.

On August 6, 1731, the Sisters at Scala took the new habit, and thus the Redemptoristines began. St Alphonsus, working with Bishop Falcoia, and at the wish of the Bishop of Scala, had carefully rewritten the rule that had been received in basic form from private revelations and committed to writing by Sister Maria Celeste.

Two months later the same Sister had another revelation.

It was the eve of the feast of St. Francis of Assisi, October 3, 1731. Our Lord Jesus Christ was shown to her in the light of glory, and with Him were the seraphic St. Francis and Father Alphonsus Liguori. Then the Lord said to the religious [Sr. M. Celeste speaks of herself in the third person]: "This soul [designating St. Alphonsus] has been chosen to be the head of My Institute: he will be the first superior of the Congregation of men." The religious, however, gave little heed to the thing she had seen. The next day was the feast of St. Francis of Assisi, to whom the religious had great devotion. She received Holy Communion entirely forgetful of what had happened the evening before. Suddenly there shone upon her soul a brilliant light from the Lord, in which she understood that she should write in the plan of the Institute the words of the Gospel: "Go ye and preach to every creature that the kingdom of God is at hand"; and through these words she was made to understand that she was to take down in His name the rule of life [for the new Institute] He had given her. The daily spiritual exercises would be the same as those incorporated in the rule already written [for the Redemptoristines] . . . (*Irish Ecclesiastical Record*, Vol. 53, pp. 449-459).

Other Sisters there had similar revelations.

St. Alphonsus Founds the Redemptorists

The revelations of the Sisters were the occasion of St. Alphonsus' seeking the advice of Fr. Falcoia and others, and of searching his own soul. He did not accept these revelations in the spirit of unquestioning credulity, but as possible indications of God's Will, which he could not ignore. Nor did he rush into the founding of a new institute; very carefully trying to do God's Will, he took a vow of obedience to Fr. Falcoia. Opposition was violent, coming from those who did not want to lose him at the Chinese College and the Neapolitan Congregation of Apostolic Missions. His great-uncle, Canon Gizzio, accused him: "You are not guided by God but by the fanciful dreams of a nun . . . You have lost your mind."

On Sunday, November 9, 1732, the Congregation of the Most Holy Redeemer, whose members would be familiarly known as the Redemptorists, was formally founded at Scala. Just three other priests besides St. Alphonsus formed the first community in the visitors' house on the convent grounds.

A second house opened at Villa *degli Schiavi* in 1733, and a third at Ciorani in 1735. Ciorani became the first permanent house because the first two were ultimately abandoned. The early companions of St. Alphonsus left him. He met rebuffs and an I-told-you-so attitude when he returned temporarily to Naples from Scala. "Suffering and trial will be the lot of those who engage in this work for God" had been the prophecy concerning the founding of the Redemptorists.

St. Alphonsus returned to the nearly hopeless-looking task of building his congregation, and gradually the work progressed. Houses were founded at Pagani, Iliceto and Caposele. On February 25, 1749, Pope Benedict XIV approved the Congregation of the Most Holy Redeemer, known before this as the Society of the Most Holy Saviour. St. Alphonsus was made major rector for life.

A Great Disappointment in His Old Age

The Kingdom of Naples kept up a constant harassing and hostile attitude toward the Redemptorists on the grounds that there were already too many religious Orders and a new one would deprive the others of donations and members. The chief agent of the trouble was Tanucci, the powerful prime minister, who from 1734 to 1776 controlled the king and the government. St. Alphonsus needed all his legal skill to save the Congregation. In 1752 he kept it from dissolution only by agreeing to the royal decree which gave all its revenue to the various bishops in whose territories the houses were located. He looked therefore for the chance to start a house outside the Kingdom of Naples, and founded several in the Papal States.

In his old age St. Alphonsus suffered the heaviest trial of all regarding the Redemptorists when Pope Pius VI decided that the Redemptorists in the Kingdom of Naples had made an agreement that went counter to the papal approval given by Benedict XIV. St. Alphonsus, nearly blind and suffering from headaches, had been tricked into signing a document that he had not fully examined. That had been in September, 1779. The papal decree of September 22, 1780, coming after a year of tremendous struggle by St. Alphonsus to right things, finally cut off Alphonsus and his fellow religious in the Kingdom of Naples from the Congregation he had founded.

A priest named Fr. Francis de Paula, following a selfish ambition, had worked to make the split in the Congregation. After the papal decree, only he and the Redemptorists outside the Kingdom of Naples were considered by the Pope to be members of the Redemptorist Congregation. The breach was not healed till after the death of St. Alphonsus, when the Regolamento he had signed was abolished in 1790. In 1793 a single major rector, Blasucci, would be elected for all the Redemptorists. Thus, St. Alphonsus spent his last years and died outside the Congregation he had founded. (The same Pope who issued the painful decree would declare Alphonsus Liguori "Venerable.")

As we notice in the beginning of so many religious Orders and other great works of religion, the powers of Hell seem to do their utmost to create confusion, to pit good people against one another, generally doing everything possible to destroy the good before it can get underway.

At the time of St. Alphonsus' death, the Redemptorists numbered about 200 in 15 houses. At the Congregation's second centenary in 1932, there were about 360 houses and 6,000 members, and these were located in almost all the countries and on most of the continents of the world.

The Redemptorists came to the U.S. in 1832 at the invitation of Bishop Fenwick of Cincinnati. Their first work was with the Germans in northern Ohio and the Indians in Michigan and Wisconsin. In 1839 they took charge of the Germans in Pittsburgh at old St. Philomena's. The courage and perseverance of St. Alphonsus through the darkest of his troubles paid off in the great good done by his followers in years to come.

The Redemptorist Spirit

St. Alphonsus described the spirit of his Congregation as well as of his own life when he said:

> The end of the Institute of the Most Holy Redeemer is to follow as closely as possible the footsteps and example of Jesus Christ, whose life in this world was one of detachment and mortification, full of sufferings and contempt.

St. Alphonsus was certain that one who lived his rule would be saved.

> Know that I am not grieved, my dear brothers, when God calls one of us to another life; I weep because I am flesh and blood, but I am consoled when I reflect that he has died in the Congregation, for I hold it certain that anyone who dies in the Congregation will be saved.

Pope Benedict XIV said: "Anyone keeping this rule will be a saint."

The chief aim of the Redemptorists, according to St. Alphonsus, is "to imitate as closely as possible, with the help of divine grace, the life and virtues of Our Lord Jesus Christ." A distinctive feature of the rule is the practice of a special virtue for each month of the year. These virtues as a whole should stamp the Redemptorist in the image of Christ. The twelve virtues are: Faith, Hope, Charity, Love of Neighbor, Poverty, Chastity, Obedience, Humility, Mortification, Recollection, Prayer, and Self-denial and Love of the Cross.

Following Christ, the Redemptorists were to preach the Gospel to the most abandoned. Originally this meant the poor in the country districts. Redemptorists have been called "the Salvation Army of the Church." Their symbol is a hill surmounted by a cross and flanked by the instruments of the Passion. This symbol was seen originally in a consecrated Host at Scala by a number of those present at Exposition of the Blessed Sacrament; this phenomenon happened several times.

The Redemptorists' characteristic work was the giving of parish "missions." These consisted of sermons, Confessions and spiritual exercises over a period of several days—all with the aim of bringing souls face to face with the realities of Heaven and Hell, turning them away from sin and lukewarmness and setting them firmly (or confirming them) on the path to salvation.

Bishop of St. Agatha of the Goths

Despite the opposition to the Congregation by the civil authorities in Naples, despite the lawsuits brought against it, and despite its internal troubles, its essential work of giving missions went on. Great success attended them as St. Alphonsus and his men went about from town to town during nine months of the year. He spent the time left over in a daily routine of praying, writing and administering to the affairs of the Congregation, and in forming the young members by conferences, admonitions and teaching. He also gave spiritual advice to many who came in person or asked for it by letter. Early in life, St. Alphonsus had made a vow never to waste time, and to judge by the accomplishments of his life, he succeeded in keeping it.

On March 9, 1762, the messenger of Pope Clement XIII startled St. Alphonsus with the announcement that he was chosen to be the bishop of St. Agatha of the Goths. St. Alphonsus wrote an immediate appeal to be excused because of age and health. He was 66, asthmatic, lame, bent over, partly blind and partially deaf. "Now, don't come back to me with any more of your 'most illustrious lordship' because it would be the death of me," he told the messenger. But Clement XIII insisted. Alphonsus still hoped that when the Pope saw him in person he would let him off. "When the Pope with his own eyes beholds these old bones, he will understand that nothing is to be got out of them, and he will send me back to die in the midst of my brethren."

Adding weight to his plea, St. Alphonsus developed such a

severe illness that he received the Last Sacraments. Still, the Pope merely said that if he recovered he should come to Rome. Thus, St. Alphonsus made his one and only trip to Rome and was consecrated a bishop at the end of April, 1762. Despite his wide influence, St. Alphonsus passed his own life in a narrow geographical area, chiefly within the Kingdom of Naples.

The Pope was right in insisting he accept a bishopric, for St. Alphonsus renewed the practice of the Faith in a difficult diocese. One of his first acts was to arrange for a general mission throughout his jurisdiction. Prudently, he used missionaries other than those of his own Congregation, of which he still remained the Rector Major. He reorganized the seminary, built a new building for it and took a personal hand in examining candidates. Much to the dissatisfaction of relatives, he refused many who applied. He himself taught the art of preaching, and he presided often at the defense of theses. In time the seminary attracted candidates also from other dioceses.

After a few months as bishop, a report of St. Alphonsus' way of life was made by a confrere. On August 2, 1762, Father Majone wrote:

> . . . Everybody admires his unwearied devotion to his work, his patience with applicants for favors, his kindness with the little ones, his charity towards all, his readiness to go down to the church to listen to one, to go up to the reception room to answer another, to go anywhere to render service to anyone who asks for it. All his time is spent in preaching and working, and in the organization of this poor diocese, without any respite or pity for himself. One delinquent he summons for a reprimand, another he recommends to the care of his parish priest, to another he writes a personal letter.

In his own report to the Holy See in 1765, St. Alphonsus gives a good picture of the direction his efforts had taken.

> Abuses, corrupt morals and superstitious practices are found neither in the city nor throughout the diocese. I take great pleasure in mentioning a laudable custom that has of late been introduced throughout the diocese . . . It is this: every day, at a fixed hour, the bells are rung and the faithful repair to the principal church . . . the door of the tabernacle is opened, and those present adore the Most Blessed Sacrament, reciting prayers for this purpose or making pious meditations. I never

absent myself from this public adoration in the cathedral . . . Since my coming, the practice of making mental prayer during the early Masses and the devotion to the Blessed Virgin, particularly on Saturdays, have been everywhere propagated.

St. Alphonsus received Viaticum four times and was anointed twice while serving as bishop. His petitions for release from governing the diocese were twice refused. Pope Clement XIII said: "His shadow alone is enough to govern the diocese." In 1772 Clement XIV (the Pope who sorrowfully was forced to suppress the Jesuits) refused again to replace St. Alphonsus as bishop, saying, "It is enough for me if he governs the diocese from his bed . . . His prayers will do as much good to his flock as all the activity in the world."

In his letter of April, 1775 to Pope Pius VI, St. Alphonsus listed his reasons for resigning:

I am in extreme old age, for in the month of September I enter on my eightieth year. Besides age, I have many infirmities which warn me that death is near. I suffer from a weakness of the chest which several times has reduced me to the last extremity, and from palpitation of the heart, which has also several times nearly put an end to my life. At present I am suffering from such constant headaches that sometimes they make me like one deprived of the use of his faculties. Besides these evils, I am subject to various dangerous attacks, which I have to remedy by blood-letting, blisters and other remedies, and so during the time of my episcopate I have four times received Viaticum, and twice Extreme Unction . . . My hearing fails me very much, so that many of my people suffer, who, when they wish to speak in private, cannot make themselves heard unless they raise their voice. I am paralyzed to such an extent that I can no longer write a line. With difficulty I sign my name, and so badly that it is scarcely understood. I am become so crippled that I can no longer walk a step, and have need of two assistants to move at all. I pass my life on a bed or alone in a chair. I can no longer hold ordinations nor preach, and what is more serious, I can no longer go round and hold the visitation, and the diocese is suffering positive loss thereby . . . in the state that I am in, I see that I am wanting to my duty and the government of my flock. I hope with confidence that your Holiness, considering this my state so miserable, will compassionate me and console me by accepting my resignation, first of all to relieve my flock who are little helped by a pastor who has become unable to aid them, and also to free me from the scruples which torment me when I see that I am unable to rule my diocese.

In the summer of 1775, Pope Pius VI released him from the active government of the diocese. St. Alphonsus was 79 and had governed his flock for 13 years.

Return to the Monastery at Pagani

St. Alphonsus thought that he was returning to Pagani to die. He had lost his teeth in 1762, the year he was made bishop. He had become severely crippled seven years before, in 1768, and did not say Mass for a whole year, until he was advised that he could sit on a chair to drink the Precious Blood. As a result of his illness, his neck had become so bent forward that his chin rested on his chest and caused an open wound. When he preached, no one could see his face. During the acute part of this attack he was, as he said, "like a log of wood" that had to lie on the bed in the position he was placed. Returning to the monastery at Pagani, he tried to play the piano, but could not. When someone kindly suggested that he compose a piece instead, he joked, "I had better compose a good *Libera* for my funeral, which cannot be far off." But he was to live for another 12 years.

He continued to lead a full life, devoting his time to prayer, writing and giving spiritual direction. Until the end of 1784, he wrote to his niece, Teresina, who was a nun. She was the daughter of his brother Hercules. Hercules had married twice; his first wife died having borne no children. The second wife bore four children, but lost her mind after much suffering from scruples. In one of his last letters to her he asked for prayers.

Do not forget to say three *Hail Marys* to the Madonna that she may give me peace of conscience, in the midst of so many scruples with which the devil continually torments me. I bless you and pray Most Holy Mary that she may give you holy peace. Every day say a *Salve* to the Madonna that she may make you enjoy peace of mind. (*Life of St. Alphonsus de Liguori*, by Austin Berthe, C.SS.R., 2 vols., B. Herder, St. Louis, 1906, Vol. 2, p. 575).

His Last Years

On August 1, 1783 St. Alphonsus gave up the office of Rector Major of the Congregation. On November 25, 1785, he offered Mass for the last time. It was feared that due to his weakness, he might have some accident at Mass. This was a very grievous sacrifice for him to make, but St. Alphonsus accepted it at the wish of Fr. Villani, his spiritual director.

He could get about only on a roller chair, and worried that this was making too much noise in the corridor. When he was wheeled outside, children gathered around, and he blessed them. "They are like a flock of young sparrows looking at an old owl," he commented. Even in the midst of so many privations, he found a way to do penance. He would remain motionless in his chair, suffering the discomfort of not moving. When he was told to straighten up, he answered: "It is no use for me to straighten myself. I am crooked anyway." Another penitential trick of St. Alphonsus at this time was to lie on his rosary in bed. However, he had a passion for obedience, and by merely mentioning the word, the attendant Brother could readily secure his cooperation.

Being forgetful at times, St. Alphonsus had Brother Francis Anthony write down the acts he wanted to make before going to sleep:

> Ten acts of love, ten acts of confidence, ten acts of contrition, ten acts of conformity to the will of God, ten acts of love for Jesus Christ, ten acts of love for the Madonna, ten acts of love for the Blessed Sacrament, ten acts of confidence in Mary, ten acts of resignation in suffering, ten acts of abandonment to Jesus and Mary, ten prayers to do the will of God. (*Berthe,* p. 585).

Even in his sleep St. Alphonsus used to repeat his favorite aspirations, such as "O my Jesus, how ravishing is Thy loveliness!" and "How beautiful thou art, O Mary!"

He used to say the Rosary with the Brother who wheeled him up and down the corridor. One day there was a doubt about whether they had finished the Rosary. The Brother thought they had. "You think, you think, but are you sure?" said St. Alphonsus. "Do you not know that my salvation may depend on this devotion?" At another time, when the Brother wanted to hustle him off to dinner before the Rosary was finished, St. Alphonsus told him to wait: "Just a moment, my dear Brother; remember that one *Ave Maria* is worth all the dinners in the world."

For about three years near the end of his life, St. Alphonsus was tormented by scruples, by worries over his salvation, by doubts against every article of the Creed, by many temptations, including despair and impurity. The Brother, knowing that he was wrought up over scruples, told him: "You must be quiet, or you will die mad, and what would the world say if Monsignore de Liguori were to die mad?" St. Alphonsus showed a perfect resignation in his reply: "Brother, and if God wishes me to die mad, what have you to say against it?" The courage of this reply is amazing, since in his immediate family his sister-in-law had lost her mind. St. Alphonsus' one salvation was blind obedience to his director. When incapable of judging, he followed blindly the judgment of his spiritual adviser. (*Berthe,* p. 592). Satan at times visited him in the visible appearance of a priest and tried to lead him astray. (*Berthe,* p. 594). Or again, the devil physically seized him with great violence.

Various people who came to visit St. Alphonsus in his last weeks of sickness were cured of diseases. One such was Fr. Samuele of Naples, a former Provincial of the Capuchins. Not being able to make himself understood when he asked for a blessing, he took St. Alphonsus' hand and touched it to his ear. He was instantly cured of a painful, long-standing malady of the ear.

On July 28, 1787 Alphonsus received Holy Communion for the last time. He drifted into a state of semi-stupor, but always roused to consciousness when anyone spoke of God, the Blessed Virgin or one of the Saints. About 7:00 in the evening of July 31, his face lit up and became full of color; he smiled as he looked for about 15 minutes at a picture of the Blessed Virgin. A little later this same thing happened, lasting still longer. Then he lay back as before, pallid and nearly lifeless. Many Masses were said in his cell in the early morning of August 1st. As the monastery bell rang the noon *Angelus,* St. Alphonsus quietly breathed his last.

His great biographer and confrere says: "Alfonso Maria de Liguori died full of years and merits on Wednesday, the 1st of August, 1787 at the sound of the *Angelus Domini,* having lived ninety years, ten months and five days."

His View of the Incarnation

"The first and most dominant characteristic of the personal sanctity of St. Alphonsus Liguori was undoubtedly his deep and tender love for Jesus Christ. This love for the Redeemer was at the root of all his other characteristics; like a motive running through a musical composition or the pattern in a tapestry, it gave tone and color and design to all the internal and external actions of his life." (*Letters of the Redemptorist Generals,* 3).

St. Alphonsus' *Way of the Cross* and *Visits to the Blessed Sacrament* give familiar testimony to his devotion to the sacred humanity of Christ. These are his works most published in English, and in fact in all languages. According to a count made in 1933, the *Way of the Cross* had at that time been published 63 times in English and 890 times in all; the *Visits* had been published 54 times in English and 2,009 times in all.

It has been said that St. Alphonsus Liguori was the St. Francis de Sales of Italy in meekness and spirit, but that unlike St. Francis he followed the Thomist view of the motive for the Incarnation. St. Thomas considered the coming of Christ as altogether remedial. Christ would not have come otherwise, "so far as God's present decrees are concerned," in the phrase of Fr. Faber.

St. Alphonsus does speak plainly of holding the Thomistic view: "Christ came on earth only to suffer and, by His death on the cross for us, to draw us to His love." (*Reflections on the Truth of Divine Revelation,* 1773). St. Alphonsus considered that in the decree of Providence, the Incarnation was due to the *mercy* of God. Had man not sinned, Christ in the present decree would not have come.

He Sings of Mary's Mercy . . .

This viewpoint had a determining effect on St. Alphonsus' basic thinking about the Blessed Virgin. Her divine maternity was decreed *dependently* on God's pre-vision of man's sin, since Christ, in the same present decree, came only after this pre-vision. Therefore, Mary's children can turn to her with unbounded confidence, since she holds her greatest privilege because of God's mercy in giving us a Redeemer. As sinners, we may approach her as the Mother of Mercy.

The stories St. Alphonsus tells of Mary's love for sinners have struck some as exaggerated. It is true that each story cannot be historically proven. But together they illustrate that Mary does love sinners, and that, in dependence on her Son, she is "suppliant omnipotence."

"What St. Alphonsus is saying for the religious mind behind which is lurking a warm heart (as well as for the individual with good sense) is simply that in God's providence Mary represents the concrete form of God's infinite mercy. Millions of devout souls have gotten this message from *The Glories of Mary.*" (F. X. Murphy in *Catholic World,* 197:140).

In his Introduction to *The Glories of Mary,* St. Alphonsus states that during missions it was the sermon on the mercy of Mary that was the most profitable for souls and that produced the most compunction. "For this reason I here leave other authors to describe the other prerogatives of Mary, and confine myself for the most part to that of her mercy and powerful intercession . . ."

. . . And of Her Glories

St. Alphonsus had been gathering material for his work on *The Glories of Mary* since his ordination to the priesthood. He only published the work in 1750, when he was 54 and thought he was near death. The immediate occasion was the publication in 1747 of Muratori's work, *The Well-Regulated Devotion of Christians,* which attacked Mary's mediatorship.

In defending his praise of Mary, St. Alphonsus quotes St. Augustine, who declares

> that whatever we may say in praise of Mary is little in comparison with that which she deserves, on account of her dignity of Mother of God; and moreover, the Church says, in the Mass appointed for her festivals, "Thou art happy, O sacred Virgin Mary, and most worthy of all praise."

The Glories of Mary "is probably the most widely read book on the Blessed Virgin in the world." (F. J. Connell in *Thought,* Fordham U. Press, 7:279-287). As of 1933, *The Glories of Mary* had been published 32 times in English and 736 times in all.

On the Immaculate Conception

"Due to the effort of this popular Mariologist—the most influential in the history of modern Catholicism—the way was made easy for the ultimate triumph of the dogma of the Immaculate Conception." (Albert Hauck in *Realencyclopedie,* Vol. XII, p. 326, quoted in *Irish Ecclesiastical Record* 82:391). St. Alphonsus entered the lists against Louis Muratori, Father of Italian History, who denied the Immaculate Conception, and defended it vigorously. Pope Pius IX asks:

> Are not the things we have solemnly approved concerning the Immaculate Conception of the Blessed Mother of God and the infallibility of the Roman Pontiff when teaching *ex cathedra* . . . found and most clearly explained, and demonstrated with the strongest arguments, in the works of Alphonsus? (*Decree conferring the title of Doctor of the Church*).

In the days before the definition of the dogma of the Immaculate Conception, St. Alphonsus found the principle, *Lex orandi, lex credendi* ("As one prays, thus he believes"), to strongly bolster it. "The truth of the Immaculate Conception," he said, "is borne in on me more especially by the common Christian instinct of the faithful, who have it rooted in the innermost recesses of their minds . . ." (Quoted by Culhane in *IER* 82:391).

All that St. Alphonsus wrote about the Immaculate Conception was brought together in one volume and translated into Latin by Fr. William Van Rossum in 1904. In the early days of the Redemptorists, St. Alphonsus asked the members to vow defense of the Immaculate Conception, not then defined as a dogma. He chose Mary, under her title of Immaculate Conception, as the patroness of his Congregation.

On Mary as Mediatrix

St. Alphonsus was not the first to teach that Mary is the "Mother of All Graces," but he did much to spread the idea. According to Fr. F. J. Connell (*Thought* 7:279-287), St. Alphonsus "regarded Mary's participation in the dispensation of graces as one of the elements of the divine plan that decreed that a man and a woman—Christ and Mary—should collaborate in repairing the damage inflicted on humanity by another man and woman—Adam and Eve."

St. Alphonsus held this not as an argument of congruity, but as a "principle of partnership" (*principium consortii).* He said there is a twofold mediatorship: that of justice and that of grace. The first belongs only to Christ by condign merit. Mary's mediatorship of grace is dependent entirely on the merits of Christ and is exercised by way of intercessory prayer.

Fr. Connell explains Mary's mediatorship of grace: "In calling Mary the Mediatrix of All Graces, we mean that the *acquisition and the bestowal* of all the supernatural favors conferred on mankind depend in some measure on her participation with her divine Son in the accomplishment of human salvation. The adequate concept of her mediation embraces two elements—first, her active cooperation with Christ in the work of the Redemption, accomplished 19 centuries ago; secondly, her concurrence in the communication to individual souls of the grace merited by the Redemption, which will continue until the end of time. By reason of the former element, Mary is called the co-redemptrix; by reason of the latter she is designated the dispensatrix of all graces." (*Thought,* 7, 283).

His Own Marian Devotion

One who reads *The Glories of Mary* cannot help noticing that this work mirrors the soul of the author. It was the loving work of many years.

> Having collected as far as I was able, and with the labor of many years, all that the holy Fathers and the most celebrated writers have said on this subject; and as I find that the mercy and power of the most Blessed Virgin are admirably portrayed in the prayer, *Salve Regina* . . . I shall divide and explain this most devout prayer in separate chapters. (Introduction to *Glories of Mary).*

St. Alphonsus felt the love of Mary and put absolute trust in her. The great saints, he says, were inflamed by the love of God to do much for their neighbor. Yet Mary loved God more than any of them. So she loves us more and will do more for us. We are dear to her also because of the great suffering we have cost her and because, more than anyone else, she knows the suffering her Son has endured for us. (*Glories of Mary,* ch. 1, no. 3).

"Be devout to the Blessed Virgin and she will save you," he

used to say. He shortened the customary afternoon Italian siesta so he could recite the five psalms of St. Bonaventure in honor of the Blessed Virgin. He made a vow to preach about Mary every Saturday and did this even at the age of 80 after retiring from his bishopric. He also fasted on Saturdays in her honor. He required the Redemptorists to preach a sermon on Mary's mercy at every mission.

The two decisions that cost him the most pain, St. Alphonsus tells us, were his deciding to be a priest against his father's wishes and the accepting of his bishopric. Before making these and other important decisions, he fervently besought the aid of the Blessed Virgin Mary. On the way to Rome before his consecration as a bishop, he went aside to spend three days at the Shrine of Loreto. The Blessed Virgin Mary appeared to him a number of times, or unmistakably made known her wishes to him in some manner.

When the tomb of St. Alphonsus Liguori was opened years after his death, Pope Pius VII asked that the three fingers of his right hand be sent to Rome. "Let these three fingers that have written so well for the honor of God, of the Blessed Virgin, and of religion, be carefully preserved and sent to Rome." ("Some Preliminary Observations," by the editor, *The Glories of Mary*, Grimm ed., p. 20).

In the Church of St. Alphonsus at Rome is the celebrated miraculous picture of Our Lady of Perpetual Help. The picture came from Crete in the thirteenth century.

In accordance with a vision in which the picture was ordered to be placed between St. Mary Major's and St. John Lateran's, it was in 1499 placed in the church of the Augustinian Fathers dedicated to St. Matthew, which was in the required position. When St. Matthew's was destroyed by the French in 1811, the picture disappeared from public view. In 1866, by the Pope's command, it was placed in the Church of St. Alphonsus, which had been built in 1855 hard by the ruins of St. Matthew's. (*Berthe*, Vol. II, p. 886).

The coming of the picture to St. Alphonsus' Church in Rome can be seen as a special token of Mary's love for this devoted servant, the fervent proclaimer of her mercy and power. The Redemptorist sons of St. Alphonsus have been noted for their devotion to Mary and for spreading devotion to her as the Mother of Perpetual Help. Celebration of the centenary of the placement of this famous picture in St. Alphonsus' Church took place in 1966.

A Practical Writer

Canon Sheehan said that St. Alphonsus was outstanding in the practical guidance of souls. "What St. Thomas Aquinas is to Christian philosophy, what Bellarmine is in controversy, that St. Alphonsus is in the practical department of ethical science and the guidance of souls." (Quoted in *IER*, 56). His practical sense showed itself even to the point of his asking the printer of his writings to use a good grade of paper and to avoid bulky looking books. "Spiritual books especially ought to be handy for reading," said Alphonsus. Another writer comments:

> All the works of St. Alphonsus are pre-eminently practical. The reason for this is that, *Doctor Zelantissimus* (Most Zealous Doctor) that he was, he set himself a pre-eminently practical object in writing . . . We cannot better define the general comprehensive practical object of St Alphonsus' writings than by saying that they were meant to be what in fact they have been, a safe and secure spiritual bridge from time to eternity, from earth to heaven, for men and women in every state and stage of life. (R. Culhane in *IER*, 56: p. 510-511).

Because of his driving zeal as well as his natural carefulness, St. Alphonsus was what would be called today a "bleeder" (one who covers his paper with ink). He wrote carefully, and then changed, and re-wrote, filling his paper with many marginal notes. He found it hard to be satisfied. "My original manuscripts," he said, "are entirely covered with marginal notes and erasures, as I am never contented, not even with myself." When he had a feverish, throbbing headache, he held a piece of cold marble to his head and continued to write. "God knows how much effort and fatigue I have experienced in that work," he said of his *Moral Theology,* on which he labored for 30 years through eight editions.

The Prince of Moralists

St. Alphonsus did his basic work on the *Moral Theology* from 1743 to 1748, digging through some 800 authors in finding opinions on various questions. He used the 300-page work of Herman

Busembaum, S.J. as a handy guide, building his commentary on its subject matter and outline. His final revision of *Moral Theology* (the 8th) culminated in a 4,000-page work.

In a letter of September 21, 1748, St. Alphonsus describes the book, and also the labor it cost:

> . . . The book itself, I believe, should come to be most useful. Not very voluminous, but full of matter most substantial, it covers the whole moral field, especially with regard to matters of practice. I have included a brief "Practice for Confessing the Ignorant" . . . But enough. These are but trifling though bothersome matters in respect to a book which has cost me years and years of labor—especially these last, when for practically five years continuously, I have been at it for 8, 9, and 10 hours a day, until I really have become disgusted with it.

The work probably came off the press in early October, 1748.

St. Alphonsus is justly called the "Prince of Moralists." In his own time, his *Moral Theology* caused a revolution in the manner of confessional practice; in succeeding years, it has had many imitators. Although very strict with himself, St. Alphonsus advanced the theories of equi-probabilism and probabilism, both of which were considered lax by many at the time, and both of which were opposed to the heresy of Jansenism, which was very strong at the time and which demanded following always the safest opinion.

In his original *Moral Theology* St. Alphonsus Liguori favored equi-probabilism, but the following year he published a treatise favoring a moderate use of probabilism. "We conclude," he says,

> that it is allowable to follow a probable opinion occurring against a more probable one, but only when the former is based on solid motivation, whether intrinsically from reason or extrinsically on the authority of learned authors. (F. X. Murphy, *Thought,* vol. 23:605-620,).

In 1846 a work appeared whose title shows the trend of some of the criticism against St. Alphonsus: *Awful Discourses of the Iniquitous Principles Taught by the Church of Rome; Being Extracts from the Moral Theology of Alphonsus Liguori,* by P. Blakeney, London. Adolph Harnack even paired St. Alphonsus with the irreligious Voltaire as having had a supreme influence on 18th-century European life by favoring an out-and-out probabilism, thus leading the Church to a breakdown in moral principles.

In 1831, however, Pope Gregory XVI had "decreed it safe to follow St. Alphonsus' opinion, even if you do not know the reason behind it—a badge of honor Rome has given no other saint." (Joseph Maier, C.SS.R in *The Priest,* Vol. 19, Sept. 1963).

St. Alphonsus has been given much credit for defeating Jansenism in southern Italy.

> The real importance of Alphonsus and his *Moral Theology,* however, lies not so much in his having been instrumental in destroying the inroads of Jansenistic severity, or even in his attempt at balancing the scales in his famous "equi-probable" system. His most pressing claim to consideration as a first-class moralist lies in the fact that he insisted so strongly upon an empirical approach to the discipline of absolving, guiding, and saving souls. (Francis X. Murphy, *Thought,* vol. 23, p. 617).

He considered passions, impulses, temptations, actual graces, psychological construction, anything that might influence action and judgment. "For this service the Church honors him as Doctor and Prince of Moral Theologians."

The Best-Selling Author of All Time

In 1933 a Belgian Redemptorist, Fr. Maurice de Meulemeester, published a folio volume of 370 pages listing all the printed works of St. Alphonsus and naming his translators and publishers. According to this, there had been 4,110 editions of St. Alphonsus in the original language, which was either Italian or Latin. Altogether there had been 17,125 traceable editions in 63 languages. Besides his books and booklets, 1,451 letters of St. Alphonsus have been published.

In figures given in 1961 for Shakespeare, the number of languages into which he had been translated was 77. But in editions of his works, Shakespeare, with a head start of 150 years, trails St Alphonsus by some 7,000 editions. (An edition here means a publication containing one or more of his works.)

In August, 1962, an article by R. J. Miller, C.SS.R. in *The Liguorian* estimated that there had been some 21,000 editions of the various works of St. Alphonsus. This would mean that, as of that time, one or other of his works had been put out in a new edition somewhere in the world every three or four days for the previous 200 years! Fr. Miller says that St. Alphonsus Liguori, as a published author, has no competitors.

> The most popular author who ever lived was St. Alphonsus Liguori, and he never wrote a novel. No other writer, sacred or profane (we are not speaking of the Holy Bible, which is in a class by itself), ancient or modern, has had so many different editions of his works published as St. Alphonsus.

In the 1980's, O. B. L. Victory Mission of Brookings, South Dakota reprinted St. Alphonsus' main ascetical works, except *Visits to the Blessed Sacrament,* in an inexpensive pocketbook format, using the old Redemptorist edition edited by Rev. Eugene Grimm, thus achieving widespread distribution in a few years' time. The titles included *Preparation for Death; The Way of Salvation and Perfection, The Great Means of Salvation and Perfection; The Incarnation, Birth and Infancy of Jesus Christ; The Passion and Death of Jesus Christ; The Holy Eucharist; The Glories of Mary; The Victories of the Martyrs; The True Spouse of Jesus Christ;* and *The Dignities and Duties of the Priest.* Most of these volumes included several shorter works by the Saint.

Declared a Doctor of the Church

The first book published by St. Alphonsus was the *Visits to the Most Blessed Sacrament and the Blessed Virgin Mary.* This was in about 1745, when he was already 49 years old. His last work came out in 1777, and concerned the fidelity of vassals. For about 30 years he poured out his literary work, to the total of 111 distinct titles. Some of these were of pamphlet size. But many also were sizable books. His *Moral Theology* alone was 4,000 pages, and the above-mentioned volumes run 400 to 900 pages each (usually including more than one work in a volume). For a man who started writing rather late in life, St. Alphonsus' output was tremendous.

But his influence has been even more tremendous. His writings, which prominently showed the love and mercy of God, broke the back of the Jansenist error, which emphasized God's justice to the neglect of His mercy and which demanded a stern, rigorous approach to religion, with infrequent use of the Sacraments—just the opposite of what St. Alphonsus called for as being the actual traditional practice of the Church. His devotional works have helped millions of readers to practice the love of God, to imitate Christ, to honor the Blessed Virgin and to have confidence in her.

The Catholic Church recognized the wide influence of St. Alphonsus Liguori by declaring him a Doctor of the Church on July 7, 1871, as proclaimed in the Apostolic Letter of Pius IX. This was done 32 years after St. Alphonsus' canonization, which took place on May 26, 1839, and less than a century after his death.

> St. Thomas Aquinas had to wait for three centuries, St. Robert Bellarmine and St. Peter Canisius for more than three centuries. St. Albert the Great was not declared Doctor of the Church until seven centuries had passed. St. Alphonsus, however, received the title in less than a century after his death. (*IER*, vol. 53).

By way of reference for American readers, St. Alphonsus Liguori was still alive during the American Revolutionary period. The earlier Doctors that were closest to him chronologically, but still more than a century and a half earlier, were St. Francis de Sales (died 1622) and St. Lawrence of Brindisi (died 1619).

The Patron of Confessors

The 13 Popes preceding Pius XII had all in some way especially recommended St. Alphonsus' *Moral Theology*. Pope Pius XII, on the occasion of the second centenary of the first edition of this greatest work of St. Alphonsus, designated him as the "Patron of Moralists and Confessors." Pope Pius XII referred in his declaration of April 26, 1950 to the hearing of Confessions as the principal work committed to the Redemptorists by their founder. "Indeed, he committed to his companions, gathered into the Congregation of the Most Holy Redeemer, as its principal duty, the hearing of Confessions."

The Redemptorist constitutions declare: "Nothing shall be dearer to the members than the hearing of Confessions, for there is no work better calculated to procure the glory of God and the salvation of souls." In his diocese, St. Alphonsus as bishop advised all pastors to have a visiting priest hear Confessions in their parishes once a month. He was a strong promoter of frequent discussion of moral cases among the priests in the diocese, and he also wanted weekly discussions of moral cases among his religious. He wanted the ablest men to be chosen as teachers of moral theology.

St. Alphonsus based his moral system on two principles. 1) He would leave the conscience free where the law was doubtful, so as to prevent sin; and 2) where sin was certain, he would urge severity to remove it, since Christ said that an eye, hand or foot should be lost rather than commit a sin. From these principles it follows that a confessor following St. Alphonsus as a guide will be lenient in not urging doubtful laws, but stern in demanding the giving up of occasions of definitely known sin. (*Circular Letters of Redemptorist Generals,* Bruce Publ. Co., 1933, p. 160).

St. Alphonsus summarized these principles in practical points for confessors and preachers: 1) Their primary purpose is to eradicate sin; 2) they must get the penitent to remove occasions of sin; and 3) they should insure perseverance in living in grace by laying the foundation of a genuine Christian life. (*Circular Letters,* p. 17).

People flocked to St. Alphonsus for Confession. He was unfailingly kind, following the principle that

> the deeper a soul has fallen into sin, the more it is bound down by the powers of Hell, the greater should be the kindness of the confessor in order to win it to repentance, to snatch it from the devil, and to bring it to the arms of Jesus Christ. (*St. Alphonsus Mary de Liguori,* by D. F. Miller, C.SS.R. and L. X. Aubin, C.SS.R., Quebec, London, 1940; TAN, 1987, p. 39).

St. Alphonsus says,

> If all preachers and confessors would discharge their duties as they should, the whole world would be holy! Bad preachers and bad confessors are the ruin of the world; and every preacher and every confessor is bad who is not devoted to his office, who does not study to improve himself in it, who does not fulfill it to the very best of his ability. (*Circular Letters,* p. 12).

The saying that St. Alphonsus never refused absolution is, however, not true. "It is beyond doubt that St. Alphonsus often deferred absolution, and for a period exceeding 15 days," concludes a documented study made in 1943 by J. H. Cleary, C.SS.R. (*IER* 62:389-391). The error of saying that St. Alphonsus never refused absolution crept in, says Fr. Faber, from an anonymous lady translator who used a French translation of Fr. Tannoia for her English text.

Tannoia does say that in his old age St. Alphonsus used to say he did not remember sending anyone away without absolution. But Tannoia, in his complete text, gives an explanation. He writes:

> When he was old, he used to say that he did not remember having ever sent away anyone without absolution, and much less had he dismissed them with unkindness and asperity. Not that he used to absolve all indiscriminately, both those with proper dispositions and those without them; but as he explained on another occasion, he would welcome sinners with kindness and inspire them with confidence in the Precious Blood of Jesus Christ, indicating to them the means by which they could rise from the state of sin. And thus encouraged, they used to *come back* to him, penitent and contrite.

On November 12, 1990 Pope John Paul II went to venerate the remains of St. Alphonsus in the Basilica of Pagani, and there he gave an address entitled *Con Animo*. In the address he recalled his Apostolic Letter of August 1, 1987, *Spiritus Domini* ("The Spirit of the Lord"), in which he had commemorated the second centenary of the death of St. Alphonsus. The Holy Father reminded his hearers that on April 26, 1950, Pope Pius XII had proclaimed St. Alphonsus the "Patron Saint of Confessors and Moral Theologians." The ferverino *Con Animo* asks all confessors to have a profound spirituality themselves so that they can more fully exercise their roles in the Sacrament of Penance as father, physician and judge, and thus bring healing to the penitent. (*The Pope Speaks*, vol. 36, no. 4, pp. 197-200).

A Composer of Music

Once, in St. Alphonsus' boyhood, his father locked him and his music teacher in a room for three hours. Like most children, St. Alphonsus found practice to be trying. But he not only developed considerable skill in playing the harpsichord, but became a music composer of some merit. Had he taken the time, he could have produced outstanding music, as is reflected in the *Duetto*, the manuscript of which was found in the British Museum after having been lost for a century. The *Duetto* is a conversation, set to music, between Christ going to Calvary and the Christian soul. The soul also addresses reproaches to Pilate.

Don Lorenzo Perosi, director of the Vatican Choir, called St. Alphonsus a "professor's professor of music." Alphonsus showed his approach to music when he said: "Music is an art which must be practiced in its perfection—otherwise it does not produce pleasure, but disgust." (*Berthe*, Vol. 1, p. 592).

As a bishop, St. Alphonsus restored Gregorian chant to the diocese and issued a pastoral letter on Church music. He was interested in composing music chiefly as a help to religion. He knew the power of song over the mind and heart of the people, and he dreaded the influence of the erotic songs common among the people. He composed hymns, both words and music, to bring out the truths of faith, and to stir up the love of Jesus and Mary in hearts. His melodies are simple and catchy.

St. Alphonsus used to sing his hymns with the people; his missionaries were also trained to do this. His own singing voice was clear and sweet, and with his exact pronunciation, carried through the largest churches, so that all could understand. Usually the people would keep repeating the same refrain while the missionary, as leader, developed the theme, using many different stanzas. For example, the priest would sing:

> My Jesus, say what wretch has dared
> Thy sacred hands to bind?
> And who has dared to buffet so
> Thy face so meek and kind?

The people would reply:

> 'Tis I have thus ungrateful been,
> Yet, Jesus, pity take,
> Oh, spare and pardon me, my Lord,
> For Thy sweet mercy's sake.

Then the priest would continue with various stanzas describing the individual sufferings of Christ. After each, the people would respond as at first.

Other compositions of St. Alphonsus, besides the above that are familiar through English translations are: "O God of Loveliness," "O Bread of Heaven, Beneath this Veil," and "Look Down, O Mother Mary, from Thy Bright Throne Above."

On Christmas Eve in 1955, Vatican Radio produced a story

entitled "Italy's Favorite Christmas Carol." It told about the hymn, "From Starry Skies Descending" (*Tu Scendi Dalle Stelle*), which St. Alphonsus had written during a Christmas mission in Nola in 1755. (*Cecelia* 85:389-390). His original purpose was to leave the people with a reminder of the mission that would make its fruits continue. Another favorite Italian hymn is the touching and simple "Your Will and Not My Own" (*Il Tuo Gusto*). It was composed by St. Alphonsus on the death of an outstanding early Redemptorist and friend, Fr. Paul Cafaro.

Altogether St. Alphonsus wrote about 50 hymns. Since they were for the people, the words are in Italian. Nicola Montani, founder of the Society of St. Gregory, included many hymns of St. Alphonsus in the *St. Gregory Hymnal*. In 1932 Fr. DiCoste, C.SS.R., published a collection of the "traditional melodies" and the celebrated *Oratorio* or *Duetto* of St. Alphonsus. The music for these hymns had never been printed, but had been preserved by the people who sang them. DiCoste presented 20 hymns in 28 pages of music. (*Cath. Mind*, 32:33-40, translated from a *Civilta Catolica* article of May 20, 1933).

St. Alphonsus, the Man

Fr. Anthony Tannoia, novice master of the Redemptorists in the early days and St. Alphonsus' admiring biographer, has left us this description of the man.

Alfonso was of middle height, but his head was somewhat large and his complexion fair. He had a broad forehead, a beautiful eye a little blue, an aquiline nose, a small mouth pleasant and rather smiling. His hair was black, and his beard, which he cut short with scissors but did not shave, well-grown. An enemy of long hair and affectation [as being] unworthy of the minister of the altar, he used to cut his hair himself. Being near-sighted he used spectacles, which he took off when preaching or speaking to women. His voice was musical and clear, and however large the church or long the mission, it never failed him, nor did it even fail him in extreme old age. His appearance was very dignified, with a manner both grave and weighty, yet mingled with good humor, so that he made his conversation pleasant and agreeable to all, young and old. His gifts of mind were admirable. His intellect was acute and penetrating, his memory ready and tenacious, his mind clear and well arranged, his will effective and strong. These are gifts which upheld the weight of his literary undertakings and did so much for the Church of Christ. (*Berthe*, Vol. II, p. 612).

A Complex Man

We can call St. Alphonsus a complex man because he was highly intellectual, yet very ardent in nature; he was a master moralist, yet himself troubled by personal scruples; he wasted no time at all, yet cultivated the arts; he prophesied and worked miracles, but often felt completely inadequate and unworthy; he searched authors ancient and new and weighed their opinions carefully, yet his judgment was quite independent; he came from the nobility, but cherished the poor and lived as one of them. At the same time St. Alphonsus was a completely simple man in the sense that complete honesty about himself and in his dealings with others was always in evidence. He was a very direct man, whose words and actions were simple and heartfelt and went directly to the minds and hearts of others.

The question has been raised that St. Alphonsus may have been somewhat neurotic.

> A strain of what we now call the neurotic in the Saint's character is not to be denied. The nature of the malady—was it rheumatic arthritis?—which made the closing years of Liguori's long life so painful may repay study when more is known of these matters, for psycho-pathology has its word to say even in the interpretation of Saints, though not of their sainthood. (*Month*, by Reginald Dingle, 13:21-31).

Concerning this question in general, it should be said that sanctity is not incompatible with neurosis. The adage that grace builds on nature has been overworked. It does not explain all sanctity historically, and it is a half-truth, an over-simplification. The other side of the coin is that grace builds to heroic heights as it overcomes the obstacles of nature by a will clinging to God. The artist in holiness, the champion of God, is often like the artist in music or oratory or the champion in sports who rises to the heights despite drawbacks that in themselves are direct obstacles to achievement in some art or sport. (Writers of Saints' Lives may, when explaining sanctity, tend too easily to be theoreticians rather than candid historians or psychologists.) The Saint may have had a harder time than others would have had, to climb up to his pedestal.

The Grace of Perseverance

A basic idea that influenced St. Alphonsus' type of spirituality and character was his emphasis on the truth that perseverance is an entirely separate grace, that it cannot strictly be merited. "With regard to perseverance," said St. Alphonsus, "I differ with St. Augustine. Perseverance is a grace distinct from the love of God. God wished it so; and when, therefore, my love assures me that I shall be faithful to God today, it does not give me the same assurance for tomorrow." (CL, p. 6).

It was this view which made St. Alphonsus, to the end of his life, dread falling from grace; it was this view which made him so emphasize prayer. More than other spiritual masters, he emphasized the prayer of petition. We must pray for the grace of continuing to pray; we must pray for the gift of prayer!

This view led him also to emphasize the need for renewing the mission in a parish by having his priests return after some months to stir the people to perseverance. It led him also to stress the work of the local pastors in confirming the good work begun at the time of a mission.

His great awareness of man's complete dependence on the free gifts of God led him to cling more and more to the merciful love of Jesus and Mary. "O Jesus, my Love; O Mary, my hope!" This was his constant sentiment.

A Very Busy Man

St. Alphonsus allowed himself no time to miss receiving the grace of final perseverance. He was one of the busiest and most productive of men. St. Alphonsus made and kept a vow not to lose a single moment of time. He divided his day into periods, and in this way he found time for everything. Even his most crowded schedule included three half-hour periods for meditation, besides the time set aside for daily Mass, thanksgiving afterwards, Divine Office, Rosary and a visit to the Blessed Sacrament. Writing books, preaching missions and retreats, composing music, administering his Congregation and bishopric, answering letters and hearing great numbers of Confessions, receiving many visitors, visiting the sick and poor—all these received a full share of his time. As a bishop, he would not touch the piano. At other times in his life, he played; he also found time to paint pictures, a few of which are still extant.

A Poor Man

St. Alphonsus had a great love for the poor and practiced personal poverty to an unusual degree. As a bishop, he made it a rule to accept no personal gifts. As an author, he wanted no profit from his books. His ring was quietly parted from its diamond and re-set with a glass mounting. His room, even when he was a bishop, was practically bare of furniture and ornament. His table fare was very meager, and for many years he ate only once a day. On one occasion, in his younger days as a missionary, he went upon arrival at the parish for a visit to the Blessed Sacrament. The young priest at the place, noting his much-patched clothing, mistook him for a vagrant and decided it was time to lock the church. Despite a request to stay, Alphonsus was told the church had to be locked.

The description he gives of his horses illustrates his poverty as well as his fine sense of conscience. He wrote to the Brother who was to sell the horses which had been long used for the daily carriage ride ordered by the doctors:

> I do not want to have any scruples about the horses I am sending you. You will therefore let intending buyers know that one of them suffers in its jaws and cannot chew either straw or oats, and that the other, the older of the two, suffers from lunacy and throws himself on the ground from time to time. To make him get up, you must pull his ears. Explain all this clearly so that I may be at ease.

The Brother evidently explained quite clearly, as the sale brought a total sum of just about five-and-a-half dollars.

When somebody objected that he was giving alms to unworthy people, St. Alphonsus would reply: "It is more than likely, but what does it matter after all? It is better to be cheated into giving too much than to lose one's soul by giving too little."

An Ardent Nature

St. Alphonsus had a very ardent nature. Tears are frequently mentioned by his biographers. When the people wept at his departure from his bishopric, he too began to weep, and went among them giving out alms. When a cousin left him and his brother Hercules 60,000 ducats, St. Alphonsus ceded his share to his brother, who was not too well off and needed money for his children. When Hercules died suddenly in 1780 (September 8), St. Alphonsus wrote to the lawyer Gavotti: "If the death of my brother, Don Hercules, whom may God have in His glory, has brought me no slight grief and distress, it also filled my mind, as soon as I heard the news, with a thousand painful thoughts about the care of my nephews . . ." St. Alphonsus was deeply attached to his family. He had much personal feeling, too, for the members of the Congregation, and took a detailed interest in their well-being. "While your illness lasts," he wrote to a young novice, "do not apply your mind to things too much. Look after your health, go for a walk in the morning, obey the doctor, and pray every day for me." (*Berthe*, Vol. I, p. 486).

When he was a bishop, people would at times leave their babies at the episcopal residence when they went in groups to work. The bishop must really have been a man of good heart for people to have found him so neighborly.

His writings, especially on the Blessed Virgin, the Passion and the Holy Eucharist, as well as the prayers he composed, are full of devotion and feeling. They tell, by the orderly way in which they are composed, of a man of intellect; they tell, in their tenderness and sweetness, of a man of heart. More than any other Doctor of the Church, St. Alphonsus Liguori has been read by the common man because he expresses the things the common man often feels but cannot say. He touches something deep within his readers because he wrote from an overflowing heart.

St. Alphonsus was an apostle to all, the "Most Zealous Doctor," because his heart went out to each one. At the age of 81 he even wrote to Voltaire when a false report came out that Voltaire had converted.

> I was grieved indeed and wept to see that truly great intellect you received from God so misused by you these many years, and times without number, most unworthy though I am, I begged God in prayer that the Father of mercies would free you from your errors and draw you altogether to His love.

The letter was not sent, as the rumor was quickly denied.

Against the coldness and rigor of Jansenism, "the subtlest heresy ever woven in the devil's loom," St. Alphonsus brought warmth and humanity to religion. On one occasion, against a book censor infected with Jansenism, he strongly upheld the opinion that unbaptized infants do not suffer, and he was ready to forego publication rather than change the opinion.

It is too bad that the great biographer, Tannoia, stressed St. Alphonsus' own sternness and mortification so much—perhaps in an effort to clear him of the common charges of laxity—that the popular picture of St. Alphonsus is overdrawn on the strict side. St. Alphonsus had an early upbringing that was somewhat rigorous, an acute legal mind, a tenacity for details, a strong tendency to scruples and a strong sense of justice, including its punitive form. Yet the predominating side of his character and his mind was characterized by an unfailing love and sweetness. This quality is what keeps cropping up in his ascetical works, and even more in his letters.

A Man of Forgiveness

St. Alphonsus was the most forgiving of men. His expression, "God make you a saint," often used when he was disturbed or angry at someone, shows instantaneous forgiveness. Francis Maffei persecuted the Redemptorists in the courts to such an extent that he died deeply in debt. Since the debts weighed on Maffei's children, Alphonsus arranged through Fr. Tannoia to have them paid.

Some of St. Alphonsus' closest fellow religious were responsible for causing him the deepest grief. Fr. Angelo Majone set up the Regolamento and, by deceit and with the connivance of Fr. Villani, obtained St. Alphonsus' signature. In excuse, it may be said that they wanted to do good, but were short-sighted. But his signature put the holy Founder in the position of bargaining away to the civil government the most essential features of the rule he had written. The very thought caused St. Alphonsus the utmost distress. He removed Majone from the office of Proctor, but kept him as a consultor. He wrote:

> I on my part will love you as before . . . As for your reputation, it will be my constant thought to defend it both before our company and strangers . . . I bless you and beg Jesus Christ to fill you with His holy love and make you all His own as He desires.

Later, St. Alphonsus was so broken by news of the Pope's order separating the Redemptorists in Naples from those in the Papal States that he almost despaired and had to be comforted like a child. But when he had regained control of himself, he said: "God be praised. The will of the Pope is the will of God." Soon he sat down to write to Fr. de Paula, who had thus maneuvered things—serving ambition—to bring about this schism in the Congregation. "My dear Francesco," he wrote, ". . . I rejoice that all of you are brought under the authority of the Pope, and that Your Reverence is made interim superior . . ."

It almost makes one angry that St. Alphonsus could write so kindly to Fr. de Paula. He rejoiced in the good work done by the houses of his Congregation in the Papal States, for the Congregation had progressed there after they were cruelly separated from his jurisdiction, though he was at the same time and by the same maneuver cut off from his Congregation.

In his dying hours, after those around had asked for various blessings, St. Alphonsus said of his own accord: "I bless the King, princes, generals, ministers and all the magistrates, in order that they may rule with justice." This was despite the fact that the weakness of the King and the stubbornness and ill-will of the minister, Tanucci, had caused incessant trouble for St. Alphonsus and his Congregation.

Success and Failure

Many miracles attended the life of St. Alphonsus Liguori. There were miracles of conversion, as well as cures from illness. He often saw into the future and prophesied; he levitated in the pulpit, to his great embarrassment; the Blessed Virgin appeared to him a number of times. Once he even blessed Mt. Vesuvius and an impending volcanic eruption died down and never took place. On one occasion he laughed off a report of a miracle, saying that if he were able to cure someone, he could cure himself.

Despite his great graces, he often felt utterly cast down; despite his miracles, he could not overcome the opposition of the civil government to his Congregation. When the first member of the Congregation died eight years after its founding, St. Alphonsus counted just eight companions. When the King of Naples made a minor concession to them, the Saint termed it a "mighty miracle."

He failed, too, on at least one recorded occasion, after making a strong appeal to a dying, fallen-away Catholic to win him back. It seems to be a characteristic of all the Saints that they feel the full weight of helplessness along with the greatest of graces and the working of miracles. In some respects they are like the popular heroes of the stage and sports arenas, who have long hours of work, moments of glory and days of failure.

If St. Alphonsus were alive today, he would again have the task of making adaptations to moral theology in the light of modern advances in medicine and psychology, heightened social consciousness and increased inter-dependence. Perhaps his task today would be to safeguard us from a tendency opposite to Jansenism—that is, from over-emphasizing the goodness of human nature. He would again have the very necessary job of bringing back simple, solid piety. This last he can do yet for any-one who will read a few of his works of asceticism and devotion. They contain many formal prayers, and they breathe the spirit of piety. If anyone says he cannot pray, let him read St. Alphonsus Liguori.

St. Alphonsus' feast day is August 1 (August 2 in the 1962 calendar).

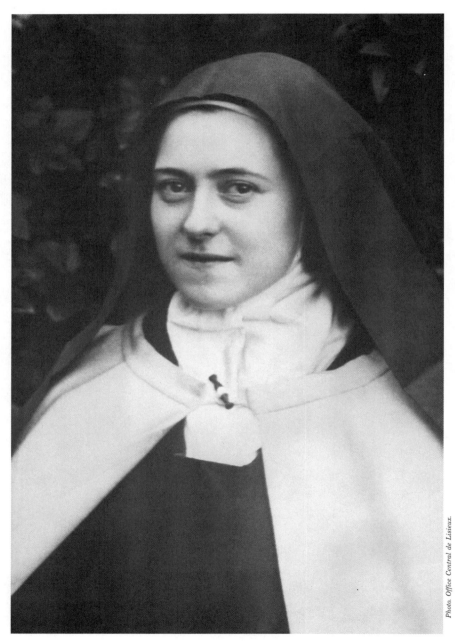

Saint Thérèse of Lisieux

33

SAINT THERESE OF LISIEUX

Doctor of The Little Way of Spiritual Childhood

Doctor of Merciful Love

1873-1897

"**H**UMBLE and poor, Therese shows the 'little way' of children who confide in the Father with 'bold trust.' The heart of her message, her spiritual attitude, is for all the faithful. Her eminent teaching deserves to be considered among the most fruitful." Pope John Paul II spoke these words during his Angelus talk on August 24, 1997. St. Therese the Little Flower, he said, would be made a Doctor of the Church on October 19, 1997, World Mission Day.

The Holy Father made this announcement to the hundreds of thousands gathered in Paris for World Youth Day. The occasion was well chosen. Therese, who died at age 24, would become the 33rd person in the long history of the Church to be given the unique title of Doctor, surely the youngest of this august group of thirty men and two women who preceded her. She is the first chosen since 1970, when Pope Paul VI chose St. Teresa of Avila and St. Catherine of Siena as the first women Doctors.

Long, Quiet Background

The Holy Father's dramatic announcement had a long, quiet background of preparation. The first suggestion that St. Therese be made a Doctor had come in 1932. At the United States Bishops' Meeting in November, 1993, Auxiliary Bishop Patrick Ahearn of New York addressed the assembly and received a unanimous voice vote of approval that the Conference petition the Holy Father to declare St. Therese a Doctor. The petition of the U.S. Bishops Conference had been preceded by those of ten other National Conferences.

Bishop Ahearn gave the reasons why St. Therese should be named a Doctor.

Neither her holiness nor her popularity qualify her to be a Doctor of the Church. What justifies the doctorate for her is the depth of her doctrine and the clarity and simplicity with which she expresses it. (Quoted in *Spiritual Life*, vol. 40, pp. 118-120, ICS Publications, Washington, D.C.).

The Bishop made clear that, rather than promoting St. Therese, he was addressing a critical need of the Church.

We are asking for a contemporary Doctor who taps into the mainstream of the mysticism that is our birthright, one who is universal, a teacher who walks the journey with us and makes us feel her presence, a teacher who like us had neither visions nor ecstasies—none of that; who teaches with artless skill in plain speech and unforgettable anecdotes, in the manner of the Gospel with its timeless stories and parables. (*Spiritual Life*, Vol. 40).

In an interview in 1995, Bishop Ahearn related that the American Bishops had received his talk with enormous applause, and that he had sent a copy of his speech to all the episcopal conferences of the world. Almost unanimously they had responded in favor of the idea of having St. Therese made a Doctor of the Church. (*The Family*, October, 1995, Daughters of St. Paul, Boston, pp. 10-12). He summed up by saying that St. Therese is the major Saint in the Catholic Church today.

Her Writings

The best known of St. Therese's writings is her "autobiography," *The Story of a Soul*. It was first published the year after her death and has been a powerful tool of spiritual development ever since. It has been translated into more than 50 languages. *The Story of a Soul* has helped profoundly to bring souls closer to the good God to whom Therese refused nothing from the age of three.

Editions of *The Story of a Soul* before 1956 followed the editorial format and content of Therese's sister, Pauline (Mother Agnes). St. Therese had given Mother Agnes permission, had even asked her, to correct and change the manuscript as she thought best. What Therese left to her sister was really a first rough draft, in need of editorial attention and even of collaboration. Mother Agnes, sister of the Saint, was the ideal person to do this. On July 16, 1897, St. Therese had given the delegation:

> Little Mother, you must revise all I have written. If you think
> fit to delete anything, or to add anything I have said to you
> personally, it is as though I did it myself. Remember this in
> the future and have no scruple in the matter. (Quoted by Bishop
> Francis Picaud, *Collected Letters of Saint Therese of Lisieux,*
> ed. Abbe Combes, transl. by Frank J. Sheed, Sheed & Ward,
> New York, 1949, p. vi).

The original manuscript does not differ in essentials from the
edited version, but the latter (Mother Agnes' edition) did lead
to some controversy and charges of "cover up." A good, balanced
discussion of the pros and cons is given in the early chapters
of *The Search for St. Therese* by Peter-Thomas Rohrbach, O.C.D.
(Hanover House, Garden City, NY, 1961). The Mother Agnes edition was the one that was instrumental in bringing St. Therese
to fame and in obtaining the "shower of roses" that she had
promised to send from Heaven. An edition from Therese's original manuscripts has since been published by the Institute of
Carmelite Studies in Washington, DC.

St. Therese's original text definitely needed editing to make it
presentable as a book. It was not planned as a book, and there
was no intention of publishing it. The text consisted of three
pieces of writing. The first part was in a simple copybook (85
pages) and was written at the request of her own sisters to preserve memories of family life. The second part, quite short, was
in response to a request by Therese's sister Marie (Marie of the
Sacred Heart in religion) to write something about "the secrets
Jesus had revealed to her." It was written in four days in September,
1896 on separate sheets of paper. The third part was written in
the early summer of 1897. It was addressed to the Prioress,
Mother Marie de Gonzague, and gives information about St.
Therese's later years in religious life. This last part was not finished, as St. Therese became too weak to continue and could not
write anymore. Therese wrote the last words in her copybook in
July, 1897: "I fly to Him through confidence and love . . ."

A Remarkable Amount of Writing

Saint Therese's poems and her prayers have been published
in English. (Institute of Carmelite Studies). She also wrote plays,
as well as directing and acting in plays. These were for festive

occasions in the convent: Christmas, the feast day of the Prioress, St. Martha's Day (to honor the lay Sisters), the Holy Innocents (to honor the novices). Her eight plays combine prose and verse. Some of the verses were sung to current popular melodies. Two of the plays are about St. Joan of Arc; the last one is about St. Stanislaus Kostka.

In her plays, as in her other writings, Therese shows a surprising independence of judgment and thought, especially for one who was so exact and obedient and who strove to be hidden. Her plays reflect, contrary to the more rigorous ascetical ideas of her time, her projection of God as the "divine beggar" seeking a return of love. "The relationship between God and us is best described as beginning in God who first loved us. The divine initiative, which Catholic tradition views as the center of an authentic and biblically rooted story of grace, has a prominent place in St. Therese's plays." (John Russell, *Experiencing St. Therese Today,* p. 55, ICS).

Remarkably, despite the fact that she lived to be only 24, Therese's collected writings are greater in volume than those of St. John of the Cross, Carmelite Doctor of Mystical Theology who lived to be 49. St. Therese's prime message is her Little Way of Spiritual Childhood. The full picture of this *Way*—and her own growth in it—comes out in glowing insights in the autobiographical *Story of a Soul* and in her letters, prayers and poems.

Added to these writings are the many quotes from St. Therese recorded by her sisters. Mother Agnes carefully took down many things Therese said during the last three months of her life. These *novissima verba* or "last words" give us a precious legacy of the thinking of a saint in her last stage of spiritual growth. In effect, what Mother Agnes took down verbatim is the "dictated" work of St. Therese. (*St. Therese of Lisieux—Her Last Conversations,* trans. John Clarke, O.C.D., ICS). Sister Genevieve of the Holy Face (Therese's sister Celine, the sister closest to her in age) at a later date (1951) published *her* account of the teaching of St. Therese. This account also gives many remembered quotes and possesses a unique value in explaining the Little Way, considering the fact that Celine was a novice under St. Therese. ([*A Memoir of*] *My Sister Saint Therese,* Gill, Dublin, 1959; TAN, reprint, 1997).

A Close-Knit, Loving Family

"God was pleased all through my life to surround me with *love,* and the first memories I have are stamped with smiles and the most tender caresses." (*Story of a Soul,* trans. John Clarke, O.C.D. from the original manuscripts, ICS, p. 17). Therese's family was close-knit and loving. Her upbringing prepared her for that spiritual growth which led her to discover her vocation. She was called to be "love in the heart of the Church." (*Story of a Soul,* p. 194.) The supernatural builds upon the natural. Therese was the last of the nine children of Louis and Zelie Martin. She was "the Benjamin" of the family, the baby, called by her father his "little queen." The four older sisters, Marie, Pauline, Leonie and Celine accepted without jealousy that she was the favorite. Yet she was brought up with a demanding discipline and was meticulously obedient. She was not a spoiled child or one who insisted on having her own way.

Therese's Parents

Therese's parents, Louis Martin and Zelie Guerin, had met on a bridge in Alençon, a small town in Normandy where their parents had settled. It seemed a chance encounter, but it is not hard to see it as planned by Divine Providence. Both had tried to enter religious life, Zelie at the convent of the Sisters of Charity in Alençon and Louis at an Augustinian Monastery in the Alps. When they met, Louis was 34 and Zelie 26. They married three months later. Louis continued his watchmaking and jewelry business, and Zelie her lace-making. In 1870, Louis sold his business and gave full time to the sales work and managing of Zelie's lace business. Zelie was a woman of much energy, totally devoted to her family, her work and her religion. She and Louis went daily to an early Mass.

Both parents were very generous to the poor. When Zelie died at age 45, after a long, heroic, and at first hidden bout with cancer, Louis retired from business. He was comfortably well off. Louis was of a quiet, contemplative nature. When the family moved from Alençon to Lisieux after the death of Zelie, he reserved a room at the top of their home, which they named Les Buissonets. Here he could have time to read and reflect and pray. He also liked to fish and to travel.

The chief reason for moving to Lisieux was that Zelie's brother

Isidore Guerin and his family lived there. The Martin and Guerin families were very close, and living near the Guerins would provide support in bringing up the two youngest Martin daughters, Celine and Therese. For Therese, "Uncle" meant Isidore Guerin and "Aunt" meant Celine, his wife. Their children, Jeanne and Marie, were just a few years older than Therese. Communication and visits were frequent between the families. Jeanne later married and Marie entered Carmel as Sister Marie of the Eucharist, becoming one of St. Therese's novices.

Her Childhood

The last child of the Martin family was born January 2, 1873 and was baptized Marie Françoise Therese. She almost died when two months old, but was given to be nursed by Rose Taille, who lived near Alençon. She remained there for a little over a year and came home healthy and vigorous. Therese had blue-grey eyes and blonde hair and spirit enough to be obstinate at times. Her mother wrote in a letter that once Therese had said *no*, nothing could move her to say *yes*.

> As for the little imp, one doesn't know how things will go, she is so small, so thoughtless! Her intelligence is superior to Celine's, but she's less gentle and has a stubborn streak in her that is almost invincible; when she says "*no*," nothing can make her give in, and one could put her in the cellar a whole day and she'd sleep there rather than say "*yes*." But still she has a heart of gold; she is very lovable and frank; it's curious to see her running after me making her confession: "Mamma, I pushed Celine once, I hit her once, but I won't do it again." (*Story of a Soul,* p. 22).

As her use of reason awoke, however, Therese became open to moral persuasion, knowing the difference between right and wrong. In her last illness she said that she had never refused the good God anything from the time she was three years old. Her intelligence was bright and her memory unusually retentive. She was an affectionate and happy child, open, playful and ready to meet all.

The picture changed with the death of her mother when Therese was just four-and-a-half. She became very sensitive and cried a great deal. Her sister Celine said that "when she had finished crying, she cried for having cried." (Quoted in Rohrbach, *The Search for St. Therese*, p. 72).

At the age of eight Therese began as a day student at the Benedictine Abbey in Lisieux. Here she found it very difficult to adjust, but she excelled in her studies. She did not care for math, but liked French composition and history. This difficult period of childhood was apparently God's way of bringing her to early spiritual maturity. The shock of her mother's death brought a sense of the changing nature of earthly things and helped Therese to yearn for the joys that do not end. Despite her emotional struggles, her mind and will remained in control. She leaned on her sister Pauline and obeyed her as a mother. And Pauline trained Therese in a strong program of prayer, sacrifice and obedience. For instance, even if her father asked her to go on a walk, she first made sure that Pauline approved.

Childhood Crises

When Pauline entered the Carmelite convent in 1882, Therese's sense of loss deepened. She had lost another mother. A half year later she fell very seriously ill. Dr. Notta, who treated her, could not determine the nature of her malady, and her father and sisters feared for her life. She had hallucinations and convulsions and seemed to be delirious. The family made a novena to Our Lady of Victories. When Therese turned away from a drink that was offered her, saying, "They want to poison me," her sisters dropped tearfully to their knees before a statue of the Blessed Virgin, pleading. Therese too turned her face toward the statue. It was then that Therese saw the statue as though it were alive. Our Lady looked at Therese with a most beautiful smile, and Therese was cured.

Writers have tried to analyze Therese's strange illness. She says in her autobiography that she thinks it came from the devil. Her sister Marie testified at the ecclesiastical inquiry that Therese interiorly knew what was going on at the time and fought against it, but could not control the hallucinations. Priest-psychiatrist Thomas Verner Moore has offered a possible diagnosis of a kidney infection known as pyelonephritis, which causes similar symptoms. (*The Search for St. Therese*, p. 99). Pope Pius XI, who beatified and canonized St. Therese, seems to lean to the opinion that the sickness was caused by the devil, "who foresaw the harm she would do him . . ." (*Search*, p. 103).

Therese made her First Holy Communion on May 8, 1884; it was a moment of special grace for her. Her more intimate union with Jesus brought her the desire to suffer with Him and to be detached from earthly things. Therese's constant reading of the *Imitation of Christ,* which she eventually largely memorized (she could entertain her family by reciting whole chapters from memory), helped this spiritual growth, ever a hard but happy path.

Beginning in May, 1885, after a retreat at the Abbey, Therese developed scruples. They caused her much suffering. She tells us that she explained her spiritual and moral worries to her sister Marie but did not mention them in Confession, a good sign that she was struggling not with decisions about right and wrong, but about good and better. The scruples lasted a year and a half, ending when she earnestly prayed to her four departed brothers and sisters for help. Good spiritual writers (e.g., St. John of the Cross) say that God at times allows scruples—not a good in themselves—as a way of purifying a soul.

In her early teens Therese also suffered frequent headaches. Her father removed her from the Abbey school because of this and also because Celine had finished there and Therese felt still more alone at school. She was placed under Madame Papineau, who tutored her at home.

Christmas, 1886

In her autobiography Therese speaks of her "conversion," meaning the attainment of a sudden maturity and the end of her childhood sensitiveness. The change was so sudden that it amazed her sister Celine. It took place right after the family had returned from Midnight Mass on Christmas, 1886. Therese overheard her father remark that he hoped this would be the last time they had to put out shoes stuffed with candy and gifts for Therese. Instead of crying and having her day spoiled, Therese received the grace of new insight and acceptance of her approaching adulthood. She regained the early spirit of spontaneity and joy she had had before her mother's death. It was a new beginning. She calls it a "glorious night."

Therese divides her years before entering Carmel into three parts. The first is the time of her happy childhood till the death of her mother, when she was four-and-a-half. The second, the most painful of the three, was from her mother's death until that Christmas night in 1886 when she was a week away from fourteen years old. It was then that the third part began. "I found once again my *childhood* character, and entered more and more into the serious side of life." (*Story of a Soul,* p. 34). This rather paradoxical statement of finding childhood again and yet becoming more serious can be understood to mean that she had found her true self and had become more able to cope happily with the real world. A book that gave her strong spiritual help at this time was that by the Abbé Arminjon entitled *The End of the Present World and the Mysteries of the Future Life.* "This reading was one of the greatest graces in my life," Therese wrote. (*Story of a Soul,* p. 102). She copied passages from this book and repeated them to herself over and over.

Missionary Desires

Little things often made a deep impression on Therese. She used them as a starting point for reflection. When a holy card showing the hand of Jesus pierced on the Cross slipped from her prayerbook one Sunday at Mass, she began to think of His Blood dripping to the ground: It should be gathered up and applied to souls. From that time on she had an intense desire to help save souls.

The famous case of St. Therese praying for Henri Pranzini, a notorious murderer, is often recounted. She and Celine prayed for him with great fervor. He kept refusing any help from a priest, though condemned to death. Therese asked God for a sign. The morning after the execution, she stole a look at the newspaper. Reading the newspaper was forbidden by her father, but she judged that this was a legitimate exception. In the paper Therese read that just before he was executed, Pranzini had reached for the crucifix held by a priest and kissed it three times. She was overjoyed at this sign of God's great mercy, and throughout her life, she continued to pray for Pranzini's soul.

Jesus said on the Cross, "I thirst." Therese's union with the thirst of Jesus for souls was at the root of her vocation to enter Carmel. With Him she thirsted for souls, and her own soul expanded to embrace the work of priests and missionaries. While she was waiting to enter Carmel, this desire found immediate expression in teaching catechism to some poor children and in denying herself candy and giving it to the children. When Therese was asked in a formal way before her religious profession why she wanted to be a Carmelite, she answered, "I came to save

souls and especially to pray for priests." (*Story of a Soul,* p. 149).
Her idea was that, by a hidden, contemplative life, she could do
more good than by an active life, for the hidden life would support the work of priests at home and missionaries abroad who
were working for the salvation of souls.

St. Therese's missionary desires propelled her through the
trying adventures of making known her wish to enter the
Carmelite convent: first to her father, then to Mother Marie de
Gonzague, the Prioress; to her protesting Uncle Isidore; to the
redoubtable Abbé Delatroette, Superior of the Lisieux convent;
to Bishop Hugonin, Bishop of the Bayeux Diocese, and finally
to Pope Leo XIII.

Trip to Rome

When giving Therese his permission to enter Carmel, Therese's
father had plucked a tiny flower, roots and all, from where it
grew in a crevice in the garden wall and had presented it to
her. The little white flower represented his own sadness at losing his "little queen" and became for her a symbol of herself,
soon to be "transplanted" to Carmel. Therese kept the flower
throughout her life. Divine Providence has allowed her to be
known and loved as the "Little Flower."

On November 4, 1887, feast of St. Charles Borromeo, Louis
Martin and his two youngest daughters, Celine and Therese,
caught an early morning train from Lisieux. They met other pilgrims in Paris and continued on their pilgrimage to many famous
holy shrines and places of cultural renown in Paris, Milan, Loreto,
Venice, Pompeii, Bologna, Padua, Rome, Naples, Assisi, Florence,
Pisa and Genoa. Therese gives vivid descriptions of scenery and
sidelights on this month-long trip. (She regretted she could not
watch from both sides of the train.) One of the priests along
was Father Reverony, secretary to Bishop Hugonin. His forbidding presence almost drained her courage in carrying out her
plan to ask the Holy Father directly to allow her to enter Carmel
at age 15. Her autobiography gives the details. (*Story of a Soul,*
pp. 134-135). However, Therese did ask, saying: "Holy Father, in
honor of your Jubilee, permit me to enter Carmel at the age of
fifteen." After he told her to do as the superiors decided, she
reminded the Pope that if he would give permission, all would
agree. Pope Leo XIII kindly blessed her, saying, "You will enter
if God wills it."

Carmel—God Did Will It

Three days after Christmas, on the feast of the Holy Innocents, Therese received a letter from Mother Marie de Gonzague. Bishop Hugonin had given his consent, leaving to the Prioress the decision about the time of entry. She set the date for Annunciation Day, which because of Lent would be celebrated that year after Easter, on April 9, 1888.

On that memorable day, fifteen-year-old Therese Martin and her relatives attended Mass together in the convent chapel. Therese received the blessing of her father and the embraces of the others, then walked through the enclosure doorway, her heart beating wildly, to meet the Prioress, her two Carmelite sisters and the other nuns. She was taken to her nine-foot-square room with its straw mattress, plain wooden cross, jug and basin, chair and table. "I am here forever and ever," she told herself. (*Story of a Soul,* p. 148).

The Prioress, Mother Marie de Gonzague, had been the one who made it possible for Therese to enter. She had treated her kindly. But her kindness took a different turn after Therese became a postulant. Perhaps it was a case of "tough love" overdone. In her letters and in speaking to others, Mother de Gonzague praised Therese. She had a genuine liking for her and respected her spiritual qualities. But "Therese the postulant" and "Therese the novice" received rebuff and correction day by day. Therese was scolded for being slow at work and inattentive at community prayer. When she missed a cobweb in a corner when sweeping, Mother de Gonzague's voice carried so all could hear: "It is easy enough to see that our corridors are swept by a child of fifteen. Sweep away that cobweb and be more careful in the future."

Therese tried to be the same to all, including her two sisters, Pauline and Marie. This involved keeping silent, not looking to them for sympathy, and avoiding that happy companionship they had enjoyed together at home. As a postulant, Therese also experienced aridity, dryness in prayer and the lack of feeling close to Jesus. When she made a General Confession to Fr. Almire Pichon, a Jesuit priest who gave retreats at the convent in 1887 and 1888, he assured her that she had never committed a mortal sin. But he told her to give thanks to God for His graces to her, for without God, "instead of being a little angel, you would have become a little demon." (*Story of a Soul*, p. 149).

Her Father's Illness

On January 10, 1889, Louis Martin led his "little queen," dressed like a queen in a flowing bridal gown, to the "Clothing" ceremony in which she received the brown habit and white veil of a Carmelite novice. A month later he suffered his third stroke, and with it loss of memory and powers of mind. He needed care until his death on July 29, 1894. Part of this time he was cared for in a hospital at Caen and part of the time by his daughters, Leonie and Celine. His time of suffering was a great trial for his children. But as he had confided to them, he had made an offering of himself to God in return for God's favors to him. He considered himself highly blessed in work, family and the religious vocations of his daughters, and he had offered himself to God in the church of Therese's Baptism at Alençon.

Therese understood now the reason for a strange vision she had had when a child of six. Her father was away from home at the time. About two in the afternoon, Therese looked out the window and saw a man dressed like her father, of the same height and way of walking, but he appeared older and stooped. She could not see his face. It was veiled. Her cries of "Father! Father!" brought her sisters running. They went into the garden, but nobody was there. The strange man had just simply disappeared. The memory of this unusual and vivid vision stayed with Therese. She now saw it as a warning of her father's final illness, which while a great suffering to her, would also be a source of grace.

Therese's life was, with few exceptions, free of anything out of the ordinary. That is the way she wanted it. She did not want visions. Her study of the works of St. John of the Cross confirmed this natural bent.

Occasionally Therese asked for a sign. She did this after her father's death, asking that—as a sign that her father had gone straight to Heaven—a nun who opposed her sister Celine's entry into Carmel would change her mind. The nun was opposing on the ground that the convent already had three sisters from the Martin family. Therese made her request during thanksgiving after Communion. Shortly after Mass, the nun in question told Therese that she now had no objection. Therese joyfully thanked Our Lord for clearing the path for Celine and for giving her the sign.

First Vows Delayed

A new suffering awaited Therese when it was time to make her profession after her year as a novice. Canon Delatroette opposed her profession and insisted that the date be postponed eight months. This was a crushing blow for a young person, especially one so eager as Therese. But she turned it into a victory over herself and bore the humiliation on the basis that it was not her wishes but what God wanted for her that counted. In the meantime, she meditated on the works of St. John of the Cross—especially *The Living Flame of Love*—and of other spiritual writers. She grew in the way of unselfish giving to Jesus.

But on the eve of her profession, Therese had the darkest trial of all. She was seized by a doubt, thinking that making profession was not God's Will for her, that everything was a mistake, and that she was deceiving her superiors. She knew she must speak to the novice mistress immediately. When she did so, the novice mistress completely reassured her. Therese's doubts left, but Therese, to make her act of humility more perfect, then went to confide her strange temptation to Mother Marie de Gonzague, the Prioress. She simply laughed. (*Story of a Soul,* p. 166). Therese's religious name was Sister Therese of the Child Jesus—to which would later be added the words "and of the Holy Face."

"Borne away on a flood of peace," Therese made her profession on September 8, 1890. But within the following year, she experienced great interior trials "of all kinds, even to the point of asking myself whether heaven really existed." Fr. Alexis Prou (1844-1914), a Franciscan from Caen, preached the community retreat in October of 1891. Ordinarily, retreats were painful to Therese, but she felt moved to confide in Fr. Prou. He told her that her faults "caused God no pain and that, holding as he did God's place, he was telling me in His name that God was very much pleased with me." Therese says, "He launched me full sail on the waves of *confidence and love* which so strongly attracted me, but upon which I dared not advance." (*Story of a Soul,* pp. 173-174).

Therese's idea of God's mercy expanded, but her dryness in prayer continued. She had an abiding inner peace, but found it hard to be recollected during community prayers. She had prayed the Rosary faithfully since childhood, but now found it trying. Therese presented a cheerful and smiling face to everybody, not only in mastering the familiar annoyances and adjusting to the conflicting personalities and faults of the nuns, but in keeping hidden the deeper interior trials of her soul. At recreation she entertained by storytelling and mimicry, a trait inherited from her father.

Of her interior trials, Therese wrote:

> During the next five years this way [of suffering] was mine. But there was no exterior manifestation of my suffering, and the fact that only I knew about it made it even more bitter. What surprises there will be at the end of life when we find out what really happened to some souls. Some people will be astonished at the way of suffering by which God led my soul. (Quoted in Rohrbach, p. 164).

Act of Oblation to Merciful Love

Therese did have one special experience of a significant mystical nature on Friday, June 14, 1895. She was making the Stations of the Cross. She explains what happened:

> All at once I felt myself wounded by a shaft of fire so strong that I thought it would kill me. I do not know how to explain it; it was as if some invisible hand had immersed me in a fire. O what fire and sweetness at the same time! I was burning with fire and I thought that one minute, even one second more, its intensity would kill me. (Quoted in Rohrbach, pp. 179-180).

Such an event, according to St. John of the Cross, is a spiritual action of God on the soul. Its purpose is to bring about a giant leap forward in the soul of a person already very close to God. Writers on mystical theology cite it as the beginning of the state of union with God after preliminary periods of purification and illumination.

On Trinity Sunday, June 9, a few days before this favor Therese had been thinking about how Jesus wants to be loved. Her prayer then was to be consumed as a victim of Divine Mercy. She wanted to save sinners in the manner of those who offer themselves as victims to Divine Justice, but she had a new way of helping them. It was to give herself to Jesus to be consumed by Love. She makes a definite distinction between an offering to Divine Justice and an offering to Divine Love. Therese asked Mother Agnes (her sister, Pauline, who was Prioress) for permission to compose and make an Act of Offering. She made it with Celine on June 11th. It begins and ends thus:

> O my God, O Most Blessed Trinity, I want to love You and make You loved. . . . O my Beloved, I desire to renew this oblation with every beat of my heart, an infinite number of times, until the shadows fade away and I can forever tell You my love face to face. (Rohrbach, p. 179).

Therese placed the paper with the Act of Offering in the copy of the New Testament which she always carried with her and which in her last two years was almost exclusively the book she used for meditating. (Therese did not have a full Bible, just the New Testament and copies of parts of the Old Testament which Celine had given her, including *Isaias* and the *Song of Songs.* Both these books she studied intently.) She often repeated the Offering.

Work in the Convent

In the course of her two years as a postulant and novice and her seven years under vows, Therese performed a variety of jobs. She worked in the laundry for nine months and in the refectory for two years; she painted pictures and frescoes; she was portress and sacristan. During much of the time she was adviser to the novices, and after Mother de Gonzague's re-election in 1896, she was made assistant novice mistress. In effect she was the novice mistress, although Mother de Gonzague held the title.

In all her assigned tasks, Therese practiced devotion to others and much self-sacrifice. As sacristan she delighted in the privilege of handling the vestments, altar linens and sacred vessels. It was a joy based on devotion to the Mass and the Blessed Sacrament.

When influenza swept through the convent in the winter of 1891-1892, Therese was one of the few who were able to stay on their feet and help the sick and the dying. The redoubtable Canon Delatroette, observing her work at this time, was converted from his long-standing opposition to become her admirer.

Therese was also appointed as correspondent to two seminarians who had asked for some "special Sister" to pray for their needs and their work. These became her spiritual adopted brothers: Paul Francois Troude (1873-1900) and Adolphe Roulland (1870-1934). Both celebrated Mass in the Lisieux convent—Fr. Troude, when Therese was in her last illness, July 16, 1897, and Fr. Roulland shortly after ordination before he left for China in July, 1896. Therese's letters to these two spiritual brothers help to bring out the depth of her daily union with the work of priests and missionaries.

In connection with her work and the daily routine of the convent we have the oft-told stories of Therese's patience and silence. She did not complain when the nun in the laundry splashed soapy water on her, nor when the nun in choir scraped her fingernail along her teeth, nor when the old Sister complained that Therese was too fast or too slow in leading her to the refectory. Often Therese felt nausea when standing during the long chanting of the Divine Office. (This and her chronic fatigue at prayer could possibly be symptoms of a heart defect. Therese's mother had noticed in childhood that her heart made an audible sound under exertion.) She did not ask for permission to sit down or to be excused. Once, at the beginning of her last illness, she was sitting down, but rose when a nun told her to stand up. She had learned to accept not only the superior, but any of the nuns to help her find the minute-by-minute will of God. Therese's silence sprang in some part from her admiration of the silence of Mary, who waited for God to make things clear to St. Joseph.

Daily Routine

The daily schedule of the Lisieux Carmelite convent began with rising at 5 a.m. (6 a.m. in the winter). A wooden clapper awakened the Sisters. There was an hour of mental prayer in choir, followed by Mass and the Little Hours of the Divine Office. Breakfast was bread and coffee. A work period ended with the main meal at 11:00 a.m. and an hour of recreation, when the Sisters were officially allowed to talk. (They often did sewing or made rosaries during the recreation time.) Vespers came at 2:00 p.m., then spiritual reading and a second hour of mental prayer at 5:00 p.m. After a light supper and a second recreation period, Compline was said at 7:30 p.m. Matins and Lauds were chanted at 9:00 p.m., and the nuns retired about 11:00 p.m. (Rohrbach, p. 140).

A glance at this schedule and a little thought about living within the walls of a convent and garden enclosure, with no outside trips or functions, with the same group of twenty or twenty-five women, day by day and year on end, must bring the conviction that this was a life of sacrifice, making demands on the human spirit. The Lisieux convent in Therese's time was not ideal. There were factions, and Mother de Gonzague was a person of both charm and contradictions. For a person who always tried to be exact, to give God all, to put neighbor before self, to make every act an act of love, as Therese did, it was a life of quiet heroism. It provided the tools and the setting for her Little Way, a way of happiness in being little and hidden, so that other souls near and far might blossom in the fullness willed for them by God their Creator.

Did the young Therese of fifteen understand what she was getting into? Some writers have said that she was disillusioned with convent life. Therese said herself that she found religious life exactly as she had expected it.

> God gave me the grace *not to have A SINGLE ONE* [illusion] when entering Carmel. I found the religious life to be *exactly* as I had imagined it, no sacrifice astonished me, and yet, as you know, dear Mother, my first steps met with more thorns than roses! Yes, suffering opened wide its arms to me and I threw myself into them with love . . . (*Story of a Soul*, p. 149, emphasis in original).

Mother de Gonzague, who constantly corrected Therese, nevertheless wrote at the same time in a letter: "Never would I have believed that a child of fifteen could possess such mature judgment: there is nothing to criticize in her, everything is perfect." (Rohrbach, p. 141).

Therese came to Carmel to lead a life of sacrifice. She was much attracted to the life of a missionary, but considered the quiet, hidden life of prayer a stronger way of helping to save souls. Her outlook was other-centered in the purest sense of loving Jesus in such a purified way that, in the hidden ways of grace, other souls would be made ready to receive His love. This primacy of the little, hidden way was highlighted in one of Therese's last conversations with Mother Agnes, when Therese offered her the advice that it is better to pray for a spiritual brother than to write to him.

> Any Sister could write what I have written and would receive the same compliments, the same confidence. But it's only through

prayer and sacrifice that we can be useful to the Church. Correspondence should be very rare, and it mustn't be permitted at all for certain religious who would be preoccupied with it, believing they're doing marvels, and would be doing nothing really but harming themselves and perhaps falling into the devil's subtle traps. Mother, what I've just told you is very important; I beg you not to forget it later on. At Carmel, we should never make any false currency in order to redeem souls. And often the beautiful words we write and the beautiful words we receive are an exchange of false money. (*Last Conversations,* p. 82).

Therese . . . of the Holy Face

We can better understand St. Therese's outlook and early spiritual maturity when we think of the second part of her religious name. She asked for the addition, "of the Holy Face," and received this permission early in religious life. Her devotion to the Holy Face, symbol of Jesus suffering, had begun in childhood.

She wrote to her sister Celine on July 18, 1890, enclosing various texts on which she meditated during her father's suffering. The texts included *Isaias* 53:1-5 and 63:1-5. In her last illness, she told Mother Agnes that the texts of *Isaias* had been the foundation of her devotion to the Holy Face and of her whole piety.

In her memoir of St. Therese, Celine writes very plainly:

> Devotion to the Holy Face was, for Therese, the crown and complement of her love for the Sacred Humanity of Our Lord. This Blessed Face was the mirror wherein she beheld the *Heart* and the *Soul* of her Well-Beloved. Just as the picture of a loved one serves to bring the whole person before us, so in the Holy Face of Christ, Therese beheld the *entire Humanity* of Jesus. We can say unequivocally that this devotion was the burning inspiration of the Saint's life . . . Her devotion to the Holy Face transcended—or more accurately, embraced—all the other attractions of her spiritual life . . . (*My Sister St. Therese,* p. 111).

Celine sums up by stating that Therese's virtues, her detachment, her love of suffering, her seraphic love yielding fruits a hundredfold came from her devotion to the Holy Face. Therese told her novices, Celine says, that the Holy Face was the book wherein she had learned the science of love and the art of practicing virtues. Celine also says that all Therese's writings are impregnated with love of the Holy Face. Mother Agnes testified at the beatification process: "As tender as was her devotion to the Child Jesus, it cannot be compared to her devotion to the Holy Face." (*Last Conversations,* p. 13). Therese herself, in thanking Mother Agnes for helping her to enter into the mysteries of love hidden in the Face of Jesus, writes:

> He whose Kingdom is not of this world showed me that true wisdom consists in "desiring to be unknown and counted as nothing," and in "placing one's joy in the contempt of self." (*Imitation of Christ*). Ah! I desired that, like the Face of Jesus, "my face be truly hidden, that no one on earth would know me." (Cf. *Isaias* 53:3). I thirsted after suffering and I longed to be forgotten. (*Story of a Soul,* p. 152).

A few weeks before her death, Therese said,

> These words of Isaias: "Who has believed our report? . . . There is no beauty in him, no comeliness . . ." have made the whole foundation of my devotion to the Holy Face, or, to express it better, the foundation of all my piety. I, too, have desired to be without beauty, alone in treading the winepress, unknown to everyone. (*Last Conversations,* p. 135).

In the summer of 1896, Therese composed a prayer of consecration to the Holy Face. It was signed by herself, her sister Marie and Sister Marie of the Trinity. All had, with permission, added "of the Holy Face" to their religious names. Their own photos were mounted with the Face of Jesus Suffering above theirs on the back of the script of the prayer. The prayer asks:

> Souls, Lord, we need souls . . . above all the souls of apostles and martyrs, so that through them we might inflame all poor sinners with Your Love. O Adorable Face, we shall gain this grace from You!

The last part of the prayer reads:

> O beloved Face of Jesus! As we await the everlasting day when we will contemplate Your infinite Glory, our one desire is to charm Your Divine Eyes by hiding our faces too so that here on earth no one can recognize us . . . O Jesus! Your Veiled Gaze is our Heaven! (*The Prayers of Saint Therese of Lisieux,* ICS, 1997, p. 92).

It is interesting to note, too, that it was shortly after St. Therese's death, that the first photos were taken of the Shroud of Turin and the startling discovery made that the image of Our Lord's face and body on the Shroud is in effect a photographic negative—and that the film negative itself comes out as a positive image. Perhaps this discovery was one of the bigger "roses" which St. Therese had promised to send from Heaven—and did send—after her death. This photo of 1898 was the inspiration for Celine (Sr. Genevieve of the Holy Face) to paint her much-printed portrait of the Holy Face. Since 1898 there has been ongoing study of the Shroud, and the Face has become familiar to the world.

Little Mortifications

In accord with her Little Way, Therese did not practice extreme forms of penance. However, her acts of self-denial would add up to real self-mastery and penance. Her only penance when in the world, before entering Carmel, was to refrain from leaning back against her chair. But because she tended to stoop, she was told to lean back. She says that in the convent the penances she was allowed consisted in mortifying her self-love, which did her much more good than corporal penances. (*Story of a Soul,* p. 159). Not to look at the clock during prayer, not to ask what news was told by a visitor, not to interrupt another's story with a witty remark or another story, to refrain from rubbing cold hands or putting them in the sleeves her habit, to eat the less flavorful food, the leftovers; such and similar acts of self-denial were parts of her Little Way.

One quite unique act of self-denial Therese explained with a touch of whimsy. Although flies were bothering her, she did not kill them. "I always give them freedom," she said. "They alone have caused me misery during my sickness. I have no enemies, and since God recommends that we pardon our enemies, I'm happy to find this opportunity for doing so." (*Last Conversations,* p. 119).

Mother Agnes was astonished to hear Therese say in her last illness: "I've suffered from the cold in Carmel even to the point of dying from it." Mother Agnes remarks: "Not even in the coldest weather did I see her rub her hands together or walk more rapidly or bend over more than was her usual habit, as all of us do naturally when we are cold." (*Last Conversations,* p. 258).

Therese had her own silent ritual at table. She imagined herself in the home of the Holy Family.

> If, for instance, I am served salad, cold fish, wine or anything pungent in taste, I offer it to the good St. Joseph. Hot portions, ripe fruits and the like are for the Blessed Virgin. To the Infant Jesus goes our feast-day fare, in particular, puddings, rice and preserves. Whenever there is a wretched dinner, however, I think to myself cheerfully: "Today, my little one, it is all for you!" (*My Sister St. Therese,* p. 169).

She Did Not Ask for Suffering

It is easy to see that Therese knew well the meaning of the grain of wheat which must die before it brings forth fruit. (*John* 12:24). She quoted this saying of Jesus when her sister Pauline (Mother Agnes) was elected Prioress in 1893, thus consoling her for the pain that had accompanied and would follow the election. Therese saw that suffering alone gives birth to souls, but she did not ask God for suffering. She told her cousin, Sr. Marie of the Eucharist, in late August of 1897:

> Fortunately I didn't ask for suffering. If I had asked for it, I fear I wouldn't have the patience to bear it. Whereas, if it is coming directly from God's Will, He cannot refuse to give me the patience and the grace necessary to bear it. (*Last Conversations,* p. 290).

Her distinctions may seem to be fine, but they hit true center in her Little Way of humble trust in God.

The prayer Therese carried on the day of her religious profession, September 8, 1890, sums up the way in which she gave herself completely. She had written it the day before.

> O Jesus, my divine spouse! May I never lose the second robe of my Baptism; take me before I can commit the slightest voluntary fault. May I never seek nor find anything but Yourself alone. May creatures be nothing for me and may I be nothing for them, but may You, Jesus, be everything . . . Never let me be a burden to the community, let nobody be occupied with me, let me be looked upon as one to be trampled underfoot, forgotten like Your little grain of sand, Jesus. May Your will be done in me perfectly, and may I arrive at the place You have prepared for me. Jesus, allow me to save very many souls; let

no soul be lost today; let all the souls in Purgatory be saved. Jesus, pardon me if I say anything I should not say. I want only to give You joy and to console You. (*Story of a Soul,* p. 275).

(The "grain of sand" refers to a grain hidden in the mortar around cut stones, which are beautiful to be seen and admired.)

Therese, the Sinner

St. Therese had a unique way of thinking of herself as a sinner whom God had forgiven in advance. This kind of outlook fitted in with her Little Way. She says Jesus knew she was too feeble to be exposed to great temptations, so He saved her from them. Else she would have had to be forgiven as was Mary Magdalen.

I know that without Him, I could have fallen as low as St. Mary Magdalen, and the profound words of Our Lord to Simon resound with a great sweetness in my soul. I know that "he to whom less is forgiven, loves less" (*Luke* 7:47), but I also know that Jesus has forgiven me more than St. Mary Magdalen since He forgave me in advance by preventing me from falling. (*Story of a Soul,* p. 83).

She then gives the example of a doctor whose child has stumbled over a stone and gotten hurt. The doctor binds up the wound and tends the child until all is healed. Then Therese says that if the doctor had removed the stone from the path in advance, without the child's knowing it, the child would not be as grateful and would not love her father as much as would the one he had healed. But if the child then came to know about the danger avoided and the hurt prevented, she would love her father even more than the injured child who had been healed. Therese says,

I am this child, the object of the foreseeing love of a Father who has not sent His Word to save the just, but sinners . . . I have heard it said that one cannot meet a pure soul who loves more than a repentant soul; ah! how I wish to give the lie to this statement! (*Story of a Soul,* p. 84).

Great Trial of Faith

Saint Therese's final transforming union with the suffering Christ began on the night between Holy Thursday and Good Friday, 1896. She describes what happened:

> I returned to our cell [shortly after midnight], but I had scarcely laid my head upon the pillow when I felt something like a bubbling stream mounting to my lips. I didn't know what it was, but I thought that perhaps I was going to die and my soul was filled with joy . . . It seemed to me that it was blood I had coughed up. (*Story of a Soul*, p. 210).

It was blood indeed, as she verified in the morning. Therese told Mother Marie, the Prioress, but begged for no special attention. A second hemoptysis took place the next night. Therese was not frightened; just the opposite. She hoped soon to be with the One she loved in Heaven. At this time she had such a clear, living faith that the thought of Heaven made up all her happiness. She could not even imagine how unbelievers could think there was no Heaven.

But during the joyful Easter season,

> Jesus made me feel that there were really souls who have no faith, and who, through the abuse of grace, lost this precious treasure, the source of the only real and pure joys. He permitted my soul to be invaded by the thickest darkness, and that the thought of Heaven, up until then so sweet to me, be no longer anything but the cause of struggle and torment. (*Story of a Soul,* p. 211).

This great trial of faith was to last through her illness. Her last year and a half of increasingly severe bodily pain was overshadowed by the cloud that obscured the joy of faith. She compared it to traveling through a dark tunnel. When she tried to get a glimpse of that land she had pictured and longed for, it seemed that the darkness grew thicker. It even hurt her to hear someone talk about Heaven.

> The darkness, borrowing the voice of sinners, says mockingly to me: "You are dreaming about a light, about a fatherland embalmed in the sweetest perfumes; you are dreaming about the eternal possession of the Creator of these marvels; you believe that you will one day walk out of this fog which sur-

rounds you! Advance, advance; rejoice in death which will give you not what you hope for but a night still more profound, the night of nothingness." (*Story of a Soul,* p. 213).

The more Therese felt the loss of a sense of faith, the more she continued to make acts of faith. Her understanding of persons who have turned away from God increased. In the last lines of her autobiography she wrote:

> Even though I had on my conscience all the sins that can be committed, I would go, my heart broken with sorrow, and throw myself into Jesus' arms, for I know how much He loves the prodigal child who returns to Him. (*Story of a Soul,* p. 259).

A week after writing these lines, she said to Mother Agnes: "Mortal sin wouldn't withdraw my confidence from me; don't forget to tell the story of the sinful woman! This will prove that I'm not mistaken." (*Last Conversations,* p. 104). The sinful woman referred to was a public sinner, in a story from the desert fathers, whose sins had scandalized a whole country. She was converted, touched by grace, and planned to do a rigorous penance. But she died on the first night of her journey into the desert to carry out her plan—not from illness or accident, but from the vehemence of her sorrow and her love for God. The holy man who had converted her saw her soul go straight to Heaven. This story was a favorite of Therese.

She Maintained a Cheerful Exterior

In the midst of this severe testing of spirit, the increasing pain of her tuberculosis and its concomitant ravages of her whole system, Sister Therese presented a cheerful exterior to the other Sisters. In fact, for many months she continued the usual routine of the convent. Her duties were taken away only in mid-May, 1897. Only in the last months of her life did the severity of her illness become known, and she was then given full treatment and care. The best record of that time was kept by Mother Agnes in a yellow notebook which has been published as *Last Conversations* (ICS) or as *Novissima Verba.*

The remedies of the day, prescribed by Dr. Alexandre DeCorniere, added to her suffering. These were, among others, vesicatories (hot plasters to induce blistering) and "pointes de feu" (repeated puncturing of the skin with hot needles). Therese had a humorous nickname for the doctor. With permission, she also had one for her sister Celine, reverting to a playful name they had used in childhood, "Bo-Bonne."

A letter from Sr. Marie of the Eucharist (Therese's cousin, Marie Guerin) on July 8, 1897 says:

> We find her very much changed, very emaciated, but she's always calm, always ready to joke. . . . If you were to see our dear little patient, you wouldn't be able to stop laughing. She has always to be saying something funny. Ever since she has become convinced she is going to die, she has been as gay as a little finch. (*Last Conversations,* p. 274).

St. Therese's poetic tribute to the Blessed Virgin, "Why I Love You, Mary," was written during May, 1897. In June and early July she wrote the third part of her autobiography (Manuscript C). This was done partly in a wheelchair in the garden.

Therese's union with Jesus is reflected in a statement she wrote on May 15:

> As for me, with the exception of the Gospels, I no longer find anything in books. The Gospels are enough. I listen with delight to these words of Jesus which tell me all I must do: "Learn of Me for I am meek and humble of heart," then I'm at peace, according to His own promise: "And you will find rest for your souls." (*Matt.* 11:29).

Then she added: "and you will find rest for your *little* souls." (*Last Conversations,* p. 44).

Pain and Astonishing Peace

"My soul is exiled, Heaven is closed for me, and on earth's side, it's all trial too," Therese said after a bad day on June 29. (*Last Conversations,* p. 68). On July 30, when it seemed she was about to die, constantly coughing up blood and feeling suffocated, Therese was anointed by Fr. Alexandre-Charles Maupas, who had succeeded Fr. Delatroette as Superior of the Carmel. Her last Communion took place on August 19. She offered it for Fr. Hyacinthe Loyson, a priest who had lost the Faith. Therese's sufferings continued, with inability to retain food, fevers and increasing feelings of suffocation. She was at times unable to bear the slightest noise or movement around her, the rustling of a paper, a whisper. Dr. Francis LaNeele, cousin to Therese through marriage, visited her in the absence of Dr. DeCorniere. He said that the right lung was completely diseased, as well as the left lung in its lower part, and that intercostal neuralgia was causing much pain.

On September 22, Therese said: "Yes! What a grace it is to have faith! If I had not had any faith, I would have committed suicide without an instant's hesitation. . . ." (*Last Conversations,* p. 196). She did not have any foreknowledge of the exact day of her death. "I know nothing except what you know; I understand nothing except through what I see and feel. But my soul, in spite of this darkness, is in an astonishing peace," Therese confided to Mother Agnes on September 24.

Even in the last days of her final suffering, Therese did not want the others to watch through the night at her side. She preferred and asked that they take their rest. Once when a Sister had fallen asleep, leaving Therese holding a glass, she waited until the Sister awakened, though her hand trembled with the effort.

"My God . . . I Love You!"

On the last day of her life, Therese said: "Never would I have believed it was possible to suffer so much! Never, never! I cannot explain this except by the ardent desires I have to save souls." At 7:20 p.m., September 30, she looked at her crucifix and said, "Oh! I love Him! . . . My God . . . I love You! . . ."

Mother Agnes describes the scene.

> Suddenly, after having pronounced these words, she fell back, her head leaning to the right. Mother Prioress had the infirmary bell rung very quickly to call back the community. . . . The Sisters had time to kneel down around her bed, and they were witnesses to the ecstasy of the little, dying saint. Her face had regained the lily-white complexion it always had in full health; her eyes were fixed above, brilliant with peace and joy. She made certain beautiful movements with her head as though someone had divinely wounded her with an arrow of love, then had withdrawn the arrow to wound her again. . . . After her death, she had a heavenly smile. She was ravishingly beautiful. She was holding her Crucifix so tightly that we had to

force it from her hands to prepare her for burial. . . . (*Last Conversations,* pp. 206-207).

Celine (Sr. Genevieve of the Holy Face) adds that Therese in her ecstasy fixed her gaze a little above the miraculous statue of Our Lady of the Smile. (Celine had brought it with her when she entered Carmel.) After many years of trying to analyze the shades of expression that passed over St. Therese's face during her last ecstasy, Celine concluded:

> At first, her expression had an air of *confident assurance* combined with a *joyful attitude of expectancy*: as the story of her soul unfolded, she might have been asking God what He thought of it. And when she had His answer her expression changed to one of *profound astonishment and then to overflowing gratitude.* (*My Sister St. Therese,* pp. 241-242).

St. John of the Cross would say that the ultimate cause of Therese's death was the final wounding of her soul with a shaft of divine love.

Therese's last poem, written during the night of July 12-13, is a prayer of preparation for receiving Holy Communion. It is also a prayer that she might die of love. (*Poetry of Saint Therese,* p. 233). Therese wrote:

> You who know my extreme littleness,
> You are not afraid to lower Yourself to me!
> Come into my heart, O white Host that I love,
> Come into my heart, it longs for you!
> Ah! I wish that Your goodness
> Would let me die of love after this favor.
> Jesus! Hear the cry of my affection.
> Come into my heart!

Abbe Louis-Aguste Youf (1842-1897), who had been chaplain of the convent and ordinary confessor of Therese through her years in Carmel, heard the convent bell toll from his sickbed and said: "What a loss for Carmel. She is a saint." (Rohrbach, p. 197). (Abbe Youf died one week later.) Then, "Wrapped in her big white cloak, a chaplet of white roses on her head and a palm branch in her hand, the body of Sister Therese lay with face uncovered behind the chapel grating, where her relatives and friends, known and unknown, could see her for the last time."

(*The Secret of the Little Flower,* by Henri Gheon, trans. by Donald Attwater, pp. 234-35, Sheed & Ward, 1934).

Some pressed rosaries or medals to her feet. A few shared the chaplain's opinion that Sister Therese was a saint. Most did not. A small group of priests, relatives and townspeople followed the coffin up the hill to the new city cemetery. She was the first nun to be buried in the plot reserved for religious. Before her death, Therese had promised that she would "let fall from Heaven a shower of roses." Within two years, letters of thanks and of petition and various mementos had accumulated on her grave. The promised shower of roses had begun.

The first favors came to Therese's own convent, and its members soon came to realize the quiet holiness of their departed little sister. Even before the burial, a lay Sister who had been unfriendly, feeling remorse at Therese's death, embraced her feet in the coffin and was cured of anemia. Mother de Gonzague said that nobody knew how much she owed to Sister Therese. She also reported that Therese had appeared to her as she was praying before her picture.

A few years previous, Mother de Gonzague had written her opinion of Therese on the back of a photo. Therese was twenty at the time.

> The jewel of Carmel, its dear Benjamin. She has the office of painter in which she excels without having had any lessons other than observing our Reverend Mother, her sister, at work. Mature and strong, with the air of a child, and with a sound of voice and manner of expression which veils the wisdom and perfection of a woman fifty years old. A soul which is always calm and in complete possession of itself at all times. A completely innocent saint, who needs no repentance to appear before God, but whose head is always full of mischief. Mystic, comic, she can make you weep with devotion and just as easily die with laughter at recreation. (*The Photo Album of St. Therese of Lisieux,* Christian Classics, Westminster, MD, 1990, p. 18).

Therese's Mission Begins

Mother Marie de Gonzague, instead of sending the usual obituary to Carmelite convents, arranged to have 2,000 copies of Therese's three manuscripts printed in the form of a book edited by Mother Agnes. *The Story of a Soul,* with an added account of Sister Therese's death, was sent out in October, 1898. Its effect was electrifying—first, among Carmelites, then, as it was reprinted and translated many times, among millions who were thus introduced to the Little Way, the Way of Spiritual Childhood of St. Therese.

In his Apostolic Letter *Divini Amoris Scientia* ("The Science of Divine Love") of October 19, 1997, Pope John Paul II wrote:

> The reception given to the example of her life and Gospel teaching in our century was quick, universal and constant—as if in imitation of her precocious spiritual maturity, her holiness was recognized by the Church in the space of a few years.

Before she was canonized, Pope St. Pius X had called Therese "the greatest saint of modern times." Pius XI, who canonized her, referred to her as "the star of my pontificate." Pius XII said, "She rediscovered the Gospel, the very heart of the Gospel."

Only after she had written her story for her own sisters, and while writing the third part for the Mother Prioress, did St. Therese come to understand that there was a hidden, Divine plan for its future. Only in her last illness, too, did she come to know and to prophesy about her future mission of helping from Heaven. On July 13 she said to her sister Marie: "If you only knew the projects I'll carry out, the things I shall do when I'm in Heaven. . . . I will begin my mission." (*Last Conversations*, p. 238). On Saturday, July 17, Therese said to Mother Agnes:

> I feel that I'm about to enter into my rest. But I feel especially that my mission is about to begin, my mission of making God loved as I love Him, of giving my little way to souls. If God answers my desires, my heaven will be spent on earth until the end of the world. Yes, I want to spend my heaven in doing good on earth. . . . (*Last Conversations*, p. 102).

She unpetaled a rose over her crucifix on September 14, and when some petals were falling to the floor, she said: "Gather up these petals, little sisters, they will help you to perform favors later on. . . ." (*Last Conversations*, p. 190).

Many volumes recording miracles and favors are on file in the convent at Lisieux. Many miracles and favors are recorded only in the minds and hearts of people St. Therese has helped, or in letters from friend to friend and relative to relative. We might say that the publicity for her book was not advance publicity, but follow-up publicity. The countless favors obtained through her intercession kept leading to new demands for *The Story of a Soul*. During World War I, Therese was in the foxholes and in the planes, as attested by soldiers, especially of the French army. Thousands of soldiers claimed they owed their lives to her, and more claimed they kept their faith through her.

Often people pray to St. Therese, saying: "Send me a rose." In the 1970's, the widow of a parish choirmaster and organist in St. Louis, Missouri prayed with such a request. She asked St. Therese to send her a rose if her recently deceased husband was in Heaven. Perhaps she recalled that St. Therese herself had asked for a sign that her father was in Heaven. The woman followed the request by making a novena. On the fifth day of the novena, she received a dozen roses from an unexpected source, a priest. He had been a fishing partner of her husband.

The Cause

The Cause for the canonization of St. Therese went through its various stages with unusual speed. The home diocese of Bayeux opened the proceedings in 1910. Therese's body was exhumed from its grave and placed in a cement vault in the Lisieux cemetery later that year. Her writings were approved by the Sacred Congregation of Rites in 1913. On June 10, 1914, Pope St. Pius X signed the decree to introduce the Cause in the Roman Court. On August 14, 1921, Pope Benedict XV declared Therese Venerable. In 1923 her body was removed to the chapel of the Carmelites, and on April 19 she was beatified. Pope Pius XI canonized her May 17, 1925—his first saint. Her feast day was originally October 3, but is now observed on October 1. Further honors on December 14, 1927 made her Patron of all Missions along with St. Francis Xavier, and on May 3, 1944, secondary Patroness of France along with St. Joan of Arc. The Basilica of St. Therese at Lisieux was opened and blessed on July 11, 1937 by Cardinal Eugenio Pacelli as legate of Pope Pius XI, whom he was to succeed as Pope Pius XII.

The Little Way

She found a way of holiness . . . in the exact observance of the Rule, and followed it steadily, weaving her life thread by thread out of insignificant actions that were too small for notice or record. But God saw them and, as each was weighted with love, valued them equally with the martyrdom of St. Cecily, the foundations of St. Teresa, or the triumphs of St. Francis. The very fact that they were too small to be an object of self-satisfaction increased their worth. (Gheon, p. 165).

The Little Way of St. Therese made an appeal to millions who came to understand better that we can all weave a tapestry of beauty from the threads of everyday life. All is precious: our work, our taking nourishment, our words of cheer, our smile in the face of annoyance, pain or trouble, our prayers done in weariness and distraction, as were those of Therese. All are precious because done with love for God.

We might compare the value the Little Way brings to small deeds to the value assumed by objects given with special love and care. A flower brought by a child with stumbling eagerness and perhaps dirty hands and torn clothes as a result of going into the mud to get the flower, is treasured by the father or mother receiving it. The flower is touched with the perfume of their child's love. This is the way Therese thought of her daily acts and sacrifices, including those that may have "dirtied" her a bit in the sense of bringing down reproof or criticism. Even when she recognized a fault in her act or manner, it just added to her sense of littleness and made her more dependent on God's complete help.

She used the example of an elevator—fairly modern in her day—to convey the idea that rather than climb the steps to the mystical Mt. Carmel, she needed to be lifted up as a child is lifted by its father. Therese told the novices,

> The most trivial work, the least action when inspired by love, is often of greater merit than the most outstanding achievement. It is not on their face value that God judges our deeds, even when they bear the stamp of apparent holiness, but solely on the measure of love we put into them . . . And there is no one who can object that he is incapable of even this much, for such love is within the reach of all men. (*My Sister St. Therese,* pp. 74-75).

Therese gave another apt example to her sister Celine. As children they had been intrigued by playing with a kaleidoscope. Therese examined it and found out that the fascinating moving colors had as a base just scraps of paper and bits of wool. But three mirrors inside the kaleidoscope imparted to them their marvelous beauty. Therese said the scraps of paper and cloth were our actions, and the mirrors she compared to the Blessed Trinity, which gave them their beauty. (*My Sister St. Therese,* pp. 75-76).

Therese's pursuit of the *little* extended even to physical size.

> Soeur Therese was rather tall, about five-foot-four, whereas Mere Agnes (our sister) was very short. One day, when I asked Therese whether—if she had her choice—she would prefer to be short or tall, she answered unhesitatingly, "I should prefer to be short in order to be *little* in every way." (*My Sister St. Therese,* p. 44).

Celine summed up the value of Therese's Little Way: "I have always maintained that Therese's greatness stems from the multiplicity of her microscopic acts of virtue, if I might express it in this way." (*My Sister St. Therese,* p. 166).

Pope Benedict XV said on August 14, 1921, when proclaiming Therese's heroic practice of virtue, "The more the knowledge of this new heroine is spread abroad, the greater will be the number of her imitators giving glory to God by the practice of the virtues of spiritual childhood." (*Last Conversations,* p. 10).

Cardinal Pacelli (later Pope Pius XII) summed up the Little Way when he blessed the Basilica in Lisieux:

> St. Therese of the Child Jesus has a mission, a doctrine. But like everything else about this Carmelite Saint, her doctrine is humble and simple and it is summed up in these two words: *Spiritual Childhood*—or in their equivalent: *The Little Way.* (*My Sister St. Therese,* p. 45).

When Pope John Paul II visited Lisieux on June 2, 1980, he said:

> Her "little way" is the way of "holy childhood." There is something unique in this way, the genius of Therese of Lisieux. At the same time there is confirmation and renewal of the most basic and most universal truth. What truth of the Gospel message is really more basic and more universal than this: God is our Father and we are His children? (Quoted in his Apostolic Letter, *The Science of Divine Love,* October 19, 1997, no. 10).

Therese Chooses All

One day Therese's sister Leonie had brought a basket containing her doll and doll clothes to her two younger sisters, Celine and Therese, and told them to choose what they wanted. (Leonie was the middle sister of the five who lived. She entered the Visitation convent in 1899, taking the name Françoise-Therese.) Celine chose a few items. Therese announced: "I choose all," and took the entire basket. Therese says of this childhood incident:

> This little incident of my childhood is a summary of my whole life; later on when perfection was set before me, I understood that to become a *saint* one had to suffer much, seek out always the most perfect thing to do, and forget self. I understood, too, that there were many degrees of perfection and each soul was free to respond to the advances of Our Lord, to do little or much for Him, in a word, to *choose* among the sacrifices He was asking. Then, as in the days of my childhood, I cried out: "My God, *I choose all!* I don't want to be a *saint by halves,* I'm not afraid to suffer for You, I fear only one thing: to keep my *own will;* so take it, for '*I choose all*' that You will!" (*Story of a Soul,* p. 27, emphasis in original.).

"Therese found grace everywhere. Holy pictures, personality quirks, smiles, frowns, letters, poems—and especially the persons who touched her life—were all epiphanies of the divine breaking through, out of the immense love the good God/Jesus bore her . . . St. John of the Cross, her spiritual father, uses the nada; St. Therese chooses the todo. But the spirituality is the same. It is the radical option for Jesus as the center of one's existence, as the most important person in one's life with no exceptions or reservations." (Redemptus Valabek in *Experiencing St. Therese Today*, ICS).

When Therese was trying to formulate in a simple way what her vocation was, she found the answer in St. Paul. "*Yet strive after the better gifts, and I point out to you* a yet more excellent way." (*1 Cor.* 12:31; 13:1).

> And the Apostle explains how all *the most PERFECT gifts* are nothing without *LOVE* . . . I understood that LOVE COMPRISED ALL VOCATIONS, THAT LOVE WAS EVERYTHING, THAT IT EMBRACED ALL TIMES AND PLACES. . . . IN A WORD, THAT IT WAS ETERNAL! . . . my *voca-*

tion, at last I have found it. . . . MY VOCATION IS LOVE! Yes, I have found my place in the Church and it is You, O my God, who have given me this place; in the heart of the Church, my Mother, I shall be *Love.* Thus I shall be everything, and thus my dream will be realized. (*Story of a Soul,* p. 194, emphasis in original).

In short, Therese found her place at the center. Her kind of wholeness must embrace Jesus and His Mystical Body, the Church, in the most complete way possible. Nothing by halves. She chooses all. Her love must be pure, burning, consuming. She recognized God's gift to her. Therese, who has been called a "ravishing miniature of the Blessed Virgin," received God's gift in the spirit of Mary's *Magnificat.* "My soul magnifies the Lord and my spirit rejoices in God, my Saviour, because He has regarded the lowliness (*littleness*) of His handmaid. . . . He who is mighty has done great things for me." (*Luke* 1:46-49). She also recognized that, as St. Paul said, there are many gifts in the Mystical Body, many parts. God freely gives. "But all these things are the work of one and the same Spirit, who allots to everyone according as He will." (*1 Cor.* 12:11). "Therese received particular light on the reality of Christ's Mystical Body, on the variety of its charisms, gifts of the Holy Spirit, on the eminent power of love, which in a way is the very heart of the Church where she found her vocation as a contemplative and missionary." (*Science of Divine Love,* no. 8).

The Little Way Invites All

St. Therese says that her Little Way is for everybody. But she also says each one can follow the Little Way according to his own gifts and his own degree of responding love. She recognized that love can be love only when it is freely given. She also recognized very strongly the gift of God which gives the soul that initial push that disposes the right use of free will. God Himself must be free to give in different measures. Therese had learned early that God, infinitely loving to all, is also infinitely free to bestow larger gifts or smaller gifts.

I wondered for a long time why God has preferences, why all souls don't receive an equal amount of graces. I was surprised when I saw Him shower His extraordinary favors on saints who had offended Him, for instance, St. Paul and St.

Augustine, and whom He forced, so to speak, to accept His graces. When reading the lives of the saints, I was puzzled at seeing how Our Lord was pleased to caress certain ones from the cradle to the grave, allowing no obstacle in their way when coming to Him, helping them with such favors that they were unable to soil the immaculate beauty of their baptismal robe. I wondered why poor savages died in great numbers without even having heard the name of God pronounced.

Jesus deigned to teach me this mystery. He set before me the book of nature; I understood how all the flowers He has created are beautiful, how the splendor of the rose and the whiteness of the Lily do not take away the perfume of the little violet or the delightful simplicity of the daisy. I understood that if all flowers wanted to be roses, nature would lose her springtime beauty, and the fields would no longer be decked out with little wild flowers.

And so it is in the world of souls, Jesus' garden. He willed to create great souls comparable to Lilies and roses, but He has created smaller ones and these must be content to be daisies or violets destined to give joy to God's glances when He looks down at His feet. Perfection consists in doing His will, in being what He wills us to be. (*Story of a Soul*, pp. 13-14).

Once [as a child] I was surprised that God didn't give equal glory to all the Elect in heaven, and I was afraid all would not be perfectly happy. Then Pauline told me to fetch Papa's large tumbler and set it alongside my thimble and filled both to the brim with water. She asked me which one was fuller. I told her each was as full as the other and that it was impossible to put in more water than they could contain. My dear Mother helped me understand that in heaven God will grant His Elect as much glory as they can take, the last having nothing to envy in the first. And it was in this way that you brought the most sublime mysteries down to my level of understanding and were able to give my soul the nourishment it needed. (*Story of a Soul*, pp. 44-45).

In later years, meditating more and more on the Gospels, Therese could find God's freedom in giving confirmed by the parables of the laborers in the vineyard (*Matt.* 20), the unequal number of talents (*Matt.* 25:14-30) and the favored prodigal son (*Luke* 15:11-32). In fact, the essence of her Little Way is the loving recognition that all comes from God and that we can but grow in humility, gratitude, trust and littleness, the more we realize His absolute freedom in choosing to favor us. If we have any gifts that attract Him, we have them only because He gave them to us in the first place.

St. Therese's reverence for God's absolute freedom had its special quality when she prayed for temporal favors.

> Whenever she did ask for relief or some other temporal favor, it was only to please others. Even then, she would make sure to ask through the Blessed Virgin because "to ask through the Blessed Virgin is not the same as asking directly from the good God. She knows very well how to take care of my little desires and whether or not to mention them to God . . . I leave it to her to see that He will not be forced, so to speak, to grant my prayers, but rather that He be left entirely free to do His Will in all that concerns me." (*My Sister St. Therese,* p. 55).

Therese's Little Way was heroic because she chose to do all the little things and to purify her thoughts and intentions and motives, as motivated by the highest degree of her love and God's grace. Little things became important to her in a sense that most of us pass over.

Her sensitiveness to little things was acute even in early childhood. As a child she once offered a coin to a cripple, which he refused. She thought she had offended him and felt very sad about it. Then she remembered that she had been told to ask for anything on the day of First Communion, and it would be granted. She remembered this for five years and prayed for the poor cripple when she made her First Holy Communion.

In Therese's letter to her sister Marie the year before Therese died (Manuscript B of *Story of a Soul),* Therese shows how her desire for everything possible—and, were it possible, even *beyond* the possible—had remained constant.

> Ah! my Jesus, pardon me if I am unreasonable in wishing to express my desires and longings which reach even unto infinity. Pardon me and heal my soul by giving her what she longs for so much!
>
> To be Your *Spouse,* to be a *Carmelite,* and by my union with You to be the *Mother* of souls, should not this suffice me? And yet it is not so. No doubt these three privileges sum up my true *vocation: Carmelite, Spouse, Mother,* and yet I feel within me other *vocations.* I feel the *vocation* of the WARRIOR, THE PRIEST, THE APOSTLE, THE DOCTOR, THE MARTYR. Finally, I feel the need and the desire of carrying out the most heroic deeds for *You, O Jesus.* I feel within my soul the courage

of the *Crusader,* the *Papal Guard,* and I would want to die on the field of battle in defense of the Church.

I feel within me the *vocation* of the PRIEST. With what love, O Jesus, I would carry You in my hands when, at my voice, You would come down from heaven. And with what love would I give You to souls! But alas! while desiring to be a *Priest,* I admire and envy the humility of St. Francis of Assisi and I feel the *vocation* of imitating him in refusing the sublime dignity of the *Priesthood. (Story of a Soul,* p. 192, emphasis in original).

Saint Therese and Mary

The last lines Therese wrote were written on September 8, 1897, a few weeks before she died. They were written on the back of a treasured holy card of Our Lady of Victories to which she had attached the little white flower which her father had plucked and given her along with his permission to enter Carmel. "O Mary, if I were Queen of Heaven and you were Therese, I should want to be Therese, that you might be Queen of Heaven." Such an unusual and striking thought shows a very tender intimacy with the Blessed Virgin. (*Prayers of Saint Therese,* p. 119). On August 31, after looking a long time at the statue of the Blessed Virgin, Therese expressed another unique thought: "Who could ever invent the Blessed Virgin?" (*Last Conversations,* p. 177).

In the last May of her life, Therese wrote her twenty-five-stanza poem: "Why I Love You, Mary." Of this poem she said to her sister Marie: "My little Canticle expresses all I think about the Blessed Virgin, and all I would preach about her if I were a priest." (*Last Conversations,* p. 235). Marie had asked her to write her thoughts about the Blessed Virgin, and the poem was Therese's response. Therefore, the poem makes a ready summary of St. Therese's way of thinking and showing love for the Blessed Virgin.

Therese follows only what the Gospels tell of Mary, saying nothing directly of the Resurrection or the other glorious mysteries of the Rosary. She wanted to view Mary here on earth as one of us, following Christ in faith and suffering. To see her glory could wait for Heaven. (Cf. *The Poetry of Saint Therese,* pp. 215-220).

> If I gazed on you in your sublime glory,
> Surpassing the splendor of all the Blessed,
> I could not believe that I am your child.
> O Mary, before you I would lower my eyes! . . .
> If a child is to cherish his mother,
> She has to cry with him and share his sorrows.
> O my dearest Mother, on this foreign shore
> How many tears you shed to draw me to you! . . .
> In pondering your life in the holy Gospels,
> I dare look at you and come near you.
> It's not difficult for me to believe I'm your child,
> For I see you human and suffering like me. . . .

Only one mention is made of personal experience, and that near the end of the poem. Therese recalls the Virgin of the Smile. Often during her last illness she repeated these two lines:

> You who came to smile at me in the morning of my life,
> Come smile at me again . . . Mother . . . It's evening now.

Mary Lived by Faith

Pope John Paul II saw St. Therese as being in advance of the Second Council of the Vatican, which presented Mary as a woman of faith, united as the first of Christians with all who followed Christ. Therese did not like sermons that presented Mary as doing extraordinary things. She wanted Mary to be presented as one we can imitate. Therese said that Mary lived by faith, just like ourselves and that priests should show proofs of this fact from the Gospel, such as, "And they did not understand the word which He spoke to them." (*Luke* 2:50). The Pope said:

> Among the most original chapters of her spiritual doctrine we must recall Therese's wise delving into the mystery and journey of the Virgin Mary, achieving results very close to the doctrine of the Second Vatican Council in chapter eight of the Constitution, *Lumen Gentium,* and to what I myself taught in the Encyclical Letter, *Redemptoris Mater,* of March 25, 1987. (*The Science of Divine Love,* no. 8).

On August 21, five weeks before her death, Therese gave to her sister, Mother Agnes (Pauline), a digest of all her thinking about the Blessed Virgin. (*Last Conversations,* pp. 161-62).

> I must see her real life, not her imagined life. I'm sure that
> her real life was very simple. . . . We know very well that the
> Blessed Virgin is Queen of heaven and earth, but she is more
> Mother than Queen. . . . She was exempt from the stain of
> Original Sin; but on the other hand, she wasn't as fortunate
> as we are, since she didn't have a Blessed Virgin to love. . . .

Therese said that if she were a priest, "One sermon would be sufficient to say everything I think about this subject. I'd first make people understand how little is known by us about her life. We shouldn't say unlikely things or things we don't know anything about! . . ." (*Last Conversations*, p. 161). Therese's aim was simplicity and truth, not apocryphal stories or exaggerated claims.

Fr. Eamon Carroll, O.Carm, says that Therese is "indeed a saint for a faithless age." She showed this in a special way by writing her best words about Mary when she was having her great temptations against faith during her final illness. Therese realized then how deep was the faith of Mary in the midst of the contradictions that surrounded the life of Jesus.

Fr. Carroll also points out that Therese's writing is filled with the Blessed Virgin: "the autobiography in all three parts, the letters, the poems, the dramatic pieces, the last conversations." He quotes St. Therese in regard to her autobiography:

> Before taking up my pen, I knelt before the statue of Mary
> (the one which has given so many proofs of the maternal pref-
> erences of Heaven's Queen for our family), and I begged her
> to guide my hand that it trace no line displeasing to her.
> (*Experiencing St. Therese Today*, 1990, pp. 83, 86).

St. Therese's personal devotion to Mary was a part of herself, woven into her very being through her upbringing. Her parents gave the name Mary to all their nine children, including the two boys and two girls who died in infancy or early childhood. At her first Communion, Therese promised to pray the *Memorare* every day. At her first Confession several years earlier, the priest had encouraged her to be devoted to Mary, and she promised to redouble her tenderness. She had great reason for personal gratitude to Mary for her cure from her long and strange illness when the statue of Our Lady took on the appearance of a living person and smiled at her. ". . . What penetrated to the very depths of my soul was the ravishing smile of the Blessed Virgin. . . .'' Throughout her life Therese attributed many favors to Our Lady, including her entrance into Carmel at age 15. She said that the Blessed Virgin was not slow in answering prayers, as some saints are, but always answered right away. (Cf. *Last Conversations,* p. 235).

Doctor of Merciful Love

The reasons why St. Therese qualifies as a Doctor of the Church were summarized in a talk by Bishop Patrick Ahearn on March 1, 1997, during a symposium on St. Therese held at Alhambra, California. He said that St. Therese will be known as the Doctor of Merciful Love. He quoted her: "God is nothing but mercy and love." Then he continued: "Everything else in the Little Way and in her spiritual doctrine follows from that profound intuition."

He also saw influence by St. Therese on contemporary spiritual themes, including: her attitude of faith and trust, her insistence on the universal call to holiness, her emphasis on Holy Scripture, her notion of Heaven as a place of helping, and finally, her clear idea of Mary as a woman of faith.

In a homily at a Mass in the National Shrine of the Immaculate Conception on September 27, 1997, Bishop Ahearn concluded with these words:

> She is the amazing saint whom God sent to light up the dark sky of the twentieth century. . . . The doctorate will canonize her doctrine, summoning us to learn our religion all over again, to learn the plain truth about God . . . that He is nothing but mercy and love.

The Bishop also pointed ahead, saying that Therese is a saint for the next millennium.

In late 1999 and early 2000, a reliquary of St. Therese containing some of her bones toured the United States for almost four months. Great crowds turned out to venerate the relics and express their devotion to the youngest Doctor of the Church. The tour was sponsored by the five Carmelite provinces of the United States. Before visiting the U.S., St. Therese's relics had already traveled to France, Belgium, Luxembourg, Germany, Italy, Switzerland, Austria, Slovenia, Brazil, Holland, Russia, Kazakhstan and Argentina. The relics were also present beside

Pope John Paul II at St. Peter's Basilica in Rome on October 19, 1997 when he proclaimed St. Therese a Doctor of the Church. A brochure announcing the travel schedule for the relics featured this short but incisive quote from St. Therese: "My way is all confidence and love."

Teacher of Holiness

Coming to the third millennium as the newest Doctor of the Church, Therese has a new importance and dignity as teacher. In her lifetime her official teaching was directed to the novices in her convent, especially in the final year when she was, in effect, the novice mistress. She was very firm with them, and at the same time she allowed them to speak freely to her about what they considered her mistakes or failures. In the words of her sister Celine (also one of her novices), Therese was never influenced by external appearances but always maintained a universal respect and reverence for the soul for its own sake. Therese said of her method:

> As for reprimands, our intention in giving them must be directed first to the glory of God and must not spring from a desire to succeed in enlightening the novices. Moreover, in order that a correction bear fruit, it must *cost* in the giving, and the heart must be free from the least shadow of passion. (*My Sister St. Therese,* p. 6).

A wonderful piece of advice not only for a religious superior, but for anybody in authority.

St. Therese's advice for those under authority was to go slowly. She urged the novices to wait until they had regained self-possession before coming to her to confide a grievance.

> Never speak about any unpleasant situation, even to our Mother, for the sole purpose of having it remedied. Open your heart, rather, through a spirit of duty and detachment of soul. Whenever you realize that you are not in this frame of mind, it would be better to wait until your soul is at peace. To speak out, even when it is only a tiny spark of resentment that you feel, will only serve to add fuel to the fire. (*My Sister St. Therese,* p. 199).

Therese quoted St. Alphonsus Liguori: "Charity consists in

bearing with those who are unbearable." In *The Story of a Soul*, she writes:

> I understand now that charity consists in bearing with the faults of others, in not being surprised at their weakness, in being edified by the smallest acts of virtue we see them practice. But I understood above all that charity must not remain hidden in the bottom of the heart. Jesus has said: *"No one lights a lamp and puts it under a bushel basket, but upon the lampstand, so as to give light to ALL in the house."* (*Matt.* 5:15). It seems to me that this lamp represents charity, which must enlighten and rejoice not only those who are dearest to us but "ALL *who are in the house"* without distinction. . . . But when Jesus gave His Apostles a new commandment, HIS OWN COMMANDMENT (*John* 15:12), as He calls it later on, it is no longer a question of loving one's neighbor as oneself, but of loving him as *He, Jesus, has loved him,* and will love him to the consummation of the ages. (*Story of a Soul,* p. 220, emphasis in original).

To avoid envy of others, Therese offered this advice:

> When faced by our limitations, we must have recourse to the practice of offering to God the good works of others. That is the advantage of the Communion of Saints. Let us never grieve over our powerlessness but rather apply ourselves solely to the science of love.

After quoting from Tauler on the subject, she continued: "We are told that the love uniting all the elect in heaven is so great and so pure that the happiness and merit of each individual saint makes for the happiness and merit of all. . . ." (*My Sister St. Therese,* p. 71).

Much human misery comes from avoiding the truth about self, others and God. On July 20, during her last illness, Therese said:

> I've never acted like Pilate, who refused to listen to the truth. (*John* 18:38). I've always said to God: O my God, I really want to listen to You; I beg You to answer me when I say humbly: What is truth? Make me see things as they really are. Let nothing cause me to be deceived. (*Last Conversations,* p. 105).

Her diligent pursuit of the truth in everything and her intuitive way of grasping the truth supported her Little Way of complete humility and complete dependence on God's generosity and goodness.

Pope John Paul II opens his Apostolic Letter on St. Therese by recalling the gift of God who reveals to the little and the humble what is hidden from the learned and the wise. (*Luke* 10:21-22 and *Matt.* 11:25-26). He continues:

> Mother Church also rejoices in noting that throughout history the Lord has continued to reveal Himself to the little and the humble, enabling His chosen ones, through the Spirit who "searches everything, even the depths of God" (*1 Cor.* 2:10), to speak of the gifts "bestowed on us by God . . . in words not taught by human wisdom but taught by the Spirit, interpreting spiritual truths in spiritual language." (*1 Cor.* 2:12-13). In this way the Holy Spirit guides the Church into the whole truth, endowing her with various gifts, adorning her with His fruits, rejuvenating her with the power of the Gospel and enabling her to discern the signs of the times in order to respond ever more fully to the will of God. (*The Science of Divine Love,* no. 1).

For those who want to avoid Purgatory, St. Therese lends encouragement in the form of a little poem she put in the slipper of Celine on Christmas, 1894.

> Jesus Himself your crown shall weave.
> And if you seek His love alone,
> If all for Him you gladly leave
> Near His, some day, shall be your throne.
> After the night of life, the day
> With light eternal shining through
> You shall behold! *With no delay,*
> *The Triune God shall welcome you.*

On gratitude, St. Therese said:

> It is the spirit of gratitude which draws down upon us the overflow of God's grace, for no sooner have we thanked Him for one blessing than He hastens to send us ten additional favors in return. Then, when we show our gratitude for these new gifts, He multiplies His benedictions to such a degree that there seems to be a constant stream of Divine grace ever coming our way. This has been my own personal experience; try it out for yourself and see. . . . (*My Sister St. Therese,* p. 97).

Everything Centers on Jesus

Pope John Paul II stated:

> As it was for the Church's saints in every age, so also for her; in her spiritual experience Christ is the center and fullness of Revelation. Therese knew Jesus, loved Him and made Him loved with the passion of a bride. She penetrated the mysteries of His infancy, the words of His Gospel, the passion of the Suffering Servant engraved on His Holy Face, in the splendor of His glorious life, in His Eucharistic presence. She sang of all the expressions of Christ's divine charity, as they are presented in the Gospels. (*The Science of Divine Love,* no. 8).

St. Therese had an incarnational bent of mind. Everything is related to Jesus and His love. She used to keep March 25, the Feast of the Annunciation, with special devotion, saying that Jesus was never so small as He was on the day of His Incarnation in the womb of Mary. (*My Sister St. Therese,* p. 46). This insight fits her whole emphasis on being little and also introduces her incarnational way of thinking. For St. Therese everything centers on Jesus, whose life began in a tiny, hidden way. Her devotion to Jesus and her love for Him led to her love for those who loved Him most: Mary and Joseph.

> Ever since my childhood I had a devotion to him [St. Joseph], which easily merged with my love for the Blessed Virgin. I recited each day the prayer in his honor: "O St. Joseph, Father and Protector of virgins. . . ." (*Story of a Soul,* p. 124).

St. Therese's interest in the Saints had the same source. They were the ones who loved Our Lord unto death as martyrs, or who loved Him through the years of white martyrdom in the cloister, or in fidelity in the lay state as had her father and mother (fit candidates for beatification). Study of St. Therese can help to shape our thinking along incarnational lines, adding to our love of the Saints and to deeper appreciation of the world's beauties, made more beautiful because Jesus walked on earth as a man.

Therese, Doctor of the Church

The twentieth century saw conflict between the teaching authority of the Pope and the Bishops united with him (the

Magisterium) on the one hand, and theologians on the other. Theologians are needed helpers in the ongoing discovery of the riches of Christ and all Divine Revelation. Catholic theologians are scholars who must be free to think, to be creative, but who must also work within an ecclesial dimension that ensures order, orthodoxy, continuity and harmony. In a sense their horizons are not restricted but widened because of the guidance of the Holy Spirit, who works not only through the teaching authority, but through the wisdom of God's little ones. Their study of St. Therese's incarnational way of thinking can draw new insights from her Little Way of Spiritual Childhood. Her Little Way itself can do much to prevent conflict.

Many miracles and favors have supported St. Therese's doctrine. The fact that Therese was made a Doctor of the Church provides incentive for theologians to study the underlying roots of her greatness. In times to come, new study of her writings by theologians may well generate new interest among all Christians, and even among those outside the Faith revealed by Christ.

In making St. Therese a Doctor of the Church, Pope John Paul II projected her as a model both for theologians and for the young.

> Therese of the Child Jesus and the Holy Face is the youngest of all the Doctors of the Church, but her ardent spiritual journey shows such maturity, and the insights of faith expressed in her writings are so vast and profound, that they deserve a place among the great spiritual masters. (*L'Osservatore Romano*, October 22, 1997).

The fact that St. Therese is so young to be named a Doctor of the Church, taking her place with such giants as St. Augustine, St. John Chrysostom, the Gregorys and others who have helped chart the intellectual path of the Church, should give new courage and assurance to young people. It may lead them to greater interest in the fact that the Church is not static. The young like movement, progress. Doctrines do not change, but insight into them and their ramifications does extend our vision of the riches of Christ.

In his Apostolic Letter, *The Science of Divine Love,* Pope John Paul II gives three special reasons why making St. Therese a Doctor of the Church has significance for our time.

First of all she is a *woman*, who in approaching the Gospel knew how to grasp its hidden wealth with that practicality and deep resonance of life and wisdom which belong to the feminine gender. . . . Therese is also a *contemplative*. By her life Therese offers a witness and theological illustration of the beauty of the contemplative life as the total dedication to Christ, Spouse of the Church, and as an affirmation of God's primacy over all things. Lastly, Therese is a *young person*. She reached the maturity of holiness in the prime of youth. As such she appears as a teacher of evangelical life, particularly effective in illumining the paths of young people, who must be the leaders and witnesses of the Gospel to the new generations. (No. 11).

Her Way Brings Heaven Closer

For Therese there was just a thin veil between Heaven and earth, between those on earth and the souls in Purgatory and Heaven. She saw from childhood that the things of earth were passing, and she set her heart in Heaven. It was an indescribable trial when, in the last year and a half of her life, her thin veil between Heaven and earth changed into a wall.

Still Therese continued her usual intimate and down-to-earth way of talking to the Blessed Virgin and the Saints. She asked, when in much pain: "And all the saints whom I love so much, where are they 'hanging out?'" (*Last Conversations,* p. 150). Therese had a horror of spiders. She worried about this in her weakened state. "I wonder what would become of me if I were to see a huge spider on our bed. Well, I still want to accept this fear for the sake of God. But would you ask the Blessed Virgin not to let this happen?" (*Last Conversations*, p. 153). The next day she confided: "Last night I couldn't take any more. I begged the Blessed Virgin to hold my head in her hands so that I could take my sufferings." (*Last Conversations,* p. 154).

Late twentieth-century piety tended to become too abstract, estranged from simplicity, more involved in words than in symbols and attitudes of faith and reverence, almost devoid of Therese's kind of piety that has warmth, strews flowers before the Blessed Sacrament or unpetals a rose to sprinkle a statue of St. Joseph or a crucifix. During her last illness she stroked a picture of one of her favorites, Ven. Theophane Venard. Asked why she did so, she replied, "Because I can't reach him to kiss him." (*Last Conversations*, p. 154). As sacristan, Therese rejoiced in seeing the reflection of her face in the chalice that would hold the Blood of Christ, or in the bottom of the ciborium before she placed in it the hosts to be consecrated into the Body of Christ. She even found a bond with Jesus in knowing her face was reflected in the eyes of Pope Leo XIII, His chief representative on earth.

Therese's Love Embraces Everybody

In her abandonment to Jesus, Therese understood and accepted that He would not always make her Little Way smooth. As a child she had offered herself to the Child Jesus as a little plaything for Him to throw on the ground, pierce, let lie in a corner or press to His Heart—whatever He wished. She says, "He heard my prayer." (*Story of a Soul*, p. 136).

One of the characteristics of Therese's Little Way was that she rejoiced in each new realization of her littleness. It made her know she was all the more dependent on God's help. This kind of thinking also lent a universality to her love for others in Jesus. In her great trial of faith, she came to understand even the thinking of atheists and of people turned away from God. In the excess of her pain she came to embrace all the sick, suffering and dying, even those who wished to take their own lives. Her Little Way led to love for all God's people and to a compelling interest in helping them.

St. Therese had a fine sense of balance. She understood that souls are as different as snowflakes. She chided a novice who neglected her duties. On the other hand, she told her sister Celine, who was exact about duties: "The goal of all our undertakings should be not so much a task perfectly completed but the accomplishment of the will of God." (*My Sister St. Therese*, p. 173). She who ate leftovers mused ruefully and honestly when unable to eat: "It's quite unbelievable! Now that I can no longer eat, I have a desire for all sorts of things, for example: chicken, cutlets, rice, tuna fish." (*Last Conversations*, p. 148). At other times in her last months, she expressed a longing for chocolate eclairs, and she advised Mother Agnes to be sure to have good food served to the Sisters if she again became Prioress. And she who sought no relief from the cold, advised Mother Agnes to have good, warm blankets for the nuns during winter. (The Lisieux convent was drafty and not well heated).

The Little Way, a Gospel Way

In his homily at the Mass on Mission Sunday (October 19, 1997) when celebrating the declaration of St. Therese as a Doctor of the Church, Pope John Paul II said that the Church is missionary by nature.

> Jesus Himself showed her how she could live this [missionary] vocation: by fully practicing the commandment of love, she would be immersed in the very heart of the Church's mission, supporting those who proclaim the Gospel with the mysterious power of prayer and communion. Thus she achieved what the Second Vatican Council emphasized in teaching that the Church is missionary by nature. Not only those who choose the missionary life, but all the baptized are in some way sent *ad gentes* (to the nations).

The Holy Father made plain why he chose Mission Sunday to declare St. Therese a Doctor of the Church.

> St. Therese is presented as a Doctor of the Church on the day we are celebrating World Mission Sunday. She had an ardent desire to dedicate herself to proclaiming the Gospel, and she would have liked to have crowned her witness with the supreme sacrifice of martyrdom.

The Pope also made plain that her Little Way can be followed by everybody.

> The way she took to reach this ideal of life is not that of the great undertakings reserved for the few, but on the contrary, a way within everyone's reach, the Little Way, a path of trust and total self-abandonment to the Lord's grace. It is not a prosaic way, as if it were less demanding. It is in fact a demanding reality, as the Gospel always is. But it is a way in which one is imbued with a sense of trusting abandonment to Divine mercy, which makes even the most rigorous spiritual commitment light. (*L'Osservatore Romano*, October 22, 1997).

St. Therese was declared a Doctor of the Church in these solemn words:

> Fulfilling the wishes of many Brothers in the Episcopate and of a great number of the faithful throughout the world, after

consulting the Congregation for the Causes of Saints and hearing the opinion of the Congregation for the Doctrine of the Faith regarding her eminent doctrine, with certain knowledge and after lengthy reflection, with the fullness of Our apostolic authority, We declare Saint Therese of the Child Jesus and the Holy Face, virgin, to be a Doctor of the Universal Church. In the name of the Father, and of the Son and of the Holy Spirit.

The closing prayer of the Holy Father's homily is itself a summary of why St. Therese is now a Doctor of the Church and of how her Little Way calls everyone to new vitality in living the Gospel.

Yes, O Father, we bless You, together with Jesus, because You have "hidden Your secrets from the wise and understanding" and have revealed them to this "little one" whom today You hold up again for our attention and imitation. Thank You for the wisdom You gave her, making her an exceptional witness and teacher of life for the whole Church!

Thank You for the love You poured out upon her and which continues to illumine and warm hearts, spurring them to holiness. The desire Therese expressed to "spend her heaven doing good on earth," continues to be fulfilled in a marvelous way.

Thank You, Father, for making her close to us today with a new title, to the praise and glory of Your name forever and ever.

St. Therese of Lisieux's feast day is October 1 (October 3 in the 1962 calendar).

BIBLIOGRAPHICAL NOTES

Story of a Soul. Translated by John Clarke, O.C.D. Copyright © 1975, 1976, 1996 by Washington Province of Discalced Carmelites, ICS Publications, 2131 Lincoln Road, N.E., Washington, DC 20002-1199, U.S.A.

St. Therese of Lisieux: Her Last Conversations. Translated by John Clarke, O.C.D. Copyright © 1977 by Washington Province of Discalced Carmelites, ICS Publications, 2131 Lincoln Road, N.E., Washington, DC 20002-1199, U.S.A.

Appendix I
FEAST DAYS

DOCTOR	TRADITIONAL CALENDAR (1962 "Tridentine" Calendar)	REVISED CALENDAR (1970 "Novus Ordo" Calendar)
1. St. Athanasius	May 2	May 2
2. St. Ephrem	June 18	June 9
3. St. Cyril of Jerusalem	March 18	March 18
4. St. Hilary of Poitiers	January 14	January 13
5. St. Gregory Nazianzen	May 9	January 2
6. St. Basil the Great	June 14	January 2
7. St. Ambrose	December 7	December 7
8. St. Jerome	September 30	September 30
9. St. John Chrysostom	January 27	September 13
10. St. Augustine	August 28	August 28
11. St. Cyril of Alexandria	February 9	June 27
12. Pope St. Leo the Great	April 11	November 10
13. St. Peter Chrysologus	December 4	July 30
14. St. Gregory the Great	March 12	September 3
15. St. Isidore of Seville	April 4	April 4
16. St. Bede the Venerable	May 27	May 25
17. St. John Damascene	March 27	December 4
18. St. Peter Damian	February 23	February 21
19. St. Anselm	April 21	April 21
20. St. Bernard of Clairvaux	August 20	August 20
21. St. Anthony of Padua	June 13	June 13
22. St. Albert the Great	November 15	November 15
23. St. Bonaventure	July 14	July 15
24. St. Thomas Aquinas	March 7	January 28
25. St. Catherine of Siena	April 30	April 29
26. St. Teresa of Avila	October 15	October 15
27. St. Peter Canisius	April 27	December 21
28. St. Robert Bellarmine	May 13	September 17
29. St. John of the Cross	November 24	December 14
30. St. Lawrence of Brindisi	July 21	July 21
31. St. Francis de Sales	January 29	January 24
32. St. Alphonsus Liguori	August 2	August 1
33. St. Therese of Lisieux	October 3	October 1

Appendix II
OFFICE OF READINGS

This table gives a handy guide to the writings of the Doctors of the Church as they appear in the Office of Readings from the Divine Office (1971). The Readings have been arranged by their season in the Church year, the date of a feast, and the Commons. The abbreviations for days of the week are: S–Sunday, M–Monday, T–Tuesday, W–Wednesday, Th–Thursday, F–Friday, Sat–Saturday.

ST. ATHANASIUS (297-373)

Lent:	Wk4-F; Wk5-S
Ord. Time:	Wk1-Th; Wk1-F;
	Wk6-T; Trinity Sunday;
	Wk13-Th; Wk23-Sat
Feast Days:	Jan. 1; Jan. 17; May 2

ST. EPHREM (306-373)

Advent:	Wk1-Th
Easter:	Wk3-F
Ord. Time:	Wk6-S
Feast Days:	June 9

ST. CYRIL OF JERUSALEM (315-386)

Advent:	Wk1-S
Easter:	Octave-Th; Octave-F;
	Octave-Sat; Wk7-M
Ord. Time:	Wk4-Th; Wk13-Sat;
	Wk17-W; Wk17-Th;
	Wk31-W; Wk31-Th
Feast Days:	Mar. 18

ST. HILARY OF POITIERS (315-368)

Easter:	Wk4-W; Wk7-F
Lent:	Wk2-Th
Ord. Time:	Wk4-M; Wk25-Sat
Feast Days:	Jan. 13
Common:	Of Pastors

ST. GREGORY NAZIANZEN (329-389)

Advent:	Wk1-T; Bap. of Lord
Lent:	Wk1-M; Wk3-Sat;
	Wk5-Sat
Ord. Time:	Wk31-F
Feast Days:	Jan. 2

ST. BASIL THE GREAT (329-379)

Advent:	Jan. 2 to Epiph-M
Lent:	Wk3-M; Wk7-T
Easter:	Wk4-M; Wk7-T
Ord. Time:	Wk1-T; Wk3-T; Wk17-T

ST. AMBROSE (340-397)

Advent:	Dec. 21
Lent:	Wk2-Sat
Ord. Time:	Wk5-W; Wk6-Th;
	Wk10-F; Wk10-Sat;
	Wk14-Th; Wk15-S;
	Wk15-M; Wk15-T;
	Wk15-W; Wk15-Th;
	Wk15-F;Wk15-F;
	Wk15-Sat; Wk16-Th;
	Wk20-F; Wk20-Sat;
	Wk26-F; Wk27-M;
	Wk31-Sat
Feast Days:	Dec. 7; Dec. 13; Jan. 20;
	Jan. 21; Oct. 9; Nov. 2

ST. JEROME (342-420)

Ord. Time:	Wk7-W; Wk13-Th;
	Wk21-F
Feast Days:	Sept. 30

ST. JOHN CHRYSOSTOM (347-407)

Lent:	Wk2-M; Holy Wk-F
Ord. Time:	Wk16-Sat; Wk17-S;
	Wk20-S; Wk21-T;
	Wk34-Th
Feast Days:	Jan. 25; Jan. 26; May 14;
	July 25; Aug. 24; Sept. 13;
	Nov. 30
Common:	Memorial of BVM (Sat);
	Holy Men; Underpriv-
	ileged; Teachers

ST. AUGUSTINE (354-430)

Advent:	Wk2-W; Wk3-S; Wk3-F; Dec. 24; Dec. 27; Jan. 2 to Epiph-T; Jan. 2 to Epiph-Th; Jan. 2 to Epiph-Sat;
Lent:	Wk1-S; Wk2-T; Wk3-S; Wk4-S; Wk5-W; Holy Wk-M; Holy Wk-W
Easter:	Octave-S; Wk3-T; Wk4-Th; Wk5-Sat; Ascension; Wk6-Sat
Ord. Time:	Wk5-S; Wk5-Th; Wk6-F; Wk8-T; Wk8-W; Wk9-S; Wk13-M; Wk13-T; Wk13-F; Wk14-S; Wk14-T; Wk14-Sat; Wk16-F; Wk19-W; Wk20-W; Wk22-S; Wk24-S; Wk24-M; Wk24-T; Wk24-W; Wk24-Th; Wk24-F; Wk 24-Sat; Wk25-S; Wk25-M; Wk25-T; Wk25-W; Wk25-Th; Wk25-F; Wk28-Th; Wk28-F; Wk29-S; Wk29-M; Wk29-T; Tk29-W; Wk29-Th; Wk29-F, Wk33-S; Wk33-W; Wk34-T; Wk34-Sat
Feast Days:	Dec. 6; Dec. 11; Jan. 22; Feb. 3; Apr. 30; May 12; May 26; June 24; June 29; July 29; Aug. 10; Aug. 27; Aug. 28; Sept. 19; Sept. 26; Nov. 21; Nov. 22
Common:	Dedication of a Church; One Martyr; Holy Men

ST. CYRIL OF ALEXANDRIA (376-444)

Advent:	Epiph. to Bap.-Th
Easter:	Wk3-Sat; Wk4-Sat; Wk5-T; Wk6-S; Wk6-T; Wk7-Th
Ord. Time:	Wk28-S
Feast Days:	June 27; Aug. 5; Oct. 28

POPE ST. LEO THE GREAT (400-461)

Advent:	Dec. 17; Dec. 31
Lent:	Ash-Th; Wk2-S; Wk4-T; Wk4-Th; Wk5-T
Easter:	Wk2-W; Wk6-W; Wk6-F
Ord. Time:	Wk5-F; Wk22-Th; Wk22-F; Wk22-Sat; Wk23-S; Wk23-M; Wk34-M
Feast Days:	Christmas; Epiphany; Feb. 22; Mar. 25; July 16; Nov. 10; Nov. 18
Common:	Of Pastors

ST. PETER CHRYSOLOGUS (406-450)

Advent:	Wk2-Th; Epiph. to Bap.-M
Lent:	Wk3-T
Easter:	Wk4-T
Ord. Time:	Wk29-Sat
Feast Days:	July 4; July 30

ST. GREGORY THE GREAT (540-604)

Lent:	Wk3-F
Easter:	Wk4-S
Ord. Time:	Wk8-S; Wk8-M; Wk8-Th; Wk8-F; Wk9-W; Wk9-Th; Wk20-M; Wk27-S; Wk27-Sat
Feast Days:	Feb. 10; May 27; July 3; July 22; Sept. 3; Sept. 29; Oct. 18
Common:	For Religious

ST. ISIDORE OF SEVILLE (560-636)

Feast Days:	Apr. 4

ST. BEDE THE VENERABLE (673-735)

Advent:	Dec. 22
Easter:	Wk3-M
Feast Days:	May 31; Aug. 29; Sept. 21

ST. JOHN DAMASCENE (676-749)

Feast Days:	Dec. 4; July 26

ST. PETER DAMIAN (1007-1072)

Feast Days:	Feb. 21; Apr. 23; June 19

ST. ANSELM (1033-1109)

Advent:	Wk1-F
Feast Days:	Dec. 8; Apr. 21

ST. BERNARD OF CLAIRVAUX (1090-1153)

Advent:	Wk1-W; Dec. 20; Dec. 29
Ord. Time:	Wk3-W; Wk6-M; Wk20-T; Wk23-T
Feast Days:	May 12; Aug. 20; Sept. 15; Oct. 2; Oct. 7; Nov. 1

ST. ANTHONY OF PADUA (1195-1231)

Feast Days: June 13

ST. ALBERT THE GREAT (1206-1280)

Feast Days: Nov. 15

ST. BONAVENTURE (1221-1274)

Ord. Time:	Wk5-M
Feast Days:	Sacred Heart; July 15

ST. THOMAS AQUINAS (1225-1274)

Ord. Time:	Wk9-Sat; Wk21-M; Wk33-Sat
Feast Days:	Jan. 28; Corpus Christi

ST. CATHERINE OF SIENA (1347-1380)

Ord. Time:	Wk19-S; Wk30-Sat
Feast Days:	Apr. 29

ST. TERESA OF AVILA (1515-1582)

Ord. Time:	Wk13-W
Feast Days:	Oct. 15

ST. PETER CANISIUS (1521-1597)

Feast Days: Dec. 21

ST. ROBERT BELLARMINE (1542-1621)

Feast Days: Sept. 17

ST. JOHN OF THE CROSS (1542-1591)

Advent:	Wk2-M
Ord. Time:	Wk18-F
Feast Days:	Dec. 14

ST. LAWRENCE OF BRINDISI (1559-1619)

Feast Days: July 21

ST. FRANCIS DE SALES (1567-1622)

Feast Days: Jan. 24

ST. ALPHONSUS LIGUORI (1696-1787)

Feast Days: Aug. 1

ST. THERESE OF LISIEUX (1873-1897)

Feast Days: Oct. 1

If you have enjoyed this book, consider making your next selection from among the following . . .

Life and Revelations of St. Gertrude the Great. 24.00
School of Jesus Crucified. *Fr. Ignatius* 13.50
Devotion to the Holy Spirit. 3.00
Pope Pius VII. *Prof. Robin Anderson* 16.50
Shroud of Turin. *Fr. Guerrera* 15.00
Ven. Francisco Marto of Fatima. *Cirrincione,* comp. 2.50
Ven. Jacinta Marto of Fatima. *Cirrincione* 3.00
St. Philomena—The Wonder-Worker. *O'Sullivan* 9.00
The Facts About Luther. *Msgr. Patrick O'Hare* 18.50
Little Catechism of the Curé of Ars. *St. John Vianney.* 8.00
The Curé of Ars—Patron Saint of Parish Priests. *Fr. B. O'Brien* 7.50
Saint Teresa of Avila. *William Thomas Walsh* 24.00
Isabella of Spain: The Last Crusader. *William Thomas Walsh* 24.00
Characters of the Inquisition. *William Thomas Walsh* 16.50
Blood-Drenched Altars—Cath. Comment. on Hist. Mexico. *Kelley* 21.50
The Four Last Things—Death, Judgment, Hell, Heaven. *Fr. von Cochem* 9.00
Confession of a Roman Catholic. *Paul Whitcomb* 2.50
The Catholic Church Has the Answer. *Paul Whitcomb* 2.50
The Sinner's Guide. *Ven. Louis of Granada* .15.00
True Devotion to Mary. *St. Louis De Montfort* 9.00
Life of St. Anthony Mary Claret. *Fanchón Royer* 16.50
Autobiography of St. Anthony Mary Claret 13.00
I Wait for You. *Sr. Josefa Menendez* 1.50
Words of Love. *Menendez, Betrone, Mary of the Trinity* 8.00
Little Lives of the Great Saints. *John O'Kane Murray* 20.00
Prayer—The Key to Salvation. *Fr. Michael Müller.* 9.00
Sermons on Prayer. *St. Francis de Sales* 7.00
Sermons on Our Lady. *St. Francis de Sales* .15.00
Passion of Jesus and Its Hidden Meaning. *Fr. Groenings, S.J.* 15.00
The Victories of the Martyrs. *St. Alphonsus Liguori* 13.50
Canons and Decrees of the Council of Trent. *Transl. Schroeder* 16.50
Sermons of St. Alphonsus Liguori for Every Sunday 18.50
A Catechism of Modernism. *Fr. J. B. Lemius* 7.50
Alexandrina—The Agony and the Glory. *Johnston* 7.00
Life of Blessed Margaret of Castello. *Fr. William Bonniwell* 9.00
The Ways of Mental Prayer. *Dom Vitalis Lehodey* 16.50
Catechism of Mental Prayer. *Simler* 3.00
Fr. Paul of Moll. *van Speybrouck* 13.50
St. Francis of Paola. *Simi and Segreti* 9.00
Abortion: Yes or No? *Dr. John L. Grady, M.D.* 3.00
The Story of the Church. *Johnson, Hannan, Dominica* 22.50
Reign of Christ the King. *Davies* 2.00
Hell Quizzes. *Radio Replies Press* 2.50
Indulgence Quizzes. *Radio Replies Press* 2.50
Purgatory Quizzes. *Radio Replies Press* 2.50
Virgin and Statue Worship Quizzes. *Radio Replies Press* 2.50
Holy Eucharist—Our All. *Etlin* 3.00
Meditation Prayer on Mary Immaculate. *Padre Pio* 2.50
Little Book of the Work of Infinite Love. *de la Touche* 3.50
Textual Concordance of The Holy Scriptures. PB. *Williams* 35.00
Douay-Rheims Bible. *Hardbound* 55.00
The Way of Divine Love. *Sister Josefa Menendez* 21.00
The Way of Divine Love. (pocket, unabr.). *Menendez* 12.50
Mystical City of God—Abridged. *Ven. Mary of Agreda* 21.00

Prices subject to change.

Prices subject to change.

Prices subject to change.

Prices subject to change.

Prices subject to change.

At your Bookdealer or direct from the Publisher.
Call Toll-Free 1-800-437-5876   *Fax 815-226-7770*

Prices subject to change.

NOTES

NOTES

NOTES

Since 1970 Fr. Christopher has been active in the St. Joseph Medal Apostolate and its related group for the laity, The Workers of St. Joseph, both of which he founded. This work includes fostering devotion through a medal of St. Joseph and its literature, making available materials on Our Lady of Guadalupe and arranging retreat-pilgrimages to her shrine in Mexico City. The combined effect of this devotion to Joseph and Mary is directed to a flowering of new devotion to Jesus present in the Blessed Sacrament. The "Joseph way of life" is well expressed in the Workers' "Sum-up Prayer":

May Joseph with hammer-blow my soul re-make
In pleasing pattern of Mary's choice.
So all I do is done for Jesus' sake,
And echoes clear the Father's voice.

Since its founding in 1979 by Bishop Jerome Hastrich, Fr. Christopher has been a board member of the Queen of the Americas Guild. The Guild's office is in St. Charles, Illinois.

Fr. Christopher is stationed at St. Francis Friary (Capuchin College) in Washington, D.C. His current apostolates include ministering to nursing home residents and helping with hearing Confessions at the nearby National Shrine of the Immaculate Conception.

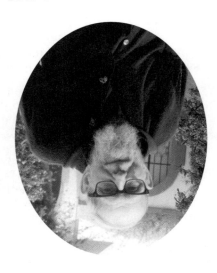

Fr. Christopher Rengers, O.F.M. Cap.

Born in Pittsburgh in 1917, Fr. Christopher received his elementary education at parochial schools in Pittsburgh and then attended Capuchin seminaries for high school and theology. He entered the Capuchin novitiate in Cumberland, Maryland in 1936, made his first vows in 1937 and final vows in 1940. He was ordained in Washington, D.C. on May 28, 1942. He obtained an M.A. in history from St. Louis University, taught four years at St. Joseph College and Military Academy in Hays, Kansas, then served as a chaplain and did parish work for over 50 years on various assignments in Kansas, Missouri, Ohio, Maryland and Washington, D.C.

Fr. Christopher's writings include books entitled *The Youngest Prophet* (on Jacinta Marto), *Mary of the Americas*, *Words from the Cross* and *They Played in Calvary's Drama*, and magazine articles in *Our Sunday Visitor*, *Soul*, *Priest*, *Pastoral Life*, *Homiletic and Pastoral Review*, and *Extension*. During his time in St. Louis, Fr. Christopher organized The Capuchin Troupe to put on pageants of Our Lady of Guadalupe and the Passion of Jesus: *Mary of the Americas* and *The Week of Redemption*. The songs and narration of these are obtainable on audio tape.

Fr. Christopher first became interested in the Doctors when the Capuchin St. Lawrence of Brindisi was made a Doctor of the Church in 1959. Fr. Christopher says, "Writing on the Doctors has been a big grace in my life. The study and reflection needed have supplied a new fulness to my understanding of the Church and of how God raises up new prophets to explain and make clear the legacy of Scripture and divine Tradition . . . Their lives and works are also a treasury for spiritual direction of self and others."

(Continued)